STRETCHING THERAPY

FOR SPORT AND MANUAL THERAPIES

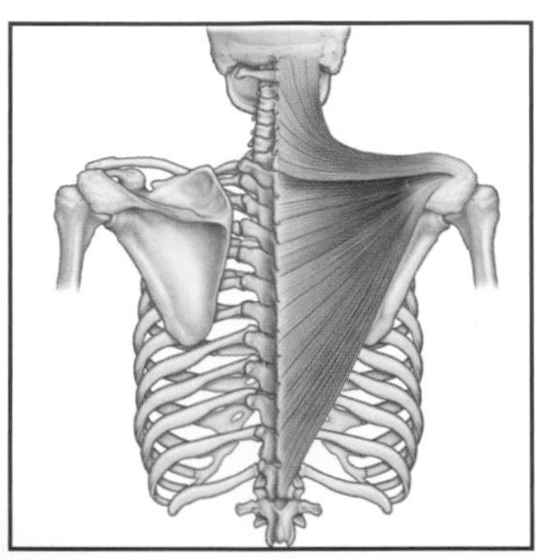

Jari Ylinen MD PHD MLCOM DO

Head of Department of Physical and Rehabilitation Medicine,
Jyväskylä Central Hospital,
Jyväskylä,
Finland

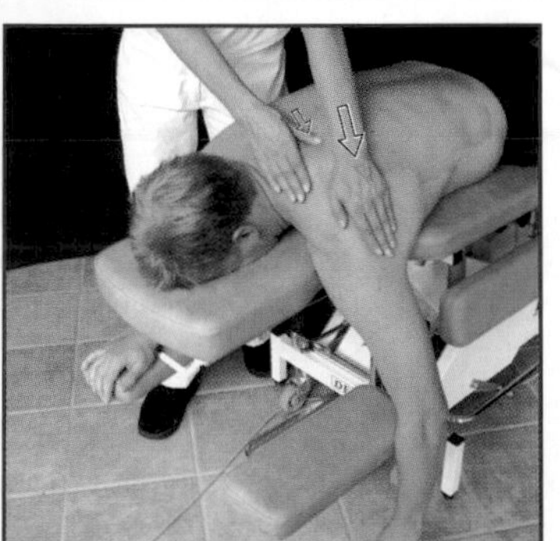

FOREWORD BY
Leon Chaitow

TRANSLATED BY
Julie Nurmenniemi

ILLUSTRATIONS BY
Sandie Hill

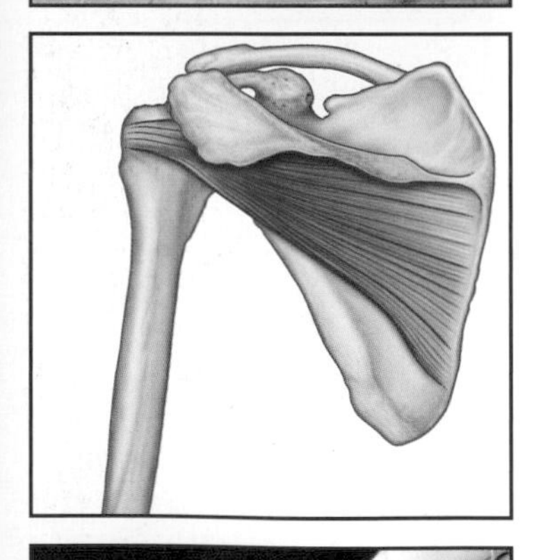

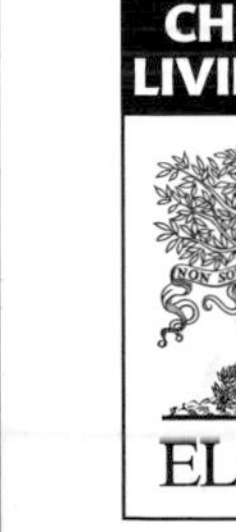

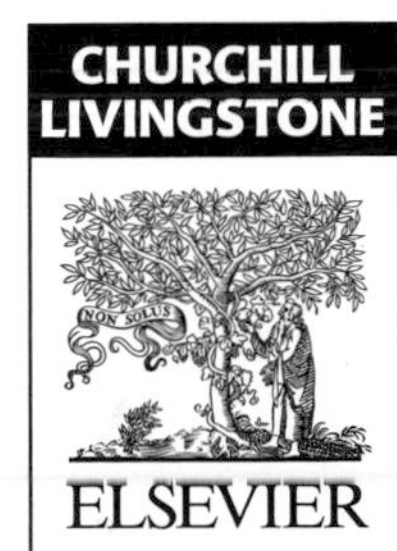

Edinburgh London New York Oxford Philadelphia
St Louis Sydney Toronto 2008

STRETCHING THERAPY
FOR SPORT AND MANUAL THERAPIES

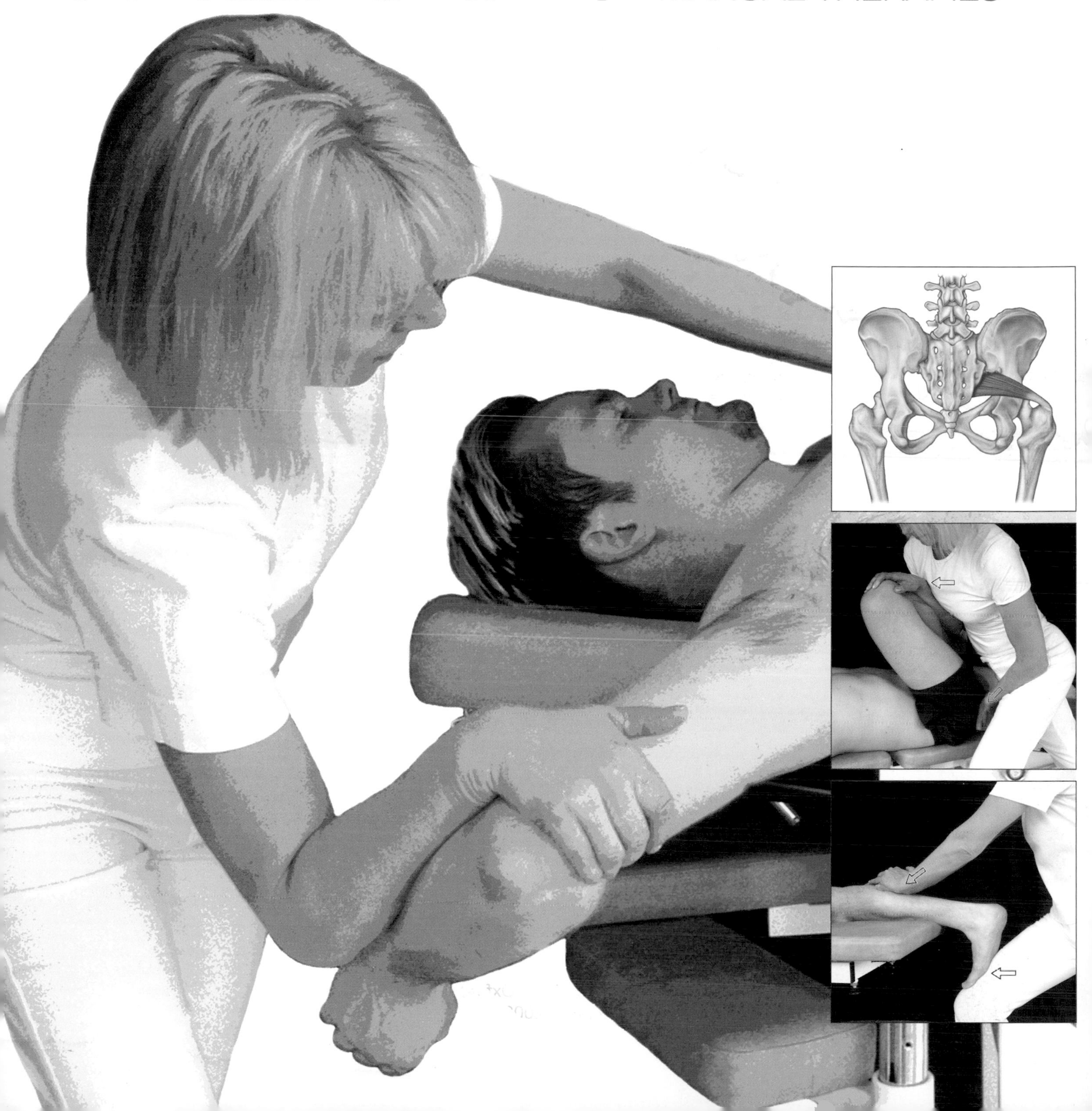

CHURCHILL
LIVINGSTONE
ELSEVIER

First Edition published in Finnish under the title *Manuaalinen terapia [illegible]*

First edition published in English

First edition 2002
English edition 2008

ISBN 10: 0443 101272
ISBN 13: 978 0 443 10127 4

British Library Cataloguing in Publication Data
A catalogue record for this book is available from the British Library

Library of Congress Cataloging in Publication Data
A catalog record for this book is available from the Library of Congress

Note
Every effort has been made by the Author and the Publishers to ensure that the descriptions of the techniques included in this book are accurate and in conformity with the descriptions published by their developers. The Publishers and the Authors do not assume any responsibility for any injury and/or damage to persons or property arising out of or related to any use of the material contained in this book. It is the responsibility of the treating practitioner, relying on independent experience and knowledge of the patient, to determine the best treatment and method of application for the patient, to make their own evaluation of their effectiveness and to check with the developers or teachers of the techniques they wish to use that they have understood them correctly.
The Publisher

The publisher's policy is to use **paper manufactured from sustainable forests**

Printed in China

For Elsevier

Senior Commissioning Editor: Sarena Wolfaard
Development Editor: Claire Wilson
Project Manager: Andrew Palfreyman
Design: Erik Bigland
Illustrations Manager: Bruce Hogarth

Section 1 STRETCHING THEORY 1

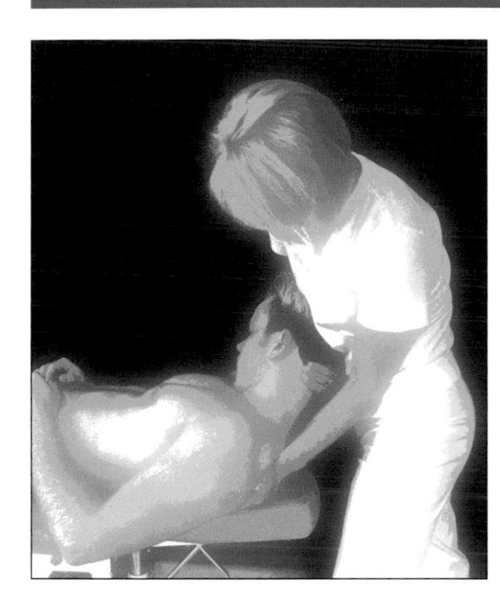

Section 2 STRETCHING TECHNIQUES 91

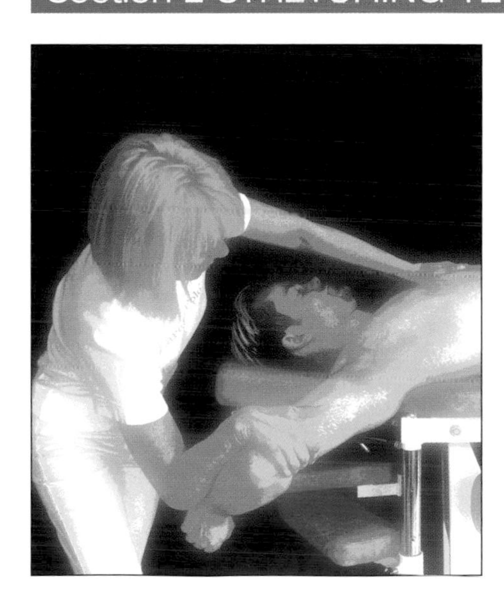

This text is important because, arguably for the first time, the topic is covered comprehensively (and well) – incorporating as it does all essential features including anatomy, physiology, methodology, safety, variations, effects and research evidence, together with excellent muscle-by-muscle illustrations and clearly described protocols.

Stretching may appear a simple enough procedure, however it is deceptively complex, and there are a great many ways of getting it wrong, and/or of producing potentially harmful outcomes, as well as a variety of different ways of stretching correctly – depending on the effects that are required.

What this excellent text has managed to combine is a broad overview of the physiology, neurophysiology and methodology of stretching, with discussion of contexts as varied as application of stretching during immobilization, trauma, post-surgery, cramp, joint inflammation and restriction, as well as in relation to specific conditions such as back and neck pain, tennis elbow, carpal tunnel syndrome, disc problems, neural damage and hypermobility.

Most importantly the preventive features of appropriate stretching are dealt with in relation to sport, body type, age, gender, inherited factors (hypermobility for example), and even the best times of day to stretch!

The effects of stretching on mobility, flexibility, strength, muscle length, tendons, fascia, ligaments, nerves are all evaluated.

Essential topics covered include motivation, preparation for stretching (including topics such as heat, cold, massage and vibration), circulatory effects, after-effects (soreness), and vitally, how to avoid complications.

A variety of different stretching methods and systems are covered, including passive, active, active assisted, dynamic, ballistic, static, Proprioceptive Neuromuscular Facilitation (PNF), Muscle Energy Techniques (MET), Contract-Relax (C-R), Contract-Relax, Antagonist-Contract (C-R A-C), as well as stretching in the context of physiotherapy practice.

A great deal of information is provided as to the research evidence of the effects and benefits relative to different types of stretching. INowadays, where there is an increasing demand for evidence relative to both safety and the therapeutic value of the use of techniques such as stretching, the many pages devoted to research evidence is very welcome.

What emerges is a sense that we now know a great deal more about the subject than previously, including important features such as the value of minimal effort, the ideal amount of time stretch should be held, the most appropriate number of repetitions, and the importance – in therapeutic terms - of the phenomenon of increased tolerance to stretch, and viscous and elastic behaviour of connective tissue, and how these features influence stretching (with clear evidence that sufficient, but not excessive, force is needed, over time – with tissues at the right temperature - for optimal effects) .

As can be seen from the comments above, the information provided is satisfyingly comprehensive and current, and the layout of the book aesthetically pleasing,

An important feature is the regular placement of self-assessment concepts/questions, a useful *aide-memoire* of key features of the preceding text, as well as being invaluable for students and practitioners/therapists who are new to these methods.

And then we have the presentation of the techniques themselves.

The illustrations are quite simply excellent, with anatomical detail and technique clearly demonstrated. Even experienced practitioners will find the illustrations helpful as many embrace unusual and clearly effective positioning, both of the patient and the practitioner. Whether the positions illustrated are used passively, or with the inclusion of isometric contractions, during one phase of the process or another, is clearly a matter of choice and previous training.

Each muscle is illustrated, with information provided as to its nerve supply, origin, insertion and function – and the technique for stretching is concisely described and beautifully photographed, with superimposed arrows to make absolutely sure that there is no misunderstanding as to what is required. Cautions are offered wherever any risk might be involved – for example in stretching sternocleidomastoid.

Stretching in clinical practice can only be safer and more effective if this exceptional text is used as designed.

Leon Chaitow ND DO
Honorary Fellow,
University of Westminster,
London

The purpose of this book is to provide a comprehensive volume of clinically well-tried stretching techniques in clear form and systematic order so that they can be easily adopted in studying and also used as a quick reference book in the clinic.

Like joint manipulation which may be unspecific and treat the whole spine or specifically directed to single joint, stretching can also be directed to the bulk of muscles or focused to a specific part of the muscle. Thus, the aim of this book is to provide more advanced stretching techniques.

I also hope that this book will awake interest in the study of manual therapy, as it shows the importance of a thorough knowledge of human anatomy for students, and thus inspires learning.

Since the knowledge of physiologic mechanisms of stretching has changed greatly during the past decade as a result of scientific research, the theory section is interesting reading for professionals having not been on the school bench lately. Thus, the first chapter is devoted to theory and research in stretching. It also includes recent recommendations about how stretching should be applied.

This textbook has been written with the intent to provide detailed study material for physiotherapy as well as the manual therapy professions: chiropractic, naprapthy, and osteopathy. However, this book is also essential reading in professions of physical education like coach, personal trainer and PE teacher.

Stretching is one of the oldest therapy forms practiced among all ancient cultures. Manual therapy including manipulation, massage and stretching has a long standing tradition in medical education. In Greece, Hippocrates (460–377 BC), the father of medicine, even prescribed its use in his writings, which I discovered during a course of medical history at the University of Turku. In the University library I found German medical textbooks from the beginning of the 1900s describing basic manual treatment techniques. In Finland, as well as in many other European countries, these techniques were also taught to medical students, which they then commonly practiced to finance their studies. After the Second World War, studies of manual therapy were replaced by chemistry and pharmacology as well as constantly growing studies of many special fields made possible by the advancement of medicine.

However, old customs inspired me to study in private massage school, Juntunen at Lahti, and thus I become a registered remedial masseur. Thanks belong to deceased Kauko Juntunen, who was the director of the massage school as well as the enthusiastic fellow students with whom training often took place past ordinary hours. There I found a good basis for studies in manual therapy, anatomy and dissection studies for which I thank all my teachers and especially Professor Risto Santti.

After this course I was able to obtain many good results in musculoskeletal disorders by treating patients with only hands using soft tissue massage and stretching techniques. After graduation as medical doctor I worked for a few years but still wanted to learn more about manual therapy and so I entered the London College of Osteopathic Medicine. There I learned further joint mobilization and manipulation techniques as well as soft tissue techniques used by osteopaths, which differed very much from Finnish and Swedish massage techniques. I become also familiar with muscle energy and positional release techniques, which gave me new insight to stretching techniques. We had many brilliant teachers from different parts of Great Britain and even some from USA. I thank them for their devoted teaching, as broad arsenal of techniques is important in practice which one only fully realizes when one knows them.

Since returning to Finland I have specialized in physical and rehabilitation medicine as well as pain treatments. Due to side effects of drugs I have become more and more convinced that manual therapies should be tried in many conditions before relying only on the long-term medication for pain. I have also devoted myself to teaching manual therapy techniques to others. My students suggested that it would be easier to memorize techniques if they are written. This induced me to write this book, and although manual therapy cannot be learned wholly from books I thank my students for the initiation of this one.

The aim is of this book is not only to show a selection of stretching techniques, but to systematically present the techniques found to be most effective during three decades that I have taught and studied manual therapy. As manual therapy is not 'alternative medicine' but original medicine the scientific basis of the therapy is important. Thus, research in the area has been dealt with extensively. Although, there is still much to be done in research, we now know physiologic effects of stretching better than many medications. I want to thank all those researchers, who have put much effort into evaluating physiologic mechanisms as well as the effects of stretching.

Finally, I also want to thank Julie Nurmenniemi for translating this book, originally written in Finnish and called 'Venytystekniikat', to English; Hilkka Virtapohja, PT, MSc, specialist in manual therapy, who is the therapist performing the stretching techniques throughout the book, and models Jouni Leppänen, Juuso Sillanpää and Vesa Vähäsalo.

Section 1

STRETCHING THEORY

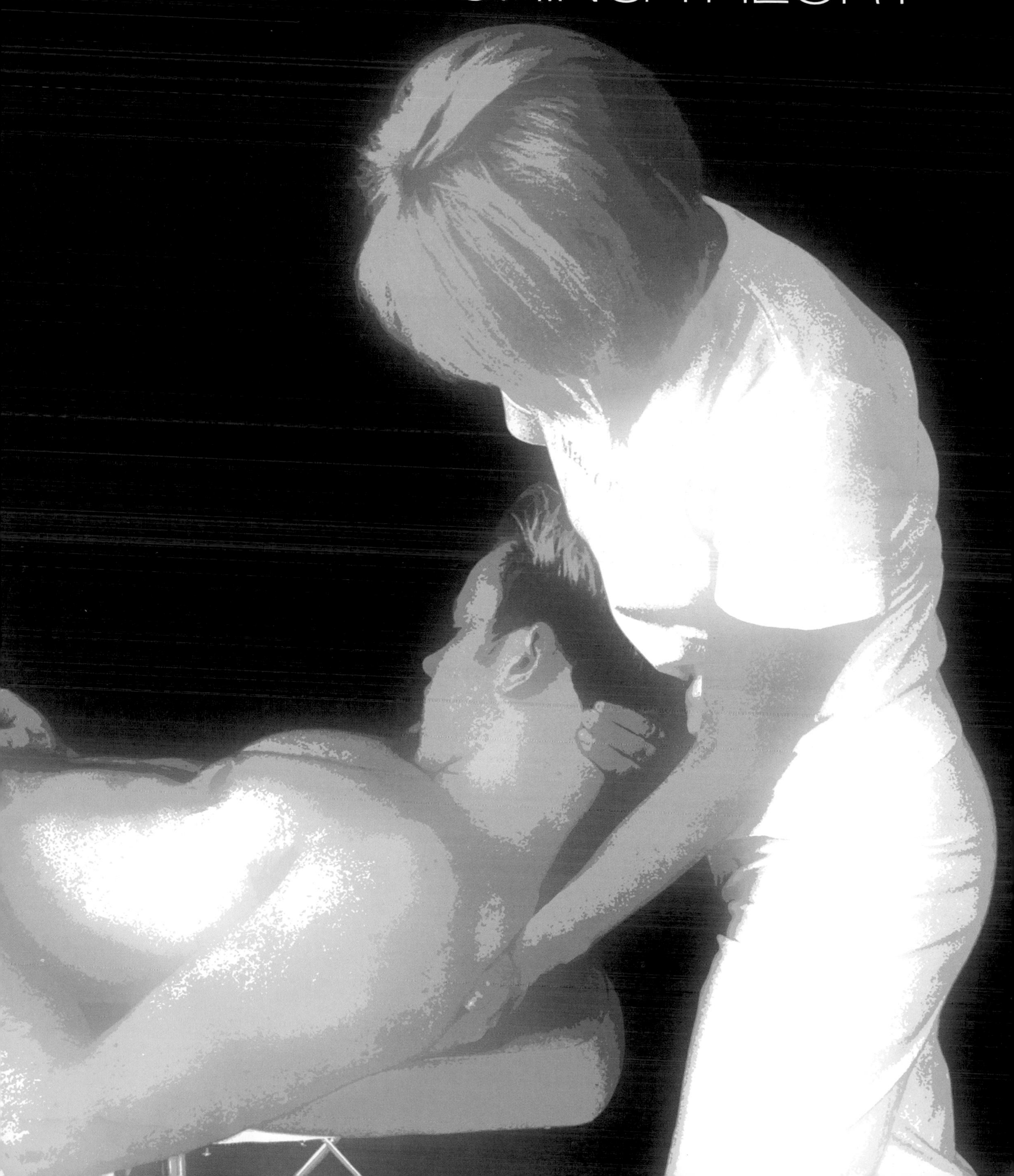

INTRODUCTION

Flexibility is considered to be an important factor affecting physical health. Range of movement (ROM) is a fundamental part of normal function of the musculoskeletal system (Figure 1.1). A certain amount of flexibility is necessary for the success of all physical movements. Individual differences in physical condition and range of joint movement can largely be due to innate, hereditary factors. Flexibility can, however, be significantly increased with intensive training of the elastic connective tissues, even in 'naturally stiff' persons. Many sports require special flexibility of the spine and extremities. People with these capabilities usually choose to practice such fields of sport from early in their life.

The general understanding of the importance of flexibility is in regard to the prevention of injury. A decrease in mobility may cause changes in function, which puts abnormal loading on the muscle–tendon system and joint structure. Thus, stretching is commonly included in the warm-up process in both training and competition situations. Furthermore, stretching is important in recovery following intense training and competition.

The purpose of stretching is usually to increase joint mobility, muscle length and flexibility, as well as to relax muscles in general. Metabolism is less efficient in stiff muscles because of increased intramuscular pressure and decreased circulation of fluids. Stretching, therefore, is also used to improve metabolism. Increased flexibility achieved by stretching will help to prevent injury to muscles, tendons and joints as well as improving performance capability.

Physical education in schools is limited, and classes seldom systematically concentrate on the maintenance and/or increase of joint mobility. Already at adolescence there are some children with signs of muscle tension and limitations in ROM of peripheral joints as well as decreased spinal mobility. Thus, problems involving joint motion may already appear prior to the end of the growth period and attention to this is important during health and posture examinations.

Many modern professions are not physically demanding nor do they require even normal end ROM. Exercise during leisure time has decreased with a noticeable increase in watching television and sitting at a computer. Physical hobbies are often unilateral, and do not emphasize increase in flexibility nor the general maintenance of joints. The development of stiffness in muscles and joints is thus common.

Naturally flexible people enjoy stretching exercises, which they find easy. People with an innate stiffness will find stretching distasteful and will most likely avoid it. Consequently, those in most need of stretching seldom practise it regularly.

In particular, many physically demanding jobs require not only stamina and muscle strength but also good mobility in the extremities and spine. The decrease in mobility becomes noticeable in the increasing difficulty in performing normal tasks. Strain-related pain due to limited ROM can be considered to be a warning sign, and one should start to do stretching exercises to restore the full ROM. However, joint mobility may have become quietly limited in those people unaccustomed to performing any exercises with full ROM. This may be because any pain and discomfort may be minimal or there has been no pain at all, until the condition is so severe that even movements in normal daily activities can no longer be performed. The decrease in mobility may even have become so serious that it is too late to restore full range of movement. Thus, regular stretching exercises become increasingly important with advanced age, not only to keep fit, but also to monitor the condition of muscles and joints.

Stretching exercises are commonly the primary focus of physiotherapy in rehabilitation and thus a specific stretching programme is often prepared for the patient. With the rise in average life expectancy, an increase in muscle and joint disorders can be expected in the future. Joint disease and injury involve a decrease in the elasticity of connective tissue surrounding joints and joint mobility in general. Muscle strength begins to weaken after middle age at about a 1% rate per year, while muscle tightness increases. This is a noticeable challenge to professional therapists. Ideally, they should have skills to preserve mobility, as well as methods of treatment to address existing limitations of movement.

GENERAL JOINT PHYSIOLOGY

The movement of any given joint is specific and depends upon joint anatomy and connective tissue structure. In addition to hereditary factors, mobility will be affected by nutrition and physical activity during growth. Physical stress during growth will substantially effect the development and characteristics of connective tissue. On the other hand, the growth period is relatively short in comparison to one's entire life, and therefore activity is also important throughout adulthood and old age for maintenance of musculoskeletal function.

Changes in flexibility may cause biomechanical problems in function of the locomotor system. Shortening of muscles will restrict ROM and cause less efficient movement patterns, resulting in unnecessary stress, which can often lead to inflammation and pain. Early detection of decreased mobility is important in the prevention of physical disability. With restricted mobility for an extended period of time, elastic connective tissue will gradually be replaced by fibrous tissue. Extensive infiltration of less elastic fibrous tissue will result in permanent restriction of mobility; then the only means of restoring normal movement are manipulation while the patient is anaesthetized or surgery.

A decrease in mobility may be caused by a variety of factors such as: non-participation in physical hobbies; repetitive and intense stress upon a small area of the body; sprains, strains and inflammation; degenerative changes with age; and neurological disease. The reason may also be iatrogenic such as excessive scar formation after radiation therapy and infected wounds. Long-standing immobilization with a cast can lead to a decrease in mobility.

Decreased movement is not always caused by changes in tissue structure, but often the activation of pain receptors in connective tissue will also cause considerable limitations by activating motor neurons and thereby increasing muscle stiffness. Joint disorders like degeneration, inflammation and trauma may also cause activation of motor neurons, even though there is no sensation of pain, and cause increased muscle tone.

Limitations of mobility can be caused by a variety of changes in connective tissue:

- tightening of connective tissue fasciae, for example following trauma, surgery, radiation damage or burns
- oedema in and around joints due to acute trauma and infection, and an increase in connective tissue in chronic conditions
- changes in joint structure resulting from fracture
- separation of the 'mus articularis' i.e. cartilage and/or bone from the joint surface
- disc damage; rupture, protrusion and/or prolapsed discs
- pinched nerves, as in sciatica
- central nervous system damage causing muscular rigidity and shortening of muscle length
- shortening of muscle length due to prolonged immobilization accompanied by splints and/or plaster casts
- general deterioration of tissues of joint ligaments and capsule with the degenerative process of aging
- exaggerated muscle tone and pain following unusually intense workout i.e. delayed muscle soreness (DOMS)
- activation of pain receptors located in connective tissue and the muscle–tendon system of joints due to trauma and inflammation
- activation of pain receptors in the connective tissue surrounding joints following overly long-lasting stretch or stretch with excessive force.

Mobility can be affected with rehabilitation. Excellent exercises for improving joint mobility include active and passive stretching as well as dynamic exercises involving broad ranges of movement (Figure 1.2).

The purpose of stretching is to increase the elasticity of muscles, tendons, fasciae, joint ligaments and joint capsules. Furthermore, stretching exercises aim to relax the neuromuscular system in general. An increase in muscle tone will often lead to pain caused by the irritation of nerve endings or the increase in pressure in and between muscles, which causes slowing of the metabolism. Symptoms of pain can be reduced with the relaxation of muscles by stretching exercises.

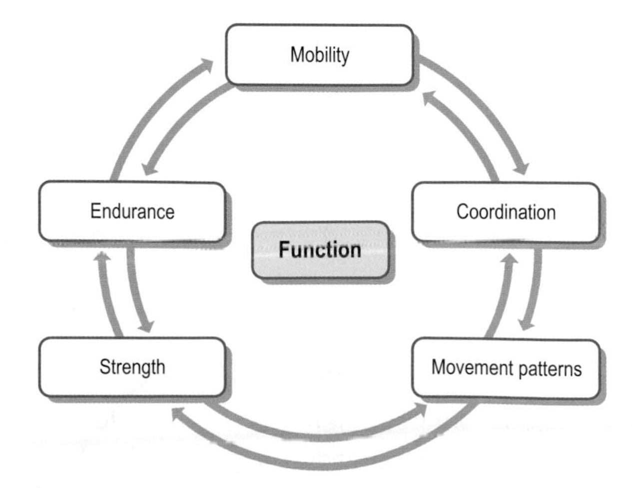

Figure 1.1 Function of the locomotor system depends on several characteristics, which essentially depend on each other.

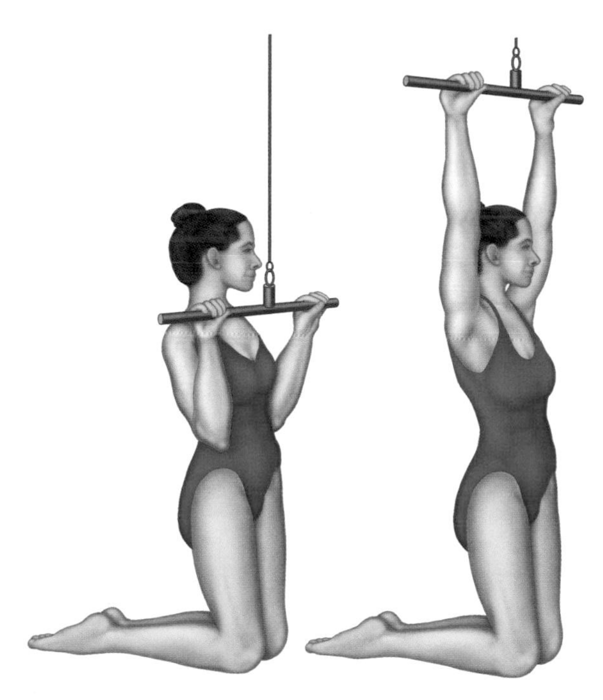

Figure 1.2 Overhead pulley system effectively stretches the muscles of the shoulder area and shoulder joint.

Stretching is especially important to physically demanding work, and competitive, as well as intensive, hobby sports, when trying to preserve muscle balance and prevent the shortening and tightening of muscles. Stretching is equally important in the prevention of trauma in people with stiff muscles. Prior to intense training or work, stretching assures optimum ROM, by increasing joint mobility in the required area of movement.

Effective stretching may not entirely remove the risk of injury as it affects only certain specific tissue characteristics and has several practical limitations, which are discussed later in this book. Sudden, violent loading, for instance in slipping or collision, may overextend normal ROM and/or overstress tissues causing rupture damage. It is important that occupational and other environmental conditions are examined and controlled for the prevention of such accidents.

Self-assessment: mobility

- Why does mobility differ between individuals?
- How does physical loading affect mobility?
- What are the factors causing commonly decreased mobility?

CONCEPTS

With stretching one can actively affect the functioning of the locomotor system. Changes in the length of muscles and tendons will subsequently cause anatomical, biochemical and physiological changes, which will affect both the biomechanical function of joints and metabolism of soft tissues.

The vast number of terms to describe joints and their functions are often used carelessly, without full understanding of their meaning. In kinesiology these terms are clear and specific. Range of movement (ROM) can be divided into active and passive ROM. Active mobilization refers to that movement made possible by the primary muscles involved in the mobility of a particular joint (Figure 1.3). Passive mobilization involves a broader area of movement with stretching of a given joint, to and past the furthest point achieved by active mobilization. It requires the use of muscles other than those directly involved in the mobility of a joint or the assistance of another individual.

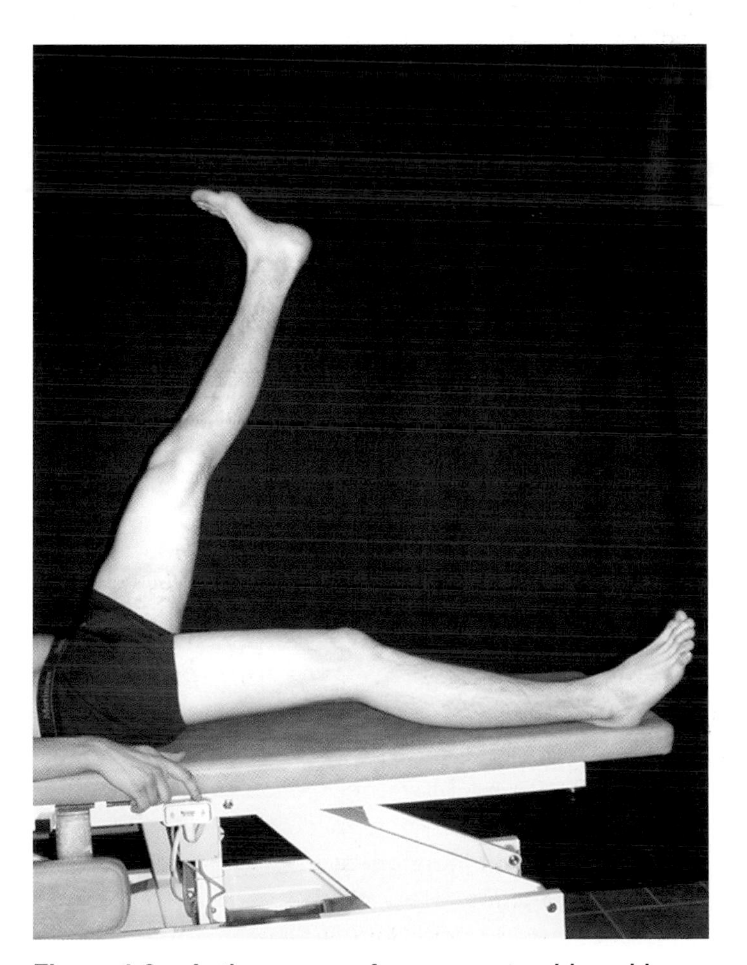

Figure 1.3 Active range of movement achieved by contraction of agonist muscles.

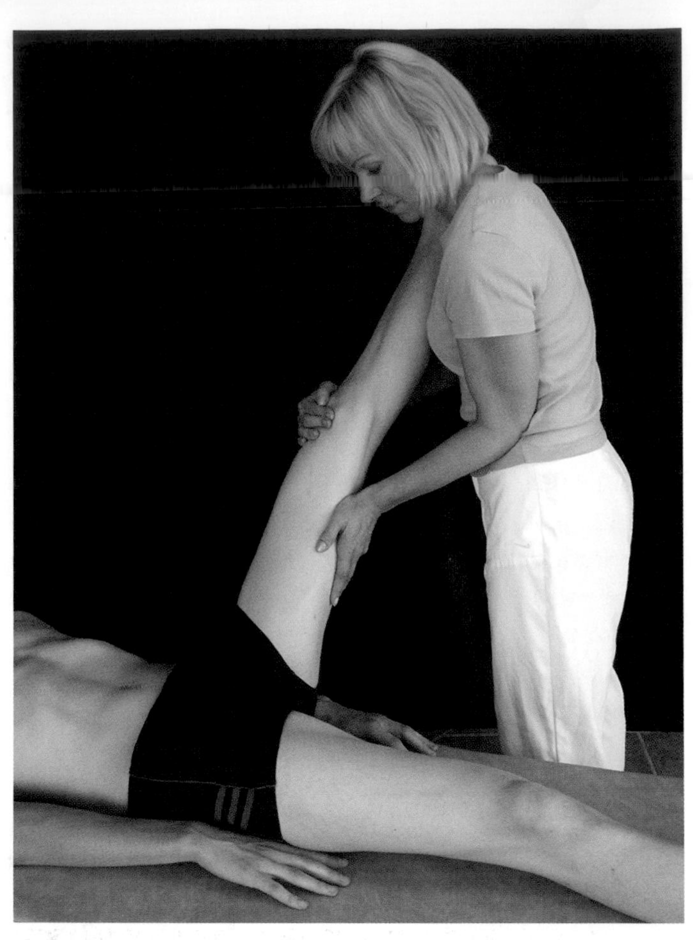

Figure 1.4 Passive range of movement achieved by static stretching.

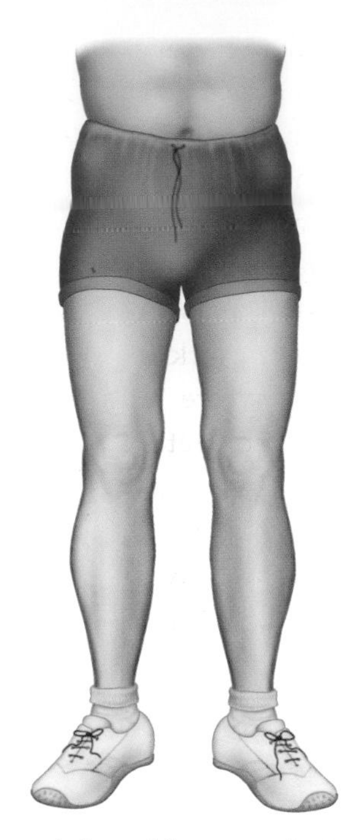

Figure 1.5 Knee joint with normal structure.

Mobility involves joint structures, their surrounding connective tissues and activity of the nervous system. The term in question is used frequently in biomechanics and is essentially the same as joint flexibility. *Flexibility* refers to the extent at which a given joint can move in different directions and is greatly dependent on the function of the neuromuscular system. A decrease in joint flexibility, or resistance caused by the surrounding soft tissue of a joint, is referred to as stiffness and results in both active and passive restriction of joint mobility. Once again, restriction is of a biomechanical nature. The term 'stiffness' is often used to describe any type of difficulty in achieving normal movement, and may involve only the individual's subjective impression of the tense state of bodily tissues, yet may not actually involve any physical restriction in mobility.

Dynamic flexibility refers to the ability to self-actively move a joint using those muscles surrounding it. In this situation, the agonist muscles contract to produce movement in the same direction, while the opposing muscles or antagonists relax to allow movement yet remain active enough to preserve joint integrity. Dynamic movement, therefore, does not only depend on potential joint mobility and limitations of muscle tension, but also, and more importantly, on the ability of the assisting muscles to achieve movement regardless of tissue resistance. *Static flexibility* refers to the extent of stretch attainable, passively, while muscles are fully relaxed; muscle force in this case has no bearing on the results.

Joint stability is equally important in joint function, as is flexibility. For example, walking and running would not be possible if the joints of the lower extremities were unable to support the movement. Flexibility and stability do not work against each other, but are both normal characteristics of joint function. Healthy joint function requires both good flexibility and adequate stability to withstand load. *Passive stability* involves joint surface anatomy, as well as joint capsule and ligament structure, strength and tightness. Passive stability depends usually on joint positioning and the load involved. *Active stability* involves the combined forces of both the movers and the stabilizers of the muscle–tendon system of a joint. Functional joint stability essentially depends on function of the neuromuscular system. Many injuries and disorders of the central nervous system involve symptoms of increased muscle tone known as spasticity. In healthy people, stiff muscles are often wrongly referred to as spastic. However, *spasticity* is a condition directly related to nerve damage or nerve diseases involving the upper motor neuron system. Damage will be located in the pyramidal corticospinal nerve pathways: the spinal cord, brain stem or the cerebral cortex. Minor damage will appear as minimal spasticity towards the middle phase of a given action while extremities are moved quickly back and forth while in a relaxed state. More severe spasticity will involve the entire joint area. Intense stretching may suddenly release spasticity and is known as the clasp-knife effect. Spasticity will affect either the muscles of extension or flexion depending upon which area of the nervous system has been damaged. *Hyper-reflex* is the term used to describe the over-active nature of spasticity. In the clinical examination, the muscle–tendon system is stretched with minimal force to check if the reflex response is exaggerated. Repetition of reflex response contractions often leads to lesser jerking movements, known as *clonus*. Damage to the pyramidal corticospinal nerve pathways may also involve a change in the Babinski reflex from negative to positive. Applying pressure to the heel with a blunt object and drawing it swiftly along the outer edge of the foot towards the toes will cause the big toe to flex. Violent extension of the big toe is an indicator of pyramidal pathway damage. This reaction, however, is normal in children under the age of 7 years.

Damage to the extrapyramidal nerve pathways of the central nervous system will result in *rigidity*. It affects the entire joint area involving both the flexor and extensor muscles. Stiffness is felt with slow movements and does not depend to the same degree on the speed of movement as it would with spasticity. Reflexes are not oversensitive and the Babinski reflex is negative. During passive flexion and extension of a joint, muscle tension repeatedly increases and decreases rapidly, causing jerky movements. The degree of resistance depends on how quickly the joint is bent and the muscles are stretched. Mild rigidity, for example in the early stages of Parkinson's disease, may be undetectable except as a stuttered resistance to fast movements.

Disease of the central nervous system may only involve spasticity of certain muscles and involuntary movement known as *dyskinesia*. *Spasmodic torticollis* is an example of spasticity that often affects the muscles on only one side of the neck, resulting in exaggerated rotation that can be temporarily relieved with stretching for a few seconds but the neck will then quickly return to the same position.

Tension with spasticity and rigidity is not always entirely the result of nerve damage. Changes in muscles will appear, as use will concentrate on slow motor neurons. The rapid motor cells are not activated and they will tend to shorten, atrophy and become less frequent. Minimal use of joint range will lead to shortening of joint connective tissue as well as in muscles. The changes become gradually permanent, as normally elastic fibres will be replaced by tougher fibrous tissue. Care should be taken to preserve mobility with regular active and passive exercises at the onset of disease in order to minimize the extent of movement limitation.

Spontaneous activation of individual motor neurons may cause a twitching effect, *fasciculation*, but may not produce actual movement. This occurs most often with partial paralysis and in spastic muscles. A mild form of a similar phenomenon occurring in healthy people is commonly called a twitch or *myokymia*. The most typical form of twitching occurs in the upper eyelid, but it may appear in any muscle and the affected muscle may vary.

Damage to lower motor neurons, i.e. those nerves exiting the spinal cord, will result in flaccidity. Muscles will become partly or completely paralyzed. Limb muscles also have reduced tone, i.e. they are hypotonic. This suggests that these patients should have good range of movement in the affected joint. However, mobility often becomes restricted in joints, because they may not have been moved regularly throughout whole ROM.

Instability refers to the occurrence of abnormal joint mobility due to lack of support normally supplied by the surrounding tissues to maintain the integrity of the joint; testing can reveal laxity of joint ligaments. *Hypermobility* refers to an exaggerated mobility in ROM but movement remains in the normal line of joint action (Figure 1.10).

Hypermobility may appear in one or more joints, and may indicate hypermobility syndrome. Instability and hypermobility are often confused with one another. Hypermobility involves exaggerated ROM within the normal function of a joint. Instability, on the other hand, can be classified as a symptom of disease involving the pathology in the joint stabilizing system. A hypermobile joint is more vulnerable to trauma and thus hypermobility may lead to joint instability more readily, compared with a joint with normal ROM and stability.

Instability may also appear in joints with normal ROM, and/or even limited ROM. Hypermobility and instability have also been defined according to type of movement (Figure 1.9). Arthritis and rheumatism, over

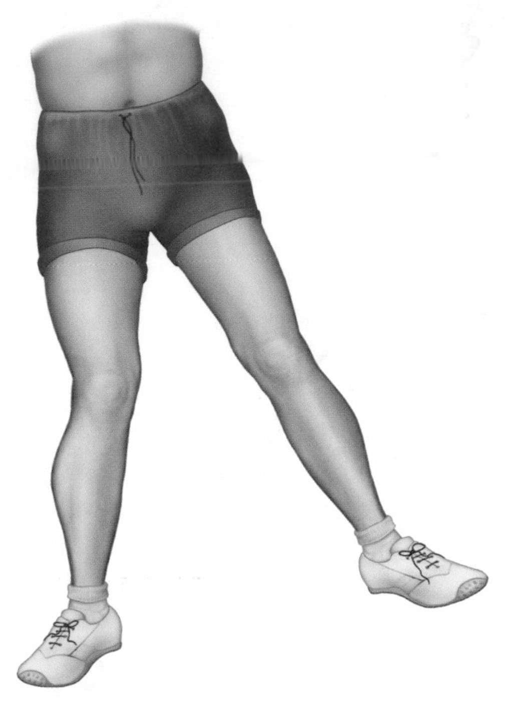

Figure 1.6 Instability of the knee due to inward deviation: *valgus deformity.*

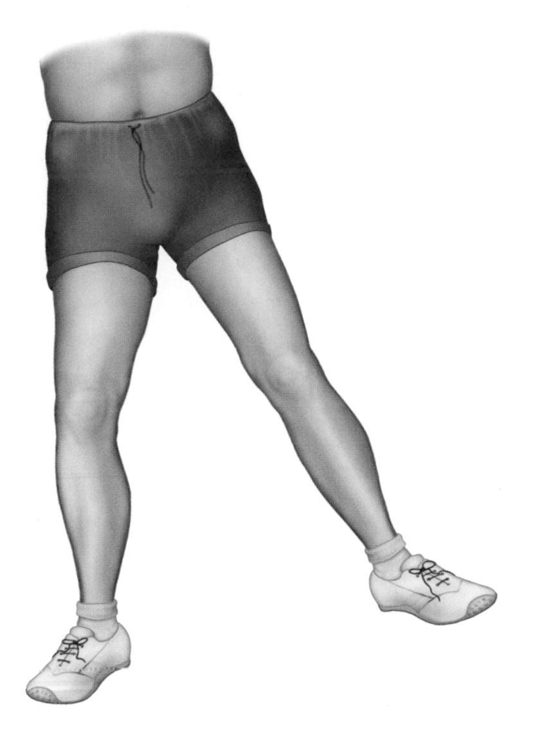

Figure 1.7 Instability of the knee due to outward deviation: *varus deformity.*

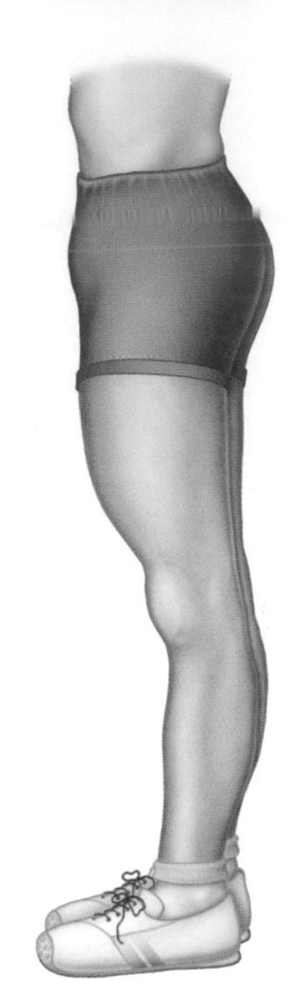

Figure 1.8 Instability of the knee due to exaggerated bending of the back: *hyperextension.*

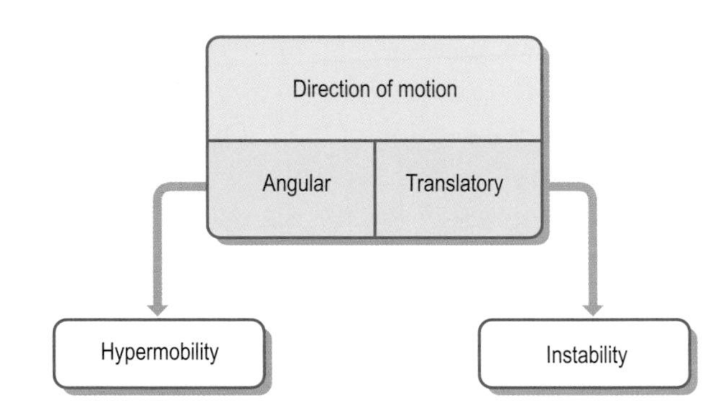

Figure 1.9 Instability in relation to type of motion.

time, may cause degeneration, which can lead to restricted *angular movement,* which may considerably limit both flexion and extension. Despite this, there may be additional *translatory movement* at the joint surface, which may stretch the stabilizing joint capsule and ligaments, causing pain and dysfunction (Figures 1.6–1.8). Some consider hypermobility as excessive angular movement, and instability as excessive translatory movement, at the joint surface.

Subluxation refers to partial joint separation from its normal position, but a part of joint surfaces are still in contact with each other (Figure 1.11). *Luxation* involves complete displacement of joint surfaces. A decrease in joint mobility is referred to as restriction, and anchylosis is complete stiffening of a joint with no or very little movement at all. In this case, decreased mobility will involve structural changes in the joint and surrounding tissues.

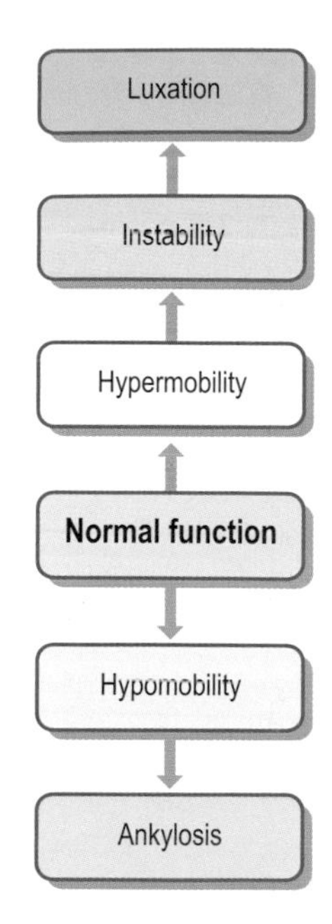

Figure 1.10 Function in relation to range of motion.

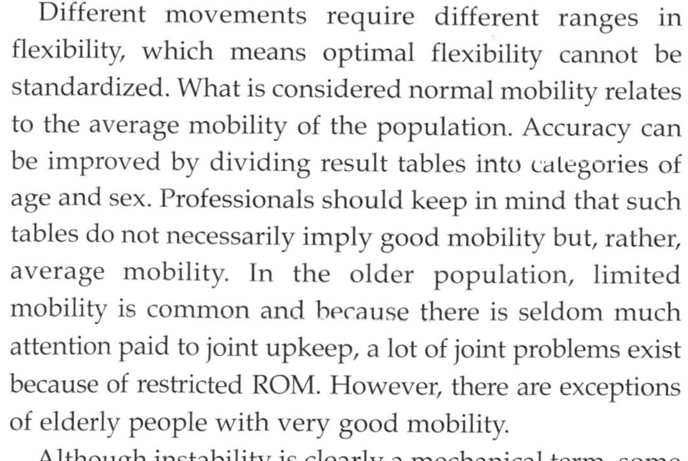

Different movements require different ranges in flexibility, which means optimal flexibility cannot be standardized. What is considered normal mobility relates to the average mobility of the population. Accuracy can be improved by dividing result tables into categories of age and sex. Professionals should keep in mind that such tables do not necessarily imply good mobility but, rather, average mobility. In the older population, limited mobility is common and because there is seldom much attention paid to joint upkeep, a lot of joint problems exist because of restricted ROM. However, there are exceptions of elderly people with very good mobility.

Although instability is clearly a mechanical term, some consider joint instability to be a defect in activation and coordination, in which pain or hyperactive mechanoreceptors inhibit synchronous function of support muscles.

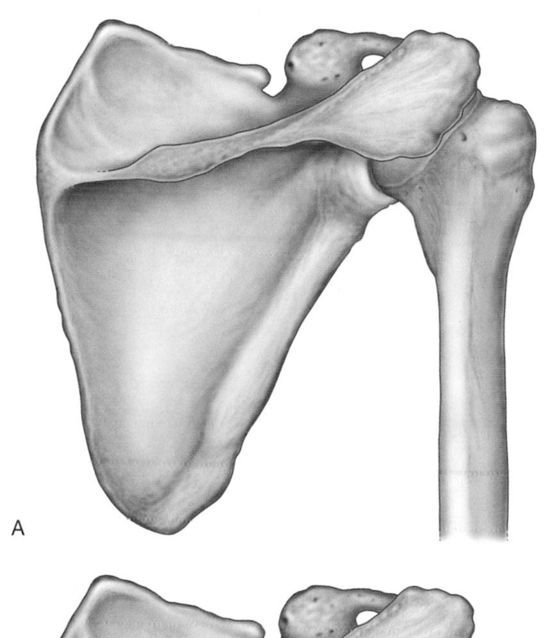

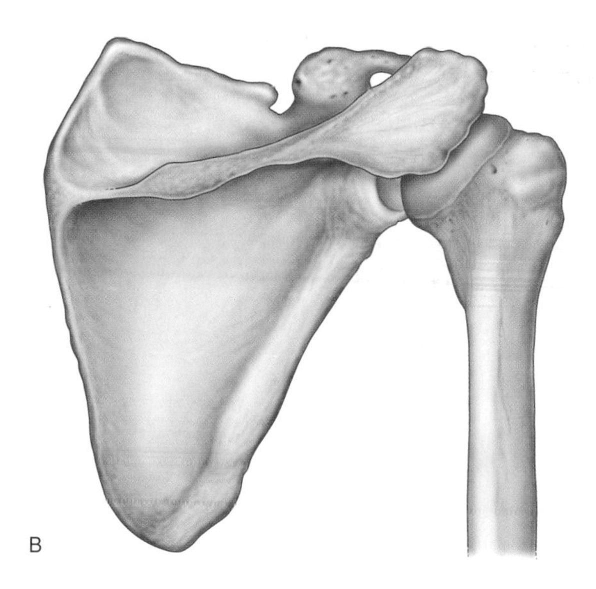

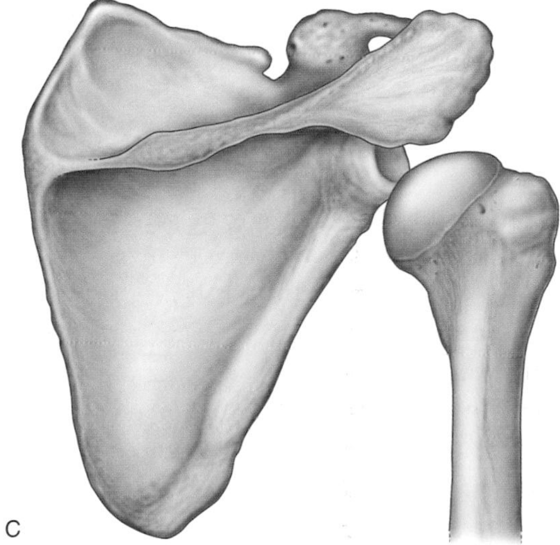

Figure 1.11
A: Shoulder joint in tack, joint surfaces in opposition to each other and joint shows maximal stability, which depends on muscle activity and support of other connective tissues.
B: Subluxation of shoulder joint with joint surfaces only partially opposite each other. Orthopaedic instability, this may often correct itself with the active movement of the upper arm.
C: Dislocation of shoulder joint; joint surfaces without any contact to one another. Manipulative repositioning is commonly needed to correct the displacement.

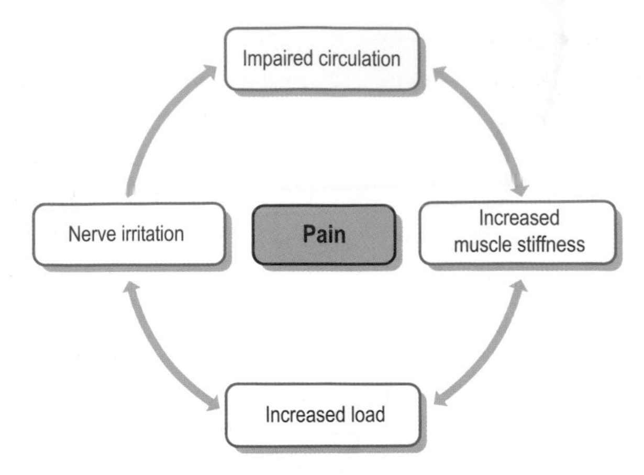

Figure 1.12 A vicious circle may develop as nerve irritation caused by pain leads to muscle tension, which leads to increased loading and impaired circulation, which again increases muscle tension.

Typically in this case, stretching of the supporting connective tissue in certain movements will induce flinching and a strong painful reaction. If this is repeated several times, it will become a constant painful condition (Figure 1.12). Joint instability, according to this definition, is more a functional than a structural problem. Examinations should not only include joint ROM but joint function in various movements, because a joint may be found to be unstable due to dysfunction of muscles, despite normal or even reduced flexibility.

Self-assessment: concepts

- During a bench press, the triceps (agonist) muscle contraction withstands an increase in the load with the increase in weight. How does this affect the activity of the biceps (antagonist) muscle?
- Into which two functional parts is flexibility divided?
- What is the difference between hypermobility and instability?
- What methods are clinically used to differentiate between pain caused by muscle tension, and joint related pain?
- What will happen to joint mobility in the rehabilitation of patients suffering from severe neurological spasticity, if regular treatments of stretching are not given?

TYPES OF JOINTS

Flexibility of the locomotor system has specific characteristics that vary, both between individuals and between joints. Joint mobility depends on physical anatomy and connective tissue structure, which are greatly determined by hereditary factors. The normal development of joints is assisted with physical activity and load. Genetic defects, deficiency disease, infection and toxins, especially during the early growth phase, as well as prolonged immobility, may cause pathologic structural changes. Excessive loading, trauma and/or inflammation of joints and their surrounding soft tissues may cause structural changes, resulting in permanent mobility limitations or instability. Joint mobility is based on joint type that involves surface shapes and structure of connective tissue.

Classification of joints according to anatomical structure and degree of motion

- *Osseus joints*: no movement
  - *Synostosis* between the sacral vertebrae
- *Fibrous joints*: little or no movement
  - *Sutures* of the skull
  - *Sydesmosis*, as in the distal tibiofibular joint
  - *Gomphosis*, as peg sutures in the roots of teeth in alveolar process
- *Cartilaginous joints*: little or no movement
  - *Synchondroses*, as in the epiphyseal plates (hyaline cartilage)
  - *Symphysis*, as in the intervertebral discs and symphysis pubis (fibrocartilage)
- Free moving *synovial joints*
  - *Ball and socket joints*, as in the shoulder and hip joints. Multiaxial movement
  - *Saddle joint* in which the structures of both surfaces are reminiscent of saddles placed together, allowing for movement in two directions. The first carpal-metacarpal joint of the thumb is an example of a saddle joint. Biaxial movement
  - *Condyloid/ellipsoid joints*, in which one surface is oval shaped and convex. The second surface is concave as in the radiohumeral and radiocarpal joints. Biaxial movement
  - *Hinge joint*, in which movement remains along one plane, as in the elbow, knee and superior ankle joints. Monoaxial movement

- *Pivot joint* allows one surface to rotate around the other as in the superior radio-ulnar and atlanto-axial (between anterior arch and dens) joints.
- *Plane joint,* in which opposing surfaces glide or slide against each other to produce movement; surfaces are flat or may be slightly curved, as in the facet joints of the spine and intercarpal joints.

FACTORS AFFECTING JOINT MOBILITY

Genetic factors form the basis of connective tissue structure and therefore will affect mobility in a number of ways. Genetic factors decide the composition, organization, shape and basic size of tissues; they also determine the shape of joint surfaces and their size. Race will fundamentally affect joint mobility. Natives to South Asia clearly have more flexible joints, and Africans have broader joint mobility than Europeans (Wordsworth et al 1987). Many other factors will affect joint mobility including exercise, hormonal factors, environment and body temperature.

Factors affecting joint mobility may be divided into two categories: internal and external. Passive extensibility refers to those internal factors affecting joint mobility including: elasticity of surrounding connective tissue; its amount and thickness; muscles; fascia; tendons; synovial sheets; aponeuroses; joint capsule and ligaments. Flexibility may be limited by any one of these structures, and may possibly involve pathological dysfunction of a particular structure.

Restriction of normal joint mobility depends on joint type and surrounding tissues. Passive resistance of the wrist joint is foremost a result of the condition of the joint capsule and joint ligaments. Restriction has been measured at 47% joint capsule involvement, 41% surrounding muscles and intermuscular fasciae, 10% tendons and 2% skin tissue (Johns and Wright 1962). That is very different from the elbow joint, as muscles and tendons have accounted for 84% of the variance in elbow stiffness (Chleboun et al 1997). Thus, factors restricting mobility may differ greatly from joint to joint depending on anatomy.

Excess fat may interfere with normal movement. Included in the category of internal factors that may limit joint mobility are the bony structure and protective layer of cartilage. Damage and inflammation following trauma or operation may limit mobility, which usually becomes evident when the cast or splint has been removed. Immobilization due to trauma often leads to shortening of connective tissue, the formation of adhesions, scar tissue, cheloids, and fibrotic contracture of muscles, tendons or other connective tissues. In these cases, stretching caused by normal movements may cause severe pain, and mobility may not spontaneously return without a specific stretching treatment.

A basic knowledge of anatomy, kinesiology, connective tissue, joint function and the nature of the pathology involved are essential in the treatment and rehabilitation of restricted joint mobility. Joint capsules and their ligaments are responsible for almost half of the total resistance in joint mobility. Both passive joint stability and joint mobility depend on the structure formed by joint surfaces, capsules, and ligaments. In cases of limited mobility, effective stretching is an important treatment method, which can usually restore normal function if applied during the early stages. Treatment should not focus only on the relief of pain with medication and passive physiotherapy. Active stability depends on muscle function: shortened and tight muscles will cause dysfunction that can be corrected with proper stretching and exercising. Prolonged immobility may, however, lead to structural changes as elastic fibres are replaced by tougher fibrous tissue to such an extent that stretching treatments are no longer effective and such tissue must be manipulated while the patient is anaesthetized.

Disease, injury and surgery will cause changes in the tissue mobility. Changes will also arise following intense stretching and as a result of prolonged immobilization. Furthermore, hyperactivity of the neuromuscular system may be involved, for instance, in the pathologic myotatic reflex, which responds to stretching, or there may be local mechanical hindrance such as in disc prolapse, causing sciatica.

During joint mobilization, it is apparent that joint position can affect restrictions in mobility. Movement is easiest in a neutral position when ligaments are most loose. Ligaments will begin to tighten and joint surfaces press against each other as joints are taken to their furthest limits of ROM. Movement in other directions will decrease or disappear completely.

Self-assessment: joint structure and physiology

- To what groups do the following joints belong: the jaw, atlanto-axial, costovertebral, radio-ulnar, interphalangeal, lumbosacral, sacroiliac joints, and the subtalar, cuneonavicular, calcaneocuboid, cuneocuboid, and intercuneiform articulations of the foot?
- Why are knowledge of muscle anatomy and their insertions insufficient for optimal muscle stretching results?
- How can joint inflammation limit muscle stretching?
- In which joints of the extremities and spine is mobility greatest?

FACTORS AFFECTING MUSCLE TENSION

Muscle balance is important to normal joint function. An imbalance between the agonist muscles and antagonist muscles of a joint can disturb joint function. This may result from hypertrophy of one or the other muscle groups due to the over-training of one side or from increased muscle tone (hypertonia) due to exercising. Or, it may be caused by muscle weakness and atrophy of one or the other muscle groups due to lack of exercising, or reduced muscle tone (hypotonia) due to same reason, which may be corrected with training. Tension can be reduced with stretching and massage. The balancing of joint forces usually involves the strengthening of antagonist muscles. For the appropriate use of stretching, one must consider structural, biomechanical, physiological, neurological, and psychological factors, which all have an impact on the neuromuscular system. An increase in muscle tone and the shortening of muscles are often involved in locomotor dysfunction. Overuse is a common cause. Joint immobilization in a flexed position over an extended period of time can lead to the shortening of muscles, ligaments and joint capsule. Problems can also arise from systemic connective tissue diseases, structural abnormalities, inflammation of connective tissue or trauma. Pain, whether internal or external, can activate motor neurons and increase muscle tension. The actual cause of any dysfunction of the neuromuscular system must be determined for an effective treatment plan. Muscle tension arising from neurophysiological disturbances can easily recur, as the system tends to react repeatedly in a similar fashion. Muscle reflex function may be conditioned with training and treatment. The change in neuromuscular system requires nerve function to adapt, creating a new balance between the muscles.

Those sections of contractile muscle fibres called sarcomeres are surrounded by an abundance of elastic fibres. The greatest resistance to stretching of a normal relaxed muscle will be due to the muscle's inner and surrounding connective tissues, not to the myofibrils. Shortening of muscles, in addition to limiting mobility for a long time, causes muscle weakness and imbalance towards joint function. Function can be restored with active exercise. The system may adapt quickly to shortened muscles, both physically and functionally. Prolonged imbalance, however, can gradually lead to pain in the muscle–tendon system, and/or the soft tissues surrounding joints; damage is even possible due to unnecessary loading. Muscle tension in itself will not always induce pain, but symptoms may arise in other tissues with continued overloading caused by joint dysfunction.

Characteristics of muscles and other connective tissues affecting their flexibility

Chronic conditions involving pain in the muscles and tendons are the most common diseases of the locomotor system. These myofascial syndromes often develop with mild but repetitive irritation on the neuromuscular system or as a result of short-term intense loading. Many factors, such as nutrition, fluids and the supply and balance of electrolytes, will affect connective tissue function. Disturbances in these factors may reduce muscle resistance to loading. Furthermore, external factors including dampness, cold and draught, are likely to disturb metabolism in the muscle and the balance of the

Factors affecting flexibility of the tissue

- Tissue water content
- Tissue chemical structure
- Relation between collagen and elastic fibres
- Complex matrix structure of connective tissue fibres
- Structures between and that bind together connective tissue fibres
- Amount and direction of connective tissue fibres
- Extent of fibres running transverse to each other
- Relation between slow and fast muscle fibres
- Shape of muscles.

neuromuscular system. Local and general inflammation can affect muscle function. Psychological factors may influence muscle function via the nervous and hormonal systems.

Muscle tension causes a rise in intramuscular pressure, which weakens circulation and metabolism in the muscle compartment surrounded by the fascia. The disturbance in metabolism accompanied by poor circulation, mechanical friction, swelling and inflammation can activate pain receptors located in muscle tissue causing compartment syndrome.

Nerves travel both between muscles and their fascia, as well as through them. They are subject to loading, stretch and irritation due to friction, especially where they enter and/or exit muscles. Irritation may cause numbness, tingling sensations or pain along the nerve. It may be felt locally, or be referred either distally or proximally from the area of irritation. Situations of prolonged irritation involving both nerve irritation and muscle pain can make it difficult to determine whether the cause is primarily due to nerves (neuralgia), or muscles (myalgia) because the entire area becomes subject to pain. In neurophysiological and radiological examinations, results are most often normal, if there are no structural problems. However, they may help in differential diagnosis of specific conditions, for example in cases of entrapment of peripheral nerves and stenosis of the spinal canal.

Intense pain that is associated with increased muscle tension may be caused by diseases of inner organs. Diseases of organs located in the upper abdominal and thoracic region, such as the liver, gall bladder, spleen, stomach, oesophagus, heart and lungs, can refer pain to the neck and shoulder area. Pain in these areas may extend to include the upper extremities. Organ disease in the mid- and lower abdomen, e.g. in the kidney, ureter, bladder, intestines, uterus or ovaries, will tend to cause back pain and may refer down the legs. Psychological factors will, in some cases, cause areas of specific, localized pain, and in others will involve the entire body. Stretching can provide temporary relief but symptoms will only return if the actual cause goes untreated. In one lifetime a variety of minor and possibly more significant trauma to connective tissue causing pain can be expected. Trauma can include bruising, stretch injuries, burns, frostbite, and chemical or radiation origins. Irritation of nerve endings in connective tissues, such as skin and joint ligaments, can stimulate a response in motor neurons responsible for muscle contraction. Shortening of muscles, and the resulting limitations of joint mobility, may lead to

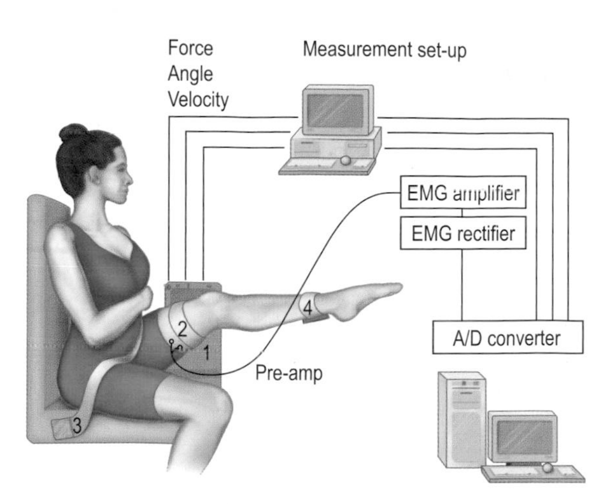

Figure 1.13 Stretching is studied with modern equipment in research. Several parameters can be measured simultaneously with the aid of computer, sensors and electrodes: stretching force – resistance by tissues; changes in joint angle; angle speed; onset and amount of electric activity of muscles during stretch. Adapted with permission from Dr Peter Magnusson from his thesis (1998).

secondary symptoms of pain. Muscles, fasciae, tendon sheaths, tendons and ligaments, as well as joint capsules, are subject to friction and overloading. Gunn (1996) hypothesized that the extra loading due to the shortening of muscles will not only cause muscle pain, but may also lead to a variety of disorders in the locomotor system such as epicondylitis tendinitis, tenosynovitis, bursitis, capsulitis and even osteochondritis. Long-term overload may ultimately lead to joint degeneration and fracture. Intense pain also interferes with the balance of the autonomic nervous system by irritating nerves of the sympathetic nervous system. Hyperactivity in the sympathetic system reduces circulation in connective tissues by constricting arterioles. Thus, muscles do not totally recover from training or work and become susceptible to overload.

STRETCHING DURING IMMOBILIZATION

Muscle atrophy caused by immobilization depends on the cell type involved. In research by Tomanck and Lund (1974) a normal soleus muscle reduced significantly in diameter during the first three weeks of immobilization, after which it remained almost the same. In comparison, atrophy of the vastus lateralis muscle was much less and considerably slower. Muscle cells of the calf are primarily of the slow type and appeared to be more susceptible to atrophy than the fast cells of the thigh muscle.

Immobilization causes not only significant changes in structure, but also affects the neural mechanisms of muscle contraction. Thus, muscle strength may weaken much more during the early stages of immobilization than changes in size may suggest. Muscle atrophy is accompanied with an increase in other connective tissues, which are not able to contract and have lower stretchability. Long-lasting immobilization also causes changes in joint structure leading to stiffness and restriction in ROM as a result of constriction of joint capsule and ligaments. Thus, early mobilization has become common practice after surgery and trauma.

Joint position and muscle tension during immobilization following surgery or trauma may cause changes in muscle length. There is an increased risk of muscle atrophy if there is immobilization of the joint with muscle in the shortened position. Muscle atrophy is noticeably faster than if the extremity is in a stretched position during immobilization with cast. Slow muscle cells will atrophy quicker than fast cells making tissue changes vary between muscles. Muscle composition also varies between individuals and thus some people may be more vulnerable to degenerative effects of immobilization than others. The initial condition of muscles is important. In muscles immobilized in a shortened position sarcomere loss can be prevented with as little as 30 min of intermittent stretching per day (Wiliams 1988).

Tabary et al (1972), Williams and Goldspink (1978) and Frankeny et al (1983) have shown in their research that the positioning of the extremities during immobilization will noticeably affect muscle structure. Positions in which muscles are slightly stretched cause an increase in the number of sarcomeres in the end portions of a muscle. The muscle adapts by growing in length. Immobilization in a stretched position for 30 min a day after 6 weeks resulted in structural changes. In addition to an increase in muscle length there was an increase in the amount of capillaries. When a muscle is stretched, the contact between actin and myosin filaments decreases, which in turn decreases maximum force of the muscle. The increase in sarcomeres will slow the muscle from weakening; this process is considered a compensatory mechanism. Muscles are suspended in long-term stretching positions in cases of bone lengthening surgery after birth defect or trauma related incidents. As muscles automatically lengthen with bone growth, there is no need to operate on them. If stretching is removed, the length and number of sarcomeres return quickly to normal, as shown in laboratory studies (Frankeny et al 1993).

Muscles adapt more readily to biochemical changes due to immobilization in a stretched position than in a shortened position. The balance between protein synthesis and the breakdown of protein has a direct affect on the growth (hypertrophy) and muscle degeneration (atrophy). Passive tension created by stretching has been shown to slow degeneration of connective tissues and reduce the breakdown of proteins in muscle tissue. In some cases, passive tension has been shown to cause muscle growth (Vandenburgh 1987).

During immobilization of a muscle in a semi-contracted position, it is possible for the amount of sarcomeres to reduce by as much as 35% while shortening in length, and muscle strength will be reduced. Muscles also adapt to changes in length mechanically by producing most force from a new resting position. Connective tissue in muscle increases with the thickening of the endomysium and the epimysium. Ultimately, muscle flexibility will be decreased with these changes.

In order to best preserve muscle integrity, immobilization in a stretched position is preferable to a shortened position. Physical trauma or surgery, however, may prevent optimal positioning. Furthermore, it is likely that while muscles are immobilized in a stretched position that the corresponding antagonists will be contracted. Optimal treatment for one muscle group may have substantial, undesired effects on another. To compromise, immobilization is usually in a position in which all muscle groups are as close to neutral or a resting position as possible. In some cases, it is possible to vary positions throughout the treatment of immobilization so that all muscle groups are in a stretched position for some of the time.

Self-assessment: immobilization and mobilization

- How does joint position during immobilization affect muscle structure and function?
- List structural and environmental factors affecting stretch ability of the connective tissues.
- Describe factors that may cause muscle imbalance and how the balance should be restored.

PHYSIOTHERAPY TREATMENTS PRIOR TO STRETCHING

Prior to static stretching (SS) methods, many different physiotherapy methods have been used to induce maximum relaxation. It has been suggested that stretching of tense muscles requires more effort and increases the risk of trauma. Thus, adequate relaxation has been considered to be important to the success of stretching and in the prevention of possible complications. If motor neuron activity is abundant, relaxation during stretching will be more difficult. Pain, in particular, can present a problem by stimulating motor neuron activity, causing muscle contraction and, in the worst case, preventing any stretching at all.

SUPERFICIAL HEAT TREATMENTS

Application of heat has been the most common method used for releasing muscle tension prior to stretching. Heat treatments are also used to produce local or systemic analgesia, hyperaemia and hyperthermia. Normal body temperature is approximately 37°C. Heating the hands to 45°C reduces metacarpophalangeal joint stiffness by approximately 20% (Wright and Johns 1961). A temperature rise of only a few degrees causes a clear increase in blood flow and nerve conduction velocity.

Superficial treatments may also raise temperatures of the deeper tissues, as a result of the increased circulation and direct conduction in tissues. There is a natural response within the body to actively balance the local rise of tissue temperature by transferring heat to other areas of the body with circulation.

Methods of superficial heat treatments include heat lamps, hot packs, paraffin, parafango, clay, hydrotherapy, and sauna to broader areas of the body. With heat lamps, the treatment time depends on the wattage of the lamp and the distance between the skin and lamp. An infra-red heat lamp is placed about 40–50 cm from the subject.

Hydrocollator packs are suspended on racks in 70–80°C water to avoid colonization of bacteria. When removed from the bath, water is drained off and the pack is wrapped in an insulating towel. The pack cools slowly and it is commonly applied for 30 min.

Paraffin baths are commonly used for the hands. The bath consists of a mixture of mineral oil and paraffin (1:7) and its temperature is 52–54°C. High temperatures are well tolerated, because of the minimal heat conveying property of the bath. Hands are immersed in the bath and removed to allow the wax to solidify, and this is repeated 5–10 times. Hands are then wrapped in a towel for 15–20 min before mobilization and stretching.

The temperature of parafango is 40–50°C and it is also applied directly to the skin. It may be covered with a blanket and treatment time is commonly 20–30 min. Opened circulation in the skin increases heat loss by the body in general; heat is released by evaporation at the skin surface. Covering body surfaces can prevent heat loss. Furthermore, room temperature and dampness will affect the loss of heat.

Hydrotherapy is one of the oldest relaxation and treatment methods. Full body immersion is usually restricted to 39–40°C, while limited portions of the body may be immersed in water with a temperature ranging from 43–46°C. Treatment time depends on the condition of the subject.

In a sauna, the optimum temperature for maximum perspiration and for speeding up circulation in the skin is 80–90°C. Temperatures higher than 100°C are tolerable if the air is dry, but if the heat is augmented with humidity, e.g. in a sauna by pouring water onto the hot rocks, the heat becomes harder to tolerate as moist air will greatly enhance heat convection. The temperature in a steam bath is at 40–45°C.

DEEP HEAT TREATMENTS

Three diathermy methods have commonly been used in physiotherapy: ultrasound (US), shortwave diathermy (SWD) and microwave diathermy (MWD). Microwave ovens are commonly used in households now, but microwave machines are rarely used in physiotherapy practices nowadays.

US is now the most common method of deep heat treatment. US therapy occurs at 0.8–3 MHz, which is above the frequency of human hearing (17–20 kHz). The output in physiotherapy devices is commonly up to 3 W/cm^2. Effects depend on a number of factors. Penetration of the US decreases as the frequency increases. There should be sufficient amount of coupling gel between the applicator and the skin. The compression force is important and should be 0.6–0.7 kg, if the surface area of the applicator is 4.0 cm^2. The beam penetrates several centimetres in fat and muscle, but only a few tenths of a millimetre in bone. The applicator is moved slowly, 1–2 cm per sec, and in order to cover an area of 100 cm^2 the treatment should last about 5–10 min. A significant problem in US therapy is that with identical US treatment parameters, different devices produce different intramuscular temperatures (Merrick et al 2003). Thus, the results from a clinical study obtained with the device of a certain make cannot be applied generally, as a device produced by a different manufacturer may produce different results.

A SWD (Short Wave Doathermy) machine is a radio transmitter producing radio frequency electromagnetic waves. It may cause electrical interference and therefore shortwave therapy machines are restricted to operate at 27 MHz. There are several types of inductive applicators, which are placed over the treatment area for 10–20 min. Continuous output is used when the goal is heating and pulsed output when nonthermal treatment effects are the primary aim. The average output power may be the same. Continuous output tends to heat more water-poor substances such as fatty tissue, and it is possible to overheat subcutaneous fat tissue, if the layer is thick.

Heat is released by evaporation at the skin surface. Perspiration is conductive and, if present in the electromagnetic field, heats the skin excessively. The skin must be examined prior to treatment, thus, clothes and all metal, including jewellery, should be taken off. Surgical stitches, implants, contact lenses, metallic intrauterine devices, and the menstruating or pregnant uterus should not be exposed to diathermy. Although this treatment method was popular in the past, it is now seldom used.

Heat treatments are not recommended as routine with all stretching. Inflammation or damage of nerves when combined with heat treatments only irritates nerves further, increasing pain and muscle tension. Based on clinical research, it is often impossible to determine whether pain is purely of nerve or muscular origin.

Factors affecting applications of heat

- Origin of heat
- Intensity of treatment
- Duration of treatment
- Coupling agent
- Thickness of different tissue layers
- State of tissues
- Circulation.

The suboccipital area, cervical ganglia, eyes, thyroid, heart, gravid uterus, tumours, cervical ganglia, laminectomy sites, and patients with a pacemaker and other devices should not be treated with SWD.

Contraindications to treatments of heat

- Acute compartment syndrome, inflammation, trauma or haemorrhage
- Arrythmia
- Bleeding disorders, especially haemophilia
- Bursitis
- Cardiac insufficiency
- Oedema
- Disc prolapse
- Fibromyalgia
- Heat urticaria
- High blood pressure
- Infection
- Intra-articular swelling
- Insensitivity
- Ischaemia due to weak circulation related to arteriosclerosis
- Malignancy
- Nerve entrapment
- Neuropathic pain
- Pacemaker
- Skin conditions: atrophy, eczema or skin tissue damage
- Stimulator
- Superficial peripheral nerves (peroneal nerve and ulnar nerve)
- Synovitis.

According to research by Noonan et al (1993), an increase in muscle temperature from 25 to 45°C reduces tension in the muscle–tendon system, improving the results of stretching. Muscle length increases considerably while muscle tissue temperature is raised, making applications of heat recommendable prior to stretching.

Wessling et al (1987) studied the effects of US combined with SS in healthy people. Continuous US was given for 7 min at intensity of 1.5 W/cm^2 on triceps surae. SS was applied during the last minute of treatment at a force of 23 kiloponds. The second group received the same stretch without US. A combination of US and stretching increased dorsiflexion an average of 1.2° more than the stretching, which in turn increased dorsiflexion by 1.3° more than no treatment. Both increases were statistically significant.

Studies have shown that active and passive muscles can tolerate greater stretching force at lower temperatures. Heat treatments do not decrease the risk of stretch related injury, because with an increase in stretch heat will reduce ability of tissues to withstand force.

Knight et al (2001) studied the effects of moist deep heat at 74°C applied for 15 min to the calf muscles of one control group of healthy individuals; and on a second group the effects of US with frequency of 1 MHz and intensity of 1.5 W/cm^2 for 7 min. These had been earlier proved to raise calf muscle temperature by 3–4°C, and cause changes in tissue elasticity (Draper and Ricard et al 1995). Following the heat treatment, the muscles underwent SS techniques. Treatments were repeated three times a week for 6 weeks. Passive dorsiflexion of ankle mobility increased in those who stretched without heat by 6°, in those who received superficial heat by 5°, and in those who received deep heat by 7°. A fourth group used dynamic calf muscle activity by rising up on toes 40 times prior to stretch as a warm up, resulting in a mobility increase of 4°. There was no statistically significant difference between treatment groups. The change in those who did not stretch at all was only 1°. Thus, stretching improved mobility, but heat treatments had no significant additional effect.

Ward et al (1994) studied the effect of topical therapeutic US on ROM and pain in patients with burns. In a randomized study, joints were treated with US followed by 10 min of passive stretching, while control joints received placebo US treatments and stretching. Treatments were performed every other day throughout a 2-week study period. There were no differences in ROM or perceived pain between the two groups.

Funk et al (2001) studied the effects of moist heat on hamstring stretching. Applications of moist heat for 30 min prior to 30 sec of SS technique proved more effective than stretching for 30 sec without heat.

Sawyer et al (2003) found that after application of a moist heat pack on hamstring muscles, it took 20–25 min to increase intramuscular temperature by 0.4°C in a depth of 2.5 cm. Hamstring flexibility was measured using an active knee extension test. No significant increase was found in the ROM compared to the controls.

Draper et al (2004) compared changes in hamstring flexibility after treatments of pulsed shortwave in healthy subjects with tight hamstrings. Subjects were assigned to diathermy and stretch, sham diathermy and stretch, and there was a control group. A straight leg-raise stretch was performed using a mechanical apparatus. The diathermy unit with an operating frequency of 27 MHz and the unit houses dual 200 cm^2 induction drum coil electrodes with 2 cm space plates were used for treatment. Subjects were lying down and diathermy was applied for 10 min followed by 5 min of simultaneous diathermy and stretch, followed by 5 min of stretching only with a pulley-and-weight system of 4.5 kg.

Increases in knee extension after 5 days were 16° for the diathermy, 5° for the sham-diathermy and no change in the control group. Three days after the last treatment the changes were 2°, 3° and 0° compared to the baseline, respectively. Results suggest that effectiveness of stretching can be greatly improved with SWD, but the effect is short-lived, if the stretching is not repeated soon.

These findings should be taken into consideration when using heat to increase muscle flexibility. Temperature has an effect on the mechanical properties of tissues and may thus affect the results of stretching. However, treatments of heat alone will not affect mobility and need to be used in combination with stretching. Applications of heat should be for a long enough period of time to raise tissue temperature during or immediately prior to stretching. Various stretching techniques often combine application of heat in different ways. In many studies heat has improved the elasticity of connective tissue. Heat can be used prior to or during the stretching process.

Heat and stretching prior to exercise is not advisable because, according to previous studies, it may increase injury risk. The increase in compliance of warmed muscles is associated with a reduction in their energy-absorbing capabilities. Thus a protective effect may be decreased with increased elasticity.

Heat improves the speed of sensory and motor neuron conductivity; it reduces proprioceptive sensitivity to stretch and therefore encourages muscle relaxation.

Cold Treatments

Cold decreases the speed of neuron conductivity, but increases muscle activity. Overall exposure to cold results in hypertonic muscles throughout the body and shivering.

In laboratory experiments (Lehmann et al 1970), heating (to 45°C) and stretching of muscle samples showed that increases in length were best maintained if the samples were allowed to cool down in the stretch position. Collagen fibres can stabilize a change in length during this cooling process. However, the same process has not been reproduced in individuals in vivo and thus best results remain with treatments of heat only. The practical difference between the laboratory and clinical tests is evident, in that the human body will actively regulate tissue temperature and it is thus difficult to manipulate, while temperature can be maintained and controlled in the laboratory testing of tissue sample.

CRYOTHERAPY

Applications of cold cryotherapy, are mostly associated with the first aid treatment of acute trauma. Treatment, also known as RICES, involves: Rest + Ice + Compression + Elevation + Stabilization. Cold treatments are effective in reducing inflammation and swelling. Cooling anaesthetizes the area of trauma and decreases conductivity of sensory neurons. Effective cold therapy prevents muscle tension due to pain, and speeds recovery time.

Methods of Application

Cold treatment should begin as soon as possible following acute trauma by placing an ice bag directly on the area of injury until symptoms of pain disappear, or for 15–45 min at a time, depending on tissue thickness. This should be followed by the application of a compression bandage. The colour of the skin and pulses in the extremity must be checked to ensure that the peripheral circulation remains sufficient.

Treatment can be repeated after about 1 h if the patient is mobile and 2 h if resting. Total treatment time depends on the severity of trauma. It may be continued until bedtime. The tendency for swelling to increase and broaden the trauma area can continue for 12–24 h. Cold packs of gel from a freezer are considerably colder (–20 – –10°C) than ice packs from a fridge (4–7°C); therefore, a wet cloth should be placed between the pack and the skin to prevent tissue damage. It is recommended that the local and surrounding skin temperature is checked every 5–10 min and if the wet cloth starts to freeze, the pack should be removed. Treatment time is no more than 30 min and will be affected by the thickness of tissue in the area treated and the nature of local circulation. Compression will shorten treatment time by decreasing circulation and allowing tissues to cool more quickly. However, it will also increase the risk of frostbite and so one should be even more cautious while using compression with cold treatment.

The patient should occasionally move fingers, hand, toes or ankle if they are under treatment. Weak function is a sign of motor neuron freezing and cold treatment should then be stopped. Nerve impulses will completely cease at 10°C and there is the risk of damage if treatment is continued.

Contrast baths use alternating exposure of the hands or feet to one bath at 4–15°C and to another at 43–46°C. They produce muscle relaxation, reflex hyperemia and neurologic desensitization. Initially extremities are immersed in the warm bath for about 10 min and then proceed to 3–5 cycles of alternate 1–3 min in the cold bath and 5 min in the warm bath.

Basur et al (1976) and Hocutt et al (1982) showed that immediate application of cold was more effective in the treatment of trauma than compression, heat therapy or cold treatment applied in the first 36 h after injury.

CRYOSTRETCH

Stretching combined with applications of cold can be used to speed recovery from acute trauma. Cold is used directly over tense muscles either until the patient reports numbness or for 20 min, because not everyone senses numbness. Following this, the therapist bends the joint as far as it will go until muscles obviously tighten or the patient experiences pain. The therapist lets up on force so that the joint angle decreases 1–2° and maintains position for 20–30 sec while encouraging the patient to relax. The patient is then instructed to apply force against resistance provided by the therapist for 5 sec and then relax. The therapist again increases stretch and holds for a count of 10 sec. This contract–relax (CR) technique is repeated 2–5 times. The patient may be instructed to use as much force as possible when applying active force or, as in muscle energy technique (MET), to use 20% of maximum. Treatment can be done 1–3 times a day, in which there is a 3-h resting period between applications of cold.

Cold therapy decreases tissue temperature and increases stiffness. Thus, combining stretch with applications of cold may seem paradoxical. However cold can be used effectively in cases where stretching has become impossible due to intense pain. Cold is often used in the stretching treatment of fibrous adhesions and scar tissue to improve mobility. Furthermore, it has been shown that applications of cold, combined with stretching, to areas of pain and tension following intense workout can be useful. Cooling decreases electrical activity in muscles and reduces amplitude of nerve impulses and slows down the conduction velocity in nerves. Thus, it may decrease muscle tension directly as well as indirectly by inhibition of nerve function.

Although cold primarily has a negative effect on the stretching of connective tissue, it does decrease nerve sensitivity and can increase muscle relaxation. This factor can be applied, for instance, with the use of cold sprays to the skin, brief use of cold packs, cold water or air. There are various cold gels on the market that have minimal effect on the superficial tissues and even less on the deeper tissues.

Simons et al (1999) suggests that the treatment of cold receptors located in the skin will release muscle tension and pain as a reflex response. The theory of this reflex response has become familiar from the control-gate theory (Melzack and Wall 1965), which has been used to describe the effects of acupuncture. Simons advises the use of cold spray and stretching in combination for the treatment of trigger points. Most treatments happen inside a building and the therapist will therefore inhale the gas evaporating from the area treated. To avoid exposure to gas, ice cubes or ice packs can be substituted for spray prior to stretching. Spray cools only the skin, while ice cubes and packs will also lower the temperature in subcutaneous tissues.

Application of cold to deeper layers will reduce the sensitivity of the Golgi tendon receptors and other mechanoreceptors, as well as pain receptors, by directly affecting the nerves and nerve endings. Applications of cold are noticeably better than heat in cases where pain results from stretching.

Cold-application treatments should be used to a greater extent in modern rehabilitation especially when mobility is limited by symptoms of pain. Cold therapy is excellent in the treatment of neurological cases involving spasticity. It is recommended in combination with stretch therapy following trauma or surgery, in which there are intense symptoms of pain or muscular tension.

Clarke et al (1966) and Feretti et al (1992) have studied the effects of cold on muscle contraction. Lowered temperatures will reduce maximum force and cause muscle tissue to stiffen. If cold therapy is used for a short period of time, temperature changes occur only superficially, and will not significantly alter maximum force or muscle stiffness. Cornelius (1992) found no benefit in combining cold therapy with CR stretching techniques.

Lentell et al (1992) studied the effect of SS of the shoulder joint with small amounts of weight and applications of both heat and cold. Subjects were lying supine with a weight equalling 0.5% of their total body weight strapped to their wrist. The shoulder was abducted 90° and flexed to 20°, with the elbow flexed at a right angle. Stretch time lasted 5 min and was repeated three times with 1 min between. Moist hot packs (66°C) were applied directly to the shoulder area for 10 min prior to stretching and during the first 2 min of the initial stretch. Shoulder motion in external rotation improved 11° in those treated with heat and 8° in the control group that received only stretching without heat. A third group received applications of cold during the last stretch and for 10 min after. Cold applications did not improve stretching results regardless whether or not stretching was combined with or without applications of heat. Testing of subjects after 24 h showed: in the SS group an improved mobility of 2%; in those who received heat, 9%; and in those who received both heat and cold, 6 %. Subjects were healthy, and therefore would not have benefited from the application of cold to inhibit symptoms of pain. Researchers decided that applications of heat were preferable, and that cold may be used to reduce symptoms of pain prior to stretching.

Brodowicz et al (1996) confirmed with research that cold treatments were preferable to heat when combined with SS of the hamstring muscles. Lin (2003) compared the effect of applying a hot pack followed by a cold pack with the application of a hot pack alone on the passive range of knee flexion. Subjects had restricted knee motion. Hot pack was applied for 20 min and followed by SS for 10 min. Stretching was applied in a prone lying position with straight hip joint and maximal knee flexion. The intensity of mechanical traction varied individually from 3 to 8 kg. The stretching was combined with the hot pack (70–75°) in one group and the cold pack (5°) in the other group. The ROM increased by 8° in the cold group and by 6° in the hot group. The difference was small, but statistically significant.

Stretching of tissue samples in laboratory research has shown better results with the gradual increase of stretching force while the temperature is above normal body temperature. The stretch should be maintained for enough time to allow the tissue temperature to drop or be treated with applications of cold.

Changes in tissue temperature, therefore, should occur before the stretch is released. According to this research, it is preferable to raise tissue temperature with exercise, applications of heat or sauna immediately prior to stretching. Temperature is lowered during the end phase of stretching with applications of cold. The effects of cold will quickly disappear because of physiological factors, such as circulation and heat conduction within tissues, which cause the tissues to achieve homeostasis. There is no evidence that the heat–cold therapy would be more effective compared with heat therapy alone in the clinic. Thus, it may be best to continue to use heat and cold therapies separately in suitable conditions.

See Box 1.1 for contraindications to cold-application treatments.

Box 1.1 Contraindications to treatments of cold

- Insensitivity
- Cold intolerance
- Cold urticary
- Raynaud's syndrome
- Ischaemia due to weak circulation related to arteriosclerosis
- Locally to skin conditions; atrophy, eczema or skin tissue damage (burns or frostbite)
- Not directly on peripheral nerves
  Peroneal nerve on the upper part of the fibula
  Ulnar nerve in the sulcus ulnaris/groove

MASSAGE

Basic massage techniques, which do not, for example, focus directly on stretching techniques, involve mechanical manipulation of connective tissues. Massage has been shown to affect the muscle–tendon reflex system, as well as mechanical receptors via pressure and stretching.

Crosman et al (1984) studied the effects of massage on hamstring stretching. Massage lasted for 9–12 min. Flexion of the hip considerably increased on the leg treated when compared with the untreated leg.

Wiktorsson-Möller et al (1983) compared the use of warm-up, massage and CR stretching techniques on the hip, knees and ankle mobility as well as on the maximum strength of the quadriceps and hamstring muscles. A stationary bicycle was used for warm-up, set at light load (50 W), for 15 min. Those in the massage group received massage treatment for approximately 12 min. The stretching group performed exercises systematically covering all six muscle groups of the lower leg; this procedure lasted about 12 min. Maximum muscle contraction for 5 sec was followed by a 2-sec resting period and, finally, the furthest degree of stretching without causing pain was maintained for 8 sec. In the warm-up and massage patients, increased mobility was only in the ankle. Stretching caused noticeable increased mobility in all tested joints. None of the treatments increased muscle strength.

Van den Dolder and Roberts (2003) studied the effectiveness of massage in the treatment of shoulder pain in the randomized controlled trial. The treatment group received six sessions of massage around the shoulder and the control group received no treatment while on the waiting list for 2 weeks. The massage group showed significant improvements in ROM compared with the control group, for abduction, flexion and hand-behind-back tests. The massage group showed significantly greater improvements in all variables of mobility and pain compared to the control group.

VIBRATION

Issurin et al (1994) studied the effects of static plus ballistic stretching of the hip adductors and extensors. Stretching was applied using force attained with the aid of a lever. In the second group, mechanical vibration was added with frequency 44 Hz and amplitude 3 mm. The increase in stretch was noticeably more in the second group.

Self-assessment: physiotherapy treatments

- What factors affect the warming and cooling of tissues?
- In what way do the stretching results of heat and cold therapies vary between the laboratory testing of tissue samples (in vitro) and clinical testing (in vivo)?
- In what situations may the applications of cold, heat or massage be recommended prior to stretching?

STRETCHING IN SPORTS

Stretching exercise as a way to preserve flexibility and prevent injury is based on experience. It is clear that good mobility in physically demanding work and athletics makes stretching a priority to avoid tissue damage.

Movement requires a certain amount of joint and connective tissue mobility. In many sports, exceptional flexibility will be required in order to achieve good results. Flexibility becomes of particular importance in fields of sport requiring a broad ROM. Large ROMs also require good coordination and technique.

Good flexibility will not always be of primary concern in some fields of sport. A certain amount of muscle tightness will be desired in sports requiring maximum strength in which ROM is short, as in power lifting. In weight lifting the ROM is larger and requires not only strength but also good flexibility in both the upper and lower extremities. Sport fields involving strength may, therefore, differ greatly.

According to research, muscle–tendon system compliance does not change with CR stretching techniques or with SS techniques of the same angle. Thus, an increase in the stretch angle achieved with either technique will mean an increase in the stored and then released energy of the muscle–tendon system. If full ROM of motion is used during movement, the increased flexibility can improve performance by using the available elastic energy. Stretching, therefore, can prove useful in a wide variety of sports.

Studies on athletes show that different sports demand different amounts of flexibility; for example, swimming requires flexible shoulder joints while karate requires good hip mobility. Gymnastics and aerobics, especially, require flexibility throughout the entire body. Usually, athletes practising sports that involve maximum strength and bursts of energy will have less flexibility than gymnasts and those who practise sports requiring stamina.

Hortobagyi et al (1985) studied the effects of hamstring stretching on the strength of the knee extensors. There was no increase of strength but function improved in regards to speed of movement. Researchers concluded that this was the result of decreased muscle tension.

Alexander and Bennet-Clark (1977) showed that differences in muscle function are related to muscle structure. A muscle with a long tendon and short muscle fibres can store more energy than muscles with a short tendon and long muscle fibres.

Several studies contend that trunk and lower limb flexibility affects walking and running economy. Godges et al (1989) found improved gait economy after only one stretching session in trained athletes. Improved hip extension and flexion flexibility, myofascial balance and pelvic symmetry were thought to enhance neuromuscular balance and contraction, eliciting lower oxygen consumption at submaximal workloads.

Gleim et al (1990) studied lower extremity mobility versus oxygen requirements during running on a running board. They showed that untrained subjects with greater muscle tension required less oxygen when running at speeds ranging from 3–11 km/h. This finding may be explained by the greater energy storing capacity of the less flexible muscle–tendon system at the time of foot impact with the ground, which is then released during take-off. Stiff muscles may also decrease the need for stabilizing muscular activity.

Godges et al (1993) examined the effects of a passive hip extension stretching exercise programme on walking and running economy. After six stretching sessions over 3 weeks, hip extension increased by 11°. There were no significant changes in walking or running economy. The subjects were healthy students with no specific problems with stiffness.

McNair and Stanley (1996) found that running decreased calf muscle tension after the exercise, but did not affect the hamstring muscle group. The effects of exercises will be specific to a particular body area depending on the type of activity used.

Williford et al (1986) compared joint ROM following warming of the joints by jogging and then stretching. One group performed a series of stretching exercises 2 days a week for 9 weeks. In addition to that, the warm-up group ran 5 min prior to the stretching routine. Flexibility improved equally in both groups. There was no difference in performance after 9 weeks of workout. The results do not support the idea that warming the muscles prior to stretching by jogging would improve the shoulder, hamstrings, trunk or ankle flexibility.

Kyröläinen et al (2001) found that stiffer leg muscles in the braking phase of running increased force potentiation in the push-off phase. A short and rapid stretch with a short coupling time and a high force at the end of pre-stretch increases musculotendon elasticity, which is also utilized in many other sports.

Nelson et al (2001) studied the effectiveness of stretching in runners. They performed 12 stretches assisted by another person plus three more on their own. SS was held for 15 sec and repeated three times with 15-sec intervals between. Time between different stretches was 1 min. Stretching routine was repeated three times per week for 10 weeks. Forward reaching while in a sitting position improved by an average of 3 cm while the results of those in the control group, who did not stretch, remained the same. Stretching did not affect oxygen consumption. The study does not imply that stiffer muscles do not return more elastic energy for a given length change, but rather it implies that flexibility exercises did not alter stiffness in the study group. Thus, stretching had no effect on running economy. Subjects in the study were not diagnosed as having any special problems with muscle stiffness in running, in which case there could have been positive effects on running economy.

Jones (2002) found that lower limb and trunk flexibility were negatively related to running economy in international standard male distance runners. There was a significant negative relationship between the sit-and-reach test score and oxygen consumption with submaximal running speed at 16 km/h. This does not, however, indicate that stretching would be detrimental to the quality of running. Stretching was not considered in this study, but only the physical characteristics of the individuals. Muscle tension involves the size of a muscle and the percentage relationship between fast and slow muscle fibres. These studies suggest that a certain amount of muscle stiffness is essential, which is logical as it is difficult to get good results with minimal muscles with poor compliance. However, runners should not interpret these results to mean that they should abandon stretching as part of their training programmes, as a certain amount of flexibility is required for optimal stride length, neuromuscular balance and symmetry. The step length of runners and walkers will shorten with muscle tension. This will further increase muscle tension and weaken running performance. Thus, stretching may improve results, and better function can be referred to as a direct training effect of stretching. However, there are also other important factors to consider such as muscle and tendon size, which increase the compliance and running economy. These factors should also be considered while planning training.

INJURY PREVENTION

Stretching is considered to be important in the prevention of injury. However, the scientific evidence concerning the preventive effect of stretching is still unclear. There are only a few prospective studies and contradictory findings have been reported. Ekstrand and Giliquist (1982) found that rupture traumas did occur more frequently in football players with greater muscle stiffness. Football players had more muscle stiffness in the lower limbs than non-players. Intensive and frequent exercising with high loading will inevitably increase muscle stiffness. In the randomized study Ekstrand (1982) showed that a routine of warm-up and stretching before exercise, cooling down after exercise, leg guards, special shoes, ankle taping, controlled rehabilitation, education and close supervision reduced injuries by 75% compared to the control group, which received no intervention. The prevention of muscle stiffness was addressed also by stretching. However, the importance of stretching cannot be assessed in detail, because other forms of prevention, including close supervision and correction by doctors and physiotherapists, were also used. In a randomized study, Bixler and Jones (1992) investigated the effects of a warm-up and stretching routine in high-school football players and found significant reduction in the incidence of injuries. The stretching was performed as part of a warm-up and thus the effectiveness of the stretching procedure itself cannot be evaluated.

van Mechelen et al (1993) studied the possibilities of preventing running injuries by warm-up, cool-down and stretching exercises in male recreational joggers. The results of this randomized study did not find differences between the intervention and control groups in the amount of soft tissue injuries. Similar results have been previously obtained by several other researchers (Howell 1984, Jacobs and Berson 1986, Kerner, D'Amico 1983).

Based on research, Ekstrand et al (1983) encouraged football players to give up completely ballistic stretching exercise and replace it with CR techniques. Reasons included the difference in effectiveness and muscle tension associated with ballistic stretching that could increase the risk of injury.

Hartig and Henderson (1999) showed that the number of lower leg stress injuries sustained by army recruits was fewer in those whose programme included extra hamstring stretching three times a day in comparison to a second company that followed the normal stretching programme. Hamstring flexibility increased significantly in the intervention group compared with the control group. However, research was not randomized and reduction of all traumas in the lower extremities due to stretching of the hamstring muscles is questionable and more specific analysis of data is essential. Pope et al (1998, 2000) could not show, in random testing of recruits, a difference in injury to the lower extremities between those that included stretching during pre-exercise warm-up and those who did only the warm-up.

Witvrouw et al (2001) found in a 2-year prospective study that lower flexibility of the quadriceps and hamstring muscles in physical education students are predisposing factors for the development of patellar tendinopathy. They suggested that a stiff muscle–tendon unit was a risk factor for the development of tendinopathy and that stretching might play an important role in the prevention of this condition. Witvrouw et al (2003) found in the prospective study that professional soccer players with hamstring and quadriceps lesions had lower flexibility in these muscles prior to their injury compared with non-injured players. In particular, it was noted that soccer players with hamstring muscle flexibility of less than 90° hip angle had a significantly higher risk for injuries and researchers suggested that these sportsmen should be advised to perform a thorough stretching programme.

Weldon and Hill (2003) reported a sytematic review on the efficacy of stretching for prevention of exercise-related injury. No definite conclusions could be drawn due to the heterogenity and poor quality of the studies. However, research evidence suggests that intensive pre-exercise stretching may increase the risk of injury, but indicates that prolonged stretching in the post-exercise period may increase the energy absorbing capabilities of muscle thereby reducing the risk of injury. The contradictory research results may also be explained by considering the different types of sports activity. While some activities do not rely on good flexibility like normal running, others require strength through large ROM e.g. aerobics, gymnastics, hurdle, javelin, martial arts, discus, golf, etc. Muscle–tendon unit with low flexibility may predispose to tendon and muscle damage in these sports. Thus, it is important to take the tendon–muscle system throughout the ROM and practise the sequence prior to real efforts.

Sports involving explosive type movements with high load, require a muscle–tendon unit that is compliant enough to store and release a high amount of elastic energy. Forceful stretching immediately before exercise may decrease the compliance temporarily, which is important to consider. It may also impair coordination. Thus, it is important as a prophylactic measure for injury prevention to understand the effects of stretching. When the sports activity contains only regularly repeated movements with short ROM and low or moderate load, injury risk due to peak stress is small or nonexistent and stretching exercises to improve ROM may have no beneficial effect on injury prevention.

Static mobility has less importance in many sports when compared to active mobility. Stretching has not been shown to noticeably prevent athletic injury. On the other hand, stiffness has shown to increase the risk of injury in sports requiring good flexibility. Stretching also reduces muscle tightness and associated pain, which makes movement easier.

In sports requiring good stability intensive stretching may increase the risk of injury by causing joint instability. It may also disturb or weaken the reflex response to stretch, which is important in protecting and coordinating muscles and tendons. However, research has shown that this effect quickly returns to normal after stretching. Thus, intensive stretching may be recommended, but not immediately prior to intense exercise or contest.

Changes in viscosity and the elastic components can affect performance; especially in sports requiring maximum force and speed, and therefore intensive muscle stretching should not be practised just prior to athletic performance. However, this does not mean that warm-up is not important for performance. Too often warm-up and stretching are considered to be the same thing.

WARM-UP

Prior to intense physical exertion preparation is made by actively warming up the body. This warming also aims to improve elasticity of body tissues. Preparation of the central nervous system to concentrate for particular performance is one of the key issues in warm-up exercises. Activation of the nervous system helps to coordinate movement, improve performance and reduce the risk of injury. Warm-up is especially important prior

Box 1.2 Effects of warm-up

- Increase in temperature of tissues
- Opening of microcirculation
- Increase in pulse rate
- Increase of peripheral circulation
- Stimulation of tissue metabolism
- Activation of motor neurons and synchronizing of nerve function
- Improved muscle coordination
- Reduced tissue resistance due to reduced viscosity
- Improved compliance of muscle–tendon system
- Increase elastic force stored in muscle–tendon system
- Improvement psychologically and cognitively of performance capabilities

to intense exertion requiring high speed and force to stimulate nervous and locomotor systems for optimal function.

de Weijer et al (2003) studied the effect of static stretch with and without warm-up exercise on hamstring length for up to 24 h. The warm-up was 10 min of stair climbing at 70% of maximum heart rate. A single session comprising three passive stretches for 30 sec was performed. Both stretching groups showed a significant increase in hamstring length between baseline and postintervention measurements. The active ROM in the hip joint increased in the warm-up and stretch group by 14° and in the stretch group by 13°, in the warm-up group by 1° and with no difference in the control group. The mobility remained relatively constant. After 24 h, the warm-up and static-stretch group still had an increase of 10° and the static-stretch group 8°, compared to the baseline. There was no significant difference between groups. Thus, stair climbing used for warm-up did not improve mobility alone but in connection with stretching exercises.

Warm-up and stretching routines are often considered to be the same, but are actually two different concepts, although SS is commonly part of the warm-up process. Stretching exercises are often performed slowly so that they will not raise tissue temperature. In some cases the effect may be even contrary. The objectives of warm-up are to activate the nervous system, increase tissue elasticity, improve coordination, raise body temperature and stimulate circulation (Box 1.2). Body temperature, in comfortable warm conditions, can be raised only a little, and will not affect tissue stretching. In harsh environmental conditions higher temperature of the extremities makes a great difference with regards to tissue elasticity and performance. On the other hand, in hot environments, the body temperature may already be too high and thus it would be detrimental to increase it further. The loading and stretching of warm-up, however, may be beneficial in increasing muscle activity and flexibility.

COOLING DOWN

The increase in nerve activity due to intensive physical work-out will gradually increase muscle tension during the rest period following active performance. Excessive loading will also activate pain receptors, which, via the central nervous system, increase muscle tension. The increase in muscle tension may further irritate pain receptors and cause a vicious circle. Stretching helps to induce relaxation and reduce muscle tension. Stretching will also affect muscle sheaths, lowering intramuscular pressure and improving the circulation in the surrounding tissues. Stretching will improve recovery in both the locomotor and nervous systems.

CIRCULATION IN MUSCLES DURING STRETCHING

High intramuscular pressure associated with muscle tension will decrease circulation in muscles. Increased activity of the sympathetic nervous system causes constriction of small arterioles and thus also decreases circulation. During stretching, circulation will actually decrease due to blood vessels becoming thinner while intramuscular pressure increases. Stretching 10–20% from resting position will decrease circulation 40%. There will be rebound following stretch, and circulation will respond by increasing acutely. The temporary disturbance to circulation during intermittent stretching with each stretch lasting only a few min is not detrimental to oxygen requirements or metabolism in the tissues. On the contrary, SS techniques applied in stages will ultimately increase circulation. However, continuous SS for several minutes may have deleterious effects and should be avoided.

Kjær et al (2000) found that SS applied in stages will also increase circulation in tissues surrounding tendons. The increase was up to three times more than during rest.

However, ischaemia will result if intense SS is maintained for prolonged periods. This may happen, for instance, in cases of joint immobilization using plaster cast in which the muscles and tendons are kept in a stretched position.

DELAYED ONSET MUSCLE SORENESS

Intense muscle effort may result in micro trauma causing gradual onset of pain, shortening and stiffening of muscles. Symptoms usually appear on the following day. If effort has been unusually intense, symptoms of pain may become worse after the second or even third day before beginning to ease. This is referred to as delayed onset muscle soreness (DOMS). Muscles will heal and mild symptoms will disappear in a few days, while cases involving greater damage can last for up to a week. If intensive exercising is continued despite severe pain, it may lead to permanent damage in the muscle.

High et al (1989), Wessel and Wan (1989) and Johansson et al (1999) have all shown in their research that stretching will not prevent DOMS caused by intense exertion. The only known method of preventing DOMS is the gradual increase in workout intensity, so the muscles can become accustomed to increased loading.

McGlynn et al (1979) and Buroker et al (1989) carried out research on whether postexercise SS alleviated DOMS or not, and found no significant difference compared to the controls. Thus, stretching will not reduce symptoms associated with DOMS, nor speed muscle recovery. No other physiotherapeutic methods or drugs have been shown to speed the recovery that will occur anyway, and fairly rapidly: usually within a week. However, the common clinical finding is that stretching can help to ease pain, if it is very severe and associated with movements in which very tight muscles are forced to stretch. Stretching is very painful in these cases, but moving without first stretching the tight and painful triceps muscle may be impossible.

Lund et al (1998) evaluated the effects of passive stretching on DOMS following eccentric exercise and found that it decreased maximal muscle strength. Jayaraman et al (2004) evaluated topical heat and SS as treatment for exercise-induced muscle damage by eccentric knee extension exercise. Isometric strength testing, pain ratings and magnetic resonance imaging of the thigh showed that these treatments do not reduce swelling or muscle damage and they did not affect soreness.

However, repeated, very intense stretching may itself lead to DOMS in a person who is unaccustomed to stretching exercises. Research by Smith et al (1993) showed that using only 6 min of intense stretching caused already mild amounts of DOMS. Both static and ballistic stretching techniques were used. Muscle soreness developed slightly more following static techniques.

Reasonable amounts of force and a reasonable time spent on each stretch should therefore be used and it is important to practise stretching exercises regularly and to start with a low intensity. It is also obvious that intensive muscle stretching may increase trauma after acute sprain and in these cases stretching should be avoided until healing has proceeded to the stage where tissues can tolerate mechanical stress.

EFFECTS OF STRENGTHENING EXERCISES ON MUSCLE STIFFNESS

Improvement in strength from resistance training is a product of both neural adaptation and muscle hypertrophy. After a couple of months the initial neural adaptation is commonly followed by structural changes with hypertrophy in muscles. It is commonly believed that strength training results in a disadvantageous increase in muscular 'tightness'.

Magnusson (1998) showed that strengthening exercises decreased elasticity in the muscle–tendon system immediately after workout. Using isokinetic apparatus, maximum loads in strength exercises of the knee joint in concentric activity caused resistance to SS of the hamstring muscles and tendons to decrease by 20–28% (Figure 1.13). Thus, maximum and repeated muscle contraction in concentric exercise will change the resilience in the muscle–tendon system, making it more stretchable and not more stiff.

The increase in stretchability results from changes during muscle contraction. Resistance in the muscle–tendon system did not change following eccentric exercise, even though the force used was noticeably greater. Eccentric exercises were more likely to cause muscle pain and subjective sensation of stiffness. However, viscosity compliance did not change following these exercises.

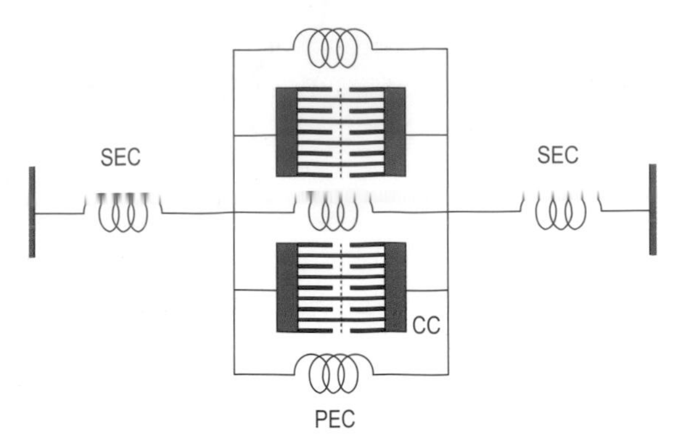

Figure 1.14 Muscle consists of numerous contractile components (CC) and parallel elastic components (PEC) plus several serial elastic components (SEC) within the muscle and in all attachments.

This is important in preserving resilience, for instance during walking, running and jumping when the calf muscles store energy during the support phase, which is freed during the push-off phase. If stretchability suddenly improved noticeably in the middle of movement, the muscle would need to work harder, because resilience would decrease causing greater demand for active muscle contraction.

Girourd and Hurley (1995) studied shoulder strengthening exercises and their effect on stretching. Shoulder mobility did not increase with combined strengthening plus stretching exercises, but did improve noticeably with only SS techniques.

Klinge et al (1997) studied effects of resistance training on passive muscle stiffness. Subjects performed isometric strength training of the hamstring muscles bilaterally 3 days per week. The load was increased gradually from 80% to the maximum during 2 weeks. On one side stretching exercises were performed in addition to the isometric training. Each flexibility session consisted of four stretches for 45 sec with a 1 min rest between repetitions. Subjects performed two sessions daily 7 days per week for 12 weeks. The maximal isometric knee flexion strength increased on both sides by 43% and remained unchanged in controls. In the stretch test, peak and final torque increased significantly on both training sides over the training period without significant EMG changes. Passive stiffness increased with no difference between sides. It is likely that the increase in isometric strength was associated with muscle hypertrophy, which may explain the increased stiffness. Increase in isometric strength and an increased passive stiffness together provide a greater potential for energy absorption of the muscle–tendon unit, which may be important in injury prevention. An increase in muscle stiffness was unaffected by daily stretching exercises used in the study.

Both concentric and eccentric strengthening exercises are known to increase muscle stiffness when tested a day later and not immediately after workout. This is related to the increased tone of muscles. Strength training increases muscle mass, and also the thickness of the tendon will increase as a result of long-standing training with great loads. Force increases with improved muscle contraction and due to greater muscle size. Muscle–tendon resilience increases with stretching and energy absorption capacity improves with dynamic movements. Muscle stiffness increases over time with increase in connective tissue, which will require more force in order to stretch. Strength training will improve tolerance to force needed for stretch. Ordinary stretching techniques may not be effective for the athlete with large muscles. Noticeable effort would be required also by the therapist to achieve any results. However, special stretching techniques with the aid of weights can provide effective results in stretching of big muscles.

EFFECTS OF STRETCHING ON STRENGTH

Stretching can increase muscle force in some situations and decrease it in others. Force is related to muscle length and the length of lever arm, which will also be affected by flexibility training. The results of many studies have shown that stretching will increase joint mobility and flexibility in the muscle–tendon system. Impaired flexibility due to stiffness in joints or muscles and tendons results in smaller ROM and decreased force potential. Limited mobility often involves pain, which will inhibit motor neuron activity and decrease force potential via the nervous system. Stretching can aid in returning normal mobility and increase pain free ROM.

Both active muscle contraction and elastic connective tissue will affect force potential. The amount of force generated by passive tissues of muscles will depend on the relationship between initial muscle length and change of length. Active stretch past the resting position before muscle contraction will greatly increase the force, due to rebound effect. In this case, muscles store the elastic energy of the connective tissue prior to the onset of contraction, and from the stretch to the next concentric contraction can produce more force and mechanical work than from a relaxed muscle or from a muscle in isometric contraction.

Stretching will also affect the automatic control of muscle tone and force production. Passive stretch may alter the muscle spindle output via Ia and II afferents to the central nervous system. Higher load will activate also the Golgi tendon organs and modulate also motor control via Ib afferents. An increased afferent drive will influence the activity of the α-motor neurons.

Hornsby et al (1987) studied the effect of resting muscle length of the soleus and gastrocnemius muscles on the force of ankle plantar flexion. Force towards plantar flexion was stronger in dorsiflexion than in plantar flexion. Tight calf muscles produced more force than in those with relaxed calf muscles. In tight muscles the connective tissues stretch sooner causing an increase in passive force production. Ankle joint plantar flexion force was 15–20% more if the knee was straight rather than bent at a right angle. The gastrocnemius muscle is shorter if the knee is bent and this position is far from the neutral position, which usually provides optimal force potential.

Rosenbaum and Hennig (1995) studied applications of heat combined with stretching on the Achilles tendon reflex and muscle contraction. Maximal force and electromyographic activity of both the gastrocnemius and soleus muscles were reduced when reflexively elicited post-stretching. The stretch reflex elicited by an Achilles tendon tap was also diminished.

Lund et al (1998) found that muscle strength was reduced immediately after stretching body parts that were suffering from DOMS. Kokkonen et al (1998) studied the effects of stretching on muscle force. Maximum strength of the quadriceps and hamstring muscles dropped 7–8% after intensive stretching. Maximum jumping potential also dropped after intensive stretching. They suggested that the stretching treatment might have influenced maximal strength through a reduction in either the passive or active stiffness of the musculotendinous unit.

Avela et al (1998, 1999) detected a loss of force in the calf muscles following stretching. Healthy subjects underwent prolonged and repeated passive stretching of the calf muscles. The stretching was applied by a motor torque device with the frequency of 1.5 cycles per sec and lasted for 1 h. Isometric maximal voluntary contraction force decreased immediately after stretching by 23% and average electromyographic activity of the gastrocnemius and soleus muscles by 20%. However total recovery was reached in 15 min. These changes were associated with even greater reduction in the stretch-reflex sensitivity. This seems to be related to a reduction in the activity of the large-diameter afferents, resulting from the reduced sensitivity of the muscle spindles to repeated stretch and unmyelinated muscle afferents III and IV. These are sensitive to metabolic fatigue and muscle damage. These receptors make an input to inhibitory interneurons. There may be also disfacilitation of the α-motor neuron pool because of a progressive withdrawal of spindle-mediated fusimotor support. Thus, fatigue may occur not only in extrafusal but also in intrafusal fibres leading to a reduction in the voluntary drive conveyed to the α-motor neurons.

Similar results were found by Cornwell et al (2001) in the study in which SS technique was applied to the quadriceps, hamstrings and buttocks muscles. Maximum jumping capacity was measured 10 min after stretching and showed an average decrease by 4%. In the other study Cornwell et al (2002) found a significant decrease by 7% in jump height after intensive muscle stretching of calf muscles. A significant decrease in muscle stiffness by 3% was noted. There was also a decrease in electrical activity of the muscles in static jumps, but not in countermovement jumps after stretching.

Fowles et al (2000) studied the effects of stretching on the force potential of the calf muscles. Intensive stretching of the calf muscles for 30 min lowered maximum force by 20%, as the force testing was carried out 5 min after stretching. A decrease in force was still evident after 1 h. The researchers suggested that a transient increase in muscle length due to stretching might negatively impact on the excitatory stretch reflex originating from the muscle spindles and thus decrease the muscle strength.

Behm et al (2001) studied the effects of intense stretching on the force potential of the quadriceps of healthy individuals. Stretching lasted 45 sec and was repeated five times with 15 sec rest periods in between. The whole stretching series lasted 20 min. Four of the subjects performed the stretches themselves while the others were assisted and all attempted to stretch as far as possible. Testing showed a significant drop in isometric maximal muscle force of 12% when measured 6–10 min following stretching. The loss in muscle force was proposed by researchers to be the result of a decrease in nervous system function and thus weaker muscle activation and contraction. In many other studies, the same results of weakened muscle force have been confirmed following intense stretching. Optimal force will not be produced by the well stretched and relaxed muscle.

Wilson et al (1994) evaluated combined dynamic and SS exercises on maximal muscle strength and stretchability of the muscle–tendon system. Experienced weight lifters stretched pectoral muscles using diagonal pushups. They lowered themselves forward as far as possible between two chairs with their hands, one on each chair, and hold the position for 8–20 sec. A second method used 5–10 kg hand weights while lying supine and allowing arms to drop as far as possible to the sides and holding the position for 8–20 sec. Both methods were repeated 6–9 times in two series. A third method stretched the chest muscles for 10–30 sec by turning the body away from the outstretched arm, which was abducted to 90° and stabilized against a wall. The technique was repeated three times on both sides. The fourth technique used a stick held with both hands, which was raised above and drawn back behind the head, keeping the arms straight. Stretching technique was repeated 6–9 times in two series. Stretches were done twice weekly for 8 weeks in place of strengthening exercises. The stiffer subjects performed significantly better than the more compliant subjects on both the isometric and concentric tests. After intervention the mobility of the shoulder joint in abduction improved by 15% and maximum bench press results improved by 5 % compared with controls. When the contractile elements of the muscle are active to a high level, more energy can be absorbed by the muscle– tendon unit. When the contractile elements of the muscle are active to a low level, less energy is absorbed by the tendon tissue and more work is required for moving. Thus, the condition of the muscle–tendon system has an effect on economy. Increasing the compliance of the muscle–tendon unit through stretching was supposed increase the contribution of elastic strain energy to movement.

In research by Kroll et al (2001), stretching of the hamstring muscles was performed daily until an improvement of 30% was achieved in mobility. No changes in maximum force were detected by isokinetic measurements compared with the control group, which performed no stretching.

Kubo et al (2002) evaluated the effects of an 8-week stretching programme on the viscoelastic properties of tendon structures. Two stretching sessions were performed daily 7 days per week. They found that training made the tendon structures significantly more compliant, which is comparable to changes in muscles. Increase in tendon compliance as an adaptation of stretching will lead to a higher ability of the tendon to absorb energy and suggests improved efficiency of the muscle–tendon system. Their findings are in agreement with previous laboratory studies that also reported an increase in tendon compliance as a result of a stretching regime (Frisen et al 1969, Viidik 1972, Wang et al 1995).

For optimal performance, it is important to improve the elastic spring characteristics of the muscle–tendon system: its capacity to store energy as well as increase strength. Subjective sensations of stiffness can be relieved with regular stretching. Differences in results between testing of muscle force can be attributed to whether the measurements were taken immediately after stretching or some time afterwards. Testing immediately after passive stretching shows a loss of force, but this effect will pass.

Force potential is related to energy stored in muscles during the stretch phase of contraction, for example in preparation to jump. During the push-off phase of the concentric contraction muscles will release the energy stored in the muscles during the eccentric muscle contractions of the buttock, thigh and calf muscles. Strong SS of one or several of these muscle groups will inevitably lower maximum force potential and reduce maximum height in jumping immediately after stretching. Stretching temporarily impairs viscosity in the muscle–tendon system, which results in less stored energy. However this does not last long and will disappear within the following hour. This is an important issue in preparing for intensive physical effort in training or athletic competition. Intensive stretching prior to performance may have negative effects on optimal speed and force. The sudden drop in force potential may also deteriorate coordination, because stretching has also a direct effect in changing the balance of the neuromuscular system.

The goals of stretching are commonly to improve muscle and connective tissue flexibility, and reduce resistance. Intensive stretching routines, however, when used as warm-up immediately prior to athletic performance may disturb coordination, reduce maximum contraction force potential and thus even increase risk of injury.

The effect of stretching on muscle force depends on the individual's personal body structure and the innate stiffness of the muscle–tendon system combined with the techniques and force used during stretching. As research has shown, intensive stretching temporarily lowers force potential but, on the other hand, dynamic stretching when combined with specific exercise, can increase force potential.

Intense stretching is not suitable for individuals with hyperflexibility and especially in cases of joint instability. Warm-up and stretching routines should be planned according to the type of sport, as well as for individual needs. Stretching routines will vary between individuals making it an important consideration for coaches when working with teams. Those with hyperflexibility should warm up with dynamic coordination and stabilizing exercises and not stretching.

It has been proven that intensive stretching noticeably affects force potential in healthy individuals without muscle tightness. Based on the research, intense stretching should be avoided immediately prior to athletic performance in sports that do not require great amounts of flexibility. Preferably, warm-up should activate nerves and increase muscle–tendon compliance rather than decrease it. It would be futile to extend by stretching during warm-up, past the required ROM needed to perform a given sport activity. Research has shown that such stretching will not prevent injury and is more likely to temporarily hinder optimal performance. Exceptions include situations in which muscle pain and shortening have developed due to intense workout, and when the activity in question requires exceptional flexibility unattainable without effective stretching.

It has been shown that stretching does not have long-term negative effects on force potential. It does encourage muscle relaxation and helps to maintain joint and connective tissue mobility. Stretching therefore, especially after workout, is important in the upkeep of good muscle condition.

INCREASING MUSCLE TENSION WITH TRAINING

Muscle tone can be quickly increased with exercise in which moderately long training series are used and repeated a few times in the training session; commonly 20–30 repetitions per series. Intense anaerobic series will cause lactic acid to accumulate in muscles and because intramuscular pressure increases, circulation decreases, thus circulation does not immediately transport all waste products away from muscles, and there is a rise in muscle tension. Increased tension will activate muscle spindles and motor neurons. Body builders use this training method to build up big muscles and, just prior to a contest, to increase muscle tone and make muscles appear larger. This effect is short-lived. When repeated regularly, muscle will start to grow, as the muscle tries to adapt to new demands and thus there will be increased production of organelles important to metabolism and an increase of capillaries. All these with an increase in muscle fibres and connective tissues will enlarge the muscles and therefore also increase muscle compliance. The reverse will happen with muscle atrophy during long-term bed rest.

Loss of salt and/or dehydration makes muscles hyperactive and muscle tension will easily go to an extreme and result in cramp. This usually occurs unknowingly while training in an exceptionally warm environment. These are pathologic conditions and need to be treated quickly.

Self-assessment: stretching and athletics

- In what ways do the goals of stretching during warm-up and cool-down differ?
- In what way should stretching techniques differ between warm-up prior to athletic activity and cooling down afterwards?
- How does stretching performed before and after an especially intense workout affect DOMS?
- How can stretching increase force potential both mechanically and via nerve function? How can it decrease force?
- What are the pros and cons of stretching for the athlete?

FACTORS AFFECTING MOBILITY

BODY STRUCTURE AND MOBILITY

Hereditary factors are significant in general flexibility. They will determine the shape of joints and the quality of connective tissues. Environmental factors may overwhelm hereditary characteristics if they disturbed the normal growth process, especially during pregnancy. The first 3 months of gestation are most critical and susceptive to external influences in the form of infection, chemical substances, radiation and nutritional deficiencies.

Anthropometric factors, such as the length of body segments, do not have a direct effect on flexibility. However, in testing flexibility, the length of the extremities in relation to the body may seem to affect results, such as with forward bending to touch the floor in an individual with exceptionally long arms. The body's basic structure (somatotype), in which individuals are categorized by body type including overweight (pyknic), muscular (athletic), and slender (asthenic, leptosomatic), is not directly related to flexibility. In all of these groups are found both stiff and flexible individuals. Mobility can be noticeably improved with exercise but even here there will be individual differences. Depending on tissue characteristics, some will achieve results quite quickly while others will require intense and extended effort.

AGE AND MOBILITY

Flexibility is greatest in small children. Their joints are very mobile because the joint surfaces are not completely formed and do not limit movement as in an adult. Joint ligaments are also more flexible and thus joints are not stable. The rate at which stiffness develops will speed up during rapid growth or usually between ages 5–12 years. Bones grow more rapidly than muscle–tendon complexes and also other connective tissue may not build up accordingly. As a result, muscle–tendon, fascia and ligament stiffness will increase during periods of rapid growth. This has been suggested as an explanation for growing pains. Schoolchildren are subject to long periods of sitting during school time and homework, but gym classes are seldom designed to compensate for this lack of regular exercise. Thus, lack of exercising has also been suggested to be the cause of decreased mobility.

Baxter et al (1988) found that symptoms of pain can be noticeably reduced with active stretching. Regular active stretching exercise can be recommended for individuals experiencing pain in the extremities during growth periods. Flexibility can increase after puberty until the age of 18. Thereafter flexibility will gradually decrease with age but not at the same rate. The change will vary individually and differences between joints in the same individual are also likely. In those over the age of 30, the X-ray will already reveal degenerative changes in the structure of many joints. Symptoms, however, will only affect a few joints in some subjects and will usually pass during the early stages. However, mobility limitations of individual joints may appear during middle age. Treatment by stretching during the early stages can effectively restore mobility. If left untreated, limitation becomes permanent as elastic tissues are gradually replaced with tougher fibrous tissue. Thus, early detection of limited ROM is important although symptoms may not yet be obvious.

Flexibility in adults will progressively decrease with age. Stiffness in general increases although the rate at which it develops may vary from joint to joint. Lack of exercise is a proven factor affecting the development of stiffness in connective tissue and poor mobility in general. Aging will weaken all aspects of muscle function: strength; speed; stamina; flexibility and coordination. Degeneration of the peripheral nerve supply in muscles and the central nervous system will weaken function, as does the shortening and depletion of muscle fibres. Muscle cells will be replaced by fat cells and fibrous connective tissue. The threshold to activate muscle will rise and thus functioning will become more demanding.

A reduction in muscle tissue will reduce resistance to stretch. Therefore, aging is not necessarily associated with increased stiffness and there may even be improved mobility. If the increased connective tissue in muscles is allowed to shorten it can cause mobility limitations. However, severely limited function is more often related to an increase of fibrous connective tissue in the joint ligaments and joint capsules.

The average loss of strength has been predicted as 1% per year after the age of 30, although changes are not consistent; the rate of strength loss will speed up after age 50. Various illnesses, operations and trauma may speed changes associated with aging and decrease mobility. Changes in function capacity are especially noticeable, if the original condition of the individual was weak and there were already restrictions in the movement of some joints.

The formation and breakdown of collagen is continuous in the tissues. Damage and degeneration of the elastic connective tissues with aging, inflammation or injury will result in repair by more fibrous connective tissue. Stretching during the repair process is important, especially in older people. Active exercise and stretching will promote the orientation of fibres along the direction of movement, limit the infiltration of cross fibres between collagen fibres and prevent excess collagen formation. Inflexible thick tissue with fibres running in all directions will more easily suffer damage under intense loading on the extremities, as well as in the neck and trunk. Stiff tissues are also supposed to increase loading on joints, restrict joint mobility and lead to structural changes in joints, such as arthrosis.

Poor general condition is often accompanied by poor flexibility. Joint stiffness can make exercise uncomfortable and training is often avoided due to symptoms of pain. The lack of exercise leads to a loss of muscle force. Arthritis of the hip, knee and ankle involves narrowing of the joint space, a reduction in the elastic tissues of the joint capsule and ligaments, which lead to limitation in joint mobility. Without effective exercising, there will be a loss of muscle force and general condition will weaken. Radiography cannot reveal the early state of arthrosis. Keeping up joint mobility with stretching and strength with active training of muscles will preserve the function, and even advanced degeneration can be symptomless while both stability and mobility have been preserved. Joint inflammation may restrict loading and in these cases emphasis in training must be on isometric strength exercises and stretching. Inflammatory phase in degenerative joints, arthritis, is commonly transient in arthrosis but it may last a long time and thus it is important to adjust rehabilitation according to that.

The early detection of limitations in movement associated with aging is important to the success of treatment with exercise. Joint mobility limitations increase with age as connective tissues are gradually replaced with tough fibrous tissue and the degeneration of joint structure. The degeneration of joint cartilage leads to reduced joint space, limiting mobility. Impaired mobility involves the reduction of elasticity in the joint capsule and especially in ligaments as connective tissue is replaced by tough fibrous tissue. Poor flexibility can disturb normal function and cause noticeable difficulties in managing daily activities.

The maximum stretching force an individual can stand before the onset of pain will usually be greater in the younger than in the older individual. Thus, the tolerance for stretching decreases with advanced age. However, it is possible for elderly people to increase tolerance with stretching exercises and to effectively improve flexibility. The maintenance of flexibility is especially important in preserving function in the elderly. The earlier one begins a regular stretching routine, the more effective it will prove to be. Stretching should begin before permanent changes occur. Joint mobility can be preserved and often the symptoms of stiffness due to degeneration can be reduced. In cases of proliferative infiltration of fibrous tissue, damage to these tissues is unavoidable in restoring mobility and intensive stretching will involve some degree of joint pain. In advanced cases, anaesthetization is needed to avoid excessive pain during mobilization.

HEREDITARY AND GENDER FACTORS AFFECTING MOBILITY

Joint flexibility varies greatly from person to person, as well as between joints of the same person.

Hereditary factors greatly determine characteristics of tissues, which affect stability, flexibility and stamina. Noticeable variations in mobility involving either excess stiffness or hypermobility may be due to hereditary tissue disorders or genetic mutations. These disorders reflect in tissue structure as it develops, making it stiff or excessively elastic. Hereditary factors will also determine the basic length and thickness of body tissues.

Gender affects mobility in a number of ways. Women tend to be more flexible than men, on average. This reflects the difference in anatomical body structure, tissue factors and hormonal function. The muscle–tendon system and joints of men are normally larger and built to be more stable. Ligaments and fasciae are also thicker and less flexible in men. Androgen dominating in men and oestrogen in women will affect differently on the development and elasticity of fasciae, muscles, tendons and ligaments. The production and release of the hormone relaxin in women during pregnancy allows joint ligaments to become loose and stretch more easily.

The difference in physical activity somewhat explains the differences in flexibility between men and women. Women often practise more sports and exercises that increase flexibility, such as gymnastics and aerobics. Men tend to join sports requiring intense force with little attention to improved joint mobility. These preferences will reflect cultural attitudes while individuals will also want to use their innate abilities by practising activities that come more naturally. However, it is recommended that men with excessive stiffness should concentrate also on improving flexibility.

CHANGES IN MOBILITY ACCORDING TO TIME OF DAY

Flexibility in the extremities and through the spine will change depending on the time of day. Stiffness gradually increases during sleep. Movement in the morning can feel stiff, but will improve with daily activity and improve more quickly with stretching.

Research has shown that temperature has a significant influence on tissue function. Flexibility can be correlated to tissue temperature. An increase in temperature will improve flexibility in the surrounding joint connective tissues and in general joint mobility. Muscle stretchiness will also improve with a rise in tissue temperature. A drop in temperature will have the opposite effect and the resulting stiffness will make connective tissue more susceptible to injury under loading. Changes in physical activity throughout the day can explain changes in tissue temperature. During sleep, energy requirements are low, circulation decreases and stiffness develops, especially in the distal joints where tissue temperature will drop the most. This is marked in conditions such as Raynaud's syndrome.

The speed of peripheral nerve conduction correlates to body temperature. Nerve function slows down with a drop in body temperature and may also cause stiffness to develop during sleep. Flexibility in the extremities when one wakes after sleep will be affected by environmental factors including: room temperature; nightwear; bedclothes type. Physical activity will increase tissue temperature and stimulate circulation.

Activity level in the central nervous system is important to movement function and coordination. During sleep this activity will slow down and when the individual wakes central nervous system functioning will take some time to return to full activity. Physical movement may feel awkward for some time upon waking, but will quickly normalize with physical activity. In cases of fibromyalgia, stiffness in the extremities related to central nervous function may persist throughout the day. Intense physical and psychological stress will tire the central nervous system, slowing reflexes and disturbing coordination. Symptoms will normally disappear with rest and sleep. However, rest alone may not be enough for complete recovery. Lack of sleep is an important accentuating factor in subjective stiffness and disturbed sleep will only partially improve condition.

The portion of spinal disc, nucleus pulposus, is made of a jelly-like substance and is 88% water. This soft part is surrounded by a tough outer covering, the annulus fibrosus. While in a vertical position the spinal discs will suffer loss of fluids and dehydration will cause an increase in joint mobility. As spinal discs are pressed together, joint ligaments loosen, and mobility in the lumbar spine will increase by about 5% from morning to evening. In a relaxed horizontal position discs will rehydrate with fluids; discs thicken and become harder with the tightening of connective tissues. Thus, the spine will be less flexible after a night's rest than after a day of physical activity. The spinal discs account for one-third of the total length of the spine. Changes in length, during a period of one day, is on average slightly less than 2 cm or about 1% of total length. Length can be quickly increased with stretching, which also helps to restore fluid in the nucleus pulposus. In a horizontal position fluid will gradually return to the nuclei pulposi and the discs will increase in size. The flexibility of the back during rest will also be affected by reduced activity in the nervous system.

Self-assessment: flexibility

- How do genotype and somatotype affect flexibility?
- How does flexibility change during different ages and what factors are involved?
- In what way does hormonal function affect flexibility?
- What factors affect mobility in regards to time of day?
- What are the differences between children and adults in the mechanisms that stretching affects in order to reduce symptoms of pain?

MUSCLE–TENDON PHYSIOLOGY

Muscle–tendon systems generate force in three ways. Mechanical work occurs during concentric and eccentric contraction of the muscle and isometric force is produced while the joint is kept unmoving. Elasticity of the muscle–tendon system plays an important role in human performance.

If an activated muscle is stretched before shortening, series elastic energy is released in spring-like motion that occurs, for example, during throwing, walking, cycling, running, jumping and weight lifting. This phenomenon is the result of strain energy stored in the elastic structures of the muscle–tendon system. The storage and subsequent release of series elastic energy is an energy-saving mechanism and is essential to good performance, especially in many fast-moving actions and in those producing high force.

DIVISION OF FUNCTION IN JOINT MUSCLE–TENDON SYSTEM

In order to understand the function of the muscle–tendon system and the mechanical effects of stretching, it is important to know the basic structure of the muscle–tendon system. Muscle cells are joined at each end by a tendon or via the aponeurosis. The musculotendon junction is heavily corrugated, increasing the cross-sectional area 10–50 times and therefore increasing stretch durability of the junction.

The seral elastic component (SEC) and parallel elastic component (PEC) represent elastic structures of the muscle (Figure 1.14). Tendons and connective tissues within the contractile proteins, are a major part of the SEC. It has been suggested that the active components, the cross-bridges themselves, are elastic structures. Parallel elastic component (PEC) consists of muscle fascia, membrane, sarcolemma and sarcoplasma. These tissues are passive elastic structures of the muscle (Box 1.3).

Box 1.3 Structure of the muscle–tendon system

A. Serial elastic component (SEC)

- muscle microfilaments consisting of actin and myosin protein fibres make muscle contraction possible - contractile elastic component (CC)
- non-contractile elastic component (NC) internal and external non-contractible protein fibres for support
- muscle–tendon junctions, tendons or aponeurosis at each end of the muscle

B. Parallel elastic component (PEC)

- **epimysium** – external membrane of muscle
- **perimysium** – membrane surrounding fasciculi, a group of muscle cells
- **endomysium** – surround muscle cells
- **sarcolemma** – covers sarcomere, which is functional unit of the muscle
- **sarcoplasma** – cytoplasm of the muscle cell

While stretching a tight muscle, tension will increase in both the SEC and PEC. During contraction actin and myosin draw over each other, increasing the number of transverse bridges. They store energy in stretching of contracting muscles (**eccentric contraction**). With an increase in length, elastic energy is stored in all parts of a tense muscle. It is freed either quickly or slowly with stretch release depending on speed of movement.

Energy will be stored noticeably more while stretching a tensed muscle than a relaxed muscle. This is because the stretch is strongly focused on the contractile parts of the muscle.

While stretching the relaxed muscle, energy is stored more evenly between the SEC and PEC. Their mutual portions are difficult to determine and depend also on the position of actin and myosin in relation to each other, i.e. to what extent they are overlapping one another, which also affects on the resting muscle tone, i.e. passive muscle tension.

Primarily, passive restriction by muscles during SS is not supposed to result from contractile fibres, but as a result of membranes and fibres connecting sarcomere, which consist of long chains of proteins possessing no contraction capabilities, but having good stretchability. Titin protein has been shown to cause most resistance in the passive stretching of muscles. It forms the internal support fibres (**endosarcomeric cytoskeletons**) by transversely joining muscle fibres. Titin joins myosin filaments at the line (M-bridge) and travels transversely to join to the Z-line located at the ends. Another important protein is desmin, which joins adjacent Z-lines together and other cell structures as well. Its transverse fibres also join Z-lines to external sections of the muscle cells (**exosarcomeric cytoskeleton**). The amount of titin and desmin depends on the muscle mass, and will rise with an increase in muscle size, while consequently also increasing resistance to passive stretching. Titin contains many immunoglobulin-like domains, which have been shown by single-molecule mechanical studies to unfold and refold upon stretch-release.

During active muscle contraction, muscles will shorten. The PEC undergoes only small changes, while SEC forming tendons will stretch. The degree of stretch depends on the intensity of contraction and external loading. The more intense the exercise, the more intense the stretch effect will be. Mobility increases noticeably immediately after workout.

Muscle consists of several muscle cells. Each muscle cell constitutes a single muscle fibre (length 1–40 mm), which is composed of many myofibrils running the length of the whole muscle fibre (Figure 1.17). Myofibril is comprised of series of sarcomeres (length 2.3 µm), which are considered to be the functional unit of a muscle. A typical muscle fibre contains about 8 000 myofibrils, which consists of 4500 sarcomeres. At the end of each sarcomere is a dense boundary called the Z-line. Between these are thin actin and thicker myosin myofilaments, which consist of proteins, which are formed by a sequence of amino acids (Figures 1.15 and 1.16).

A sarcomere is the portion of striated muscle that functions as a single muscular unit. Muscular tension depends on the contractibility of these sarcomeres containing myosin, actin and their transverse bridges. Maximum contraction is achieved when sarcomeres are at their shortest with maximum interlocking of actin and myosin forming as many transverse bridges as possible. Active resistance to stretching will depend on the number of existing common bridges formed between actin and myosin (Box 1.4).

Active muscle force decreases when a muscle is stretched beyond its normal resting position. Muscle tension against stretching is greatest when length is 1.2–1.3 times its normal resting position. Any longer and the amount of stored energy begins to decrease until it is the same as in a resting muscle. This occurs at an increase of about 1.5 times the resting position when actin and myosin form the fewest number of transverse bridges.

Although tension due to the contractile part of a muscle decreases during SS there is an increase in total tension. PEC causes an increase in tension during SS techniques as muscles lengthen. In extreme stretch positions passive tension also increases due to the SEC and compensates for the decrease of the contractile part. Tendons belonging to

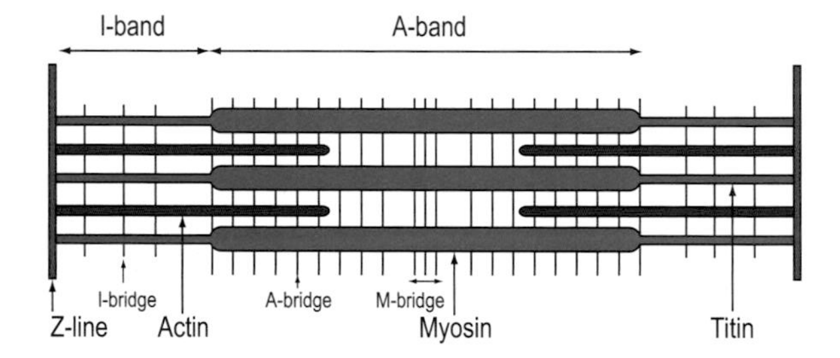

Figure 1.15 At rest actin and myosin fibres are only slightly overlapping one another with few common bridges. Stretching will further reduce the extent to which they cross over each other.

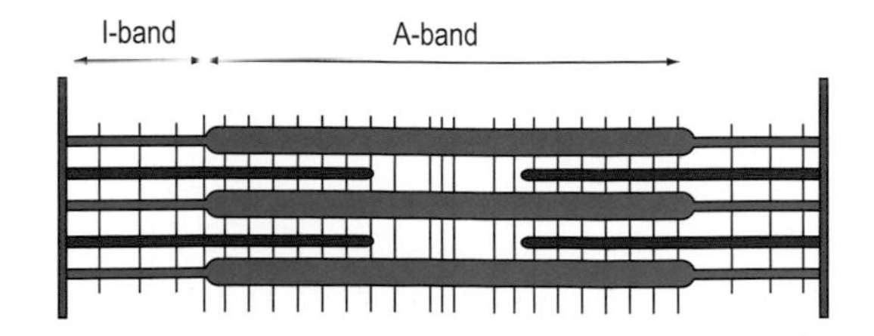

Figure 1.16 During muscle contraction, actin and myosin draw together, increasing resistance to stretching, which depends on how much they overlap one another and forming many more bridges.

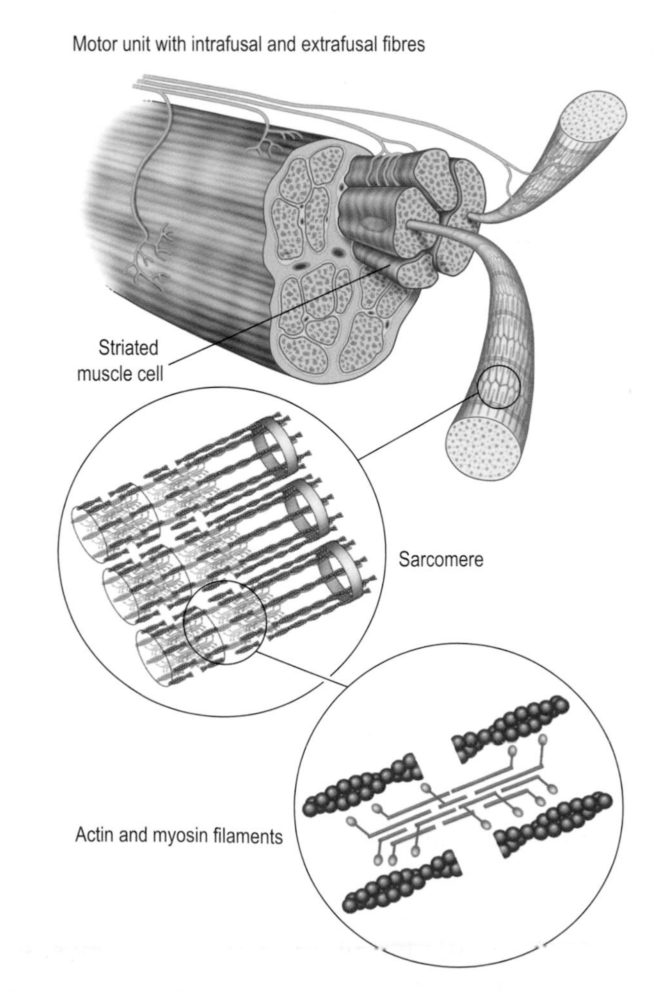

Figure 1.17 Structure of the muscle. Motor unit with intrafusal and extrafusal fibres; striated muscle cells; sarcomere; actin and myosin filaments.

the SEC stretch only slightly but are important in absorbing fast force changes in muscle tension.

Resting tension of muscles is considerably affected by the position of joints. If one end of the muscle is separated from its insertion the muscle will still be able to contract by approximately 10% from its resting length. Thus, there is constant stretch and tension also in the muscle at rest, which disappears only if it is surgically removed and allowed to contract fully. This also applies to complete tendon rupture.

The sarcomere is a contractile unit of muscle consisting actin and myosin filaments and non-contractile proteins arranged in series forming the myofibrils, which are surrounded by sarcoplasmic reticulum. Muscle fibers (*cells*) consist of myofibril bundles surrounded by a membrane (*endomysium, sarcolemma*). Fascicles consist of parallel muscle fibers enfolded by a membrane (perimysium). Muscle consists of several fascicles surrounded by fascia (*epimysium*). Examining the structure of the muscle with electronic microscope shows that during rest, the collagen of these fasciae is bunched up together. When a muscle is stretched, the collagen fibres change structure by thinning out alongside the muscle fibres. After stretching, most of the collagen will bunch back together being an important part of PEC.

The type of muscle cells will affect the amount of collagen in muscles considerably. Collagen and membrane thickness around and within the muscle will be greater in muscles that are made up primarily of slow cells (tonic muscles) in comparison to muscles made up of primarily fast cells (phasic muscles). Tonic muscles specialize in maintaining static postures and repetitive slow movements while phasic muscles are for the production of fast dynamic force. The amount of collagen affects the mechanical characteristics of a muscle to support its function. Slow muscle cells better preserve static postures and store more elastic energy in collagen structure during stretch. Thus, function in dynamic movements is more economical, increasing stamina in comparison to fast muscle cells. Fast cells can quickly produce and release energy during muscle contraction, but will tire more quickly than slow cells.

Resistance to stretch caused by muscle involves a number of factors: total length of muscle; length of, and organization of, muscle fibres; diameter of muscle; degree of active fibres; muscle tone; collagen structure; joint lever system; joint angle; and speed of stretching. Resistance to stretching in the muscle–tendon system is nonlinear and it will become even less linear as the speed and intensity of stretching increases.

Electrical activity in muscle function correlates to the production of force. Testing of muscle electric functioning by electromyography can measure the relation between electric activity and force. This relationship will be affected, however, by many factors, such as stored elastic force during stretching. However, contractile activity does not contribute to the viscoelastic response in the dynamic or static slow stretch, as shown in several studies.

A musculotendinous unit has two different viscoelastic properties. Creep is characterized by the lengthening of muscle tissue due to an applied fixed or increasing load. Stress relaxation is characterized by the decrease in force over time necessary to hold a tissue at the same particular length.

Muscle length and muscle tension will be affected by the joint position. Several muscles cross over two or more joints and thus there are several combinations of joint

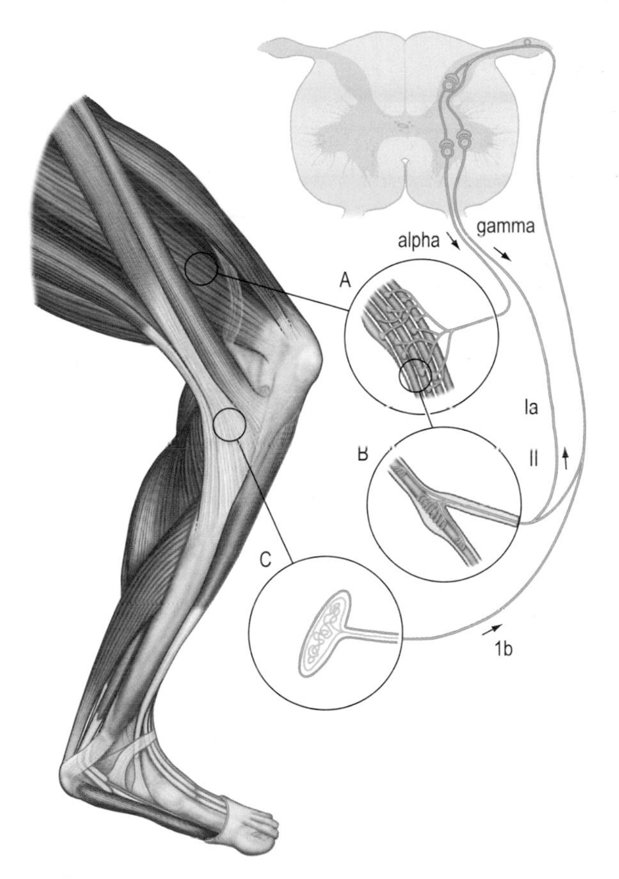

Figure 1.18 Nerve supply to muscle–tendon system. A: Extrafusal fibres with efferent α-motor nerve. B: Muscle spindle with gamma motor nerve and Ia- and II-afferent nerves. C: Golgi tendon organ with Ib-afferent nerve.

Box 1.4

- STRETCHED MUSCLES: few interlocking of filaments
- RELAXED MUSCLES: moderate amount of interlocking of filaments
- CONTRACTED MUSCLES: numerous interlocking of filaments

positions that may affect muscle tension. Movement produced in two different joints by the same muscle is achieved in two different ways. If movement in joints occurs in the same direction with regard to the muscle (**concurrent motion**) the muscle will shorten at one end while lengthen at the other end. Change in muscle length and resistance to stretch is minimal. This situation can be seen in the hamstring muscles when the knee and hip are flexed and likewise when they are both extended simultaneously. When movement in joints occurs in opposite directions with regards to the muscle (**countercurrent motion**), the muscle will shorten or lengthen at both ends. Consequently there will be a decrease or increase in stretch resistance. Knee flexion combined with hip extension will reduce tension in the hamstring muscles. If joints are bent close to their maximum, the muscle will be at its shortest. Active contraction becomes weak and the muscle cannot store elastic energy in dynamic movements. When the knee is extended and the hip flexed, hamstring muscles stretch and are able to store greater amounts of elastic energy in dynamic movement. If joints are bent close to their maximum the muscle will be at its longest and passive resistance to stretch will be greatest.

In normal movement concentric muscle contraction is often assisted by previous eccentric contraction due to stretching by external force, for instance when in walking calf muscles become stretched on the support phase during eccentric contraction and concentric contract on take-off phase while the stretch is simultaneously released.

Most movements involve the stretching and shortening cycles of the muscle–tendon system. In order to take advantage of elasticity, concentric contraction needs to follow immediately after stretching. Concentric contraction will be able to produce more mechanical work following a stretch associated with eccentric contraction than from a muscle that is relaxed or in isometric contraction. Eccentric contraction temporarily changes a muscle's elastic characteristics and contraction mechanism and will increase maximum force production, which is greater than that achieved by maximum isometric contraction. Contraction speed increases with submaximal loads compared to maximum effort as a result of stored elastic energy.

Pain and functional disturbances in the locomotor system will often involve abnormal shortening in muscle length. Changes in muscle length often cause joint pain involving overloading, degeneration and inflammation. Irritation of pain receptors in the joint capsules cause tension, and subsequently muscle contraction. Long-standing alterations in the length and function of muscles can cause structural, biomechanical and physiological changes. Changes in muscle length may be caused by inflammation, trauma or be iatrogenic, for example as a result of immobilization, tenotomy, or joint operation. Shortening of muscles around a joint can cause muscle imbalance and postural deviation, which disturb joint function leading to unnecessary loading and/or trauma. If muscles are not actively used, nor periodically stretched, their resting length will become shorter. Muscle kept in a shortened position for extended periods of time will be more difficult to stretch and irreversible changes will occur with time.

PHYSIOLOGY OF STRETCHING

Changes will occur in all tissue during stretching. The effects depend on the amount of force plus the time duration of the stretching techniques used. Blood vessels will stretch with the surrounding connective tissue and withstand stretching well in the healthy individual. Skin and subcutaneous tissue do not normally give any significant resistance in stretching; however, when using manual stretching the skin may be the structure that is stretched most if the grip gives away. After trauma, scald combustion radiation therapy or surgery, excessive scar tissue may develop in the skin or subcutaneous connective tissue, which may restrict movement and stretching.

EFFECTS ON FASCIAE

Fasciae form continuous structures found throughout the body from the skin surface to the deepest tissue. Fasciae of the locomotor system appear in three levels: below the skin (epidermis) lies the dermis, which is richly supplied with blood vessels, and under that is a thin fascia layer. The next layer of fascia is thicker, tighter and less flexible.

In many areas the superficial layer will slide freely on top of the deeper layer and skin is therefore quite pliable. Deeper layers of fascia will separate muscle groups and surround inner organs to support and stabilize them.

Connective tissue acts to support and stabilize muscles, blood vessels, and nerves. Tissue sheets direct muscle force to the whole muscle and reduce friction between muscles, fasciculus and fibres. Connective tissue sheets (CTS) accounts for 30% of the total muscle mass. Fasciae are also an important part of the structure in tendons.

Without regular stretching, CTS will gradually lose their flexibility. There can be both structural changes and dehydration. CTS, under abnormal mechanical and chemical influence, may be damaged, thicken, shorten and calcify. Tight CTS, when stretched, often induce pain-causing limitations in movement. Although stretching and exercise may be avoided due to such pain, exercise is important in order to restore normal mobility. When a muscle is not tight, but relaxed during passive movement, CTS will only slightly resist movement, while joint capsules and ligaments tend to give more resistance and limit the movement.

Box 1.5 Function of connective tissue sheets

- To keep tissue in a certain form
- To attach different tissues together
- To combine the function of different tissues during movement
- To reduce stress between different structures by providing flexibility
- To enable repetitive movement by reducing friction
- To preserve some degree of muscle tone during muscle relaxation
- To store energy for movement
- To help tissues regain normal structure during movement
- To protect tissue

EFFECTS ON TENDONS

Tendons consist of bundles of collagen fibres all running in the same direction. Tendons will vary in length and thickness. The fascia that envelops tendons is called the epitendineum. It surrounds the entire tendon and the endotendineum surrounds the tendon bundle. Bundles will often join together at various locations. The deepest layer, the peritendineum, surrounds the tendon fascicle.

Tendon fibres at rest are in a wavelike formation and will straighten out during stretch. Tendons stretched beyond capacity will suffer micro trauma and are unable to return to their original length. Tendons are susceptible to tearing and rupture even when stretched less than 1% of their length, despite laboratory research showing that tendons can stretch under constant pull up to 20% of their resting length. The elastic characteristics of tendons allow for only about 2% lengthening while still preserving their full stretching capability.

Tendons account for about 10% of passive resistance during joint movement. Healthy tendons can withstand considerable stretch force (50–100 N/mm^2). The diameter of the Achilles tendon is approximately 100 mm^2 and if healthy it can withstand loading up to 1000 kg. Tendons are more durable than bones. Their strength improves with growth and the increase in diameter. They can continue to strengthen even after an individual's growing period and are thickest between ages 25–35 years. Resistance to loading after that will gradually weaken. Because tendons withstand loading far better than muscles and bones, injury will usually affect muscles or bones before a healthy tendon. Injury and aging, however, can weaken tendon durability. Ruptures are most commonly found in the long head of the biceps and the Achilles tendons due to tendinosis. It is a degenerative process affecting tendons usually after middle age, but it may affect athletes earlier, as they experience greater strain. Extra fibrous tissue replaces original elastic tendon tissue and makes the tendon gradually thicker, although there is no inflammation as in tendonitis. The tendon will have low loading capacity and stretchability and thus it often becomes painful and vigorous loading will cause tendon rupture.

Stretchability of the muscle–tendon junction is noticeably greater compared with the tendon itself. It may be stretched up to 8% of resting length. However, the junction is most susceptible to injury in the muscle–tendon system. The second area likely to suffer tearing before tendon rupture is the tendon to bone attachment. Tearing is usually the result of sudden and over-intensive loading. Avulsion fracture is more common in younger individuals with strong, healthy tendons and strong attachments, which resist tearing and pass the stress on to the bone. In older individuals, elasticity of tendons will be less, making tendon tearing or rupture more likely under intense loading.

Tendon elasticity increases with a rise in tissue temperature and so the risk of tendon injury lessens. Decrease in tissue temperature will increase the risk of injury. Previous injuries may weaken tissue characteristics and stretchability and thus make subsequent injuries more likely. Excessive loading during the early stages of recovery from injury, while tissues are still under repair, will easily cause more damage. Tendon rupture requires an extended recovery period compared with muscles. Resistance to loading will be only 70–80% of normal even after 1 year, and thus the possibility of injury recurrence is high.

EFFECTS ON JOINT LIGAMENTS

Joint ligaments consist of collagen and elastic fibres. The amount of fibres in ligaments will vary with regard to joint mobility. In most cases, ligaments will contain more collagen fibres than elastic fibres, but exceptions include the ligaments found between the vertebral arches (**ligamentum flavum**) and the cervical ligament (**ligamentum nuchae**), which consist primarily of elastic fibres. Ligaments are fairly similar to tendons in morphology, but with a more irregular organization of fibres. Furthermore, collagen fibres in ligaments are thinner with abundant elastic fibres between them, making ligaments more flexible than tendons. Elastic fibres can stretch up to 150% of their normal length before rupture occurs.

Ligament structure changes with age as elastic fibres decrease and collagen fibres increase. Mineral and calcium deposits infiltrate ligaments and bridges of connective tissue form between fibres. Consequently, stiffness increases causing limitations in mobility. Stiff tissues will tear under loading more easily than elastic tissue, increasing the risk of trauma.

EFFECTS ON NERVES

Nerves withstand relatively strong stretching force. The risk of injury depends on force, duration and type of stretching technique (static or ballistic). Changes begin to occur when a nerve is stretched to 5% past its resting length. At this point function can often still fully return to normal. Structural changes will happen when a nerve is stretched to 10% past its resting length. Nerves stretch linearly 5–20% from resting position with increased stretching force. Flexibility weakens after that, and neither will the nerve immediately return to normal length, but consequently retains stretch for an extended period of time. Stretching to 30% past resting length will cause tearing of nerves. Damage in stretching is not concentrated to one spot, but will diffuse throughout the stretched part of the nerve, making repair by operation difficult or often impossible.

Nerves make movement in the extremities possible as:

- nerves are exceptionally loose while joints are in a neutral position
- nerves are situated such that they do not need to stretch intensely during joint movement
- nerve elasticity allows for some degree of stretch.

Resistance to stretch in nerves may change permanently with inflammation (neuritis) or as a result of injury. Disturbed function due to inflammation or trauma will make nerves susceptible to external irritants. Damage can also be caused by obstruction of microcirculation to nerves during compression or stretching. Circulation has been shown to weaken when nerves are stretched 8% from their resting position, and complete stoppage occurs at 15%. Circulation does, however, return to normal soon after stretching is stopped. The risk here is in long-term SS.

Factors that weaken nerve elasticity and flexibility

- structures under compression
- inflammation of nerve
- adhesions and scar tissue
- replacement of elastic tissue by collagen fibres
- abnormal structure of nerve
- abnormal pathways
- stitches.

Self-assessment: effects of stretching on different tissue types

- In what way do the parallel and serial components of muscles differ during active and passive stretching?
- What are the four protein molecules important to muscle function?
- How does intense stretching affect muscle force potential and why?
- What difference is there between muscles primarily consisting of slow cells to those of fast cells during the different phases of stretching?
- Which tissue structures are most vulnerable to damage during intense stretching?

NEUROPHYSIOLOGY OF STRETCHING

NERVE SUPPLY TO MUSCLE–TENDON SYSTEM

The function of the neuromuscular system is to produce and control movement and maintain the body posture and position of body parts while regulating muscle tone (Figure 1.18). Static muscle tension will preserve posture while increase in muscle tension will produce movement. Muscle spindles, Golgi tendon organs and mechanoreceptors of joints are important for muscle reflex functioning. They refer information to the central nervous system concerning muscle length, tension and position of joints. Myotatic reflexes involve the regulation

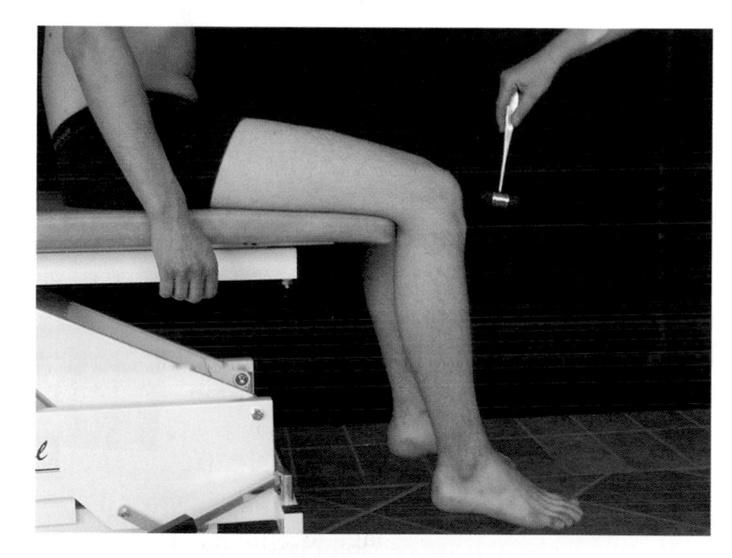

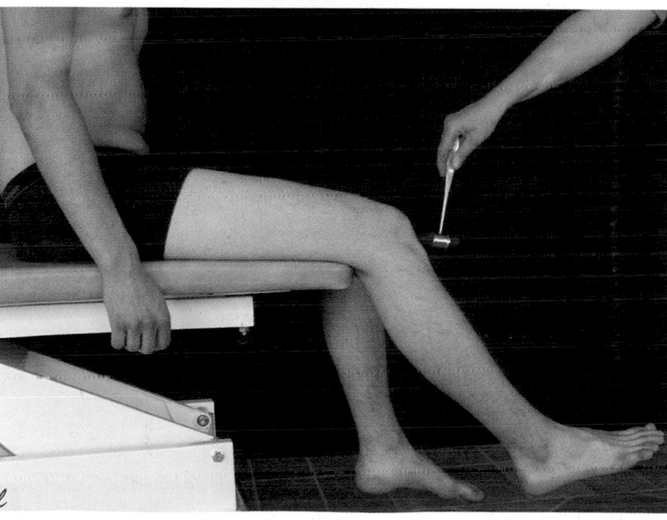

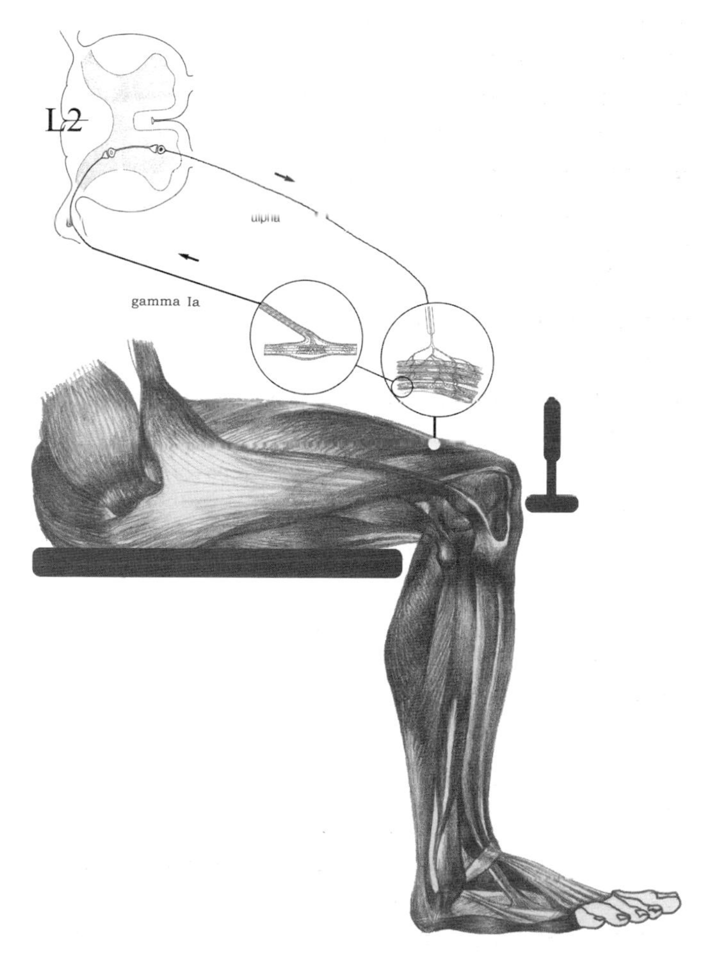

Figure 1.19 Patella reflex. The classical example of fast stretch reflex is the patellar reflex. Tapping on the tendon below the knee cap initiates an impulse activation of the primary nerve endings that is transferred along the gamma Ia-afferent nerves and impulses are carried to the posterior horn and passed via the interneurons to the second lumbar (L2) anterior horn and efferent alpha motor neurons, which carry impulses to the quadriceps muscle. The muscle contracts quickly, causing a jerking movement.

of muscle tension with the help of this sensory input. This motor servosystem functions partially at the segmental level. The information from mechanoreceptors and sensory organs such as the eye and balance organs of the inner ear are mediated via afferent nerves to the central nervous systems, which regulate muscle function and control myotatic reflexes. Thus, the supraspinal nervous system, i.e. the nervous system above the spinal cord, is essential to muscle function. Regulation of muscle tension is primarily autonomic. The neuromuscular system attempts to maintain a certain muscle tone required to proper functioning of each muscle. Motor neuron activity depends on muscle length and tension regulated by mechanoreceptors in the muscle, as well as messages sent automatically by the central nervous system to regulate movement and maintain posture (Figure 1.19). This system functions also during consciously produced movement. Higher levels in the central nervous system can thus affect reflex responses at the spinal cord level. Affects can be to stimulate function (activation) or to slow function (inhibition).

Golgi tendon organs are located in the muscle–tendon junctions and junctions between muscle tissue and aponeurosis fasciae but not directly in the tendons themselves. There will be one Golgi tendon organ associated with 3–25 muscle cells making them especially sensitive to changes in muscle tension. They will already be activated with minimal muscle contraction and continue to respond to muscle tension throughout the entire period of loading. Impulses are mediated from the Golgi tendon organs via the Iβ-afferent nerves to the posterior horn in the spinal cord. The impulse, after synapse, continues to travel up via an afferent spinal nerve to cortex in the brain and cause sensation of tension. Impulses from Golgi tendon organs are relayed in the spinal cord to the interneuron, which affect directly on the α-motor nerves decreasing motor nerve activity and therefore muscle tension (autogenic inhibition). When there is intense activation of Golgi tendons, tension will be reduced both in the corresponding muscles and in those that produce the same movement (agonist muscles, synergist muscles). This is a system designed to prevent over-intense muscle contraction, which might cause tissue damage. Intense stimulation of Golgi tendon organs will activate (excitation, facilitation) motor nerves to antagonist muscles, causing muscle tension in these muscles to increase. This mechanism stabilizes joints during loading. Golgi tendon organs are only slightly affected during passive stretching and so do not cause any significant response. Nor are they related to tendon reflex responses, which in the clinic are initiated by hitting the tendon with a reflex hammer. Although there may be some response from Golgi tendon organs at the start of passive stretching, active function will cease with sustained SS. The proper activation comes first with very intensive stretching of muscle–tendon junctions, because the irritation tolerance of Golgi tendon organs is very high. Thus, Golgi tendon receptors primarily sense muscle tension with active contraction.

Muscle spindle function involves regulation of muscle length and Golgi tendon function involves regulation of muscle tension during muscle contraction. Muscle spindle receptors are the primary sensory receptors to react during passive stretching. Passive stretching will improve mobility as a result of the mechanical stretching of connective tissues as well as stretching of the muscle spindle receptors, which adapt to new length. Activity in the muscle spindle receptors decreases which, in turn, reduces motor neuron activity. Slow passive stretching does not induce any momentary afferent response from golgi tendon organs. However, the change in length may affect on discharge during active movements. CR techniques and BS affect in different ways because active muscle contraction will activate both Golgi tendon organs and muscle spindle receptors (Box 1.6). All of these stretching techniques increase tolerance to stretch in the muscle–tendon system by raising pain tolerance. Muscles will stretch farther using more force with each subsequent stretch because of adaptation of pain sensing free nerve endings.

Extrafusal fibres form the main portion of muscle tissue and the contraction mechanism that produces the force. Lying between and parallel to these, inside the muscle, are the sensory organs called intrafusal fibres. The number of fusiform muscle spindles will vary in different muscles. A greater number of these receptors will be found in muscles requiring fast and accurate coordination, such as the small muscles of the fingers, eye and deep upper neck muscles. Fusiform cells attach to muscle cells at each end and move in conjunction with them. As muscles stretch, the contractile portion of fusiform cells located on both ends will also stretch. There are two different types of intrafusal fibres: the nuclear bag and chain fibre. In the non-contractible middle portion are located the primary nuclear bag fibres, and in the contractible ends are the secondary nuclear bag fibres. Nuclear chain fibres are spread in chainlike fashion in the middle area of muscle spindles. The ends usually join to nuclear bag fibres, which in turn join to the exterior endomysium of extrafusal fibres. Nuclear chain fibres are thinner and shorter than nuclear bag fibres. They activate dynamically even with small stretch effect.

Sensory nerves and their ends are divided into two different types: the primary annulospiral endings and the secary flower-spray endings. Primary annulospiral endings wrap around the nuclear bag fibres, and branches from the nuclear chain fibres also join them. Afferent nerves from primary endings are classified the large type Ia group. They react quickly to irritation caused by stretching by increasing discharge. They are active with both dynamic movement and under static tension. During the dynamic movement there is phasic response, as discharge noticeably increases. While the final position is maintained or the stretch is completed, nerve activity decreases and tonic response settles to the level with the new muscle length. They relay information about muscle length and speed of change in muscle length. Thus they sense both speed and force of stretch. Secondary spray endings branch out in a flowery formation and are located only in the middle part of the nuclear chain fibres. Their afferent nerve innervation is from the small type II fibre group and they refer information only about the static muscle length.

Motor innervation of fusiform cells is supplied by the gamma efferent nerves, which innervate the contractile end portions of the muscle spindles. Contraction in the ends will cause the middle area of the muscle spindles to stretch. This will change the activity in afferent nerves. Thus, the gamma efferent activation regulates activity in the sensory endings of the muscle spindles. Gamma efferent nerves to spindle cells are of two types: gamma 1 innervates nuclear bag fibres and gamma 2 innervates nuclear chain and bag fibres.

When a muscle contracts, muscle spindles shorten passively. This should remove tension in the primary and secondary endings at which point sensory information to the central nervous system about muscle length and tension should cease. To prevent this, gamma motor neurons activate automatically during muscle contraction and attain contraction of muscle spindles. The function of the gamma system is to regulate stretch receptors and preserve muscle spindle sensory detection at a certain level during contraction and lengthening of

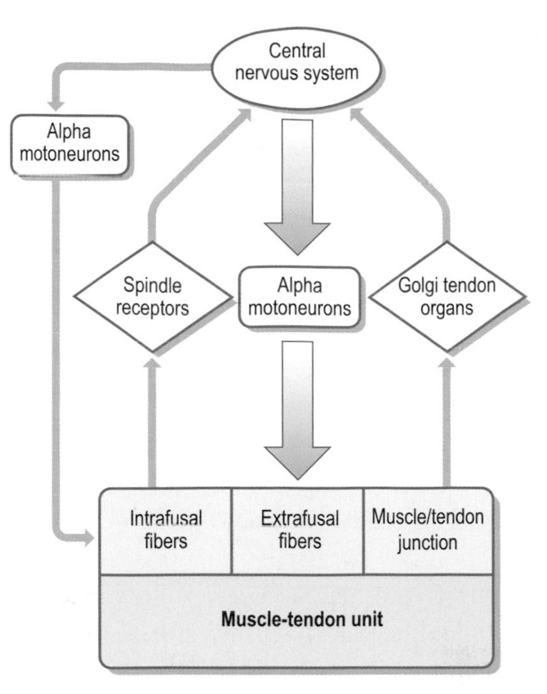

Figure 1.20 Schematic diagram about neural control of muscle function.

muscles. Activation of gamma motor neuron function occurs via the central nervous system. As the ends contract, there is passive stretching in the middle where the sensory nerve endings are located. Sensitivity increases in the primary nerve endings, located in the middle, which improve sensory reception of fast movements and preserve length detection as well.

Muscle tension increases during stretching. This is not, however, due to nerve intervention, but is a mechanical response. In comparison, the stretch reflex is relayed via the central nervous system. This reflex occurs with stimulation of motor neurons by quick stretch causing muscle contraction. The myotatic reflex involves both the sensory and motor nerves in a reflex arch. There is only one impulse junction between nerves, located in the posterior horn of the spinal cord. Thus it is also called the monosynaptic reflex. Hitting the tendon with a reflex hammer, which causes a quick stretch in the muscle, can test the tendon reflex (Figure 1.20). Muscle spindles located in the muscle react to stretch, as the length of intrafusal fibres change and activate primary endings, which send an impulse along the sensory Ia-afferent nerve to the posterior horn of the spinal cord. Stimulation transfers directly to the anterior horn to activate the α-motor neuron and sends an impulse back to the muscle. The result is a fast muscle contraction which immediately releases. If the muscle is tense, there will be no muscle jerk from activation of the motor neuron. If the muscle is relaxed in a shortened position, there will be no reflex reaction to tapping of the tendon because no stretch occurs. Thus, there should be a slight pre-stretch in the muscle–tendon system during testing while the muscle is relaxed. This monosynaptic reflex arch is not essential in the regulation of muscle function. The tendon reflex may partially or completely disappear with compression due to disc hernia, inflammation and diabetic neuropathy or simply due to degeneration of the nerve with aging.

More complex reflexes affect many of the descending tracks of the central nervous system and interneurons. There can be disturbance or even total loss of reflex control with damage to the central nervous system causing flaccidness or pathologically increased reflex activity causing spasticity. The increased muscle tone in spasticity cannot be voluntarily controlled with relaxation exercises. The increased reflex activity may be evaluated in the clinic while the accentuated tendon reflex causes clonus i.e. there will be no single muscle contraction while hitting the tendon with a reflex hammer, but the contraction will repeat several times, gradually diminishing.

During active movement while walking, the elastic energy is stored in the calf muscle during the support phase in which the contracting calf muscles become stretched. After eccentric contraction of the calf muscles, there is concentric contraction during the push-off phase and stored energy is then released. Electrical activity in the muscle increases during the support phase and continues to increase with the push-off with concentric contraction and then decreases during the swing phase when the stretch has been released.

In relaxed muscles, electromyography shows little, but not significant activity that would cause active resistance during SS. In healthy subjects myotatic reflex, or any other reflex mechanisms transferred via the central nervous system, will not directly affect rest tone or stretch resistance at rest. Thus, resistance to stretch involves mainly passive component characteristics such as viscosity. However, forceful stretching causing pain will irritate free nerve endings and increase muscle tone directly via reflex mechanisms.

Passive muscle stretching and stretch associated with movements will both affect length of the extrafusal fibres and the intrafusal fibres (Figure 1.21). There will be activation in the muscle spindles of the primary and secary mechanoreceptors which cause active potential formation in type I and II sensory nerves from which information is sent along the afferent nerves in the spinal cord to the cortex of the central nervous system. The impulses are transferred by the efferent neurons in the spinal cord back to the level of the innervation of the muscle and via peripheral motor neurons back to the muscle. If stimulation is strong enough, the muscle will reflexively contract due to activation of interneurons in the spinal column causing spinal reflexes.

Activation of planned movements will come from the motor cortex and it is also possible to voluntarily inhibit reflex activity.

Reflexes can be divided into two different types:

- Quick reaction (**fast reflex**) causes immediate short lasting irritation in muscles that increases tension in relation to stretch force and speed.
- Slow reaction (**tonic reflex**) develops gradually and lasts throughout the entire stretching period. The amount of response is in relation to the force of stretch.

Slow stretch reflexes are transferred via group IIa-afferent nerves and last throughout the entire stretching phase. When the body's gravity is moved forward while standing, the calf muscles stretch and automatically try to preserve balance by increasing activity. When walking, the calf muscles stretch on the support phase and the muscle begins to reflexively contract and it is released first in the end of push-off phase. Many muscles contract and lengthen simultaneously during movement. Regulation of movement is a highly organized and complicated system. Even simple movements involve both complex reflex systems and higher nervous control centres.

Reciprocal innervation

Muscles have both sensory afferent and motor efferent innervation. Reciprocal innervation makes coordination of muscle function possible. However, these reflex arches are often simplified hypothetical models, because the many different parts of the central nervous system interacting with each other form a complicated system to regulate body function.

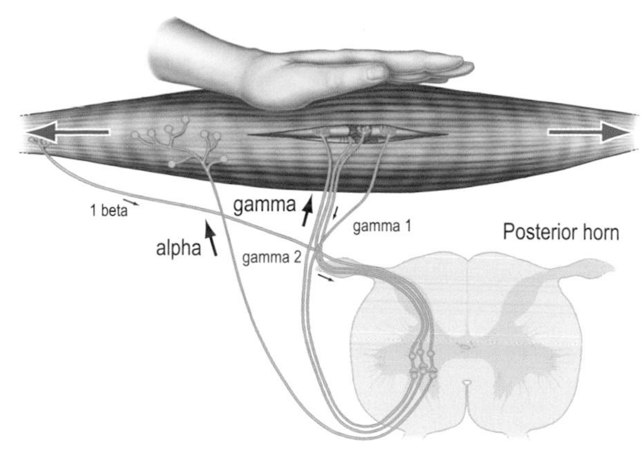

Figure 1.21 In addition to the mechanical effects on the muscle–tendon system, manual compression and stretching also affect on the muscle spindles (gamma 1 and 2). The Golgi tendon organs located in the muscle–tendon junctions are activated to a lesser extent with static stretching and considerably with techniques including active muscle contraction.

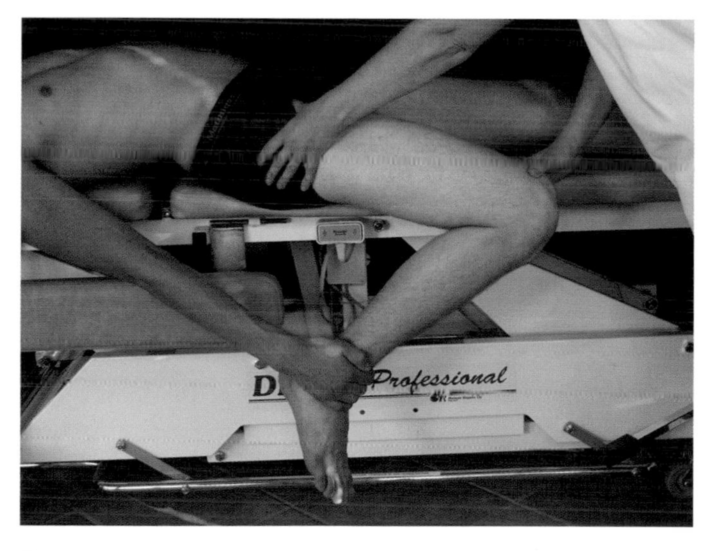

Figure 1.22 Passive stretching using gravity force and manual compression on muscle-tendon junctions of iliopsoas and rectus femoris muscle.

Muscles travelling over a joint in the same direction will usually work together as a group and muscles travelling over opposite sides of a joint form pairs in which function depends on each other. When muscles on one side contract, antagonists are supposed to relax due to reciprocal inhibition by the central nervous system, according to simplified theory of reciprocal inhibition. However, in reality the antagonists contract with the agonists (cocontraction) in order to stabilize a joint in many movements. Movement can be performed slowly under loading and it is possible to stop joint movement in a particular position or posture by balanced, combined activation of several muscle groups simultaneously, which often involves both agonist and antagonist muscles (coactivation). Thus, central nervous system is important for the regulation of cocontraction of muscles not only around one joint, but also several joints in legs, body and arm simultaneously, for example in weight lifting. Both sensory and motor innervation of muscles are needed to make coordinated movements possible while maintaining joint stability and balance of the whole body. Receiving information from muscles, joint capsules, ligaments and other sense organs, essentially from the balance organ and eyes, rapid automatic analyzing of this huge amount of information in the central nervous system is essential for adequate functioning. Depending on received information, the central nervous system may simultaneously activate some muscles to start and speed up movements and inhibit some muscles to slow down and stop.

Autogenic inhibition involves a muscle's ability to inhibit its own function. The purpose of this autogenic inhibition is related to protection from overloading the muscles. When a muscle is intensely stretched, the increased tension in muscle spindles activates the muscle's own reflex reaction. Inverse myotatic reflex will cause inhibition of motor nerve and rapid reduction of muscle tension. When stretch force reaches a particular level, resistance disappears suddenly with a subsequent clasp-knife phenomenon. This was earlier thought to be associated only with Golgi tendon organ function, but is now considered to involve muscle spindle gamma neurons and pain nerves with thin myelin sheath. Often mechanoreceptors and pain nerves in joint capsules and ligaments are involved with inhibition of muscle activity when there is excessive loading.

SS has been shown to only slightly increase electrical activity in normal muscles, which reflects minimal increase of motor neuron activity. When the stretch is maintained, this will decrease, and there will be no significant activity in afferent nerves from muscle spindles of Golgi tendon organs during passive stretching.

Approximately one-third of patients with repaired tissue damage caused by acute strains will suffer chronic functional problems. This is due to structural changes in connective tissue during the repair process, imperfection in restored proprioception and hyperactivity of pain

Box 1.6

- Muscle spindles are primarily stretch sensitive receptors
- Golgi tendon receptors primarily react to active muscle contraction

nerves. Stretching and active muscle contractions improve not only mechanical flexibility of connective tissues and other tissue properties, but also have an effect on muscle–tendon and joint reception activity in relation to sensory information (Figure 1.23). Exercising should aim to normalize nerve function. Activation of nerves with certain exercises can achieve both functional and structural changes in the central nervous system, which affect muscle activation and coordination. Improved nervous function makes the contraction and relaxation of agonist and antagonist muscles faster and more efficient.

Mechanoreceptors of joints

There are several receptors in joints, which aid in the regulation of movement and posture. These receptors are divided by structure and function into four different types. They appear in the tendons, the tendon sheaths, ligaments and joint capsules (Table 1.1). Receptors are found mostly at the muscle–tendon junction but also at the tendon–bone insertion. Joint ligaments are normally located externally to joints, reinforcing with joint capsules or completely separate from them. The cruciate ligaments of the knee are an example of exceptions to the rule, as they are located inside the knee joint. Forceful stretching of ligaments will cause a reflex tension in quadricep muscles to stabilize the joint. Pain receptors in joints protect connective tissue from excessive stress. If receptors are not functioning properly, such as with local anaesthesia in athletic competition, there is a risk that intense effort and stress may cause tissue damage.

Type I receptors are called Ruffin corpuscles or endings. They consist of nerve endings surrounded by thin capsules that are located in the exterior joint capsule layer. These mechanical receptors are found in greater quantities in the big joints of the extremities, such as the hip and knee, than in the small joints of the hand and foot. They activate easily to stretch irritation and their function decreases slowly for the duration of the stretch. Receptors are activated even with minimal loading (about 3 g) and will continue until the load is removed. These easily activated mechanical receptors are always partially activated according to joint position and thus mediate information even during rest. They refer information about joint movement, direction, range and speed regardless of whether or not movement is active or passive. They sense pressure on joints and reflexively cause muscle tension to preserve posture, assist movement and decrease activity in pain pathways. Receptors are by type, both static and dynamic.

Type II receptors are called Vater–Pacini corpuscles. They are nerve endings surrounded by capsules thicker than the type I receptors. These mechanical receptors are found more often in the small joints of the extremities than in large joints. They activate easily both with slow and fast movements of joints as with type I receptors, but their function stops quickly with static loading and stretching. They function to relay information about movement changes and are not active while joints are at rest. Receptors are by type dynamic.

Type III receptors, known as Golgi tendon organs, are thin and located in the joint capsules and in the ligaments of many joints, but they have not been found in the ligaments of the vertebral joints. They are larger than other joint receptors and their activation threshold is high. Golgi tendon organs activate only with intense irritation, when a joint nears its furthest ROM and joint ligaments are considerably stretched. The activity will gradually decrease within a few seconds while the joint stretch is maintained. Thus, they do not function while the joint is not moving. Their primary job is to refer information about direction of joint movement and reduce joint movement by protective reflexes. Receptors are by type dynamic.

Type IV receptors are free nerve endings without capsules and are divided into two categories. Type α receptors are located in the fatty tissue layer surrounding a joint, the entire joint capsule including the synovial tissue. They are not found in the joint cartilage. They are innervated by nerves without myelin sheath. Type β receptors are not associated with any particular tissue, but they are mostly found in the internal and external joint ligaments. They are innervated by thin nerves with myelin sheath. Normally these pain receptors are not active until intense stress causes mechanical damage or there is infection or chemical inflammation in the joint. They do not adapt easily and function can last for extended periods of time.

Table 1.1 Characteristics of mechanoreceptors of joints

Type	Location	Size	Nerve fibres	Irritability	Sense
I Ruffin corpuscles	Joint capsule, outer layer	100 × 40 μm	Thin myelin sheath 6–9 μm	Activate easily Adapt slowly	Position Direction Movement
II Vater-Pacini corpuscles	Joint capsule, inner layer	280 × 120 μm	Middle sized Myelin sheath 9–12 μm	Activate easily Adapt quickly	Movement
III Golgi tendon organs	Joint ligament and muscle-tendon junction	600 × 100 μm	Thick myelin sheath 13–17 μm	Require intense irritation Adapt slowly	Muscle contraction pressure Stretch
IV Free nerve endings	Joint ligament and capsule, muscle-tendon	1 μm	Without myelin sheath <1 μm Myelin sheath 2–5 μ	Require intense irritation Not adapt easily	Chemosensitive Ischaemia "Pain sense"

Function of central nervous system in regulation of muscle tension

Regulation of muscle tone during movement and rest occurs via the central nervous system in the cerebrum, cerebellum, brain stem and also in the spinal cord.

The primary motor area is located in the precentral gyrus of the cerebral cortex and in front of that is located premotor cortex. Impulses leave from these areas to travel along the corticospinal tract down to the spinal cord. This main pathway of motor impulses is called the pyramidal tract. It will end at the anterior horn from which α-motor nerve mediates impulses to the muscles and induces conscious movement.

Some descending nerves synapse with gamma efferent nerves running into muscle spindles. Nerve pathways from the cerebellum via the thalamus also run in the pyramidal tract and are important in movement control. They regulate muscle spindle activity, which affect muscle cell contraction during movement as well as during rest. Movements are finely controlled with the help of muscle spindles and gamma reflexes.

The central nervous system regulates muscle tone via muscle spindles by assessing and changing their length and, in turn, afferent information from spindles affects impulse activity to α- motor neurons. Muscle spindles are an important part of the servosystem regulating muscle tone, which is automatic to a greater extent, although it may be affected both consciously as well as by stretching. Stimulation of areas in the brain responsible for inhibition will decrease muscle tone while stimulation of areas responsible for facilitation will increase muscle tone. Normally, the function of the central nervous system is balanced.

The formatio reticularis is important, regulating several organ functions in the body as well as movement and muscle tone. Incoming information from sensory nerves is processed by the formatio reticularis. Sensation related to muscle tension from muscle spindles is regulated by the limbic system and the hypothalamus. Afferent gamma nerve activity will automatically increase activity of formation reticularis. Reticulospinal tract is a nerve pathway leaving from the formation reticularis to the spinal cord, which affect both α- and gamma motor nerves. These areas do not function alone, but are controlled by nerve connections with the cerebral cortex. The cerebral cortex inhibits gamma motor neuron activity. If the cortex is isolated from the formatio reticularis, or there is trauma or necrosis, e.g. as a result of cerebral infarct, muscle tone will consequently increase and result in spastic paralysis of muscles. The bulboreticular formation also inhibits gamma motor neuron activity, but it does not function alone and it depends on activity of the extrapyramidal tract and cerebellum. In contrast, higher centers of the bulboreticular formation independently activate gamma motor neurons. The area extends from the thalamus and hypothalamic nuclei via the middle cerebellar peduncle to the pons. This area will be activated by the dentate nucleus of the cerebellum and tracts to the thalamus, which will thus also increase gamma neuron activity. Injury to these tracts to the cerebellum can cause hypotonic paralysis of muscles and partially or completely prevent reflex reactions. When the basal ganglia, cerebellum or cerebral cortex control over movement is decreased as a result of, for example, stroke, brain haemorrhage or contusion, gamma neuron activity will subsequently increase.

Spasticity related to overactive reflex, as mentioned earlier, results from lack of inhibition of the gamma system and leads to overactive gamma motor neuron function, which in turn causes an increase in α-motor nerve activity. Although overactive gamma motor neuron function can appear with damage to higher motor centers, more significant factors causing spasticity involve the lack of activity in descending inhibitory pathways below the cortex, which maintain normal inhibitory interneuron (Renshaw cell) activity and thus decrease spinal motor neuron function. A decrease in their activity will automatically increase α-motor neuron activity and increase muscle tone and amplify reflex activity. Ib-afferent nerves from Golgi tendon organs activate inhibitory interneurons, but the effect is decreased while there is a defect in central inhibition. Furthermore, the effect of Ia-afferent nerves from muscles in preventing inhibitory interneurons is decreased and fast stretching of muscles causes a considerable increase in activity of spastic muscles. Stiffness associated with spasticity is not only due to nervous function, but also involves gradual changes in viscosity and elasticity making tissues resistant to stretch even during rest.

Formatio reticularis function affects information received from the vestibular nucleus, which mediates information from the balance organ of the inner ear. It increases muscle tone via direct reflectory nerve tracts to motor neurons. The nucleus also receives information from the eyes and mechanoreceptors, especially from the upper neck area. Vestibular nucleus function is affected by other autonomic areas, such as the basal ganglia and cerebellum, from which information decreases nucleus function. Thus, the increase in muscle tone may be suppressed.

For most of the time, lower centers of the nervous system entirely and automatically regulate body, arm and leg posture. The cortex primarily controls conscious function of the fingers. Specialized, precision movements require more guidance from the cortex than the larger movements of the arms and legs. Gamma information to the central nervous system regulates fine motor function, especially in the fingers. Thus, muscles in fingers contain more muscle spindles compared to the big muscles in extremities.

Muscle stiffness is also affected by mechanical and metabolic factors. Internal muscle stiffness is regulated by elastic deformation of the transverse bridges between fibres in the short term. However, muscles become completely flaccid if efferent motor neuron function ceases due to peripheral nerve entrapment, trauma or nerve root compression, for instance due to the pressure from disc hernia. Regulation of muscle tone during rest is an autonomic function, which depends on the activity of motor neurons coming from the anterior horn of the spinal cord. This autonomic system can also be affected consciously with various relaxation exercises and other techniques like biofeedback and hypnosis.

Self-assessment: nervous function in relation to regulation of muscle tone

- How do the mechanoreceptors of joints and muscles differ in function during static and contract–relax-stretch techniques?
- How do intrafusal and extrafusal fibres differ in function and in nerve innervation?
- How is information regarding muscle tone and movement relayed to the central nervous system?
- Why can sensory reception of muscle tone alter in different situations?
- What is the difference between stretch response and stretch reflex?
- How can stroke or brain trauma result in a significant drop in muscle tone or, in contrast, spasticity?
- How can joint receptors both decrease or increase muscle tone?

DEFINITIONS OF STRETCHING

ACTIVE STRETCHING

Usually no exterior force is applied during active stretching of muscles, which uses voluntary contraction of agonist muscles to produce active ROM. Thus the ROM will depend on the resistance of the muscle to be stretched as well as on the strength of the agonist muscle performing the stretch. Active stretching is used primarily to maintain normal mobility while passive stretching attempts to increase ROM.

PASSIVE STRETCHING

Passive stretching is a simple stretching method. It uses external force, directed to stretch the desired body tissues with the aid of an assistant, therapist, machine, weight and pulley system or without external aid by the subject pulling, for example, the legs with their own hands or using gravity and body positions to create stretching force.

Some consider stretching to be passive if another person supplies the stretch force and active if oneself performs it without help from any other person. However, if another person supplies the stretch, it is a case of assisted stretching, which may be passive or active. In passive stretching the individual receiving treatment does not directly participate in the stretching process other than as an object to be treated. The idea of being simply an object, however, is questionable. Although an assistant may apply stretching, the individual must participate by preparing with the appropriate positioning and actively relax muscles. While using CR stretching technique the subject at first contracts the muscle to be stretched against the resistance of the assistant and thereafter follows passive stretching. While using CR-AC the technique is definitely active even though there would be assistance in both antagonist and agonist contraction phases. There are several manual compression techniques used with stretching, which also fall in this category (Figure 1.22).

ACTIVE ASSISTED STRETCHING

In the active assisted stretching the therapist applies passive stretching, while the subject assists the movement by contracting the agonist muscles. This stretching technique has been used to increase mobility as well as strengthen weak muscles and improve coordination. CR stretching is an even more commonly used form of active assisted stretching.

DYNAMIC STRETCHING

Dynamic stretching implies that the muscle is stretched by moving a joint in the direction that muscle will be stretched and immediately returned in the direction that the stretch will lessen. This may be repeated several times while gradually increasing the ROM, so that the targeted tissues become gradually elongated. Stretching may be slow with a steady speed or may accelerate to high speed with deceleration near the end ROM as in ballistic stretching, which is essentially dynamic stretching. Dynamic stretching (Fig. 1.22) may be active while using antagonist muscles to produce the movement (a) or it may be passive while using the weights (b) and gravity (c) to produce the stretch. Athletes often use weight-assisted dynamic stretching.

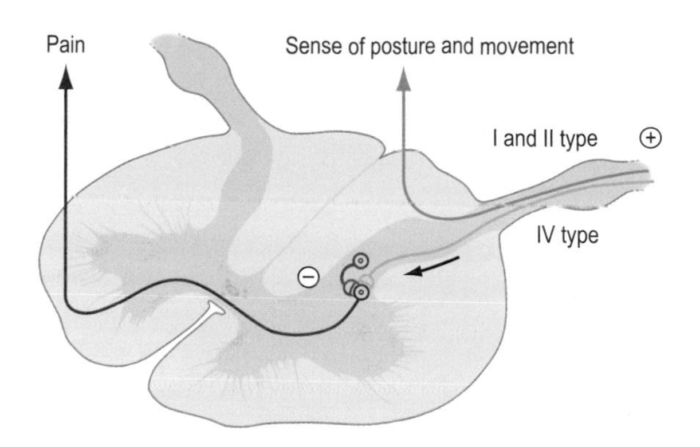

Figure 1.23 Modified drawing according to the gate control theory, the irritation of sensory nerves inhibits pain nerve activity in the posterior horn of the spinal cord (Melzack and Stillwell 1977). Inhibition has been shown to also occur in several other levels in the central nervous system. Exercises activate mechanoreceptors causing inhibition on pain pathways. However, many types of physical training, and static loading in particular, have a contradictory effect and may thus activate pain nerves, making the condition worse.

BALLISTIC STRETCHING (BS)

In ballistic stretching methods, movement is achieved with strong and repetitive muscle contraction of the agonist muscles to stretch the antagonist muscles. Movement is usually repeated a number of times without stopping and is classified as a dynamic stretching technique. Dynamic stretching techniques can also be done with a slow steady speed, in which case they would not be ballistic. Strong and fast stretching causes a reflex that activates muscles and a resistance to stretch. However, ballistic stretching is not so fast that it would initiate intense muscle contraction and prevent movement, as it slows near the end of the ROM. Muscle tension level is greater than in SS and CR techniques.

The ballistic method is an important stretching method for many athletes. It can be used to increase stretch strength and improve coordination at the farthest ROM. It is a demanding technique requiring balance, control over movements, strength and speed. As a specific training exercise for certain sports, such as swimming, weight lifting, javelin throwing and many other track events, it is a popular stretching technique. Ballistic techniques are often used during warm-up for sports requiring good mobility. The advantage of this technique is that it combines stretching with coordination exercises.

STATIC STRETCHING (SS)

SS involves moving the joint to the point in which there is considerable resistance from muscle tension. The stretch is maintained at this point until reduction of tension takes place and then the joint is returned so far that the stretch is released. SS may also be repeated several times.

SS also includes an active component, when moving to the stretch position and, again, when returning from it. Stretching by definition is essentially passive, because the joint has to be held in a stretched position for a relatively long time. Of course the antagonist muscle can also achieve this, but the force will often then be quite low and does not produce an effective stretch.

Agonist Contract Stretching (AC)

In active ROM training, extremities are actively moved into the stretch position and held there for a given amount of time. Thus, it involves static phase. Agonist muscles are used to achieve the stretch position and therefore a certain amount of strength and effort is required so that the stretch will be effective. This stretching technique is not suitable in conditions of trauma or overstrain, where contraction of agonist muscles provokes pain, or the muscles are weak.

Both active and passive stretching methods have positive and negative aspects. SS is easy to perform. Active stretching is less likely to cause tissue damage and may also increase muscle strength. Whatever technique is used, it is important that the assistant motivates the patient. The therapist can encourage the patient, which should mean the force of the stretch is gradually increased and thus results, especially in alleviating pain, will be improved. However, assisted SS involves some risk of overstretching and may cause tissue damage.

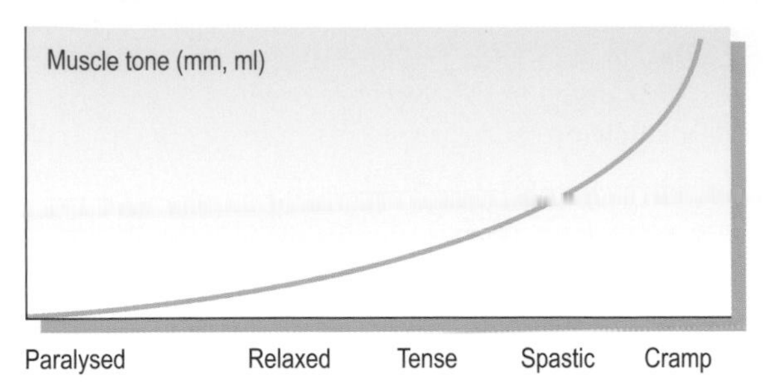

Figure 1.24 Muscle tone measured with computerized muscle tonometer and state of the muscle.

RESEARCH ON STRETCHING

During effective stretching, connective tissue is applied greater force than the force in resisting the movement. Stretching can be made more effective by increasing the force, stretch duration and amount of stretches, and reducing tissue resistance. Resistance to stretch is primarily in connective tissue surrounding joints, passive components of the muscle–tendon system and contractile components of muscles. Passive components of resistance include the viscosity and elasticity of muscles and tendons due to connective tissue, joint ligaments and capsules, subcutaneous tissues and skin (Figure 1.24). Active components of resistance include voluntary and autonomic muscle tension that involves the complex reflex mechanisms of the central nervous system. Stretching techniques attempt to reduce the degree of both passive and active resistance.

Studies have focused on determining the effects of different stretching methods:

- on range of motion
- on viscosity and elastic characteristics of the muscle–tendon system
- on stress tolerance of the muscle–tendon system
- on electrical characteristics of muscles and reflexes

VISCOUS AND ELASTIC RESISTANCE OF CONNECTIVE TISSUE DURING STRETCH

The basic structure of connective tissue is formed by the different thickness and complex direction of collagen fibres, which are surrounded by protein-polysaccharide structures. Collagen is durable in stretching and is organized in different connective tissue structures such as tendons, ligaments, tendon-membranes and joint capsules, according to their specific requirements.

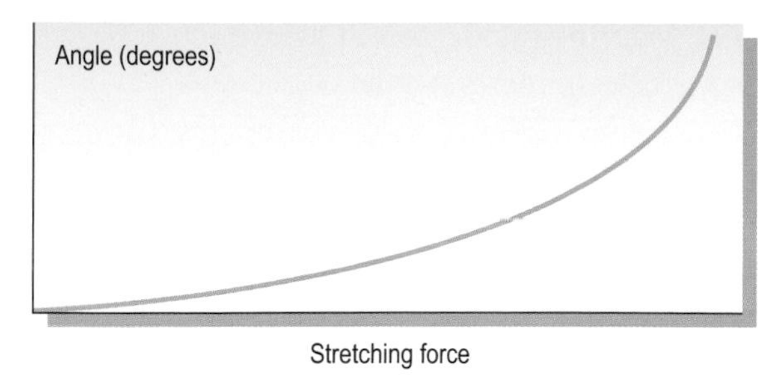

Figure 1.25 Joint angle increases rapidly with only a small increase of force at the beginning, but resistance will rise with the joint angle, and near the end of the range of motion (ROM) only a small increase in ROM can be achieved even by a considerable increase in the stretching force.

The behaviour of the viscous and elastic components of the connective tissue varies depending on the structure and amount of tissues fibres. Thus, different connective tissues will have specific viscous and elastic properties and each type will respond in its own way to stretching. Power is quickly released from elastic factors, while viscous factors react slowly. Stretching causes elastic and plastic deformation in connective tissue. After stretching elastic properties in connective tissue structure will return to their previous state, if the stretch has not been too forceful. Viscous properties will allow more long-standing changes in tissue structure. Continuous or repeated stretching with enough force will cause plastic changes due to creep phenomenon in connective tissues, in which deformity remains after stress is released. The resistance against stretch will then decrease. Plastic changes are supposed to happen primarily in myo-tendinous junctions.

Resistance, due to the pulling spring, increases linearly to a limit that the spring can tolerate. Biological material such as connective tissue resistance is not linear but increases logarithmically (Figure 1.25).

During walking, the calf muscles stretch during the push of phase then, during the swing phase, return to the original position and result in neither mobility nor elastic force changes in the next step. Therefore, this process essentially involves elastic deformation, due to eccentric muscle contraction and stretching forces, due to gravity and forward movement. Viscous deformation would mean a decrease in elastic force and walking would become clumsy, requiring much more effort in every next step.

If connective tissue is stretched intensely, there will be some degree of mechanical weakening although there is not necessarily any tissue damage. Weakness will depend on the technique and the amount of stretching. If tissue is stretched faster with greater force, or slowly with less force, the greater force will cause more structural change and the risk of tearing increases.

After repeated intense stretching, stiff, short muscles will improve joint mobility with plastic changes. The relation and degree of elastic or plastic changes will vary depending on the circumstances in which the stretching is carried out. Primary factors include force, duration and tissue temperature. A change in the elasticity of soft tissues is known as the hysteresia phenomenon; this effect is associated with progressive use of force but there will be a limit at which tissue damage can occur. Changes caused by stretching will last longer when using less force and a longer stretch duration than when using greater force to achieve changes more quickly. Slow stretching is recommended for plastic deformation; however, if the force is too small plastic deformation will not be achieved no matter how long the stretch lasts. Stretch force needs to be strong and long enough to produce plastic deformation in order to ensure sustainable improvements in mobility when flexibility has been reduced by shortness and stiffness in connective tissue. Connective tissue, however, should not be torn. Adhesions are an exception because they restrict movement due to mechanical factors and cause pain when stretched. It requires skill to apply the appropriate force when stretching in order to achieve plastic deformation without causing tissue damage. Using too great a force can damage connective tissue, muscles, tendons, joint ligaments or joint capsules. This can result in a loss of muscle power, hypermobility of joints, the formation of adhesions and scar tissue.

Garrett et al (1988) found actively contracted muscles can withstand 15% more stretching force than passive, relaxed muscles. Similarly, the energy absorption capacity of active muscles is 100% more than relaxed muscles. Therefore, muscles endure greater amounts of stress while active than when passively stretched. Tired muscles will be less durable under stress.

Self-assessment: factors affecting stretch

- How does electrical activity of muscles change during stretch?
- How long does decreased resistance due to viscosity and elasticity last following stretch?
- How many repetitions are useful with intermittent stretching to increase the effect?
- How should one perform stretching to achieve elastic deformation?
- How should one perform stretching to achieve plastic deformation?

RESEARCH FINDINGS OF SS IN HEALTHY SUBJECTS

Ankle dorsiflexion

Henricson et al (1983) studied the effects of SS on calf muscles in badminton players. The subjects performed five static stretches for 15 sec using the standard standing wall stretch three times a week over 12 weeks. All stretches were preceded by sustained heel raise for 15 sec. The average gain on active ankle dorsiflexion ROM was 5°, but it was not statistically significant compared to the controls.

Toft et al (1989) evaluated the passive tension resulting from dorsiflexion of the ankle in handball soccer players before and 90 min after single CR stretching of the plantar flexors. Stretching lowered the passive tension by 18% and for the period during which it was performed twice a day for 3 weeks the passive tension lowered by 36%. Before the measurements, no stretching was performed for 20 h or more.

Grady and Saxena (1991) studied the effects of once-daily SS of the calf muscles. Three groups performed wall daily stretches for 6 months: Group 1 stretched for 30 sec; Group 2 for 120 sec and Group 3 for 300 sec. The average gain in active dorsiflexion was 2–3° with no significant difference between groups and between the prestretch and poststretch values.

Zito et al (1997) studied the effects of SS in subjects with symmetrical limitations of ankle dorsiflexion. Four active dorsiflexion contractions for 5 sec were used as a preconditioning. One bout of two static stretches for 15 sec was performed on ankle dorsiflexion. Stretching was performed in unilateral standing with the subject's heel suspended over the edge of a platform. Measurements of passive dorsiflexion ROM were taken over 24 h, but no significant increase was noticed.

McNair et al (2000) tested the effects of SS on the ankles. While lying on their back with knee straight, each subject undertook SS for 4 × 15 sec, 2 × 30 sec, 1 × 60 sec and continuous passive motion for 60 sec, so that total stretch time was equal. The force of resistance was measured continually for 60 sec with angle speed at 5° per sec by an isokinetic machine, while the ankle was flexed to 80% of the maximum range of dorsiflexion to measure stiffness at the ankle joint. The decrease in force relaxation response of soft tissues was measured at 80% of the maximum ROM of the ankle joint.

Stiffness decreased significantly for the continuous passive motion condition only and the mean magnitude of the decrease was 16%. If decreasing stiffness is a key aim of a stretching programme, the findings indicate that continuous motion is more effective than SS. Viscoelastic resistance decreased most quickly during the first 15 sec. The decrease in tension force was 11% for the 15 sec and about 20% for the other hold times and continuous passive motion. Consecutive decreases in tension occurred for the first 20 sec.

Duong et al (2001) studied the stress relaxation of the ankle joint after long duration stretch and the time course of recovery from stretch. The ankle was stretched in a fixed dorsiflexion angle for 20 min. The ankle was then released for 2 min, during which time subjects either remained relaxed or performed isometric contractions, and then stretched again. In a second experiment the ankle was stretched for 20 min, then released for 20 min and then stretched again. During stretch the ankle torque declined rapidly. Already after 5 min about half of the maximal stress relaxation was obtained. However, resistance continued to decline after that. Torque recovered by 43% within 2 min of the release of stretch. Recovery did not depend on whether subjects remained relaxed or performed isometric contractions. The time course of recovery was similar to the time course of stress relaxation. The study suggests that long duration stretches are required in order to produce a large proportion of the maximal possible stress relaxation and that recovery is rapid when the stretch is released.

Youdas et al (2003) studied the effect of SS of the calf muscles on active ankle dorsiflexion ROM in subjects with no special tightness in the lower extremities. They performed standing wall stretches once per day. One group stretched for 30 sec, a second group for 1 min and a third group for 2 min. ROM was measured while subjects were lying prone with the knee straight. After 6 weeks' training there was still no significant increase in active ROM.

In summary, stretching has not been noticed to produce any significant increase in active ROM on the ankle joint in healthy subjects. On the other hand, there is no clear justification why the training should aim to improve ROM in healthy subjects without decreased mobility. In studies measuring resistance of tissues after stretching, significant effects could be noticed, although the effect tends to disappear rather quickly.

During stretching of the calf muscles there is an increase in passive tension with the dorsiflexion angle of the ankle joint. Passive resistance by structural factors of the ankle joint will be more significant if the knee joint is flexed. Gastrocnemius will commonly bring on most of the resistance if the knee is extended and the resistance from other calf muscles and the ankle joint will become more important factors near the end of the normal ROM. It is difficult to differentiate at which point the stretch will be directed from the musculotendinous unit more to the ankle joint. Thus, the calf muscles have not been a popular research subject.

Hip flexion and knee extension

The knee flexion muscles are most commonly used in research on the effects of stretching (Table 1.2). Most of these are also the muscles of hip extension. Known as the hamstring muscles, they run along the posterior femur bone, crossing over both the hip and knee joints. Hamstrings are a tight muscle group in many people and thus it is usually not difficult to find subjects with such short hamstring muscles that they restrict the movement far from the extreme of range of normal passive ROM of the hip joint. When the knee joint is extended, the same problem applies as with the ankle joint: the knee joint has to be straight during stretching. Several researchers have used the alternative method in stretching as well as in measurements: the hip joint has been flexed allowing the hamstrings to stretch by extending the knee joint. In healthy subjects without joint limitations, the muscle–tendon system will noticeably tighten before stretching is directed to the joint capsule. This makes it possible to focus study on the effects of stretch on the muscle–tendon system, and not have joint mobility limitations interfere, as in many other joints.

Bohannon (1984) studied the effect of hamstring stretching lasting 8 min. Measurements and stretching were carried out while test patients were lying supine by raising the leg straight up with a pulley weight. The knee joint was kept straight with the aid of a splint. Maximum force tolerated for 8 min was tested 2 weeks before treatment began and was used as stretch force. Hip joint ROM was measured 15 sec after stretch. After 3 days of treatment mobility had improved by 7° in the stretch group and 1.5° in the control group. Follow-up testing was taken 1 day later and showed that mobility had increased 4.5° in the stretch group and 0.5° in the control group compared to the baseline. Difference between groups was no more significant.

Borms et al (1987) compared the SS of hamstring muscles using different durations of stretch time. The stretch duration in the first group was 10 sec, in the second group 20 sec and in the third group 30 sec, with 8–15 sec rest periods between each stretch. Stretching was performed twice weekly for 45 min and it was continued for 10 weeks. Test measurements of hip flexion mobility were taken while the subject was supine and the leg lifted straight up. The average increase in mobility was approximately 13° in all groups. Researchers concluded that 10-sec stretch duration time is preferable, because it achieved equally good results as longer stretch duration times. Improvement was initially faster in the 20- and 30-sec groups but this levelled off at 7 weeks, with the final results the same. Stretching time in this study was especially long, whereas in most studies total stretching time has been approximately 15 min per session.

Gajdosik (1991) compared passive compliance and length of clinically short hamstring muscles in relation to muscles that were not considered to be short. The difference between groups was about 13° in straight leg raise as well as in knee extension while the hip was fixed at a 90° angle. The torque versus angle was measured during stretching and results show that the curves describing passive compliance were shifted left in stiff subjects (Figure 1.26). Stretching was stopped due to sensation of the maximal stretch by the subject or increased activity in electromyography. Maximal passive torques tolerated during stretching did not differ between the groups and because the passive compliance was greater in the group with stiff hamstring muscles, the change of muscle length was also less in the inflexible group.

Hugh et al (1992) tested effects of SS for 45 sec on the hamstring muscles. Viscosity and elastic components of

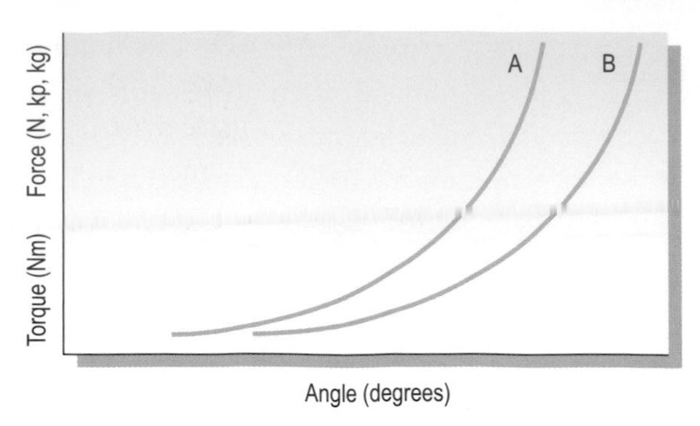

Figure 1.26 The torque-angle or force-angle curve describes the resistance caused by the muscle–tendon unit while the angle of the joint gradually increases during stretching with steady speed. A: Stiff muscle. B: Muscle with normal tone. The total area under the torque-angle curve describes the work done during stretching and the energy spent in stretching. It also describes the amount energy stored in the muscle–tendon unit during stretching.

resistance decreased 15%. However, the change had returned to the base level only 10 min after stretching. The effects of single stretches are thus significant, but last for a relatively short period of time.

Bandy et al (1997) compared the SS of hamstring muscles using different durations of stretch time in healthy subjects with short hamstrings. Stretching was performed once daily, 5 days a week for a total of 6 weeks. The stretch duration in the first group was 15 sec, in the second group it was 30 sec and in the third group, 60 sec. Hip flexion mobility only increased by 4° in the 15-sec stretch group. In comparison, the 30- and 60-sec stretch groups showed a 12° improvement in mobility. Thus, the 60-sec group did not further improve results from that of the 30-sec group.

The same subjects were divided into two groups to perform the six-week stretching programme using 30-sec and 60-sec stretch durations. Difference in the results between these two groups was not significant. Results were not affected by performing the stretch once or three times per day. The effectiveness of stretching can be improved to a certain extent by increasing stretch duration and the number of repetitions. These results suggest that 30-sec stretch duration performed once daily is recommendable.

Halbertsma and Göeken (1994) evaluated the effect of SS in healthy subjects with short hamstrings. The stretch duration was 10 min and it was performed twice a day for 4 weeks. The ROM increased by 5° in the instrumental straight-leg-raising stretching group and by 1° in the control group. The increase was due to influence on stretch tolerance and had no effect on muscle stiffness.

Magnusson et al (1995) evaluated the effects of a single SS of hamstring muscles. Subjects stretched hamstring muscles by bending forward while in a standing position. Stretch was continued to the point of pain and it was held in that position for 90 sec. Stretching resulted in a 30% reduction in resistance caused by the connective tissue. The change was greatest during the first 30 sec and continued with only minimal change thereafter. Electric activity of muscles during stretch remained constant. Thus, the effect was not caused by relaxation but primarily involved mechanical effects. However, the effects had disappeared when the measurements were repeated 45 min after the treatment.

Li et al (1996) and Gajdosik (1991) evaluated the effect of SS on hamstring muscles for 15 sec. Forward bending exercises were repeated 10 times daily for 3 weeks. The subjects achieved an increase in mobility of 12–13°. Total stretching time was significantly longer than that used by Bandy and Irion (1994), which explains the better results, although the time used in a single stretch was the same. Thus, the results are not only dependent on duration of the individual stretch but also on how often stretching is repeated. The total stretching time is an important factor for affecting the results.

Halbertsma et al (1996) studied the effect of SS on hamstring muscles. Subjects stretched the hamstring muscles by bending forward from a standing position with one leg raised in front and resting on a table. Stretch duration was 30 sec with a 30-sec rest period between and continued for 10 min daily for 4 weeks. Flexibility measurements were taken while subjects were lying supine and the leg was raised straight up by machine until pain was felt. Hip flexion improved in the stretch group by 9°, while there was no change in the control group. Thus, the ROM increased significantly, because the hamstring muscles were able to tolerate a more intense stretch force, but neither hamstring muscle length nor stiffness was affected.

Magnusson et al (1996) studied the effects of SS on hamstring muscles for 45 sec. Stretching was repeated 10 times daily. The magnitude of the initial increase in joint angle was 5° and 17° after 3 weeks' training. This study produced the largest of improvement in mobility compared to previous studies of SS. Total stretching time was also longer being 9000 sec, which emphasizes the total time spent on stretching. Results showed an unchanged torque-angle curve, which means that joint ROM increased as a result of elevated stretch tolerance rather than a viscoelastic accommodation. Thus, elasticity of tissues does not seem to change even after long-standing stretching despite increased mobility.

Bandy et al (1997) evaluated the effect of time and frequency of SS in healthy subjects with short hamstrings The groups stretched once a day 5 days per week for 6 weeks and the control group did not stretch. Group 1 performed 30-sec stretch and Group 2 one 60-sec stretch. The change in flexibility appeared to be dependent on stretching, but there were no significant differences in results between the stretching groups. No additional increase in mobility occurred, when the frequency of stretching was increased from 1 to 3 times per day. The results suggest that one stretch for 30-seconds duration is an effective amount to sustain a hamstring muscle stretch in order to increase ROM.

Magnusson (1998) studied the effects of 90-sec stretches of the hamstring muscles. Stretching was repeated five times with 30-sec intervals. Testing showed a 13% decrease in resistance due to viscoelastic properties. While the same angle was used in repeated stretches as in the initial stretch, the resistance decreased progressively with stretch repetition. However, 1 h after the stretching, the effect was gone and a new stretch required the same force as earlier. Researchers concluded that SS alone does not have long-term effects on muscle–tendon compliance, at least not if the stretch force does not pass pain tolerance. Stretching force decreased in repeated stretching, because the angle was not increased and resistance decreased temporarily.

Starring et al (1988) compared the effects of repeated and continuous SS in healthy subjects with short hamstrings. Subjects were in a sitting position and stretching was applied by machine to one leg while the other one was used for comparison. SS was maintained for 15 min daily for 5 days. Total stretching time of the repeated stretching was the same. Each stretch lasted 10 sec with an 8-sec rest interval. Mobility was measured while sitting with the hip in a right angle position. Knee mobility improved with SS by 13°. One week after stretching had stopped, the knee mobility was still 8° better than at the baseline. Repeated stretching improved the mobility 15° and 10°, respectively. There was no significant difference between the groups. Mobility increased and was preserved better in women compared to men. This was assumed to be due to differences in connective tissue structure and muscle size. Researchers suggested that connective tissue in men contains more collagen making it more resistant to stretch. This would mean that plastic changes are less likely in men.

Magnusson et al (2000) studied the effects of repeated 45-sec stretches of the hamstring muscles three times with 30-sec intervals. The final joint angle increased by 14°. Testing showed a decrease in resistance of around 20% during stretch with no significant difference between the first and third stretch. Thus, the stretching produced an instantaneous viscoelastic stress relaxation and absolute resistance and energy remained unaffected by the repeated stretches. This is essential for the muscle–tendon unit to maintain utilization of the elastic energy.

Magnusson et al (2000) compared passive resistance to stretch in the hamstring muscles of flexible and inflexible persons. Measurements were performed during slow passive knee extension to a maximal angle and followed by a static phase for 90 sec. Cross-sectional areas of the hamstring muscles were obtained with magnetic resonance imaging and there was no significant difference between groups. The peak tension at maximal angle was greater in flexible than in inflexible subjects in the final 20% of length change. There was no significant difference in viscoelastic stress relaxation in the static phase. Flexible people attained a greater angle of stretch with an accompanying greater tensile stress and energy storing capacity compared to inflexible people. This was due to a greater tolerance to the externally applied load and thus a larger change in moment arm. Moreover, absorbed energy was greater within flexible rather than within inflexible subjects also in the final 40% of length change.

Chan et al (2001) evaluated the effects of two different SS protocols on flexibility and passive resistance of the hamstring muscles. Subjects stretched the hamstring muscles by bending the back forward from the hips while in a sitting position with the leg out straight. The other leg was in flexion beside the buttocks. Force used in passive stretches did not produce pain. One group performed two series of five repetitions of 30-sec stretches with 30-sec intervals and repeated the series after a 1-min rest. Stretching was continued three times per week for 4 weeks. The second group did one series of five repetitions of 30-sec stretch with 30-sec intervals, three times weekly for 8 weeks. Knee extension with the hip flexed to a right angle, was approximately 160° in all groups. The mobility did not change in the control group. Pain-free mobility increased in the 4-week stretching group by 9° and in the 8-week group by 11°, but the difference was not significant. Improved mobility in the 4-week training group resulted from the increased tolerance to stretch, whereas relatively lower passive resistance at the end-of-range in the 8-week group was related to adaptation of connective tissues. Based on test results, increasing repetitions will not be as significant as increasing treatment duration. Researchers suggested that stretching treatment programs should last 2 months to ensure improved flexibility changes at the tissue level.

Willy et al (2001) evaluated the effects of a single SS of hamstring muscles. Subjects performed stretching in a standing position with one leg raised up in front, resting on a high surface. The back was bent forward at the hips until the stretch felt uncomfortable. This position was maintained for 30 sec with a 30-sec rest before repeating the stretch. SS was performed once daily, 5 days a week. After 6 weeks knee extension had increased by 9° when measured with the subject lying supine and the hip at a right angle. After a 4-week break from treatment, mobility had reduced to only 2° better than the pretreatment measurements, showing effects to have almost disappeared completely. A new series of treatment for 6 weeks improved mobility by 11°. Compared to the initial values.

Feland et al (2001b) studied hamstring stretching of 65-year-old subjects. Stretch duration times for different groups were 15, 30 and 60 sec and repeated four times with 10-sec intervals between. Stretching was executed four times per week for 6 weeks. Flexibility increased by 4°, 8° and 12°, respectively, in each group. Thus they recommended stretch duration of 60 seconds. Age affects muscle–tendon tissue characteristics, and elderly individuals profited more from longer stretching times than younger individuals. Measurements were taken weekly for one month following stretching and ROM gradually returned to the baseline. Thus, increased mobility cannot be maintained without regular stretching.

Cipriani et al (2003) compared the effects of two hamstring stretching protocols. Subjects performed six stretches for 10 sec with 10-sec intervals to the hamstring muscles of one leg and two stretches for 30 sec with 30-sec intervals to the hamstrings of the other leg. Stretching was continued for both legs twice daily for 6 weeks. Subjects demonstrated significant gains in ROM for hip flexion with no differences between the two protocols. The denominator was total stretch time for a day regardless of the duration of a single stretch.

After stretching, the elastic changes in connective tissue (elastic deformation) return to their prior shape, while changes in structure (plastic deformation) remain. Elastic change passes rapidly as the connective tissue stretches but completely returns to its former state with no reduction in resistance to stretch. Effective stretching uses enough time and force to achieve plastic changes to attain new length and reduce resistance to stretch. Plastic changes have been shown to occur primarily at the muscle–tendon junction area and are associated with its viscosity and elastic characteristics.

Hip extension and knee flexion

Measuring the ROM of the hip joint has not attracted many researchers, although stiffness of hip flexor muscles is almost as common as hamstring muscles.

Godges et al (1993) evaluated the effect of SS in healthy subjects with limited hip extension. The stretch duration was 6 min and it was performed twice a week for three weeks. The angle was measured with the goniometer when the pelvis started to lift while extending the hip joint. The passive ROM increased by 11° in the stretching group and no increase was noticed in the control group.

Clark et al (1999) studied the effects of CR stretching technique applied to the anterior thigh muscles and static positioning on passive straight-leg raise. Stretching was carried out with the subject lying prone. The leg was allowed to hang over the edge of the table with the hip and knee flexed and foot on the floor. The leg to be treated was on the table with the hip straight and secured to the table with strapping. The knee was flexed until resistance. In the CR technique subjects had to tense the thigh muscles for 6 sec by pressing the lower leg against the assistant. After 5 sec of relaxation, the knee joint was flexed as far as possible without producing pain. Stretching was repeated six times. In passive positioning subjects assumed the same positioning as described above, but the limb remained flat on the plinth for 2 min. Straight-leg raise increased on average by 8° in the CR group, by 5° in the positioning group and by 1° in the control group. All groups differed significantly from each other. Although stretching was not applied in the positioning group, the hip rotates slightly backwards, stretching the rectus muscle of the leg on the table due to

Table 1.2 Test results of static stretching of the hamstring muscles on healthy subjects

Changes in angle have been measured of the hip joint with the knee extended or of the knee with the hip flexed to a right angle

Researcher	Duration of single stretch (sec)	Repetitions	Frequency per day (times/week)	Duration (weeks)	Total time per week (sec)	Change (degrees)
Medeiros 1977	3	20	8	–	480	6
Tanigawa 1972	5	3	6	–	90	7
Sady et al 1982	6	2	3	6	216	11
Prentice 1983	10	3	3	10	300	9
Starring et al 1988	10	50	5	–	500	15
Bandy & Irion 1994	15	1	5	6	450	4
Li et al 1996	15	10	7	3	3150	12
Gajdosik 1991	15	10	7	3	3150	13
DeWeijer et al 2003	30	3	1	–	90	13
Halbertsma et al 1996	30	10	1	4	300	9
Hardy 1985	30	3	6	–	360	12
Bandy & Irion 1994	30	1	5	6	900	12
Bandy et al 1998	30	1	5	6	900	11
Bandy & Irion 1997	30	3	5	6	2700	10
Willy et al 2001	30	2	5	6	1800	9
Willy et al 2001	30	2	5	2 × 6	3600	11
Chan et al 2001	30	10	3	4	3600	9
Chan et al 2001	30	5	3	8	3600	11
Magnusson et al 1996	45	1	1	–	45	5
Magnusson et al 2000	45	3	1	–	135	14
Magnusson et al 1996	45	10	7	3	9000	17
Bandy & Irion 1994	60	3	5	6	5400	10
Bohannon 1984	480	1	3	–	1440	7
Halbertsma & Göeken 1994	600	2	7	4	33 600	5
Starring et al 1988	900	1	5	–	4500	13

flexion of the hip joint on one side. Stretching anterior thigh muscles changes hip position allowing a more neutral pelvic alignment and thus increases the straight leg raise.

Björklund et al (2001) studied the effects of stretching on the extensor muscles in knee joint mobility. Subjects performed isometric contraction for 5 sec, followed by 2–3 sec of relaxation and 20 sec of stretch, with the cycle repeated once. Treatment was carried out four times a week for 2 weeks. Total stretching time was 320 sec. The ROM in flexion increased by approximately 15°, but the knee flexion angle did not change when using the same stretch force. Thus, the passive stiffness of the muscle was unaffected by the stretch regimen. However, subjective stretch sensation decreased and led to improved tolerance and ROM. If force was not measured, the most likely conclusion would have indicated improved mobility due to less resistance, which has been a common misinterpretation in the past if the goniometer is the only research tool.

Hip abduction

Möller et al (1985b) studied the effects of SS of thigh adductors on the ROM of the hip joint in soccer players. Stretch duration varied for different groups with 15, 45 and 120 sec. In the control group the ROM was noticed to decrease 24 h after intensive training. ROM in all stretching groups improved significantly compared to the control group. Researchers concluded that the 15-sec stretching time is as effective as 2 min in the treatment of the hip adductors.

Madding et al (1987) studied passive stretching of the thigh adductors using only single stretch exercises. Subjects indicated when they began to feel pain at which point stretching was not increased but maintained for 15, 45 and 120 sec according to each group. No significant difference between the three groups was demonstrated. Researchers recommended the shortest stretching time especially in athletic settings.

Amount and duration of stretching

SS is achieved by turning a joint as far as it will go to lengthen the muscle–tendon unit while the individual tries to relax as much as possible. This position is then held for a while. The stretching is ideally performed without excessive stress on joint related to muscles. The preferred number of repetitions varies greatly in different recommendations and is seldom based on the acquired information from research. Much research has also been conducted on the effects of stretch duration of individual stretches, as well as on the total duration of stretching, which can be utilized in recommendations (Table 1.2).

SS has been shown to have long-term effects on improved joint mobility and a reduction in tissue resistance. It requires, however, stretching that is continued for enough time for the effects on tissue to last. Effects at the tissue level require about a 2-month stretching programme and regular exercise thereafter to preserve the acquired effects.

Stretch force is commonly applied within pain tolerance. However, this may vary depending on the subject and stretch situation. The subject may be encouraged to go on further with the stretch when the pain has just appeared and thus the force used in stretching may be considerably greater than if the subject is told to stop as soon as pain or discomfort is felt. Thus, the amount and duration of stretches does not guarantee positive effects, if the force used in stretching is too low to produce any significant effects.

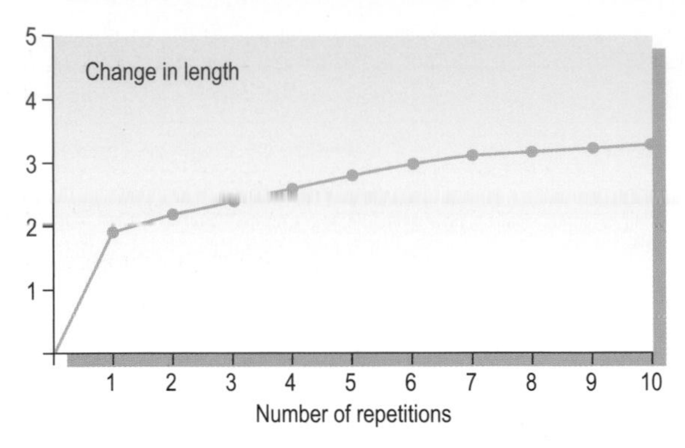

Figure 1.27 Repeated stretching with the same force achieves the greatest effect on length with the initial stretch and length will somewhat increase to the fourth repetition, but after that there will be little change.

Taylor et al (1990) showed with a laboratory specimen of muscle–tendon unit that the greatest effects occur during the first 12–18 sec of SS and 75% of changes in the viscoelastic properties of the muscle–tendon unit occur with repeated stretching during the first four stretches (Figure 1.27). This implies that a small number of stretches will lead to most of the elongation in repetitive stretching. This has also been verified by the clinical studies presented. Total time spent on stretching per week is more important than time spent on individual stretches.

The static stretching table on p. 55 appears to show a great variation in results. Thus, there must be a factor which has not been considered by most researchers. That factor is the force used in stretching exercises, which is certainly as important a factor as time.

Recommended SS routine

- 30-sec stretch time for young and middle-aged
- 60-sec stretch time for elderly
- four repetitions
- twice weekly
- progressively increasing force until the target ROM has been achieved
- stretching has to be done regularly
- in cases of disease or injury, stretching time and repetitions are increased accordingly.

CONTRACT–RELAX STRETCHING (CR)

After the SS technique, CR stretching is the next most popular technique for improving flexibility. It can be done with or without an assistant as in passive stretching techniques. A pre-stretch position is used during the initial stage by moving the joint as far as possible until resistance is significant. The subject then uses isometric contraction to tense the antagonist muscles while the therapist resists the movement for 5 sec or the body part is placed against a firm object. The subject then relaxes the muscles while the joint is stretched further until the muscle–tendon system becomes tight again. This CR stretch cycle can be repeated several times.

Medeiros et al (1977) compared SS to isometric contractions of the hamstring muscles. Stretch duration was 3 sec with 20 repetitions daily for 8 days as well as isometric contractions. The ROM improved in the isometric contraction group by 7°, in the SS group by 6° and in the control group by 1°. Comparisons between the two treatment groups indicated that the isometric contraction and passive stretch procedures had significant and similar effects compared to the control group.

Möller et al (1985a) studied the effects of CR + SS stretching on the lower extremity joints. Subjects first tensed the muscle groups that were to be stretched for 5 sec and then they allowed the muscles to relax as much as possible for 2 sec. After that, SS technique was applied in which the joint was held at its farthest ROM for 8 sec. Stretching was repeated six times and after that hip, knee and ankle movements increased from 4° to 6°. ROM was recorded as the same with measurements taken 1.5 h later. Knowing how long the effects of stretching will last is important to athletes who require good mobility during performance.

Nelson et al (2001) studied the influence of the time duration of contraction on the efficacy of the CR stretching method. Contraction times of 3 sec, 6 sec or 10 sec did not show noticeable differences in the results. This may be related to the subject's ability to achieve maximum power within only a few sec in isometric contraction. Neither did tiring of muscles improve stretch results.

Feland and Marin (2004) compared the effectiveness of submaximal and maximal contraction in CR stretching. They used healthy subjects demonstrating tight hamstrings, defined as the inability to reach 70° of hip flexion during a straight-leg raise. They were randomly assigned to one of three treatment groups performing 20%, 60% and maximal isometric voluntary contraction of hamstring muscles, and a control group. Stretching groups performed three stretches for 6 sec with a 10-sec rest between contractions, once a day for 5 days. There was no difference in flexibility gains between the treatment groups, but all treatment groups had significantly greater flexibility than the control group. It seems that using submaximal contractions is just as beneficial at improving flexibility as maximal contractions.

CONTRACT–RELAX AGONIST-CONTRACT STRETCHING (CR-AC)

This technique involves the CR stretching technique after which there is dynamic contraction of agonist muscles. Describing the technique from the beginning; the subject initially moves the muscle–tendon unit into a stretched position and tenses the muscle against therapist or an object that will resist the movement. The subject then relaxes these antagonist muscles and allows the stretch to increase by contracting the agonist muscles. The subject then preserves the new stretch position with the new position against the support and the cycle is repeated.

The complete stretch cycle includes the isometric contraction of antagonists, relaxation of antagonists and the dynamic contraction of agonists: contract–relax agonist-contract. This technique is also referred to in the literature as the hold–relax technique (HR). Passive stretching occurs while the body part is moved to the first phase and some therapists also use passive stretching at the end of active contraction. This technique makes use of active contraction in both the agonists and antagonists.

It has been suggested that muscle contraction prior to stretching will activate the Golgi tendon organs, which encourage muscle relaxation by causing inhibition of motor neurons via activation of the Renshaw cell to reduce muscle sensitivity to contraction. Another theory states that muscle contraction prior to stretching activates muscle spindle receptors, which decreases their sensitivity, reducing muscle tension and resistance to stretch. Contraction of antagonist muscles should, therefore, improve muscle relaxation and decrease resistance to stretch. However, it has been shown that active muscle contraction increases the activity of the neuromuscular system, which should make muscles more susceptible to contraction. On the other hand, according to research electrical activity is small at rest and effective muscle stretching does not require complete muscle relaxation (Osternig et al 1987).

While stretching the hamstring muscles, contraction of the quadriceps, which is an agonist muscle in relation to direction of stretching movement, has been indicated to reduce hamstring activity with reciprocal inhibition from muscle spindles mediated by Ia-nerves. However, it has been perceived that contraction of the agonists will actually increase activity in the antagonists. Active contraction of the antagonists may reduce the uncomfortable sensations caused by stretching. Thus, sensations of discomfort are more likely to arise from the antagonist muscles stretching phase than in contraction phase. An important reflex regulator during stretch is activation of the muscle spindles and Ia-afferent nerves. Muscles crossing over one or two joints will function in different ways at different muscle lengths. When a muscle crosses over two joints, both of their positions will affect muscle length and power potential. The motor control is more complicated in muscles crossing two or more joints, and it does not function in the same way as the agonist–antagonist system of muscles crossing only one joint.

Active contraction was once thought to decrease tension in the antagonist muscles. However, studies have not confirmed the old theory of reciprocal inhibition. Stretching of relaxed normal muscles in healthy people has not been shown to produce any tonic stretch reflexes. Such an increase in reflexive tension is not the norm and indicates damage in the central nervous system.

McCarthy et al (1997) studied the effects of the CR-AC method on active ROM of the cervical spine. Stretching exercises were performed twice a day for 1 week. Prior to measuring, active maximal lateral flexion and then rotation to each side was repeated five times. Overall ROM in rotation improved on average by 22 °, which was significant compared to the control group in which the mobility increased by 10°. However, the difference between groups disappeared 1 week after the stretching exercises had stopped. This phenomenon is already familiar from studies on SS.

Self-assessment: research on stretching

- What does static and passive stretching mean?
- How should age be considered while applying SS techniques?
- What are the affects of stretching, as an increaser of ROM, based on short-term and long-term exercising?
- How does the electrical activity of muscles change with CR and CR-AC methods, and how does this affect results?

COMPARISON OF STRETCHING METHODS IN HEALTHY SUBJECTS

Studies have shown that different types of stretching can alter passive stiffness and energy in muscle tissue both acutely and chronically. Stretching methods have been compared in research but the results have not indicated that one method is better than another (Table 1.3). However, there are noticeable differences between stretching methods in regard to stretching mechanics, effectiveness and risk of complication in different conditions and the purpose for which they are used.

Holt et al (1970) compared SS, BS and CR-AC stretching techniques. SS was performed in a sitting position on the floor with the knees extended. Subjects grasped the calf muscles with their hands to pull themselves forward for 20 sec. Ballistic stretching (BS) was carried out in a sitting position while attempting to touch toes with fingertips using a swinging motion for 20 sec. In both groups, subjects continued each stretching four times with a 10-sec rest period between. Total exercise time was 2 min, after which there was a 30-sec rest period and then both exercises were repeated in a standing position. In the CR-AC technique, subjects were in a supine position with legs outstretched. The subject flexed the hip joint as far as possible while keeping the knee extended. This was followed by maximum contraction of the hamstring muscles for 6 sec against resistance applied by the tester. Then the subject flexed the hip again as far as possible and this manoeuvre was aided by a slight push from the tester for 4 sec. Stretching was performed four times for about 20 sec after which there was a 10-sec rest period and then stretching was applied to the other leg. The total exercise time was 2 min. The second stretch was performed in a standing position with the legs extended. The subject first reached forward as far as possible towards the toes. Following this, the individual was instructed to try and raise the body back up slowly for 6 sec while the therapist added resistance to the movement by placing pressure against the sacrum and upper thorax with their hands. Following this, the individual was instructed to once again reach forward as far as possible. Stretching was repeated three times for about 20 sec, after which there was a 10-sec rest period, and then stretching continued for 2 min. All groups completed stretching exercises three times weekly. Each group used each stretching techniques for 1 week. Final results showed that in both exercises that involved reaching for the toes from a sitting position, stretching increased in both SS and BS methods by 2 cm. In the CR-AC group, mobility improved significantly more, by 5 cm.

Hartley-O'Brien (1980) compared six different stretching techniques on hamstring flexibility:

1. Passive stretching and actively maintaining the position. Relaxed lower limb was raised up as far as possible according to the individual's pain threshold, after which hip flexors were contracted for 6 sec while maintaining the position. Following contraction, passive stretching was applied and the whole process repeated five times within 1 min.
2. Passive stretching. Lower limb was raised up as far as possible within pain tolerance and the position was maintained for 1 min.
3. Dynamic stretch plus maintaining position. Hip joint was actively moved back and forth from a 45° angle into flexion once per sec × 4, and then the final flexed position was maintained for 6 sec. Treatment was repeated six times.
4. Relaxation–stretch. This technique is identical to passive stretching except that the subject is asked to focus on relaxing the muscles using visualization.
5. Active proprioceptive neuromuscular facilitation. The subject raised the lower limb as far as possible within pain tolerance. The assistant then maintained the position while the subject attempted to extend the leg for 6 sec. This was followed by 6 sec of passive stretching and the series was repeated five times.
6. Passive proprioceptive neuromuscular facilitation. Lower limb was raised as far as possible within pain tolerance, after which the subject contracted the extensor muscles with maximum force for 6 sec. Stretch was increased, and then the individual attempted to extend the leg for 6 sec. The series was repeated five times within 1 min.

Mobility was shown to increase in all stretching methods. SS techniques were slightly more effective than the other techniques, but there was no significant difference.

In research by Grahn et al (1981) CR methods were shown to increase mobility to a lesser extent than BS techniques. Sady et al (1982) compared SS, BR and CR techniques. The most noticeable improvements in mobility were achieved with the CR technique. Improvement in joint mobility varied considerably between different joints.

Holt and Smith (1983) compared the efficacy of three stretching techniques CR-AC, AC and SS-IC. Stretching was performed in a sitting position on the floor with the knees extended. Using the CR-AC stretching method, subjects were in a supine position with legs outstretched. The subject flexed the hip joint as far as possible while keeping the knee extended and the ankle in dorsiflexion. This was followed by maximum contraction of the hamstring muscles for 6 sec against resistance applied by the researcher. Then the subject flexed the hip again as far as possible and this manoeuvre was aided by a slight push from the researcher for 4 sec followed by 10-sec rest. Subjects in the AC group flexed the hip joint as far as possible while keeping the knee extended and ankle in dorsiflexion. This position was kept for 10 sec followed by a 10-sec rest. Subjects in the SS group flexed the hip joint as far as possible while keeping the knee extended and ankle in dorsiflexion. This was followed by maximum contraction of the hamstring muscles for 6 sec against resistance applied by the researcher, but the subjects were not allowed to flex the hip further, but followed it with a 10-sec rest. All techniques were repeated five times. The active ROM improved by 15° in the CR-AC, by 8° in the AC, by 2° in the SS and with no difference in the control group compared to the baseline. Improvement of the passive ROM were 14°, 4°, 4° and 0°, respectively. After 20 min active ROM in the CR-AC group was 9° and after 1 week 2° more compared to the baseline.

Prentice (1983) compared two different stretching techniques on the hamstring muscles (SS and CR-AC). Stretching was applied 3 days a week for 10 weeks. Subjects were lying supine while the assistant raised the lower limb with the knee extended and the ankle at a right angle. Stretching was increased until muscle tension or pain prevented further stretching. This procedure was repeated three times. SS was maintained for 10 sec with 10-sec rest intervals. Movement was resisted by the assistant while subjects contracted the hamstring muscles for 10 sec during the CR-AC technique, after which agonists were contracted for 10 sec. Then the assistant fixated the position and the process was repeated. Mobility increased on average by 12° with the CR-AC technique and 8° with SS. CR-AC was found to be significantly better.

Cornelius et al (1984) studied the effects of three stretching methods (SS, CR and CR-AC) on dorsiflexion of the ankle. Only CR and CR-AC methods showed significant increase from the initial measurements. The CR-AC method improved mobility more than the CR method, but the difference was not significant. In another test study by Cornelius et al (1992), applications of cold were included with the CR method, which showed better results than with SS techniques, whether or not cold was used.

Williford and Smith (1985) studied the effects of SS and CR. They did not find significant differences between them in the results achieved.

Hardy (1985) compared four stretching methods on the hamstring muscles (SS, AC, CR and CR-AC). The treatment series of all methods were repeated on 6 consecutive days. Stretching was performed with the individual in a supine position while the assistant performed straight leg raise until hamstring muscle tension prevented further hip flexion. In the SS group, stretching was maintained three times for 30 sec with 30-sec rest periods. In the CR method, muscle contraction of the hamstring muscles was maintained for 3 sec in one group and for 6 sec in the second group, while the assistant resisted movement. Stretch was then immediately increased until tension prevented further hip flexion and position was maintained for 10 sec. Treatment was repeated in both groups, three times, without breaks. In the AC group, the leg was flexed slowly to the limit of the ROM and then the subject performed contraction of the hip flexors for 10 sec before taking the leg to the new end point during the 30-sec rest period. In the CR-AC method subjects contracted the hamstring muscles for 3 sec, and in the second group for 6 sec while the assistant resisted movement. Then the subject attempted to actively increase hip flexion for 10 sec while the assistant maintained the new position. All groups performed three sets of three repetitions with 30-sec rests between them in one session, for 6 days. Measurements were obtained after the final stretching session and on the following day. After the final stretch mobility improved by approximately 13° in the SS group and in both CR groups. Mobility improved in the AC group by only 8°. In the 3-sec CR-AC group mobility increased by 16° and in the 6-sec group by 20°. One day later the improvement was by 10° in the SS group and by 7° in both CR groups, by 5° in the AC group and by 13° in both CR-AC groups compared to the baseline. The control group had no improvement in mobility.

Wallin et al (1985) compared two stretching methods on the hamstring and calf muscles (CR and BS). In order to stretch the calf muscles with the CR method, subjects held onto a railing for support and while leaning forward, pressed the heel of the foot down against the floor for 7 sec. Then the foot was moved half a step forward and for 5 sec the hip was pressed forward and the calf muscles were stretched for 7 sec. In BS, subjects leaned forward to alternately stretch the calf muscles of each leg. To stretch the hip extensors with the CR method, subjects stood with legs straight, one for support while raising the other up onto a chair. Pressure was applied against the chair for 7 sec, which was followed by a 5-sec rest period. Finally, by leaning forward to flex at the hip joint, stretch to the extensors was applied for 7 sec. In BS subjects bent forward and down as far as possible to stretch hip extensors. The thigh adductors were stretched with the CR method by the subjects holding onto to a railing for support while spreading the legs as far apart as possible. In this position, the soles of the feet were pressed downwards for 7 sec followed by a 5-sec rest period. The legs were then allowed to spread farther apart. In BS subjects crouched down with one leg out straight to the side. Stretching of the adductor muscles was achieved by repeatedly bending the body to the same side as the straight leg. Stretch treatment was then applied to the opposite side. CR stretching methods were repeated five times. BS continued for 1 min and 10 sec for each muscle. Both groups performed stretching exercises three times per week for a month. There was a significant difference between groups after 14 training sessions. The mobility in the CR group increased by 6–11° and in the BS group by 1–4°.

Three groups continued stretching one, three and five times a week, respectively, for another month with CR method. Stretching once a week was enough to maintain improved flexibility, but stretching three and five times a week further increased it and five times over more.

Sullivan et al (1992) compared two stretching methods on the hamstring muscles (CR-AC and SS). Subjects stood with one leg resting on the table with hip flexed to 90°. In the first SS group and the CR-AC group, stretching was performed by bending forward from the hip with the back straight. In the second SS group and the CR-AC group, the back was allowed to bend into a curve, causing the pelvis to tilt back. Duration of SS was 30 sec. The CR-AC group tried to press the leg downwards for 5 sec. After a 5-sec break the quadriceps were tensed for 5 sec and then the exercise was repeated several times. Stretch was increased during the breaks by bending the body forward and then straightening for the next contraction. Stretching sessions lasting five mins were performed once a day on 4 days per week for 2 weeks. Knee joint extension was measured while the hip was at a right angle. Those using the rounded back technique did not gain any advancement in either the static or CR techniques. Those using a straight back to bend forward from the hip with SS gained in ROM by 9° and in the CR technique by 13°. The difference between groups was not significant. Thus, posture proved to be more significant to the results than the type of stretching technique used.

Bandy et al (1998) compared two stretching methods on the hamstring muscles (AC and SS). One group actively stretched the hamstrings by lying supine and bending first the hip to a right angle and then trying to extend the knee as far as possible for 5 sec. This position was maintained for 5 sec and the return phase lasted again about 5 sec. The stretch was repeated six times per session. Total actual stretching time was 30 sec. The second group used SS for 30 sec once a day. Stretch time was ultimately equal for both groups. Treatments were carried on 5 days per week for 6 weeks. The ROM improved on average by 11° in the SS group and by 4° in the AC group. This concludes that it is difficult for the agonist muscles to supply enough force for stretching, making its effectiveness less than with SS techniques. Thus, it seems that contraction of antagonists and relaxation prior to stretching is essential for active stretching techniques.

Feland et al (2001c) compared the effects of two stretching techniques in healthy elderly subjects (CR and SS). The leg was raised to the point of mild discomfort in a straight-leg raising and the subject was asked to perform a maximum voluntary contraction of the hip extensors for 6 sec, the leg was then further raised to the point of mild discomfort for 10 sec followed by another stretch and relaxation. A total of 32 sec of stretch time was applied also in static stretch. Flexibility increased by 5° in the CR group, by 4° in the static group and by 1° in the control group. The increase was significant in both stretching groups with no significant difference between groups.

Payne et al (2003) compared three different stretching techniques of the hamstring muscles (SS, AC and CR). The first group performed SS for 30 sec. The second group performed active stretching by contracting quadriceps muscle for 30 sec and the third group performed 30 repeated 1-sec CR stretches. Stretching was performed once a day, 5 days a week for 5 weeks. A significant increase in flexion movement of the hip was noticed in all groups, but there were no significant differences between the groups.

There is a lack of studies identifying strategies capable of increasing the effectiveness of stretching exercise. Swank et al (2003) found that adding modest weights to stretching exercise (Body Recall) increased passive ROM for the elderly compared to the control group performing a stretching exercise regime without extra load.

ELECTRICAL ACTIVITY OF MUSCLES DURING STRETCHING

Using surface electromyography (sEMG) equipment, several researchers have quantitatively demonstrated the relationship between stretch and the level of muscular electrical activity, which results from active contraction of the muscle.

Moore and Hutton (1980) studied the effects of three different stretching techniques (SS, CR, and CR-AC) on electrical activity in hamstring muscles and on hip mobility. SS was achieved with controlled force by using a pulley system while subjects were lying in a supine position. Minimal activity was recorded in hamstring muscles with the SS method. Contraction of the antagonist muscles prior to stretching caused greater amounts of electrical activity during the initial stages of CR and CR-AC stretching techniques. The stretching portion of SS and CR methods was applied in the same manner. Thus, it was concluded that muscle contraction during the initial stages only affects the electrical activity in muscles at the start. In the CR-AC method, in most subjects, active contraction of the agonist muscles increased activity in the antagonist muscles because of cocontraction. Contraction of the agonist muscles did not cause a reduction of activity in the antagonist muscles due to reciprocal inhibition. Thus, resistance to stretch was greater in the CR method and greatest in the CR-AC method. Hip mobility increased noticeably in all methods. Effectiveness of treatments varied somewhat between individuals. However, average difference in effectiveness between methods was not statistically significant.

Thigpen et al (1985) studied the effect of SS on α-motor neuron irritability. The calf muscles of one leg in subjects were pre-tired by using toe-raises. The second leg was used for comparison of results. The H-reflex amplitude in the soleus muscle decreased while ankle joint moved in

Table 1.3 Results from studies comparing stretching techniques

Researcher and year	Muscles tested	Results (better > worse)
DeVries 1962	Various	SS, BS
Holt et al 1970	Hamstrings	CR-AC>BS,SS
Tanigawa 1972	Hamstrings	CR>SS
Medieros 1977	Hamstrings	CR, SS, NS
Moore & Hutton 1980	Hamstrings	NS
Hartley-O'Brien 1980	Hamstrings	SS, BS>CR, CR-AC
Cornelius & Hinson 1980	Hamstrings	CR-AC>CR>SS
Sady et al 1982	Various	CR>SS, BS
Holt & Smith 1983	Hamstrings	CR-AC>CR>SS-IC
Lucas & Koslow 1984	Hamstrings	CR-AC, CR, SS, NS
Wallin et al 1985	Hamstrings, hip adductors, calf muscles	CR>BS
Hardy 1985	Hamstring	CR-AC,CR>SS
Etnyre & Abraham 1986	Calf muscles	CR-AC>CR>SS
Condon & Hutton 1987	Calf muscles	CR, CR-AC, SS, NS
Osternig et al 1987	Hamstrings	CR,CR-AC>SS
Etnyre & Abraham 1988	Calf muscles	CR-AC>CR>SS
Etnyre & Lee 1988	Hamstrings	CR-AC>CR>SS
" "	Shoulder	CR-AC,CR>SS
Godges et al 1989	Hamstrings	SS>CR + Massage
Cornelius 1992	Hamstrings	CR-AC>CR>SS
Sullivan et al 1992	Hamstrings	CR-AC>SS
Bandy et al 1998	Hamstrings	SS>AC
Feland et al 2001b	Hamstrings	CR>SS
Payne at al 2003	Hamstrings	AC>CR>SS

AC = agonist contraction; BS = ballistic stretching; CR = contract–relax stretching technique, which involves isometric contraction of stretched muscle; CR-AC = contract–relax and agonist–contract stretching technique; IC = isometric contraction; NS = no significant difference; PNF = proprioceptive neuromuscular facilitation; SS = static stretching.

The number of subjects has been small in all studies and thus in several studies the difference in the ROM between groups has not reached statistical significance. However, the Table shows a clear trend between stretching techniques in favour of the CR techniques. Hartley-O'Brien (1980) . Godges et al (1989), found that SS increased the mobility slightly more than the active techniques.

Box 1.7 M- and H-reflexes

The M-reflex is activated directly by electrical stimulation of the α-motor nerve. The H-reflex is initiated by stimulation of the Ia-afferent gamma nerves and impulses running via the posterior horn and continues at the same level in the spinal cord to the anterior horn and α-motor nerve innervating the muscle. The H/M relation has been used in research to illustrate the irritability of the α-motor nerve.

dorsiflexion with SS. Pressure to the Achilles tendon caused the calf muscles to stretch and produced almost as much inhibition as at dorsiflexion (Box 1.7). SS significantly decreased the H-reflex amplitude when compared to the control leg in which no decrease was recorded. It was suggested that activity in the Ib-afferent nerves from the Golgi tendon organ cause inhibition of motor neuron function as well as gamma afferent nerves from muscles spindles.

Etnyre and Abraham (1986) compared the effects of three different types of stretching on α-motor neuron function using the H-reflex (SS, CR and CR-AC). The reflex decreased most following the CR-AC stretching method in soleus muscle. The CR stretching reduced reflex function more than the SS method, but the difference disappeared after less than 1 sec.

Condon and Hutton (1987) compared the effects of four different stretching methods on dorsiflexion of the ankle (SS, AC, CR and CR-AC). α-motor neuron irritability was measured using the H-reflex. Sensitivity was less in the AC and CR-AC methods than in the SS and CR methods. They suggested that contraction of agonist muscles causes a decrease in motor neuron activity due to reciprocal inhibition. However, they found no significant difference in effectiveness between the stretching techniques on ROM.

Osternig et al (1987) studied electrical activity in the hamstring muscle during different stretching techniques. They found that average activity decreased by 11% with SS. In the CR techniques CR and CR-AC activity increased by 8–43% compared to the baseline. Despite this, stretch improvement was 5% more compared to the SS exercises.

Osternig et al (1990) compared the effects of three stretching techniques on electrical activity in the hamstring muscles and knee mobility while sitting (SS, CR and CR-AC). EMG activity steadily decreased during stretching with the SS method while with CR and CR-AC methods the activity increased compared to the baseline measured before stretching. The increased activity has been thought to increase muscle stiffness. However, increase in ROM was about 5% less in the SS group than in the other two techniques. The CR technique has been criticized because it increases muscle electrical activity, which has been suggested to increase muscle stiffness and reduce the effectiveness of stretch. This theory was shown to be false.

Magnusson (1998) and McHugh et al (1998) showed in research that while stretching the hamstrings as far as possible within pain tolerance, the electrical activity of the muscles remained below 1% compared to the level of maximum voluntary contraction, when subjects attempted to keep muscles relaxed as possible. When SS is maintained, electrical activity associated with muscle function does not increase, but it actually decreases slightly. In SS lasting 90 sec and repeated five times with 30 sec between stretches there was no significant increase in electrical activity (Magnusson 1998). Magnusson also showed that the increase in electrical activity did not produce noticeable differences between SS and CR techniques during the stretch phase. Electrical activity caused by muscle contraction disappeared during relaxation and was not shown to cause increase in resistance. More power is needed in the CR technique than in SS because pain tolerance increases and the stretch can be forced further. Thus, a CR technique acutely results in greater joint ROM due to an increased stretch tolerance. This can be even more clearly found in the clinic while the passive stretching of the muscle with intense pain and sensitivity of connective tissues has to be stopped almost before it is started. However, while using CR technique, it is often possible to proceed gradually provided that the patient is able to contract the muscle actively despite pain.

Halbertsma et al (1999) studied the effects of passive stretching of the hamstring muscles using a machine that performed straight leg rise while the individual was lying supine. Subjects stopped the stretch when they began to feel pain. Thereafter ROM was still increased as long as an increase in stretch could be tolerated. The leg was let down immediately once movement stopped. Stretching was repeated at 2-min intervals four times. Mobility did not improve in repeated stretches, and tissue resistance did not significantly change. Researchers concluded that short-term stretching does not improve tissue flexibility when stretch force does not exceed the tolerance of pain. EMG activity was minor and was shown to be greatest during the middle phase of the movement and not at the full stretch position.

Carter et al (2000) found that overall electrical activity of muscles decreased following CR stretching techniques. This has also been presented as the reason for increased flexibility immediately following stretching. Isometric contraction of muscles was supposed to activate Golgi tendon receptors in relation to the intensity of the contraction; the stronger the contraction, the greater the activation. The increase in activity is supposed to inhibit motor neuron function and induce muscle relaxation. In comparison, the activity of Golgi tendon receptors will be minimal with passive stretching.

Guissard et al (1988, 2001) and Guissard and Duchateau (2004) studied spinal reflex response during passive stretching of calf muscles. The activities were recorded in the soleus muscle in response to the electrical stimulation for different dorsiflexion angles of the ankle. Both the Hoffman and tendon reflex amplitudes were reduced during stretching. The results indicated that reduced motor neuron excitation during stretching is caused by pre- and postsynaptic mechanisms, soon as the ankle joint returned to the neutral position, the reflex responses recovered. Premotoneuronal mechanisms are mainly involved in small-stretching amplitude and postsynaptic ones play a dominant role in the reflex inhibition when larger stretching amplitudes are performed. SS programme including 30 training sessions caused a 31% increase in the ankle dorsiflexion angle. The improved flexibility was associated with a decrease in muscle passive stiffness. The changes were partially maintained 1 month after the end of the stretching but reflex activities had returned to the original level. Thus, the neural effects show a different time course compared to mechanical effects, which are responsible for long-term increase of mobility. The improved flexibility was associated with a decrease in muscle passive stiffness after the first 10 training sessions.

Several researcher have found that passive stretching of the calf muscles decreases Hoffmann reflex amplitude in the soleus (Etnyre and Abraham 1986, Condon and Hutton 1987, Nielsen et al 1993). It has been shown that the inhibition increases in correlation with an increase in the stretching force (Guissard et al 1988). Passive stretching preceded by an isometric contraction of the stretched muscle in the CR method, or assisted by the contraction of its antagonists, induces greater H-reflex inhibition and ROM compared with the passive stretching technique alone. Reflex activity returns to normal immediately after stretching.

Vallbö (1974) found no significant gamma activity from muscle spindles during passive stretch. The effect of stretching may relate to the lengthening of muscle spindle, which may raise the threshold of discharge. Enoka et al (1994) suggested that the CR stretching techniques decrease muscle spindle reflex response to stretching while active contraction may change the length of muscle spindles.

CONCLUSIONS OF STRETCHING RESEARCH

The superiority between static and CR techniques has been long debated. Research results concerning the effects of different stretching techniques are somewhat contradictory and none of the methods have been shown to be clearly superior to the others in improving mobility.

The differences may be due to many factors during testing. The number of participants in all studies has been small, and for that reason individual differences in performing stretching and random variation may noticeably affect results. Stretching force, duration and repetition is difficult to standardize in clinical studies and can be performed only by using special technology. Different measuring techniques and measurement devices have been used without testing the repeatability. Several studies have relied only on manual goniometry, which is difficult to perform reliably; at least testers subjectively placing the goniometer without exact landmarks should be blindfolded. In research, stretching force, speed and angle should all be measured, not only one component of the testing parameters. The quality of testing concerning these factors has improved in recent studies performed by Chan, Gajdosik, Göeken, Halbertsma, Magnusson and some other researchers, while using sophisticated equipment which is capable of simultaneously measuring all important parameters. Also introducing EMG in stretching studies has brought to light new information on the effects of stretching.

Research studies have focused intensely on the stretching of the hamstring muscles. Muscle structure varies between muscles, and therefore these results will not necessarily apply to all muscle groups. The various muscle types will vary both in structure and function. The hamstring muscles cross over two joints. Some muscles will cross over several joints and some over only one joint, which will affect their flexibility. Several studies have concerned only triceps surae muscle while stretching the ankle joint towards dorsiflexion. However, there are also several deep muscles in the calf, which affect on the resistance and mobility, at least near the end of the ROM.

The use of the hamstrings for stretch testing has been criticized because it involves stretching of the sciatic nerve and is not an isolated muscle stretch. Furthermore, stretch length of the hamstrings will be affected by rotation of the pelvis, which is difficult to stabilize during testing.

Stretching of joint capsule and ligaments may affect resistance more than the muscle tissues. These connective tissues will react in a different manner than muscle tissue. Also response from free nerve endings mediating pain as well as proprioceptors in structures of the joints will be different and may affect mobility.

Several studies have found the CR technique to be superior and there are several theories on the superiority of the CR technique compared with SS. Commonly the effectiveness has been explained according to the neuromuscular reflex mechanics of muscle function. According to the theory of neuromuscular relaxation, contraction prior to stretching decreases motor neuron activity owing to autogenic inhibition. Thus, the muscle–tendon system can be stretched further when active muscle resistance is reduced via the nervous system. However, it has also been claimed that active muscle contraction before stretching is harmful, because it activates motor nerves and increases muscle tension. Both theories, according to research, are incorrect. First of all, subjects are able to relax muscles and it has been shown that there is no excessive electrical activity in muscles that need to be lowered prior to stretching, at least not in subjects without any neuromuscular disease. Ia-afferent function has been shown to increase following active muscle contraction. This will increase electric activity in muscles and therefore cause a minor increase in muscle tension, but this will rapidly decrease during relaxation and thus does not cause any significant increase in resistance during stretching.

Active muscle contraction has been shown to have other neurophysiological effects. Active muscle contraction causes pain inhibition. Muscles can be stretched further due to the rise in the pain tolerance level, which has shown to be the reason for improved ROM after stretching. It most likely causes elastic and plastic changes in muscles as well, which are greater in relation to the intensity of contraction.

It has been reported in many studies that the ballistic method is less effective in increasing mobility. It is also considered to be more likely to cause injury. Stretching of connective tissue is thought to require slow stretching, because speedy execution of exercises does not allow tissue enough time to adjust and thus only elastic reversible changes will happen. Activation of the stretch reflex has been thought to increase muscle tension and increase the risk of tissue damage. However, the increased muscle activity is more likely to be protective than a risk factor. BS requires considerable skill and uncontrolled use of this method can easily lead to injury.

It is possible to relax muscles during SS exercises. No sign of the stretch reflex has been noticed. Maintaining control during SS is easier than with the ballistic method, because the movements are simplified and stretching is performed slowly. Self-applied SS exercises are very safe and have been used for thousands of years, for example as in yoga. Muscle electric activity is less during SS than during BS and there will be less pain following intense sessions. With respect to some sports, SS may be criticized that it does not specifically support necessary athletic movements. Sports requiring exceptional flexibility and elastic force will need active BS exercises to improve coordination as well.

Several studies have shown the CR technique to be more effective in improving ROM than SS techniques. According to some studies, the ROM improves even further when combined with active contraction of the agonist muscles. It has been supposed that this is because of the decrease in the electrical activity of antagonist muscles due to reciprocal inhibition caused by contraction of agonist muscles during stretching. However, many studies have shown that electrical activity does not cease, but actually often increases. Subsequently, active resistance by muscles may even increase, but according to recent research, complete muscle relaxation is not necessary to improve mobility with stretching.

It is important to direct the stretch to the desired area using the correct posture and fixation techniques. Stretching programmes often advise 5–10 sec for stretch duration. However, 20–30 sec is more effective for the hamstrings. Increasing stretching time to 60 sec does not noticeably improve results in healthy young test participants, but injury, spasticity and old age are factors which may make longer stretching times useful. Stretch effect occurs primarily during the first four repetitions. To increase the amount of stretches has been shown to be of less value.

The time of day that stretching is performed does not have much effect on the final results. Stretching in the morning helps to reduce stiffness that has developed during rest especially in those with body structures prone to stiffness. On the other hand, mobility is naturally improved by the afternoon, making stretch exercises easier. Most important is that stretching is regular in order to improve and preserve mobility.

Stretching force should be such that it produces the sensation of stretch. It may feel uncomfortable if muscles are tense, but an intense pain should not be provoked. Stretching should be done slowly when trying to improve flexibility. Fast movements can lead to strain injuries and can easily induce pain. Especially so if an assistant helps to intensify stretching. When considering stretching techniques for the most ease of learning, SS techniques are considered preferable.

Communication is important when assisting in stretching exercise. Stretching should not be performed too quickly so that patients have time to inform the therapist before the stretch becomes too great for the tissue it is affecting. The effectiveness of a stretch will be related to the amount of force used. Force is increased gradually with SS, but if the force exceeds pain tolerance, it may cause tissue damage. Pain is a warning sign and stretching should be done within pain tolerance. The level of pain tolerance will vary between individuals and may vary depending on the condition and previous stress of tissue. It does not only involve the individual's physical endurance, but it is also affected by neurophysiological and psychological factors, which become evident during treatment. In pathologic conditions of hypersensitive tissues it may be impossible to do any stretching, if the rule of painlessness is followed. Thus, the therapist has to rely on their experience of estimating the proper stretching force while trying to increase the mobility. Unfortunately this may lead to an incorrect estimate with poor experience. Although force is increased gradually, it may still exceed the full stretch tolerance of tissues. Thus, the CR method may be recommended in the first instance in painful conditions. Mobility is increased gradually by the ROM, which is freed after each active muscle contraction. Thus, CR is a safe method also for inexperienced physiotherapists.

Researchers have concluded that the restriction due to spontaneous muscle activity is insignificant in passive stretching. However, to avoid active torque it requires that treatments are performed slowly and do not induce pain. In this type of stretching resistance will come almost entirely from muscle and tendon viscosity and elastic characteristics causing passive torque, when joint connective tissues do not limit movement. If stretching is carried out quickly, muscle activity increases, and there is resistance to stretch due to the active contractile component of the muscle. Its importance is greatest during the initial phases of stretching. The speed of stretching usually slows down as the joint reaches its farthest ROM and importance of passive components of connective tissue increase for resistance. Once the stretch is maintained near the extreme tolerable position there seldom remains any difference from speed of performed stretching.

The effect of stretching was earlier considered to be due to inhibition of motor neuron function. Research has indicated this assumption to be false. Electrical activity of muscles will usually diminish to a very low level when consciously trying to relax muscles. The electrical function of the active contractile component has not been shown to increase during passive slow stretching before reaching pain threshold. In contrast, fast movement at the beginning of stretch will reflexively increase muscle activity. This activity will quickly diminish, if the stretch is then maintained in the same position i.e. during static stretch.

Active muscle contraction will affect viscosity in the muscle–tendon system and increased mobility may be the result of changes in mechanical factors. Based on research of the earlier discussed SS technique, the effect of stretching on healthy individuals primarily involves improved tolerance to stretching and the CR technique raises pain tolerance in the muscle–tendon system prior to the static phase of this technique. Thus, it can be considered to be more effective and safe in many instances.

Factors to consider in the research of stretching

- The extremity to be tested and body stability during testing
- Measurement of stretch force during testing
- Effect of weight of body part on stretch force tested in different angles
- Measurement of stretching speed
- Measurement of electrical activity in muscles
- Measurement of ROM
- Temperature of environment
- Patient's ability to withstand stretching
- Environmental factors affecting concentration.

Self-assessment: stretching techniques 1

- **What do the following abbreviations stand for? SS, CR, AC, CR-AC, H-reflex, M-reflex.**
- **How does the position of the pelvis affect stretching of the hamstrings in a standing position and test results while lying on the back?**
- **What parameters should be measured in stretching studies to properly control the measurement process?**
- **Why does the risk of strain differ noticeably between SS, BS, AC and CR?**
- **How long should the contraction phase of the CR technique last?**
- **How often and long does one need to stretch in order to increase and preserve mobility?**

PROPRIOCEPTIVE NEUROMUSCULAR FACILITATION

The proprioceptive neuromuscular facilitation (PNF) method was initiated in the rehabilitation of cerebral palsy patients by Herman Kabat. He published a number of articles about this method during the 1950s and the techniques spread around the world. Kabat pointed out that movements naturally do not occur straight, but in spiral-diagonal patterns such as in throwing, and kicking. The method uses the repetition of first passive and then active ROM to improve coordination of neuromuscular function. The idea was facilitation of the nervous system, which means repeating the same movements several times, which aim to help patients to learn movement patterns so well that they become automatic. PNF technique does not use straight lines of movement because it is thought that many joint movements combined with diagonal movements activate the central nervous system more effectively. Movements are based on postures and extension reflex models, which are associated with early development and disappear with normal growth.

Movements consist of passive exercises and both active isometric eccentric and concentric exercises. This method of treatment is still used by several physiotherapists and is supposed to encourage and speed the recovery process in cases of cerebral stroke. Muscle spasticity is treated by positional and stretching exercises in which the goal is to inhibit neuromuscular hyperactivity. Initially the exercises are performed passively. As movement patterns are established and control begins to develop, exercise can be partially assisted and finally performed actively by the patient. Facilitation exercises attempt to activate the agonist muscles, while inhibition techniques attempt to relax the antagonist muscles. The PNF method aims to improve function by using both techniques to produce balance in the neuromuscular system. These techniques focus on increasing activity in the flaccid agonists and decreasing activity in the spastic antagonists, which is supposed to happen as a result of reciprocal inhibition. The intention is to reduce movement restriction caused by spasticity and improve muscle control. Tension in paralyzed muscles is thought to improve by reflexive activation via the Golgi tendon organs, which sense active tension, muscle and joint mechanoreceptors. These are thought to be activated best by extending a movement to its fullest position. However, slow passive stretching in which there is no muscle contraction does not significantly stimulate the Golgi tendon receptors. On the other hand rapid movements will activate muscle spindles or cause activation of pain receptors, which cause a reflex reaction and an increase in motor activity, which may prevent stretching. Thus, all movements should be performed slowly.

Higher centres in the central nervous system can affect the activity of motor nerves, and it is important to learn how to reduce it consciously. Active relaxation will decrease activation of the motor neurons and will help to reduce spasticity. Even partially paralyzed muscles, which suffer from spasticity, may be completely silent at rest while measuring with EMG. 'Active rest', slow passive movements and slow stretching of spastic muscles are thought to best reduce spasticity.

PNF stretching techniques use the broad diagonal exercises in order to learn control over movements. Movements are taken as far as possible. Exercises can be achieved by the therapist, passively, with total relaxation, or partially assisted as the patient actively participates and stops periodically to rest. The patient may also try to resist movement along the entire ROM, which involves eccentric contraction.

The disadvantage with the PNF technique is that all patients will require a skillful therapist to assist the process and the patient may be able to perform only some parts of the movements alone. The technique involves isometric contractions. The therapist is required to stabilize the joints during the effort phase. This can prove to be quite difficult, if the patient is quite strong. However, it should not be a problem while the therapist understands the joint function and uses the appropriate contact with techniques. Intensive effort often involves the Valsalva manouevre in which the breath is held and the epiglottis is kept closed causing blood pressure to rise during maximum effort. To prevent this, relaxed exhalation can be used during the effort phase.

Tanigawa (1972) compared PNF-stretching technique and SS. Subjects were healthy individuals with diagnosed hamstring muscle tension. The selection criteria was that hip flexion remained under 70° due to muscle tension when the leg was lifted straight up. Two classic PNF-stretching techniques based on diagonal movement were used (Knott and Voss 1968). In the first technique the subject was lying supine while the leg was raised up with the knee extended. The therapist flexed, adducted and externally rotated the hip joint. At the same time, the therapist applied dorsiflexion to the ankle joint, rotated it inwards and extended the toes. The subject tried to resist the movement. In the second technique the therapist raised the leg up with the knee extended. The hip joint was flexed, abducted and rotated internally. The ankle joint was dosiflexed, externally rotated and the toes extended. In both techniques the subject tried to extend the hip and ankle joints for 7 sec after which there was a 5-sec rest period. The leg was allowed to rest on the table this time before beginning the next stretch. Both technique was repeated a second time were performed passively at first and then repeated twice with active resistance. In the SS method the hip was maintained in a flexed position for 5 sec with a 5-sec rest period between stretching, which was repeated 4 times. Stretching was applied twice weekly for 4 weeks in both groups. Joint mobility increased by 16° in the PNF group, by 7° in the SS group and by 1° in the control group. Mobility decreased after1 week of no stretching and results were 10°, 2° and 0 °, respectively.

The title PNF has been used liberally in the literature in relation to stretching techniques of single joints in healthy subjects, and most commonly in association with the CR and CR-AR techniques, although these techniques do not involve any diagonal movements with stretching.

MUSCLE ENERGY TECHNIQUE

Muscle energy technique (MET) is a mobilization method that was developed by the osteopath Fred L. Mitchell in the late 1940s. It is defined as an osteopathic manipulative treatment in which the patient actively contracts muscles from a controlled position in a specific direction, against a distinctly executed counterforce by the therapist. Thus, the technique involves the manual stretching of joints by the therapist into a pre-stretch position and then the patient tries to forcibly resist. The patient is then advised to relax as much as possible while the therapist moves the joint into a new position. This technique is basically similar to the CR technique. However, instead of maximum force, patients are usually encouraged to use only 20–25% of maximum force in the MET. An important factor is the direction of resistance in relation to joint positioning in that the muscle to be stretched is the one to contract. During intense effort other muscles will contract as well, especially in the vertebral column, and tend to change the position which must be prevented. The MET technique includes specific positions to stretch especially back muscles (Mitchell et al 1979).

MET technique can also be used instead of CR stretching in the extremities. If the patient is very strong, the therapist may find it difficult to maintain the correct position and should remember to instruct the use of only partial strength.

STRAIN AND COUNTER STRAIN

Another interesting osteopathic technique, strain and counter strain, was developed by Lawrence Jones in the 1960s. It is based on the theory that muscle spasm caused by strain injury is a disturbed protection mechanism that prevents normal joint function (Jones 1981). The treatment aims to reduce the exaggerated muscle spindle discharge from irritated muscles, which may be located only in single or a few segments between the vertebrae of the spinal column. As a result of trauma, tender points develop in connective tissue, which are monitored by palpation. The tender points should disappear with the release of muscle spasm after successful treatment. This is achieved by moving the joint as far as possible in the direction from which the strain came. It is also the same position in which the painful muscle is at maximum contraction and in which pain clearly eases during the stretch. Muscle spindles assessing the length of extrafusal fibres are, at this time, at their shortest. The sustained over-activity of muscle spasm is released by maintaining the muscle in an intensely shortened position for 1 min and 30 sec. After that, it is important to return the joint very slowly to the neutral position so that the muscle spindles are not reactivated. Thus, the theory is that there is a hyperirritability of intramuscular receptors, which will cease if the muscle is kept in the shortened position and not in the stretched position. One and a half minutes is considered a safe time. If the stretch directly affects the joint and is sustained for a longer period of time, it may cause irritation due to stretch of ligaments and increase pain, which has been shown in several studies.

FUNCTIONAL STRETCHING

The osteopath, Harold Hoover, described the functional stretching technique during the late 1950s. The joint is placed in the same manner as in the counter strain technique, in which there is as little pain as possible. Thus, the joint is moved in the direction towards ease and comfort (Hoover 1958). However, the idea is not to move the joint into a position in which the muscle is at maximum contraction, but in a neutral position so that tension in the agonist and antagonist muscles is the same. This is called dynamic neutral position. Relaxation is indicated by checking the texture of the tissue.

Self-assessment: stretching techniques 2

- **What types of stretching techniques have been used in research and what are their commonly used abbreviations?**
- **What is meant by the PNF method and the terms facilitation and inhibition?**
- **What is the difference between PNF and MET stretching techniques?**
- **What is meant by strain and counter strain technique?**

STRETCHING IN PHYSIOTHERAPY

Stretching is used to recover and preserve normal function in the muscle–tendon system and joint mobility. Stretching can be used to treat painful conditions of the muscles, correct muscle imbalance and disturbed coordination of the neuromuscular system. It is also important for tissue condition: their stretchability and durability.

The aims of stretching are to improve flexibility and reduce passive resistance to movement. Stretch treatments need to be effectively prescribed and directed to the correct area of the body. They should not unnecessarily load joints and their surrounding tissues so that symptoms of pain develop. If limitations in movement involve the joint and not only shortened muscles, articulation, manipulation and traction techniques can be used.

Only regular movements covering the whole ROM of the joint or stretching exercise can preserve the flexible characteristics of connective tissue. Healthy joint capsules and ligaments will stretch enough so that movement is possible, but the joint remains stable. If they stretch too far, the joint will become unstable and there will excessive stress on stabilizing connective tissues around the joint. Connective tissues at joint structures do not resist movement in an unstable joint, making mobility easy. However, joint stability becomes completely dependant on muscle tension. Pain may cause excessive muscle tension restricting ROM, although the joint may be unstable.

Movement energy is stored by elastic connective tissues during walking and running, which increases force, speed and, above all, provides the most economical use of energy in movement. The muscle–tendon organ works like a spring allowing smooth movement and thus preserving joints.

Stretching will inevitably help to prevent injury. For example, in the event of an automobile accident, elasticity in the cervical area will allow the neck to bend with the force. With aging, the elastic fibres of connective tissue are gradually replaced by tougher fibrin, and there will be less flexibility. Intense trauma will be more likely to cause damage to these rigid tissues that do not stretch as easily under loading. The structure of connective tissue will affect the success of stretching exercises. There needs to be enough elastic fibres remaining for treatment to have an effect. These do not come back, if they are lost due to long-standing immobility.

MUSCLE INJURIES

Treatment to acute muscle strain includes rest, ice, compression and elevation: (RICE). Immobilization and applications of cold are necessary immediately following trauma in order to reduce inflammation and improve the recovery process. Immobilization during the initial stages will also help to limit the amount of scar tissue. Duration of treatment depends on the extent of injury. For small injuries, 24 h of immobilization will be enough, with greater amounts of damage requiring up to 2–7 days. More than 7 days of immobilization is not advisable because regeneration with the infiltration of connective tissue will begin to form in directions other that that of the healthy tissue (regeneration) disturbing normal structure. On the other hand, beginning to load muscles too early after trauma may cause further damage (Box 1.8).

Stretching becomes important to recovery after treatment of the acute stage. Stretching can begin carefully and within pain tolerance following the prescribed immobilization period. In mild cases mobilization can begin after 2–3 days. Early mobilization has been shown to improve connective tissue and capillary circulation in the area of trauma. Repair fibres form in the same direction as the original fibres and the over production of fibrous connective tissue with fibres running in all

Box 1.8 Recovery from muscle trauma

Acute Stage 0–7 days after injury
- inflammation
- synthesis of fibronectin and elastic type III collagen fibres
- division of satellite cells starts during the first 2–3 days
- specialization of satellite cells into muscle cells starts after 3–4 days
- synthesis of stronger type I collagen fibres starts after 5–7 days

Sub-acute stage 1–3 weeks after injury
- muscle cells grow and organize while connective tissue is reinforced by the formation of transverse bridges

3 weeks after injury
- tissues in area of trauma mature and strengthen under stress
- Small trauma have healed within a month, but the total recovery may take several months from big trauma

directions is prevented. Connective tissue in muscles should form in the same direction as contractile muscle fibres to improve force. Passive and active stretching, as well as isometric muscle contraction, can begin according to pain tolerance usually 1 week after muscle trauma. Dynamic exercise placing direct stress on the area of injury usually can begin after 3 weeks. The amount of load is increased gradually. Tissue can be considered healthy when strength capacity has returned to normal, which can be confirmed with simple dynamic or isometric strength testing, depending on function of the body part.

MUSCLE CRAMP

Muscle cramps usually occur with a rapid increase of loading on an already shortened muscle. Disturbances in fluid and electrolyte balance make muscles more susceptible to cramping. The same applies to energy losses after exhaustive exercising.

Muscles kept in a shortened state for prolonged periods of time are more likely to cramp without previous loading. Cramping in the plantar muscles develop usually during rest when the ankle joint is extended, and foot muscles cramp when the sole is extended. Often cramping will occur upon waking when stretching the lower leg, in which the muscles of the calf of foot contract without loading and consequently produce intense cramping. Stretching as soon as one feels the muscles beginning to cramp is the best technique for prevention. This can be done by standing up on the feet or stretching manually. Manually pressing the muscle and stretching are also often the best way to release cramps. Stretching and massage reduce the muscle tension that leads to cramping and help prevent recurrence.

The fascia covers and is fused with the muscles. In addition, it compartmentalizes the muscles. The fascia varies in thickness and density according to anatomical location and there are huge individual differences in thickness. Exercising may raise the pressure within the fascia affecting circulation and metabolism. Stretching after physical effort or athletic exercise can decrease excessive muscle tension, intramuscular pressure and improve the recovery process in the tissues. Stretching the fascial bands and ligamentous tissue relieves the compression irritation of the involved nerves running through fasciae and prevents recurrence of the symptoms

In neurological diseases there may be constant over activity in the nervous system controlling the muscle tone, which causes muscle tension to increase. Regular stretching and relaxation exercising is important in reducing muscle tension and preserving mobility. Stretching can reduce spasticity and prevent muscle cramps.

It is important to take care of muscle condition. Weak muscles will tire faster than strong muscles. Recovery following loading is also important. Tired muscles have been shown with research to be less resilient to stress and sudden loading can cause muscle cramp.

In regards to well-being, an important factor affecting flexibility is subjective muscle relaxation. Stiff joints and muscles often cause symptoms of pain that can disturb sleep. Stretching after physical effort or athletic exercise can improve the recovery process in tissues.

Intense active exercise in muscles unaccustomed to workout will more likely produce muscle tension. This may feel unpleasant and exercise is often not continued. When exercise is begun lightly, with the amount of stress gradually increased with each workout, the muscles have time to adapt and the subject will become accustomed to the new muscle tone in a few weeks. If the degeneration of connective tissues has already occurred or there is a chronic painful condition, exercise may cause overstress and pain and other forms of treatment may be needed to relieve symptoms in addition to stretching.

Self-assessment: myofascial pain

- What are the common causes of muscle pain?
- What does the vicious circle refer to in regards to muscle pain?
- What mechanism associated with heart attack involves pain and stiffness in the neck and shoulder area?
- What tests should be done before the patient is allowed to return to competitive sports after muscle injury?

FRACTURES AND SURGERY

Joint mobility decreases rapidly following trauma and surgery due to immobilization. Fingers are especially susceptible to stiffening. The most common fracture is of the wrist due to falling. Fingers are normally left free to move during immobilization with cast. Joints are kept in functional neutral position during immobilization to reduce the risk of stiffening. Severe inflammation of the tendon sheath also sometimes requires immobilization of the wrist. Patients are told to exercise their fingers to prevent stiffening of the joints. However, medical staff may have forgotten to tell this to the patient or the patient may not remember to exercise the fingers regularly. In these cases, prolonged immobilization may lead to joint stiffening even within 4 weeks. Some mobility can be restored, but full recovery may not be possible even with intensive stretching, if it is not started immediately. The risk of joint stiffening increases in fractures, if bone formation is delayed requiring extended immobilization. Furthermore, the proximal joints, in this case the elbow and shoulder, need to be actively exercised as well.

Similarly, fractures of the ankle and foot require active exercise of the toe joints to preserve mobility. Exercise is most effective if actively performed whenever possible. If active movements are not possible, passive stretching and mobilization helps to prevent stiffening of the joint capsules. Active muscle function during immobilization is important in preventing tissue degeneration, odema and thrombosis. Repeated short isometric contractions are useful when dynamic movement is not possible. The replacement of muscle cells by connective tissue can be delayed and partially prevented with external electric stimulation. However, it will not prevent shortening of connective tissue fibres of joints during immobilization.

Especially important are stretching exercises following surgery of the tendons of the hand to preserve mobility and prevent the formation of adhesions. This is especially so on the palm of the hand, where the complicated structure of flexor tendons can easily stiffen up in a flexed position due to adhesions. Local infections sometimes arise as a complication after surgery. Infection often leads to the infiltration of excessive connective tissue around tendons, which will limit mobility if not stretched regularly. Also hereditary factors may induce excessive collagen formation around tendons in the hand and sometimes in the legs. Most commonly it affects flexor tendons of the fourth and fifth finger in the hand, preventing extension. The need for surgery in cases of Dupuytren's contracture can often be prevented with regular stretching of the flexor tendons of the hand.

TRAUMA AND BURNS

Clean trauma will usually heal quickly, but soiled traumas often lead to local infections and excessive formation of connective tissue. Stretching is important to preserve the mobility. During burn recovery in hands it is especially important in encouraging the formation of elastic scar tissue to prevent tightness, which may limit joint mobility. Stretching should be performed daily, with the application of pressure bandages following treatments to reduce the formation of scar tissue.

SPASTICITY

Injuries to the head, haemorrhaging in the brain and stroke often involve muscle spasticity, which has been dealt with in the section on muscle tone. Research by Halar et al (1978) showed that spasticity affects muscle tissue, but not tendons. In the legs it will interfere with walking, and in the arms it can prevent normal function, which is needed in activities of daily living. In both the arms and legs SS can be made more effective with splinting.

Harvey et al (2000) studied the effect of SS on ankle mobility in patients with recent spinal cord injury. Ankles were stretched continuously into dorsiflexion with a torque of 7.5 Nm for 30 min each weekday for 4 weeks, while contralateral ankles received no stretches. The intervention did not change the mobility or the torque-angle curves of the ankle whether the knee was extended or flexed. Thus, the stretching procedure applied was not sufficient to produce any significant changes in patients with paraplegia or quadriplegia spasticity.

Bressel and McNair et al (2002) compared 30-min stretch duration times using static and dynamic techniques to stretch stiff ankle joints of patients with lower extremity spasticity as a result of stroke. Stretch position was 80% of maximum dorsiflexion in both tests. Angle speed was 5°/sec in dynamic stretching, moving from the stretch position to normal position, back and forth, without breaks. Ankle stiffness decreased by 35% with SS and by 30% with dynamic stretching and there was no significant difference between stretching methods. Walking speed was not influenced by the stretching treatments.

Harvey et al (2003) studied the effect of SS on extensibility of the hamstring muscles in patients with recent spinal cord injuries. Patients had no, or only minimal, voluntary motor power in the lower limbs and insufficient hamstring muscle extensibility, which prevents adequate hip flexion so that the patient tends to fall backwards when sitting with the knees extended. Hamstring muscles were stretched continuously with a 30 Nm torque at the hip for 30 min each weekday for 4 weeks while hamstring muscles of the contralateral leg were not stretched. The intervention did not produce any significant change in the mobility.

Increased ROM as a result of effective stretching has been shown in healthy people. However, the efficacy of intensive stretching therapy in people with functionally significant contracture has not yet been shown in studies, although these treatments are common practice. Interventions aimed at preventing or reversing the contractures must provide sufficient mechanical stimulus to induce tissue lengthening and remodelling. However, there are no controlled studies, as they would be unethical.

People with spinal cord injuries provide their hamstring muscles with large stretch torques when dressing and transferring weight with routine daily activities. This may explain why many such patients develop good extensibility of the hamstring muscles over time. It has been estimated that stretch torque on shortened hamstring muscles administered by body weight while sitting with the hips flexed and knees extended could exceed 144 Nm (Harvey et al 2003), which suggests that this is sufficient magnitude for effective stretching and force used in previous studies has been too low.

JOINT INFLAMMATION

Excessive stress to joints should be avoided when stretching and especially so in cases of joint inflammation. Active, intense exercise and even passive mobilization can irritate, increasing the inflammation and making symptoms worse. Treatment to preserve mobility can be used during inflammation in the form of a few gentle passive and active stretches that do not irritate the condition further. Gentle stretching once a day, i.e. extending the affected joints to their full and painless ROM a couple of times, is usually enough. Long-term inflammation can be detrimental to the tissues of the joint capsule and cartilage. Inflammation caused by bacteria can be treated with antibiotics while aseptic inflammations are treated with specific medications for gout and rheumatism, anti-inflammatory analgesics, and corticosteroids. Once pain and inflammation are under control more intensive exercising to return normal mobility can begin. Long-term inflammation may result in the replacement of elastic fibres with stiff fibrin in the joint capsule and full recovery to normal ROM may not be possible. Traction should be applied as early as possible. The longer and greater the limitations in mobility are, the more difficult full recovery will be. Long-term limitations in joint mobility will always involve shortening in the muscle–tendon system, which will also require stretching to achieve normal ROM.

Factors affecting flexibility following joint inflammation

- Age
- Gender
- Joint type
- Joint structure of articular surface
- Joint capsule and ligament structure
- Surrounding muscles
- Type of inflammation or infection
- Joint tissue trauma
- Loading
- Immobilization
- Medication
- Passive and active exercise
- Mobilization
  —technique
  —force
  —time
- Additional therapies.

LIMITATIONS OF JOINT MOBILITY

Joint degeneration usually involves the gradual onset of limitations in mobility, which does not always cause pain during the early stages. However, pain will arise when movements require a ROM which exceeds limitation. The joint capsule may also become stretched under sustained static loading in relaxed positions and pain may subsequently appear. Inflammation can cause joints to stiffen quickly with intense resting pain. Active inflammation needs to be controlled with medication before treatment to increase mobility can begin. Otherwise the treatment would only further irritate joint inflammation and increase pain. As the inflammation eases, rehabilitation can begin with ROM exercises according to pain tolerance. Once inflammation has completely subsided more intense mobilization can begin. In some cases, cryotherapy, local anaesthesia or sometimes even anaesthesia has to be administered prior to mobilization as the soft tissues are tender.

Stretching technique will depend on joint structure and the nature of the immobility. Joint limitation in the shoulder due to inflammation is often best aided by the CR technique. The frozen shoulder is stabilized at the end of the passive ROM and active muscle contraction is used to stretch the joint capsule. Contracting subscapularis will stretch the rotator cuff medially and infraspinatus laterally. ROM is increased during the relaxation phase with the freed mobility space following the release of tension; then stretching the joint capsule requires only minimal amounts of force. The technique is repeated until the desired ROM is attained. Often intra-articular injection of local anaesthetic is required to enable the stretch at the first attempt.

In cases of joint capsule inflammation SS techniques usually cause intense pain and are therefore not recommended. SS may be successfully used following immobilization depending on the patient's stretch tolerance. The use of light loading can significantly improve stretch tolerance; however, if the force used is too light, no amount of time will produce results.

Traction away from the joint surface at a right angle is often the least painful direction for stretching in cases of limited ROM due to arthrosis. In this case all stabilizing structures of the joint will be directly affected by stretch and thus require a greater amount of force compared with other directions. Stretching should be long enough to achieve permanent structural changes in the joint capsules and joint ligaments. This can be achieved with both continuous static and repetitive intermittent stretching.

Steffen and Mollinger (1995) examined the effects of long-term SS on the contracted knee joints of elderly people but they achieved no improvement in mobility. It is important that a stretching programme begins during the early stages of joint stiffening. If mobility has been limited for an extended period of time, elastic fibres will be significantly replaced by more fibrous connective tissue, which is not as flexible. In this scenario only mechanical tearing of the fibrous tissue can restore mobility, which is carried out in arthroplasty. Based on long-term clinical experience, excessive limitations in mobility can be restored and symptoms of pain relieved if stretching treatment begins early enough. Elderly people should, therefore, be encouraged to seek treatment at the earliest signs of joint stiffness. If more than half of the ROM of the joint has been already lost, there is great risk of permanent limitation.

MUSCLE SHORTENING IN LOWER EXTREMITIES

Limited mobility in the lower leg joints is not always due to arthritic changes in the joints, but may be the result of tightness in the muscle–tendon system. Pain due to inflammation or abnormal posture can activate muscle tension and cause limitations in mobility outside the joint area. Important factors include muscle type as well as how much from the full ROM is used — not every day but weekly. If posture keeps the muscle–tendon system in a shortened state for a prolonged period of time and there is significant stiffening, the elastic fibres will gradually be replaced by tough connective tissue. At this stage, mobility can only be improved with the reduction of adhesions by tenotomy. These treatments can be avoided in many cases, however, with active regular stretching, if started in the early stages of the stiffening process.

Leivseth et al (1989) studied the effects of stretch to the thigh adductors in osteoarthritis of the hip. Passive stretching was applied manually with 20–30 kilopond force directed at the adductors while the hip was flexed 45° with the knee supported against the therapist's thigh, allowing for maximum abduction. Duration of stretch was 30 sec, repeated every 10 sec for 25 min and treatment was applied 5 days a week for 4 weeks. Abduction improved by 8° and a decrease in pain was noted in all cases. The difference in glycogen levels in muscles of the arthritic side was 85% of that measured of the healthy side in the initial stages, but rose in the arthritic side to equal amounts during treatment. The diameter of type I fibres in the adductor longus muscle increased by 68% and type II fibres by 79% in the side of osteoarthritis. This may be due to improved mobility and decreased pain that encouraged subjects to move more.

Feland et al (2001c) studied the effects of SS of the hamstrings in elderly people with the average age of 85 years. The angle of knee extension was measured while individuals were lying supine with the hip flexed to 90°. Limitations in mobility occurred after 20° in the initial stages. Stretching was achieved by lifting the leg straight up while the patient was lying on their back. Treatment was repeated four times with 10 sec intervals between, 5 days a week for 1 month. Flexibility improved on average by 14° in those of the 60-sec stretch duration group, by 8° in the 30-sec group and by 4° in the 15-sec group. One month following treatments, flexibility had decreased near the original level in all groups except the 60-sec group, which was still 5° more compared to the baseline before stretching.

Increasing muscle length in stiff muscles of elderly people was shown in research to require longer stretching times than in previous studies of young people. Short muscles tend to return more quickly to their original length, if stretching is stopped completely. Thus regular stretching is needed to preserve mobility of the muscle–tendon organ in elderly people as well as resistance exercises to preserve strength.

TENNIS ELBOW

Solveborn (1997) compared the effects of regular stretching and forearm bands in the treatment of epicondylalgia. Patients met with the physiotherapist six times during the first month to receive stretching instruction. They were instructed to perform home stretching exercises twice daily. Both treatments were successful with a continuous symptom reduction, but relief of symptoms was statistically more significant in the stretching group than in the group with forearm band. Improved wrist mobility was only recorded in the stretching group.

CHRONIC BACK PAIN

Disc degeneration and spondylosis of vertebrae are associated with aging and will reduce mobility of the spine. These changes involve functional limitations and increase susceptibility to pain, especially with forward bending. Mobility can be improved in the vertebral joints, just as in the extremities, with stretching exercises. Exercise would be easy if stiffening developed at the same pace throughout the spine without symptoms of pain. However, it is more likely joint mobility will vary between vertebrae and stretching will easily be directed towards those joints which are more flexible. There may even be hypermobility, and thus stretching will not affect the stiff joints. Specific mobilization and a special exercise programme are necessary in order to improve mobility in the required areas of the spine and to avoid making the condition worse in joints with excessive laxity.

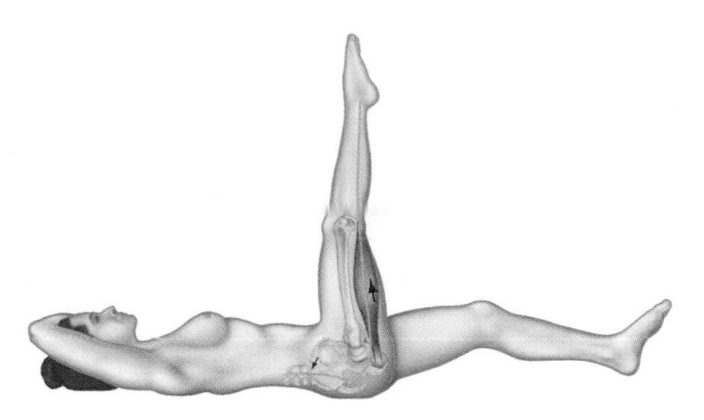

Figure 1.28 Hamstring muscles are stretched by straight leg raise. However, disc prolapse may cause sciatica, causing pressure at the nerve root and preventing further stretching. Thus, straight leg raise will be 60° or less, because of the protective muscle spasm.

Limited joint mobility will lead to degeneration of the deep intervertebral muscles and a reduction in strength of the back muscles. Muscle tissue may be replaced by tougher, less flexible fibrin and fat tissue. This can only be prevented by restoring mobility with active exercising at an early stage of the back disorder.

Tight hamstrings, iliopsoas, piriformis, quadriceps, quadratus lumborum and paraspinal muscles are usually involved in back pain as possible sources, or as complications due to pain. In physiotherapy attention is often focused on stretching the hamstrings in treatment of the lower legs. However, the iliopsoas muscle is of particular importance to back function. The iliopsoas is commonly involved in back pain and it is also often the actual cause of back and hip pain. Tension in the iliopsoas muscle may likewise be caused by pain in the lower abdomen, lower back and hip area. It may also tighten under static loading during sustained hip flexion or due to strain wound after hyperextension of the hip joint. Referred pain from trigger points in the iliopsoas muscle can affect the lower abdomen, hip and back. Tightness in the iliopsoas muscle will cause straightening of the lumbar spine, which puts more loading on the discs as loading moves off the facet joints onto them. Disc function and metabolism is disturbed in the lumbar spine due to increase of intradiscal pressure. Discs become dehydrated, which causes further stiffening of the back.

Hamstring muscle tightness will cause the pelvis to tilt backwards and normal lumbar lordosis will diminish, become straight or turn to kyphosis, which will decrease mobility. Furthermore it will lead to an abnormal posture in which the straight lumbar spine is accompanied for by bending the thoracic spine, shoulders and head forwards. Straightened lumbar spine and excessive kyphosis in the thoracic spine place an increased pressure on the front part of the lumbar vertebrae and, particularly, the inferior spinal discs. It will stretch intervertebral and iliolumbar ligaments and the posterior side of discs. The back's ability to withstand loading weakens. This process will be accentuated due to degenerative changes with advanced age, which also decrease mobility of the back. Stress on the spine may become too great and cause back problems. This postural syndrome is a common cause of chronic back pain. It becomes even more evident if work and leisure activities require repetition of forward bending or a statically held forward bent position. Both frequently repeated and chronic back pain often involves two problems: improper posture and disc degeneration. Active stretching to restore and preserve back mobility as well as exercise to restore normal posture are important before stiffening changes in the spine become permanent contracture.

Symptoms of pain in the lumbar spine of the young and middle aged will often be due to instability as well. Active stretching exercises, which are often advised for treatment for a stiff back, may increase instability and pain. Treatments should preferably be designed to increase stability to support joints by improving muscle tone and strength. Age is not necessarily a direct indication as to whether or not stiffness or hypermobility is the problem. Even school age children may have back stiffness and people in advanced age may have hypermobility, although these cases diverge from the norm in the majority of people. It is also possible for one individual to have hypomobility in some joints while having hypermobility in others. Stretching routines should be based on clinical examination in which each joint is tested for mobility. Examination of the entire spine at once with tests including only gross movements is not sufficient to reveal variations in mobility between each articulation. It may give normal results, although half of the moving segments would be hypermobile and the other half hypomobile.

Long-term periods of sitting, especially in a forward position, will over-load the spinal discs. Such loading can even affect school children, who sit a great deal and often have symptoms of pain in the lower back, chest and neck. Lack of exercise and poor posture will usually affect the thoracic spine first with stiffness developing by puberty. Mobility is normally less in this area due to the physiologically kyphosis structure of vertebrae and due to the stabilizing effect of the rib cage. Therefore, stiffening will tend to affect this area more easily while stiffness in the lumbar spine tends to develop at a later stage. Thoracic stiffness causing upper back pain is especially common during early middle age. It is also the more common cause of chest pain in advanced age compared to heart diseases.

Deep breathing is important in back function. During deep inhalation the spine will extend, while during exhalation cervical and lumbar lordosis increase, as does thoracic kyphosis. The movement causing alteration in compression on the spinal discs will improve metabolism by diffusion. This pumping system will be less efficient with poor posture. Stiffness will also limit rib cage mobility, which consequently will restrict deep respiration. Thus, lack of mobility in the spine will decrease general function in the elderly. Breathing is important for muscle function. Deep inhalation activates neck, shoulder and chest muscles and is an effective method of mobilizing the chest area. Forceful exhalation will activate the cervical, chest, abdominal and back muscles. Maximum exhalation will increase forward bending. Breathing exercises with stretching have been used effectively, particularly in yoga, to relax muscles and improve mobility.

The onset of disc degeneration in the lumbar spine has been shown to exist even in school children. This is primarily due to innate structural characteristics of the disc tissue. Problems will affect all the joint discs but due to pressure degeneration will be more prominent in the lumbar spine. Unusual and sudden intense loading may cause damage and lead to degeneration in otherwise healthy discs. Nucleus pulposa is the soft centre of the disc, which is surrounded and encased by dense connective tissue of annulus fibrosus. No nerves or blood vessels infiltrate the nucleus pulposa. Degeneration causing the breakdown and stretching of the annulus fibrosus can lead to disc rupture, protrusion or prolapse. All these conditions may cause intense neck or back pain, when they appear in the posterior side of the annulus fibrosus, which is well innervated. A strong reflex reaction associated with pain causes the paravertebral muscles to tense up. The quadratus lumborum muscle and the iliopsoas muscle are often involved as well. Intensive long-standing muscle contraction decreases circulation in muscles and they become stiff, tender and painful. Stretching and mobilization can relieve back pain caused by tense muscles and disc prolapse will disappear spontaneously in most cases.

Herniation of the nucleus pulposa through the outer layer of annulus fibrosus due to degeneration and breakdown is known as disc prolapse and causes intense pain accompanied by protective muscle spasm to prevent movement. Sciatica can be caused by pressure at the root of the sciatic nerve by disc hernia or by chemical irritation by smaller amounts of acidic nucleus pulposa. The pinched nerve will be stretched in the canal between vertebrae or spinal canal, if the straight leg is raised up while the patient is lying supine as in the Lasegue test (Figure 1.28). This will automatically cause protective muscle spasm in the hamstrings, which will prevent further stretching of the nerve root and will noticeably limit hip mobility. Hip flexion becomes difficult when raising the leg while lying or bending forward while standing. Some patients will not experience any back pain with disc prolapse, but only pain symptoms referred to the lower extremity and mobility will be limited. Rarely, there may be hamstring spasm without any pain in the leg. Intense stretching may result in nerve damage in cases of prolapsed disc. Thus, hard resistance caused by hamstring muscles, which does not give way with CR, testing is a contraindication for any stretching — including SS.

Back pain often appears before actual disc degeneration can be found with X-ray or magnetic resonance imaging. Disc degeneration may proceed symptomless and thus disc hernia may occur without prior symptoms. In many cases symptoms begin during childhood and it takes often several years before protrusion or rupture develops. Disc degeneration develops gradually with fluid reduction and the back becomes stiff. In some people back stiffness will be accompanied by pain, especially if immobility develops only in some discs and not evenly throughout the spine. The stiff area in the spine will cause via long moment arm twisting pressure on the first mobile segment and may induce pain and protective muscle spasm. Active stretching, mobilization and manipulation will be considered as forms of treatment. Hypermobility can cause similar symptoms, but does not benefit from stretching or mobilization. Treatment planning will be aided by clinical testing of mobility to determine the cause and best treatment.

Postural changes such as straightening of the thoracic spine and exaggerated kyphosis increase stiffness. In scoliosis of the spine mobility will be decreased on the convex scoliosis of the spine mobility will be decreased on the convex side of the curve, while on the concave side mobility will be increased. Straightening of the lumbar spine causes restriction in extension and lateral flexion but in some cases will also limit forward flexion. Excessive lordosis in the lumbar spine increases mobility in every direction.

Back mobility has been shown to be better in children who actively move and exercise. Postural examinations of school children should include back mobility evaluation as well as checking for possible scoliosis. Exercises to improve and preserve back mobility could be advised in cases where stiffness is detected.

Halbertsma et al (2001) studied the extensibility and stiffness of the hamstrings in patients with nonspecific low back pain. The patient group showed a significant restriction in ROM and extensibility of the hamstrings compared with healthy controls. No significant difference in hamstring muscle stiffness was found between both groups. Thus, the restricted motion in patients was not caused by increased muscle stiffness, but determined by the decreased stretch tolerance associated with back pain.

Controlled research of the effects of stretching on chronic back pain is minimal, because treatments usually include other forms of conditioning as well, making it difficult to isolate results. Elnaggar et al (1991) compared flexion and extension stretching exercises in patients suffering from chronic back pain. Treatment included repeated dynamic and SS techniques. Symptoms of pain were relieved in both groups to the same extent, but an increase in mobility was recorded only in those using flexion exercises. Khalil et al (1992) conducted research on the effects of SS techniques on chronic back pain diagnosed as being caused by muscle condition. A control group received physiotherapy, traction of the lumbar spine stretching, and strengthening exercises. In addition to that the stretching group received stretches which were systematically given by the two therapists. Local applications of cold were used prior to stretching. SS techniques were maintained, depending on the individual, from 2 sec to 2 min and repeated three times each treatment day; there was a total of four treatment days in a 2-week period. Stretches were directed to the paraspinal muscles, quadratus lumborum, the tensor fascia latae and the hamstrings. The lower back was stretched into flexion, extension and rotation. Stretching was taken as far as pain tolerance would allow. The rehabilitation programme showed a high rate of success. In the beginning, average back pain was moderate or severe, measured by visual analogue scale (VAS; 0–100). Pain reduced significantly following stretching treatment, as decreased from 63 to 16 on the VAS. In the control group pain decreased only from 71 to 53 on the, which is not clinically significant.

Self-assessment: back problems

- How do kyphosis, lordosis and scoliosis affect thoracic and lumbar spine mobility?
- In what way will disc and facet joint degeneration affect back mobility?
- Name the primary muscles commonly affecting back movement in lower back pain?

CHRONIC NECK PAIN

Chronic nonspecific neck pain is the second most common condition after the low back pain in modern industrialized countries. There has been a lack of studies to show significant long-term effects of training in chronic neck pain. Recently Ylinen et al (2003) compared in a randomized controlled study the effectiveness of isometric strength training, dynamic endurance training of neck muscles and stretching exercises in women with chronic neck pain. Both muscle training groups performed the same stretching exercises as the stretching group. All groups were given advice to exercise three times per week at home. Neck pain and disability decreased significantly in all groups during 12 months' follow-up. However, both training groups improved significantly more compared to the stretching group. Also neck ROM improved statistically significantly in both training groups compared with the control group. The change in rotation was 12° in the strength training group, 7° in the endurance training group and only 1° in the stretching group. Thus, strength training combined with stretching exercises was more effective than stretching exercises alone in improving mobility. Contrary to popular belief strength training does not restrict mobility, at least not if it is combined with stretching exercises. Winkelstein et al (2001) found that the total insertion area of deep cervical muscle fibres into the lower cervical joints covered 22% of the total facet capsule area. They estimated that the magnitude of loading to the cervical joint capsules due to eccentric muscle contraction to be as high as 51 N. This amount of stretching of joint capsules may explain the greater improvement of mobility in the strength training group. Some neck muscles attach to ligaments and fascia, which forceful contraction will also stretch, as well as non-contractile elastic components of muscles themselves. Thus, there may be several mechanisms affecting greater mobility as a result of strength training. Mechanical loading, movement, pressure and stretching of hypersensitive muscles cause pain. Regular exercising with proper intensity may decrease sensitivity of soft tissues and abolish chronic pain. Thus, it is recommendable to combine strength training with stretching in rehabilitation.

CARPAL TUNNEL SYNDROME

Carpal tunnel syndrome is a common complication of repetitive activities and causes significant morbidity. It is also the most common operative diagnosis in the upper extremity. Clinical tests often reveal the aetiology of symptoms like the Phalen sign and the Tinel sign. However, these tests based on compression and tapping of the peripheral nerve are not specific and may be normal in carpal tunnel syndrome. Thus, electroneuromyography should be used to make a diagnosis, if surgery is planned. Although surgery is a common treatment method in carpal tunnel syndrome, in mild and moderate cases stretching and mobilization should be preferred in the first instance. Conservative treatment has shown to decrease pressure in the carpal tunnel (Seradge et al 1993) and about half of the patients will improve and can avoid an operation as shown in several studies (Bonebrake 1994, Sucher 1994, Valente and Gibson 1994, Garfinkel et al 1998, Rozmaryn et al 1998, Sucher and Hinrichs 1998, Todnem and Lundemo 2000). A loose splint keeps the wrist in a neutral position while asleep and decreases the pressure in the carpal joint and has also been shown to be a useful conservative treatment method (Gerritsen et al 2002). It may also be helpful in certain working conditions. As about half of patients who have undergone surgery continue to have varying degrees of symptoms post-operatively surgery may be recommended as a first choice only in severe cases. It is important to avoid immobilization postoperatively. Stretching and active exercising have shown to be beneficial for recovery (Cook et al 1995, Provinciali et al 2000).

STRETCH AS A CAUSE OF PAIN

Stress to ligaments and capsules during prolonged and intense stretching of joints has been shown to cause pain. Harms-Ringdahl and Ekholm (1986) studied the effects of forward flexion of the cervical spine in healthy individuals. Pain was provoked when the neck was bent and sustained forward as far as possible for 3 min. Dalenbring et al (1999) examined the development of symptoms when the cervical spine was kept in a rotated position. Symptoms of pain developed on average after 3 min of passive stretching. The subjects were lying on their stomachs with the head turned to the side with a pillow under the chin to increase rotation. Symptoms of pain developed in all individuals after 7 min of stretching. Pain continually increased if stretching was not stopped. Descriptions of pain varied between individuals and included for example: squeezing, throbbing, pulling, burning and stinging. Pain receptors in the joint ligaments and capsules protect joints by preventing excessive stretching, which may cause tissue damage. Nerve receptors and connective tissue of joints in the extremities will react in the same way. The number of receptors and tissue structure will vary, however, between joints, and the time it takes for symptoms of pain to develop will differ. However, sustained stretching of joint capsule and ligaments for many minutes can increase existing, or cause new, pain and should be avoided. These studies show clearly that stretching cannot be applied for too long and recommendation for the duration of the stretch in therapy as well as in exercises should be followed.

Stretching which is either sudden and intense or slow and sustained can cause tissue damage. Pain receptors sense abnormal postures, which cause overstretching in tissues and respond by activating motor neurons, which produce an intense static contraction in order to prevent the abnormal posture causing excessive strain on connective tissues. However, this protective muscle spasm becomes often sustained.

Stretching studies have commonly used young subjects with good mobility. Joint ROM will often be reduced in older people as there is a decrease in tissue elasticity with age. Limited mobility may prevent normal stretching of the muscle–tendon system and pain may develop more quickly than in the previously mentioned studies.

Painful conditions due to stretching may be occupational. The mechanism is often prolonged forward leaning or rotation positions. Farmers commonly have to look backwards while driving a tractor and rotate both their back and neck. Similar working conditions occur for fork lift truck drivers. But as relatively few people work in this type of job, painful conditions occur much more frequently at rest. Stretching leading to a painful condition may occur, after sleeping in an awkward position; this can occur after being in the position only for a few minutes. The neck is more vulnerable to distortion in rotation while lying prone. Both the neck and back are vulnerable to side bending and rotation while lying on the side. Sleeping in the sitting position without proper support to the head often leads to a painful condition of the neck. One of the most common causes of back pain in modern society is badly designed chairs, which allow the pelvis to tilt backwards and cause stretching in the lower back ligaments and discs. Postural back syndrome is a common condition like postural neck syndrome.

MUSCLE TIGHTNESS

Krivickas and Feinberg (1996) have produced a series of tests to measure stiffness in body structure. Points based on five tests involving both lower extremities are added together to obtain muscle tightness score; the maximum score being 10, indicating extreme stiffness.

Testing the mobility of muscle–tendon unit

Iliotibial tract/band: a variation of Ober's test can be used in a prone position with the legs stretched out. One leg is abducted with the knee flexed to a right angle. The hip is extended and then adducted by lifting at the ankle. The test is given a point, if adduction does not reach the middle line.

Rectus femoris: knee flexion is measured while in a supine position with the hip flexed to a right angle and then while lying prone with hip extended. The test is given a point if the angle difference is at least 10°.

Iliopsoas: in the Thomas test the patient lies supine and flexes one hip to draw flexed knee as far as possible up to chest. A point is given if the other leg flexes as well.

Hamstrings: the angle of passive knee extension is measured while the patient is lying supine with the hip flexed to a right angle. The test is given a point if the angle is at least 25°.

Triceps surae: dorsiflexion of the ankle is measured while patient is lying supine with the hip and knee extended. The test is given a point if the angle is no more than 5°.

Factors affecting effectiveness of stretching techniques

Functional

- Stretching force
- Speed of stretching
- Direction of stretching movement
- Duration of stretch
- Repetition of stretch
- Number of stretching series
- Number of stretching days
- Time between stretching
- Method of stretching
- Temperature of tissues

Structural

- Type of joint
- Arthrosis
- Oedema
- Type of muscle
- Muscle tone — spasm
- Adhesions
- Surrounding connective tissues.

MEASURING STRETCH FORCE

Strain and pressure gauges are commonly used to measure the force of stretch. In this case, the speed of stretch will be noticeably affected by tissue resistance and needs to be standardized in research. In some studies, stretching is stopped according to pain tolerance and in this case measures stretching force which is the same as the resistance produced by the stretched tissues. When movement is stopped during stretch, resistance immediately begins to drop, allowing tissue to adapt in stretch. Time of measurement is important during stretching and often the continual measuring of force is used in research.

SUBJECTIVE AND OBJECTIVE MUSCLE TENSION

Muscle tension can normally be felt with palpation. This can not be considered objective observation although a rough estimate of muscle tension can be acquired. Clearly a better method is to move body parts to assess resistance while the patient tries to relax maximally. However, it is problematic that some patients will begin to tense muscles when they are told to relax and some will even move the extremities. Subjective muscle tension can be measured with a continuous scale. In a continuous scale the extent of stretching force may be described with a VAS from 0 to 100, in which one end represents complete muscle relaxation and the opposite end extreme muscle tension or spasm. The benefit of using a continuing scale is that even small changes can be measured.

Mark with an X along the 100 mm line to best indicate your experience of muscle tension during the past week.

No tension Extremely tense

100 mm

____

Subjective muscle tension can be measured by a categorized scale although a continual scale is often considered to be more valuable in research by statisticians (Box 1.9). On the other hand, a categorized scale may be easier, for instance elderly people, in normal clinical situations. The continual scale may be interpretated in different ways by different people. Some might consider themselves at the beginning of the line, indicating no extra muscle tension, while others associate the middle section with normal muscle tone in which there is some degree of tension. This problem will make this scale unreliable and difficult to compare with others. The only way to achieve reliable repetitions is to add a point on the scale marked 'normal'.

Mark with an X in the box the alternative that best describes your experience of tension in the neck, back, arms, legs, etc. during the past week:

Box 1.9 Measuring stretch sensation

In the assessment of stretch force, Borg's scale based on subjective sensation to stretch may be used. It will increase safety in SS techniques.

Number	Sensation
0	nothing
0.5	extremely weak
1	very weak
2	weak/slight
3	moderate
4	moderately intense
5	intense
6	
7	very intense
8	
9	
10	extremely intense

☐ normal
☐ slightly tense
☐ moderately tense
☐ very tense
☐ exceptionally tense.

Mark with an X in the box the alternative that best describes your experience of tension in neck, back, arms or legs during the past week:

☐ extremely flaccid
☐ moderately flaccid
☐ normal
☐ moderately tense
☐ extremely tense.

The form of questions will affect the quality of answers. The previous series of questions concentrate on subjective experience of muscle tension for measurement. It does not associate any feelings that muscles are flabby. Answers may vary greatly, when the questions are exactly the same, but the scale has been changed.

Mark with an X along the line to best indicate your experience of muscle tension during the past week:

Completely flaccid — Exceptionally tense

100 mm

Muscle tension can also be measured objectively. The instrumental straight-leg raising test enables simultaneous measurement of the pelvic-femoral angle, force to lift the leg and electric activity of the muscles by the surface electromyography and the extent of leg excursion at which pain or tension is experienced (Göeken 1991). These measurements provide information on ROM, extensibility of the hamstrings, muscle stiffness and activity, pain perception causing defence reactions and stretch tolerance.

Muscle spasticity often involves an increase in electrical activity that can be measured with the aid of sEMG. It describes 'active muscle tension' during movement. However, the measurement of changes in electrical activity as a result of passive stretching is not useful, because there is no electrical activity if the muscles are relaxed. Electrical activity may increase after intense exercise and may also be high in a tense muscle. Despite even this, activity can often be eliminated with conscious relaxation of the muscles. This applies also in most of the cases on spastic muscles, which may also be completely silent when evaluated with sEMG after relaxation. However, there is considerable hyperactivity even with minimal irritation in spastic muscles and in spasmodic dystonia at rest.

However, muscle tone variate greatly between different people even during complete relaxation when electrical activity is at zero and there is no active contraction. This can be evaluated by measuring visco-elastic stretch resistance with an isokinetic force measurement machine or by applying pressure directly to the muscle with a force gauge using steady speed (Fig. 1.29 and 1.30). Muscle tension at rest is not consistent, but fluctuates according to environmental factors, psychological, physical characteristics and depends greatly on foregoing physical activities.

Non-physical Muscle Tension

Patients may experience annoying muscle tension without physically demanding work, injury or pain, which would cause tension. Joint mobility may show up as normal with testing, and neither can muscle tension be measured objectively nor an increase in electrical activity be detected. Muscles may seem very soft and pliable and yet the patient still experiences excessive muscle tension. This conflict between subjective experience and objective testing involves excessive attention and psychological energy focused on the muscles creating the experience of tension. It may be only transitional, because of exceptional psychic stress or it may be severe psychic

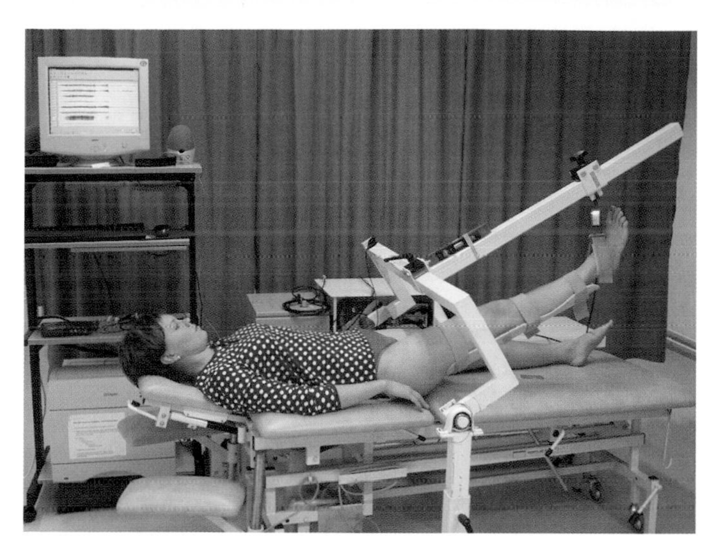

Figure 1.29 Instrumental straight-leg raising system with sEMG (Mega Electronics Ltd, Kuopio) at Department of Physical and Rehabilitation Medicine of Jyväskylä Central Hospital.

disease disturbing the patient's whole life. Stretching will not help in the case of somatization. Physical exercise can be used to increase muscle tension and help the patient to differentiate between a tense muscle and a relaxed muscle in cognitive therapy combined with training therapy. All methods to induce relaxation used in physiotherapy may be useless and may even make symptoms worse. If symptoms are shown to involve a difficult psychological disorder with conversion symptoms it is important to treat that instead of focusing on the treatment of physical symptoms, which will only complicate the condition further.

Assessment of a patient's condition usually requires thorough examination of both physical and psychological factors. In many postural and trauma-related situations, tension will affect the deep muscles, particularly in the spine and cervical area and requires specific manual testing of each individual joint. This requires techniques that physicians and physiotherapists do not learn in their normal training, although these are essential for proper

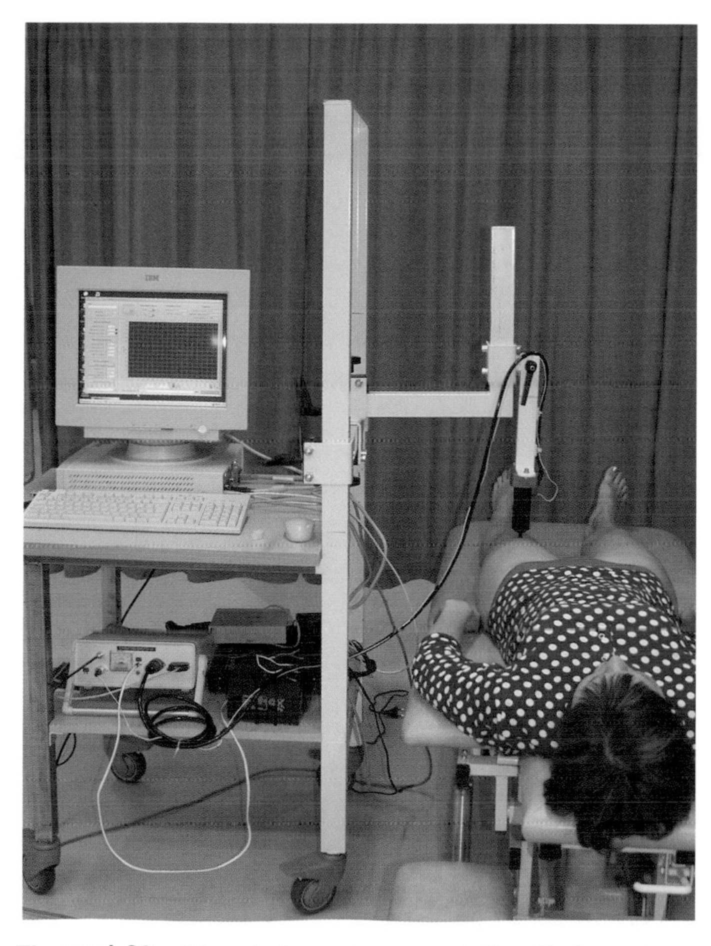

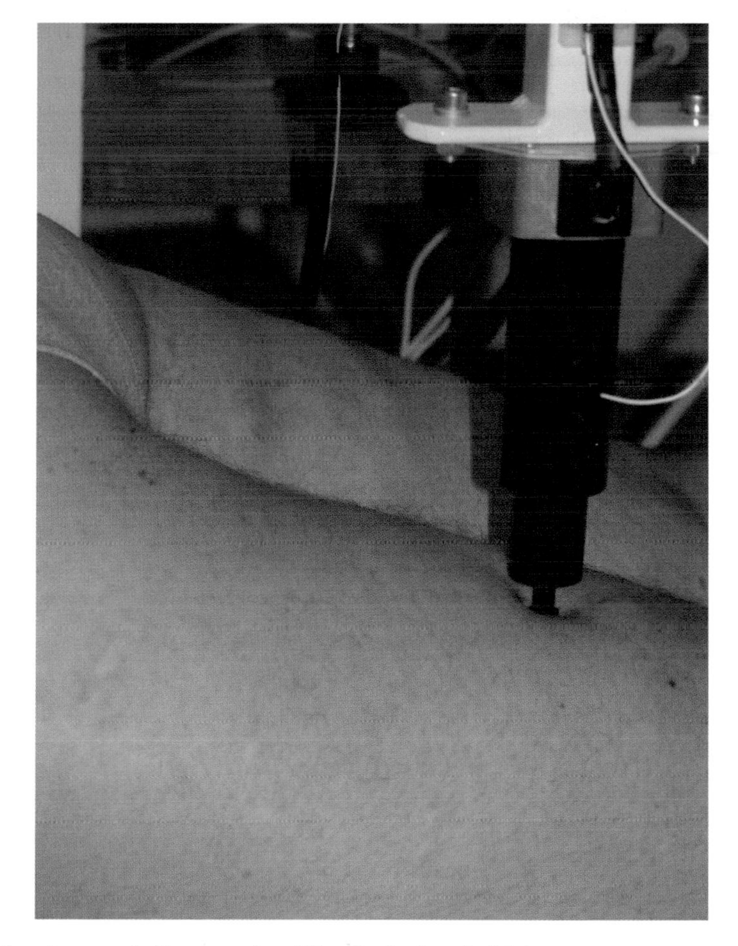

Figure 1.30 Muscle tone measured directly by a computerized muscle tonometer (Medirehabook Ltd., Muurame, Finland) at Jyväskylä Central Hospital.

clinical examination. Superficial muscles may be relaxed, and tension in the deeper layers may not be directly palpable, but cause stiffness and limit mobility in joints. There may be associated symptoms of local pain, or pain referred to other areas of the body. These cases are easily labelled as psychological, when the physical cause cannot be found due to poor examination techniques and thus remain untreated. When pathologic conditions of muscle tension and pain are labelled psychological, the patient will often suffer considerable emotional stress. This also may happen even without the condition being directly labelled as psychiatric, if no appropriate diagnosis and treatment are found for the problem.

Chronic somatic pain conditions will easily lead to psychological stress. On the other hand, psychological pathologies can cause postural problems and excess stress leading to muscle tension and pain. Muscle tension will usually involve both physical and psychological factors. The determination of which came first is not always important, because in difficult cases treatment to address both physical and psychological factors will, in any case, be required. Concentrating on only one or the other may hinder results or make results nonexistent, and treatment intervention could cause anxiety that could make things even worse.

Self-assessment: muscle tension

- **What is the difference between objective and subjective muscle tension?**
- **How can muscle tension be measured objectively?**
- **What problems are associated with measuring muscle tension in respect to physiotherapy and their results?**
- **How can somatic and psychological muscle tension be recognized?**

MOTIVATION

The most important factor preventing continued stretch exercising after instruction will be a lack of motivation. Stretching needs to be experienced as useful before it will become a routine practice. Joint mobility will vary greatly between individuals and unfortunately it is often those with the most stiffness and in most need of stretching that will refrain from it due to discomfort. Likewise, those with good flexibility are more apt to practise regular stretching as it easy and enjoyable.

Women are more likely to stretch in conjunction with other forms of exercise. Men tend to prefer strengthening exercises, which may even restrict mobility, and small ROM when training is performed with heavy weight. Men will be less flexible in general, making the need for stretching even greater, especially with age.

Regular stretching exercises often require lifestyle changes that may be, difficult to obtain. Motivation is often greater when limitations in mobility cause pain, which can be eased by stretching, but regular stretching is easily forgotten when pain subsides.

Active athletes with good body awareness will be able to detect changes in mobility. Those with less body awareness may find it difficult to notice difference in movement before and after stretching. When working with patients, changes in mobility can be measured. Observation is important in marking progress and promoting stretch exercise. Stretching is often experienced as difficult and thus, avoided. In this case, educated instruction is important and should address individual needs; not all stretches are necessary for all people. The focus when planning an exercise program is to use those stretches most suitable for improving mobility for the intended individual. Anybody might grow tired of exercise that does not produce results and too extensive exercise program.

Factors that encourage motivation

- Goals of stretching are made clear
- Written personal stretching plan
- Supervised instruction during initial stages to ensure proper execution of exercises
- Regular practice of stretching routine
- Exercise diary
- Measuring progress, ROM

HYPERMOBILITY

Hypermobility refers to ROM that extends past the normal physiological limits. It is commonly considered as a contraindication to stretching.

When an individual has several hypermobile joints, it is known as hypermobility syndrome (HMS). Generalized excessive laxity of ligaments is a hereditary condition affecting connective tissues. Connective tissue is more elastic than in normal people, which is most often due to aberration in type I or III collagen. The synthesis of collagen depends on genetic factors and the hypermobility syndrome is thus hereditary. Hypermobility is found in 5–7% of the population and affects children more than adults. It is not generally considered pathological, because it does not always cause joint problems. It may even be an asset in athletics.

When joint structures and ligaments are exposed to excessive stress, tissues can be damaged. Hypermobility can be the result of an over-stretch trauma. More commonly, hypermobility is the result of innate tissue properties due to heredity factors and tissue formation in the early years. Hypermobility can appear in only a single joint. Intense stretching exercise, especially during early bone growth can lead to hypermobility. In older individuals, hypermobility may develop with degeneration of ligament. In cases of chronic inflammation such as in arthritis there may also be degeneration of joint capsule and ligaments leading to laxity. Severe tearing of soft tissues due to joint trauma is the most common cause of single joint hypermobility in adults.

Regular, excessively intense stretching in sports or work can lead to instability in normal joints. Symptoms of pain may disperse once stretching is stopped, but long-term joint pain is common without stabilizing exercise therapy.

A hypermobile joint undergoes great stress in the extreme position. The ability of muscles to stabilize a joint weakens as a joint is taken past its normal ROM. Cartilage and the surrounding soft tissues suffer under stress, resulting in pain and possible tissue damage. Although stretching of hypermobile joints should be avoided, patients are sometimes told to stretch, because no proper manual examination of the mobility has been done. Stretching during pregnancy should be considered carefully as an increase in elastine hormone production increases flexibility in all the joints.

Joint instability allows excess stress to affect the surrounding connective tissue. Symptoms of pain will tend to develop over time without the presence of trauma. The direct influence of occupation on joints should be considered. It is recommendable that patients with hypermobile joints do not work in jobs that involve heavy loading, which require good stability of joints. Other symptoms associated with hypermobility include numbness in the extremities: (acroparaesthesia).

Box 1.10 Testing for hypermobility is commonly achieved using Beighton's (1983) system of evaluation.

Points for hypermobility:

- extension of metacarpophalangeal joint of little finger past 90°
- bending of thumb reaches forearm on the flexor side
- elbow mobility over 10°
- knee extension over 10°
- hands can be placed flat on floor while bending forward with knees locked

Points are added separately for the upper and lower extremities. If the total is at least four, with nine being the maximum, hypermobility is indicated.

Intense, static and long-standing stretching can irritate nerve endings in the joint ligaments and joint capsule causing pain that may not be relieved without therapy. Analgesics are often of poor help for this type of pain. Stretching of connective tissue can induce segmental muscle spasm causing intense local pain and stiffness in the neck and back. Mobilization and manipulation can provide relief, but further stretching often increases the symptoms.

Treatment programs for pain in the locomotor system often concentrate only on stretching. Increasing mobility by stretching in individuals suffering from pain associated with hypermobility may be harmful. If muscles are to be stretched, the therapist should be careful not to stretch joints. Treatment should include postural, proprioceptive and ergonomic exercises to prevent stretching of joint ligaments. Exercises that increase muscle strength and stabilize joints are necessary to improve body control. Regular exercise can preserve muscle tone, which is also important for passive stability of the joints.

There are also rare genetic syndromes associated with joint laxity, such as Ehlers–Danlos syndrome, which is an inherited connective tissue disorder characterized by articular hypermobility, curved bones, cutaneous extension and scarring. Joint laxity, increased luxation and fracture risk are associated also with Marfan syndrome, osteogenesis imperfecta and Larsen syndrome. These patients need special care and, especially, fragility of bones should be taken into consideration.

COMPLICATIONS DUE TO STRETCHING THERAPY

SPRAINS AND STRAINS

Sprains are the most common complication of stretch treatments. The extent of injury will depend on the amount of force and speed involved. On the other hand, it depends on the flexibility of tissues. The sarcomeres do not stretch evenly throughout the muscle. Those located near the tendon–muscle junction stretch more than those located in the middle of the muscle. Injuries will usually occur at the muscle–tendon junction or close to it. The risk of strain increases with age, because elastic fibres decrease and fibrous fibres increase in muscles.

Injury due to treatment usually happens during SS techniques. The stretch may be too forceful or it may be performed too quickly so that the patient does not have time to react with protective muscle contraction or to complain. Sometimes patients do not indicate early enough that they are experiencing pain, as perhaps they are trying to be brave and show that they can tolerate the therapy. Pain tolerance will vary between individuals. There may be also some loss of local sensation. Stretching force will be affected by the therapist's technique. If stretching is done quickly, force is noticeably greater and tissues do not have time to stretch and the risk of complication increases. There are huge differences in connective tissue properties and tolerance to stretch.

There is less risk of strain with the CR technique, because it requires active participation of the patient and pain will prevent too forceful muscle contraction and less force is needed in stretching phase compared to SS. This technique is preferable, especially when the risk of strain is greater, such as with tired muscles as they have less resilience to stress. Scar tissue due to previous injury or surgery will also increase the risk of strain and should be considered during treatment while choosing method and stretching.

Self-induced strain while stretching usually involves loss of balance while using body weight to gain pressure. This can be avoided by ensuring proper support during stretching exercises. Effective stretching also requires concentration and thus an environment with distractions is a risk factor. Patients with paresis or muscular weakness have an increased risk for loss of balance and may need assistance to perform stretching safely.

If force is continually increased during SS it will in the end lead to partial or complete tearing of tendons or muscles. The most common area to be affected is the muscle–tendon junction. Occasionally the muscle and tendon will remain unaffected but the tendon will pull a small fragment of the bone away at the insertion causing avulsion fracture. In all these cases the muscle will react with painful contraction. In addition to primary trauma, there may be secondary complications due to fear of repeated trauma. Patients may refuse to stretch and limitations in movement may develop in the future.

Rupture of large muscles and tendons can be repaired by surgery while smaller strains are usually left to recover without any special intervention. The decision is made individually depending on the extent of the trauma, the loss of function and the function remaining. Complications are relatively rare while comparing the amount of stretching treatment applied daily.

NERVE DAMAGE

The straight leg raise is used to test for possible compression of lower lumbar nerve roots. It is commonly known as Lasègue's test and if positive, it suggests irritation of nervus ischiadicus (Dyck 1984). Compression of nerve roots usually involves disc prolapse in the cervical or lumbar spine. Nerve compression in the lumbar spine often produces sciatica with pain referred from the back down into the leg. About 10% will experience only referred pain in the leg. A smaller percentage will experience no pain at all. The sciatic nerve will not stretch much, if there is compression at the root. Lasègue's test is positive if the hip flexion remains under 60° because hamstring spasm protects the nerve from stretching. Nerve compression can be suspected if resistance to stretch is not elastic, as normally in nature, but stops abruptly. Stretching is contraindicated until nerve compression is released. There is intense resistance also with CR techniques and will not allow stretching after contraction phase. Forceful SS may damage the nerve.

Flexion of the neck and trunk has been recorded to cause a stretch of the spinal cord and dura of up to 18% (Reid 1960). Thus, a slump position in sitting adds tension to the nerve tissue complex. Læssøe and Voigt (2004) found that knee joint ROM was acutely diminished in a stooping position. The nerve tissue complex was considered to be a factor to restrict the movement, because flexion of the neck and back are not directly mechanically related to the hip and knee joint. Thus, an influence from the nerve tissue must be considered to be a causative factor when the straight leg raise or knee extension in sitting position is restricted.

Nerves are normally protected from excess stretching by their elasticity, length and looseness. This looseness, however, can be lost because of compression in the foramen between the vertebrae or because of peripheral entrapment of the nerve. The effects on other tissues must be always considered when stretching is used to improve muscle and joint mobility. Intense stretching may damage nerve tissue. The sciatic, ulnar and peroneal nerves are more susceptible to damage than other nerves due to the nature of their pathways. The ulnar nerve travels superficially and unprotected at the elbow and the peroneal nerve superficially to the fibula. The nerve sheath, or epineurium, forms almost 90% of the transverse surface here, and is subject to rapid loading and stretching while sitting or in the crouching position. The sciatic nerve may be damaged at the root, if there is disc hernia combined with intense stretching of the hamstrings. Nerve compression at the root can also develop with structural changes in the spine due to spondylosis. Nerve tissue will respond to stretching in these cases before other tissues. Continuing to stretch with disregard for this type of resistance can cause nerve damage resulting in sensory changes, paralysis and a chronic painful condition.

The appearance of an autonomic hyper–reflex syndrome in sciatic nerve following stretch has been shown in patients who have spinal cord damage in the cervical or thoracic area. Symptoms include: an increase in blood pressure, headache, slowing of pulse, and sweating. The possibility of hyper–reflex syndrome should be considered with the acute onset of any of the above symptoms after stretching of the hamstring muscles.

INJURY TO BLOOD VESSELS

Growths in the bone or cartilage of the inferior femur and superior tibia have been known to cause damage to blood vessels due to pressure during stretching. Both benign and malignant tumors of cartilage are rare, making this type of complication uncommon. This should be considered a possibility if the femur or tibia is abnormally thick. If there are noticeable differences between the lower limbs in clinical testing, these should be examined by X-ray.

Myositis ossificans involves calcification of muscle tissue, caused by inflammation or injury. Stretching may result in damage to blood vessels or nerve tissue as they rub under stretch against the ossified tissue. Other changes in soft tissue are possible such as ectopic ossification and heterotrophic ossification, which can appear unexplained. Both active and passive stretching may increase pain and even exacerbate an already active ossification process. Intense stretching cannot reduce limitations in mobility that subsequently develop due to ossification. Active stretching and exercise to return normal function become important but only after surgical intervention to remove calcified tissue.

Extreme rotation of the arthritic cervical spine, especially with intense tilting of the head backwards, can block circulation in the vertebral arteries and damage to the blood vessels is also possible. In the worst scenario, stroke or bleeding can result. In arteriosclerosis the blood vessels are less flexible and stretch or pressure may cause damage. The risk of damage increases with age with hardening of the arteries and may already be significant at middle age. Stretching the head backwards should be avoided. Furthermore, extreme rotation of the neck will put pressure on blood vessels especially at the atlanto-axial level and possibly cause occlusion or embolism and subsequently brain infarction. Extension, and rotation lateral flexion combination is contraindicated with articulation manipulation and especially with stretching. The circulation will be blocked for several seconds in stretching compared to a split second in manipulation.

Examination of tissues and attention to risk possibilities is very important when treating patients with stretching. Determining the appropriate stretching force and technique for each individual requires knowledge and skill. Using only small amounts of force will be safe, but may not produce any results. Stretching force should be close to pain tolerance before mobility can be improved with an increase in tissue flexibility and positive changes in tissue structure, but excessive force can result in tissue damage. Effective, safe stretching requires skill and practical experience.

The simple stretching technique of separating muscle insertions away from each other will not always be possible due to joint structure and the normal direction of movement. While stretching muscles, extreme twisting of the joints should be avoided as it could cause overstretching of ligaments, damage to joint capsules and hypermobility. Unnecessary pressure on joints can be avoided by using stretching techniques that include fixation as shown in the stretching techniques section.

Stretching of the anterior cervical muscles requires rotation and backward tilting of the head. Research has shown that this position can block circulation of blood to the head. If prolonged, it can cause oxygen deficiency to the brain and possibly embolism and stroke. In young individuals weakness in the artery walls may lead to localized dilation — aneurysm— which under pressure can rupture. It is wise to treat superficial flexor muscles of the cervical area by using fixation at their inferior insertions, stretching with lateral flexion while tilting the head diagonally forwards and not backwards. This will allow greater ROM compared to purely lateral flexion. Stretching of the deep muscles anterior to the cervical spine should be avoided completely.

Contraindications to joint stretching

- Hypermobility
- Joint ankylosis
- Nerve compression
- Angiopathy
- Osteoporosis
- Acute trauma
- Joint inflammation
- Recent surgery
- Intense pain in stiffened joints.

INJURY TO JOINT DISCS

Disc hernia occurs most often with disc degeneration when resistance to load has weakened. Hernia is often preceded by mild symptoms of pain in the neck or back due to disc protrusion or torn discs. Muscle tension caused by pain, and disc degeneration, can limit mobility. Intense stretching of the cervical or lumbar spine towards flexion while sitting or standing places particular stress on the posterior portion of discs and can cause damage and disc prolapse. Intense twisting in the lumbar spine may also be dangerous, if the discs are under pressure such as when in a sitting position. Lateral bending will always involve some degree of rotation and there should be no extra load on the spine. In cases of difficult back pain, it is recommendable to perform stretching while lying down when there is least stress on the discs. Disc pressure is especially high when flexing the spine while sitting on the ground (Figure 1.31).

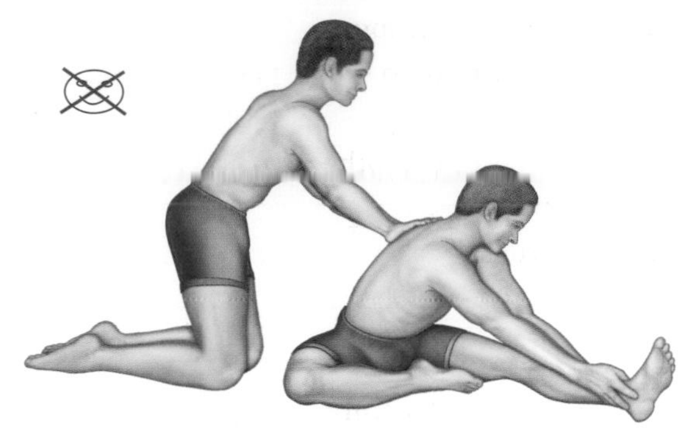

Figure 1.31 The assistant may cause more harm than benefit when trying to stretch hamstring muscles. There is a risk of disc prolapse and fracture, if too much friendly force is applied to the back. This type of stretching should not be allowed.

RISK OF FRACTURE

There is considerable risk of fracture when stretching the intercostals. The lowest rib is especially susceptible to injury under pressure. In cases of advanced osteoporosis intense stretching of the spine by bending forward can cause compression fracture to the anterior portion of thoracic or lumbar vertebrae. Those with calcium and vitamin D deficiency are at risk. Lack of calcium often appears in menopausal women suffering from lactose intolerance or milk allergies. Disturbed digestion in the intestinal tract can also prevent adequate absorption of calcium. Repeated treatments of cortisone in large doses can result in bone degeneration within only a few months. Bone degeneration can also be related to thyroid, parathyroid and adrenal gland diseases as well as many other less common diseases.

Important factors affecting stretch

- Joint biomechanics
- Muscle structure and muscle insertions
- Flexibility of muscles and tendons
- Flexibility of joint capsules and joint ligaments
- Flexibility of blood vessels
- Free pathway of nerves
- Flexibility of surrounding connective tissue and muscle involved in same movement
- Periods of immobilization
- Trauma, surgery and radiation treatments

- Adhesions and scar tissue
- Surgical intervention on blood vessels (artificial blood vessels and stents)
- Certain types of joint prothesis artificial joint
- Inflammation
- Spasticity or rigidity
- Stretching techniques
- Pain tolerance.

Ankylosis involves structural changes in tissues causing extreme stiffness. Stretching usually induces only pain and is no longer even appropriate. The tough collagen fibres will not stretch but only tear causing difficult symptoms of pain and joint instability, which are more problematic than joint stiffness.

Self-assessment: stretch treatments

- **How can stretching lead to symptoms of chronic pain?**
- **What are the most common complications with stretching of the muscle–tendon system?**
- **Why is the CR technique safer than the SS or BS technique?**
- **In which conditions can stretching techniques be life threatening?**

INTRODUCTION TO STRETCHING TECHNIQUES

Stretching of the muscle–tendon system in theory is simple; muscle insertions are separated from each other as far as possible. Joint ROM and other connective tissues, however, may limit or prevent a direct movement line between muscle insertions. Therefore, stretching is not often so simple. In some cases, stretching by separating muscle insertions from one another along a direct movement line is even contraindicated and may cause life-threatening complications, such as with the front cervical muscles.

Joint structure and flexibility is as individual as muscle size, tendons and attachments. Some individuals will have 'extra' muscles while in others certain muscles or muscle sections will be nonexistent. The differences due to hereditary factors, injuries or surgery may also demand a modification to stretching techniques.

Techniques normally found useful may not be effective in all individuals due to differences in flexibility. Painful muscles may be tense, but they may be also loose. It is noticeably easier to apply stretching techniques to short stiff muscles, while finding techniques in cases of soft relaxed muscles that easily extend will require more ingenuity on the part of the therapist. Scar tissue, adhesions and trigger points will also appear in loose muscles. While using traditional stretching the muscle will give way and stretching will focus on joints, although that was not the aim. The therapist should be prepared to deal with these conditions while stretching muscles i.e. fixation techniques should be known.

Each joint has connective tissue structures that help to maintain stability. These structures include the capsule and ligaments, and some joints have also intra-articular structures — discus and menisci — which increase the stability and maintain the integrity of synovial joints. Close-packed position refers to the extreme end of ROM, where the ligaments and capsules are taut, and thus the joint surfaces compress each other. Movement of the joint will reduce the closer it is moved to the close-packed position. In loose-packed position the largest amount of joint play occurs, because ligaments and capsules are lax. Thus it is important to be sure that the joint is in maximal or at least near maximal loose-packed position while stretching muscle–tendon units. Otherwise stretching will be applied more on the joint than on the muscle–tendon unit.

The basic stretching technique of separating attachments as far as possible from each other will often be enough to stretch muscles that cross over at least two joints, such as the hamstring muscles. However, muscles that cross only one joint, such as pectoralis major, almost always require a different stretching technique, because close-packed position commonly restricts the movement before the muscle becomes stretched at all. Stretching is ineffective or it may be even harmful if a muscle does not stretch but the joint is moved to its most extreme position and then intense force is applied; all the while the therapist believing that they are stretching the muscle. Joint pain may result from overstretching while using the basic stretching technique due to ligament and capsule damage.

SAFETY CONCERNS IN STRETCHING

Muscles are electrically silent or there is only low activity during normal stretches until the limit of the ROM nears. Many researchers have considered the low electrical activity associated with SS exercises as a benefit, which decreases the risk of injury. In comparison, the CR technique, which increases muscle electrical activity somewhat, is considered to increase the risk of injury due to the possible increase in muscle tension. However, this finding is based on theory and has not been indicated with research. Both clinical experience and recent studies have shown the situation to be the opposite to that which researchers had previously suggested.

A noticeably larger amount of force is required from the therapist during the contraction phase of the CR technique than during SS exercises. Patients apply their own isometric maximum force or a part of that against the therapist. The stretching phase in which ROM is increased comes after the relaxation phase when the electrical activity of muscles has ceased. The amount of force required to be applied by the therapist at this phase is significantly smaller than in the contraction phase, as the stretch is increased by only so much that a new barrier is reached with the same — or a slight increase in — stretching force as in the beginning. Thus, the amount of force required at the stretching phase may be significantly smaller with the CR technique than with the SS technique in which stretching force is progressively increased.

The safe stretching force with the SS technique is difficult to estimate. This does not present such a big problem in the CR technique as the stretch usually increases according to the freed amount of mobility once the muscle contraction is released and resistance ceases. Thus, there is no need to increase the stretching force so much to increase the ROM.

Harvey et al (2003) studied the magnitude of static stretch that physiotherapists apply to the hamstring muscles of people with spinal cord injury in an effort to induce lasting increases in the extensibility. The stretch force applied by different therapists to any one subject varied as much as 40-fold. Some therapists provided stretch torques well in excess of those tolerated by individuals with intact sensation.

Wide variation is not a wonder, because stretching force is not commonly practised during studies and few institutions have even equipment for that. This is an important issue, because CR techniques cannot be applied in cases of paralysis. Thus, there should also be emphasis on the teaching of SS techniques, despite the popularity of CR and MET techniques.

PRACTICAL CONSIDERATIONS

The photographs in the second section of this book (p. 00) clearly illustrate the stretching techniques so that the text could be kept as succinct and simple as possible.

Reference in the text to superior and inferior muscle attachments applies to positions in relation to a standing posture and not that which is shown in the photographs. Some muscles work in unison with other muscles and the same stretching technique can be used for all as a group. In order to avoid repetition, muscle anatomy for each muscle of one group is listed prior to instructions for their common stretching technique.

Stretching techniques based on manual compression provide the possibility of effectively stretching muscles that are not significantly shortened. Pressure applied to the body of a muscle will cause a pre-stretch that can easily be directed, for example to the muscle–tendon junction. The main stretch is performed then, following this fixation by moving the joint or joints. Compression stretching techniques are important in individuals who do not exibit much stiffness. This technique can also be use to treat specific sections of muscles such as the medial or lateral portion of the gastrocnemius, the distal or the proximal ends of a muscle. Fixation with the hand remains in place to direct the stretch and then can be moved to another portion of the muscle for the next one. Compression may be allowed to move along the muscle when successive parts of the muscle needs to be treated and is known as stretching massage technique. This technique is not explained for every muscle to avoid repetition.

Stretching of the muscle–tendon system involves stretching of nerves and is unavoidable with some muscles. Likewise, it is not possible to specifically stretch only nerves without muscle–tendon involvement. In cases of nerve root compression and inflammation, stretching to the nerve in question should be avoided as it may exacerbate pain and possibly cause permanent damage. Furthermore, advanced levels of superficial sensitivity will also make intense stretching of nerve tissue contraindicated. When stretching the extremities, numbness, tingling, pain, lack of sensation and weakened muscle force are all possible symptoms of nerve compression. These symptoms do not confirm nerve compression however, and thus consultation may be needed.

There may be protective muscle tension to prevent stretching. Protective muscle tension and increased muscle tension can be determined by using the CR technique. A protective muscle spasm will not release with treatment. Using intense SS techniques at the start of treatment may cause nerve damage because it is impossible to know for sure whether it is connective tissue or nerve tissue that is being stretched. For example, about 10% of patients suffering from cervical or lumbar disc hernia will not experience symptoms of pain in the neck or back but only in the extremities at various degrees of intensity.

It is possible, when using fixation as part of a stretching technique to various parts of the body, to use not only the whole hand but also the forearm, thenar, hypothenar, thumb and fingers. The forearm is most often used to stretch along a muscle in the same direction as fibres by leaning into the position, which makes pressure easier to achieve without causing stress to the therapist. Treatment level should be appropriate for the therapist, so they can most effectively use their own body weight. Different parts of the hand can be used to apply stretch, and pressure can be directed more specifically or to a small area by using the thumb, fingers or whole palm. Technique variations depend on desired results: whether one wants the stretch to affect the muscle as a whole or only a specific part of the muscle, which is not possible with ordinary stretching.

Some stretching techniques may appear initially to be the same, but in practice they will affect different muscles according to placement of fixation and the direction of pressure. Muscles usually appear in many layers and near joints short muscles are located under the larger muscles that pass over the joints. Joint position during stretch will determine which muscle group will be affected. Although treatment involves muscles that cross one particular joint, positions of all joints should be considered. For example, flexing the knee while the hip is partially flexed one is able to direct the stretch to the vastus intermedius, medialis and lateralis. Flexing the knee while the hip is extended will direct the stretch to the rectus femoris.

Stretching requires good knowledge of anatomy and kinesiology in order to treat specifically problem muscles or sections of muscles. Therapy can be improved and motivated by combining anatomical information with clinical practice.

Simultaneous lengthening of the muscle by moving the joint and direct manual stretching of the muscle requires more skill and practice than traditional simple stretching techniques. Thus, techniques should be practised properly. Most stretching techniques can be adapted to contact– relaxation techniques as well. There may be several techniques in each muscle as examples show.

These techniques are not described with every muscle to avoid unnecessary repetition, but they may be applied when felt appropriate and depending on the skill of the therapist.

Manual stretching may be applied in different ways:

- joint in the neutral position, as performed in traditional massage
- muscle stretched and then concentrating to increase stretch by manual compression
- muscle pre-stretched, patient tenses up the muscle for 5 sec and relaxes, and then therapist applies manual stretch or stretching massage
- muscle pre-stretched and then manual stretch is applied while increasing joint angle to simultaneously increase stretching.

To intensify stretch effect with manual stretching, it may be applied in several directions:

1. Away from the proximal musculotendinous junction towards the body of the muscle (e.g. biceps brachii and femoris muscles)
2. Away from the distal musculotendinous junction towards the body of the muscle (e.g. rectus femoris muscle)
3. Across the body of muscle (e.g. pronator teres)
4. Towards insertion away from musculotendinous junction (e.g. scalenus muscles)
5. Manual pressure to induce stretch may be applied in different ways:
   a. hand may be applied only locally on the musculotendinous junction or on the site of trigger point or fibrous tissue due to previous trauma
   b. hand may be moved stepwise from the musculotendinous junction towards the belly of the muscle to intensify stretch effect
   c. in big muscles the hand may also be moved sideways to increase stretch in the lateral and medial side of the muscle
   d. hand may be allowed to glide from the musculotendinous junction towards the belly of the muscle to intensify stretch effect in different parts of the muscle. In big muscles the direction of the glide may be changed to ensure that all parts of muscles will be stretched effectively. This technique is called stretching massage

There is usually only one stretch given for each muscle or group of muscles. For some cases, however, it was decided to provide more than one technique in order to present the possibility of alternative options. Different techniques may be just as effective in different individuals; on the other hand, differences in body structure may make some techniques preferable to some and ineffective in others.

Abbreviations

AC agonist contract
BS ballistic stretching
C Celsius, unit of temperature
CR contract-relax
DOMS delayed muscle soreness
DS Dynamic stretching
HR hold-relax
IC isometric contraction
MET muscle energy technique
MHz Megahertz, unit of frequency
N Newton, unit of force
PEC parallel elastic component
PNF proprioceptive neuromuscular facilitation
ROM range of motion
SEC series elastic component
sEMG surface electromyography
SS static stretching
W Watt, unit of work

Abbreviations

Nerve supply: C – cervical root, Th – thoracic root, L – lumbar root

Origin and Insertion: C – cervical vertebrae, Th – thoracic vertebrae, L – lumbar vertebrae

Terms

Pronation = internal rotation of forearm
lowering the medial edge of the foot
Supination = external rotation of forearm
lifting the medial edge of the foot

STRETCHING TECHNIQUES

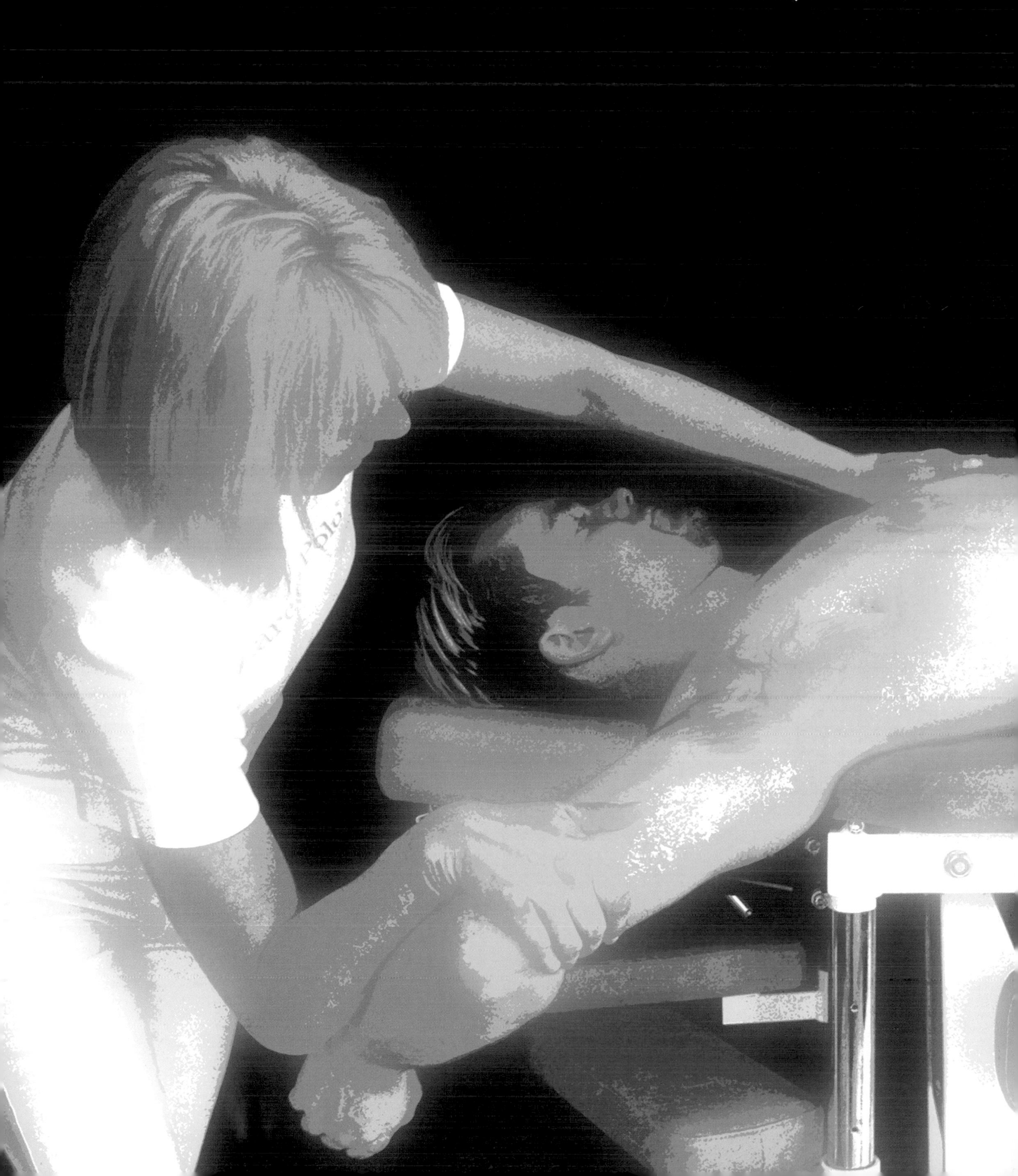

MASTICATORY MUSCLES

FRONTAL MUSCLES OF NECK

DORSAL MUSCLES OF NECK

MUSCLES OF SHOULDER

MUSCLES OF UPPER LIMB

MUSCLES OF THORAX

BACK MUSCLES

ROTATORES BREVES AND LONGI THORACIS

ABDOMINAL MUSCLES

MUSCLES OF LOWER LIMB

Temporalis

Nerve, supply: Trigeminal nerve (V cranial nerve) divides into the mandibular nerve, and finally temporal nerve.

Origin: Temporal fossa.

Insertion: Coronoid process and the interior and anterior side of the mandibular ramus.

Function: Closes mouth by elevating the mandible. It is the strongest jaw muscle.

Stretching technique:

Patient is lying on side, mouth open and head supported. Therapist presses jaw slightly downwards with one hand while stretching with the thumb of the other hand upwards towards the body of the muscle above the cheekbone.

Notice: Stretching of the muscles of the jaw is not possible if the mouth is closed.

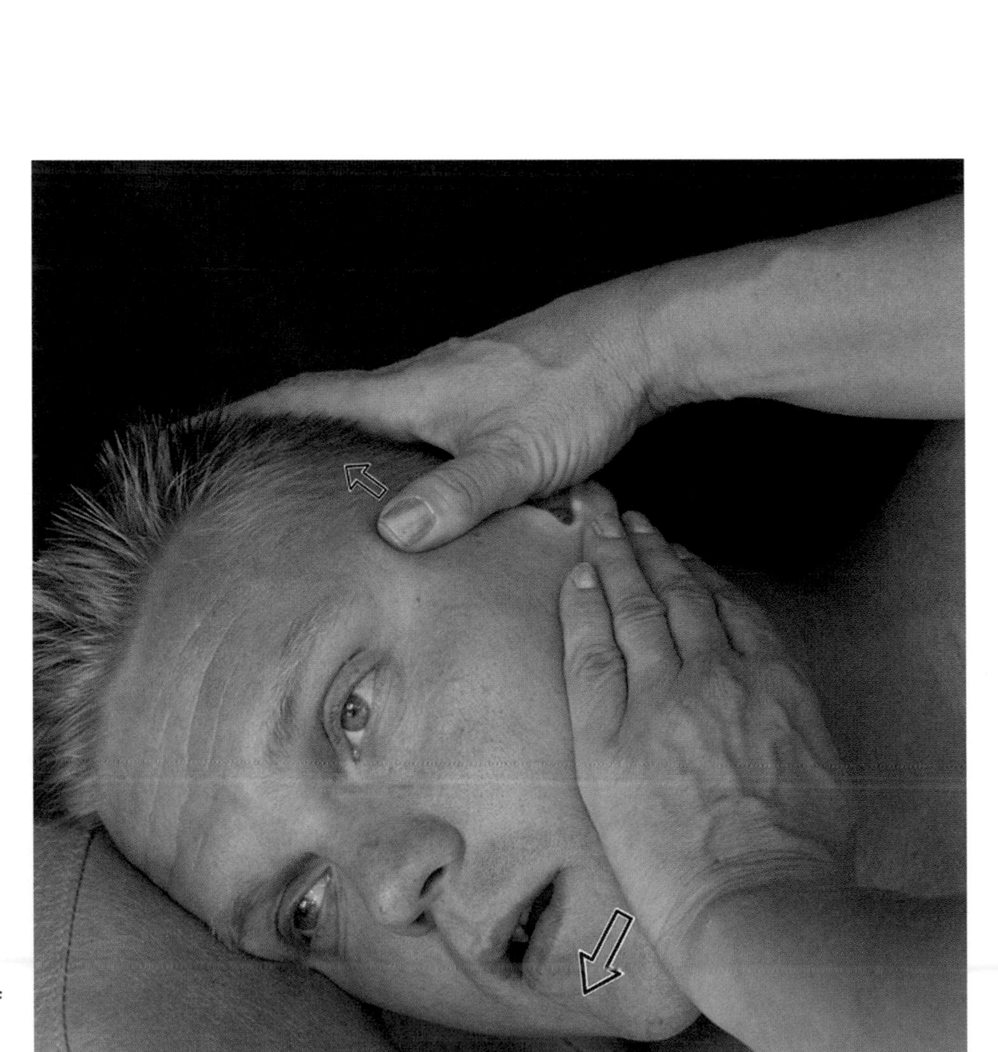

Masseter

Nerve, supply: Trigeminal nerve (V cranial nerve) divides into the mandibular nerve, and finally the masseteric nerve.

Origin: Zygomatic process and arch.

Insertion: Masseteric tuberosity on the angle of the mandible.

Function: Closes mouth by elevating the mandible.

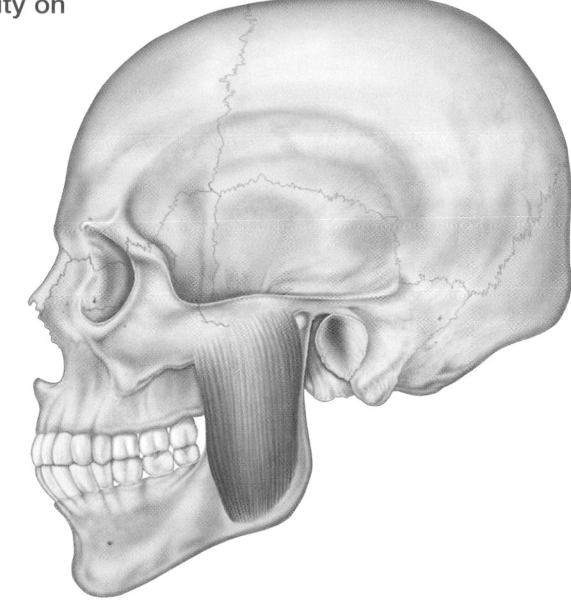

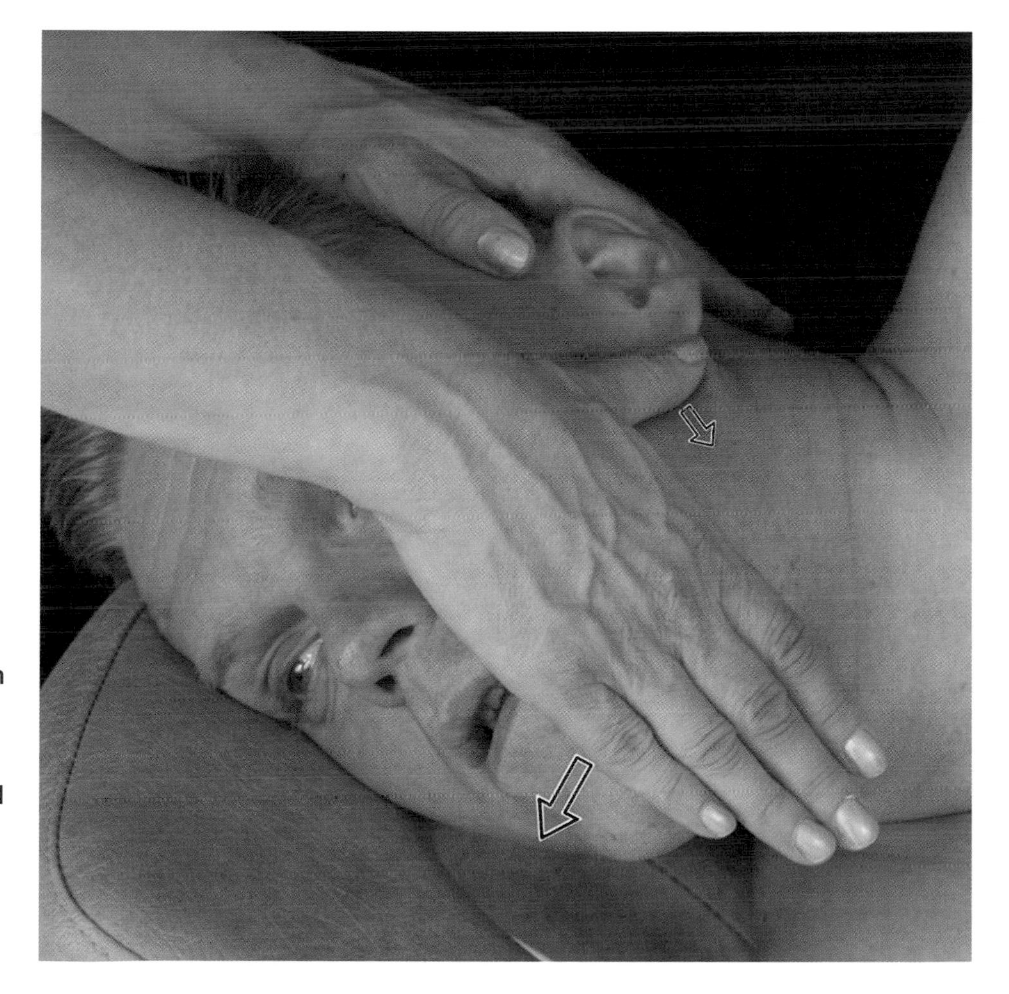

Stretching technique:

Patient is lying on side, mouth open and head supported. Therapist supports head with one hand while stretching with thumb of other hand below cheekbone, downwards, toward the body of the muscle, as the jaw is pressed slightly downwards.

Platysma

Nerve, supply: Facial nerve (VII cranial nerve).

Origin: Lower mandible and skin of throat.

Insertion: Anterior thoracic tendon sheath.

Function: Opens mouth and draws lower lip down.

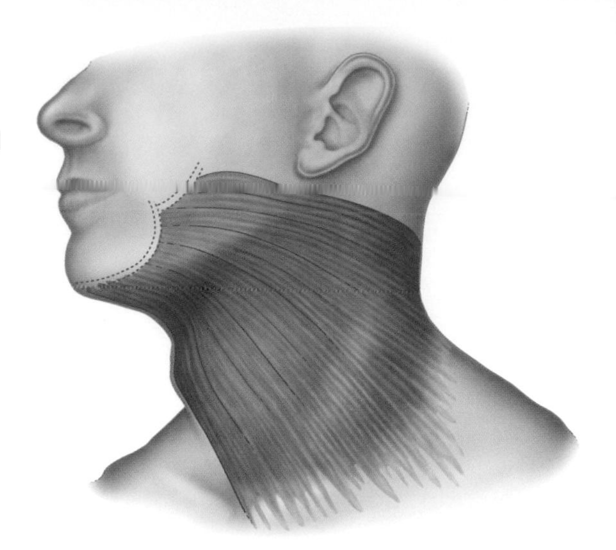

Stretching technique:

Patient is lying on back, head and cervical spine rotated and bent away from muscle to be treated. Therapist presses downwards with one hand to broad area of the chest, below the collarbone, and stretches with the other hand upwards against the chin increasing rotation and side bending.

Warning ❗ While stretching the anterior cervical muscles the head should not be bent extremely backwards: this may cause blockage in the carotid and/or vertebral arteries or embolism, if the patient has atherosclerosis and plaques from the arteries become loose. It may result in haemorrhage if there is vulnerable aneurysm, and it may occur even in young people.

Effective stretching can be performed without unnecessary risks by using manual fixation.

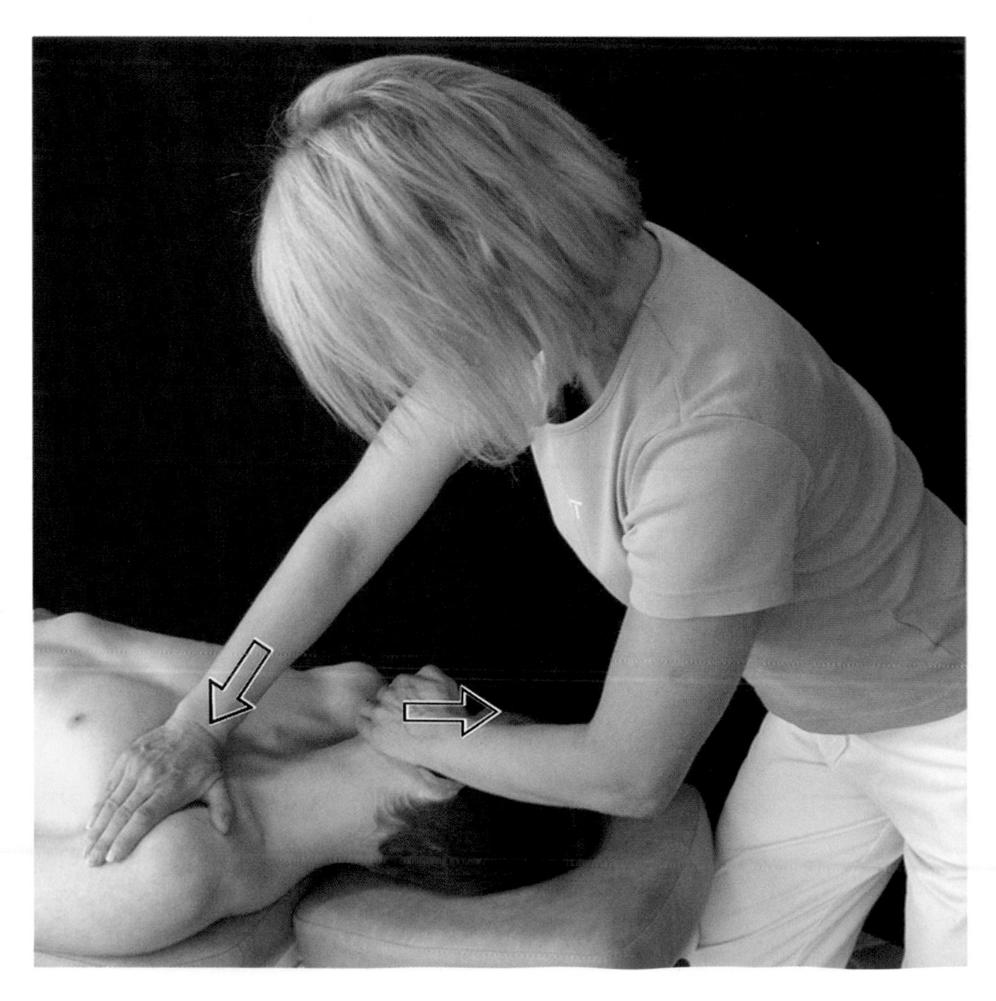

Sternocleidomastoideus

Nerve, supply: Accessory nerve (XI cranial nerve) and ventral rami of spinal nerves, C1–2.

Origin: Manubrium sterni and medial part of calvicle.

Insertion: Mastoid process and superior nuchal line of occipital bone.

Function: Unilateral action rotates the head to opposite side, bends it to the ipsilateral side and brings forward. Bilateral action protrudes the head, bends the cervical spine somewhat forwards and extends the head at the same time. Assists in deep inspiration.

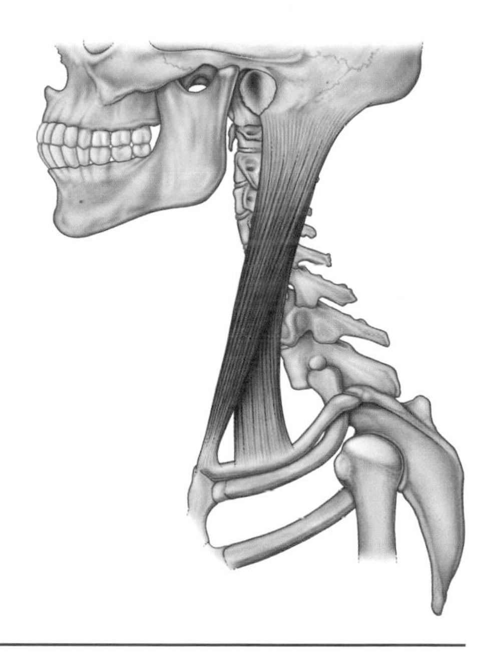

Stretching technique:

Patient is lying on back, head and cervical spine rotated to the contralateral side and lifted slightly upward to expose muscle. Therapist supports head with free hand while pulling muscle to side using broad contact with the tips of the thumb and fingers of the other hand.

Notice: Pressure on the carotid arteries should be avoided, which is more likely to happen if the head is not lifted and rotated prior to grasping the muscle. Having the patient actively lift the head will additionally help to safely define the muscle from sensitive structures surrounding it. It is even recommended that the patient continues lifting the head during the whole treatment procedure, although he/she may rest between stretches.

Warning ❗ Stretching in a position of extension, with rotation and bending of the head to one side, may damage the carotid or vertebral arteries in cases of arteriosclerosis or aneurysm. This position may also prevent blood flow to the brain on the opposing side due to pressure on the corresponding arteries. Calcification of the cervical arteries can lead to stroke and in younger people weak artery structure and the risk of rupture of the aneurysm is evident with excessive rotation of the spine. Compression over carotid sinus should be avoided, because it may cause stroke or arrhythmia.

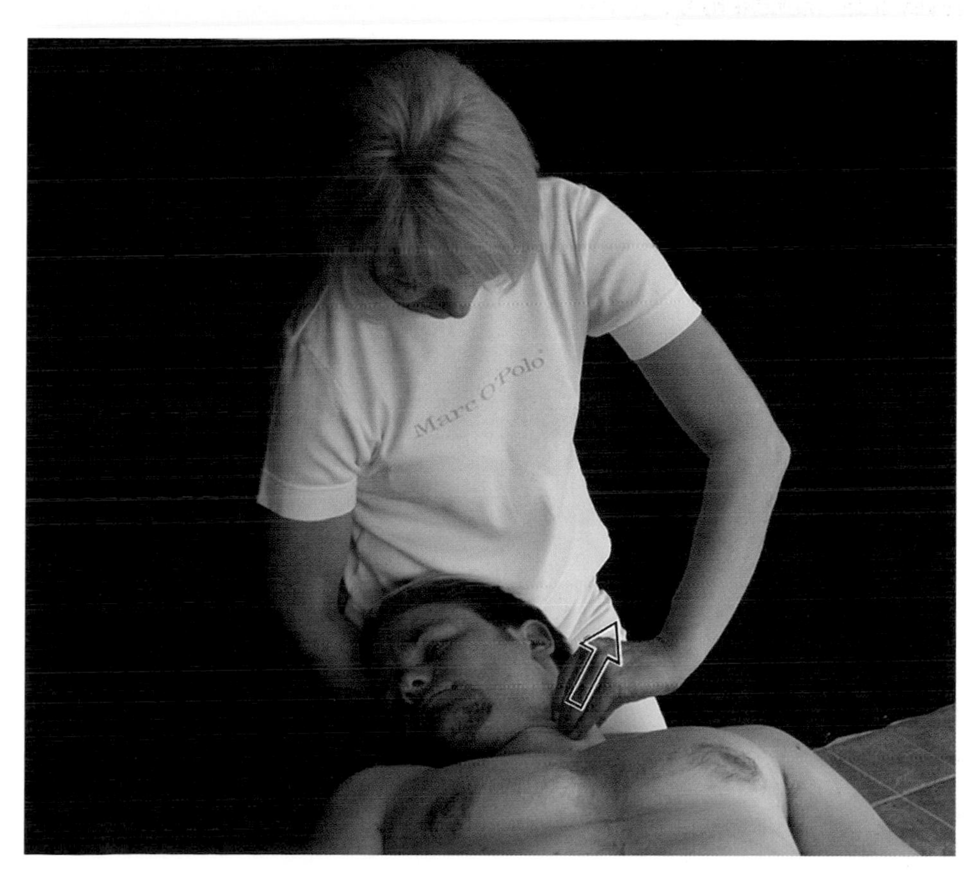

Scalenus anterior

Nerve, supply: Ventral rami of spinal nerves, C4–7.

Origin: Transverse processes of C3–6.

Insertion: Anterior scalene tubercle of the first rib and occasionally the pleural cupola.

Function: Lifts first rib and bends cervical spine forward and to same side. Assists in deep inspiration.

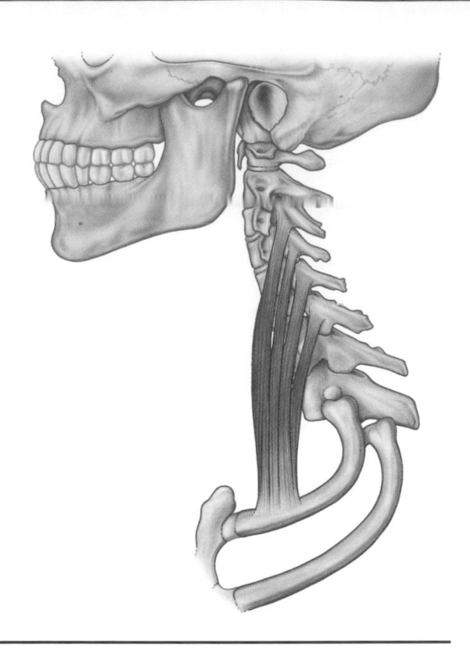

Stretching technique A:

Patient is lying on their back, therapist supports head with body contact and hand at the base of skull. Therapist applies the thumb or the first metacarpal bone of the other hand on the insertion of the muscle on the rib. Therapist lifts head and cervical spine forward, rotates and bends away from muscle to be treated. The angle of stretch and level of contact in the neck will vary slightly depending on which section is to be stretched. In changing position the cervical spine is allowed to partially straighten before the next stretch is performed.

Positioning of the cervical spine for stretching will be affected by mobility and individual posture. The optimal position must be adjusted to suit each individual.

Tension–relaxation technique: Patient attempts to bend head towards or the side of the muscle for 5 sec while therapist resists movement patient takes a deep breath in and then relaxes gradually while therapist performs stretch.

Warning ! Therapist does not apply pressure

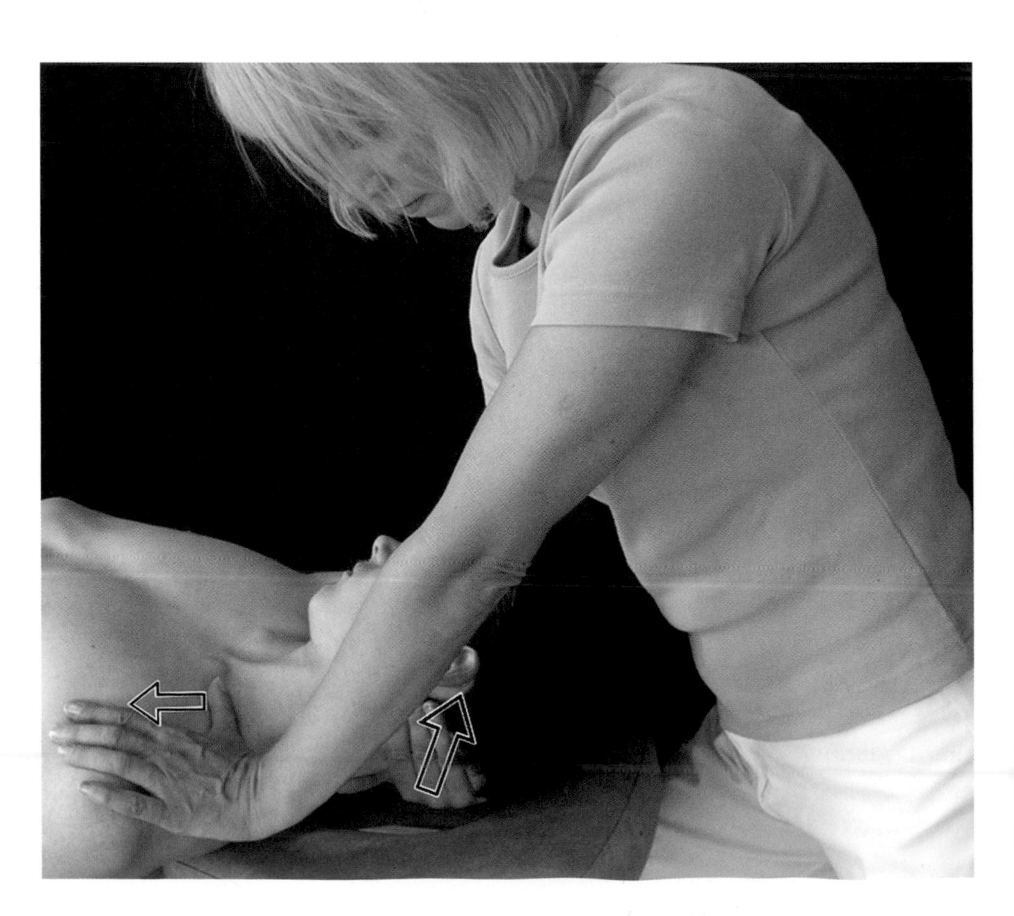

Scalenus medius

Nerve, supply: Ventral rami of spinal nerves, C3–8.

Origin: Posterior tubercles of the transverse processes of C2–7.

Insertion: First rib behind the subclavian artery groove and into the external intercostal membrane of the first intercostal space.

Function: Lifts first rib and bends cervical spine forward and to same side. Assists in deep inspiration.

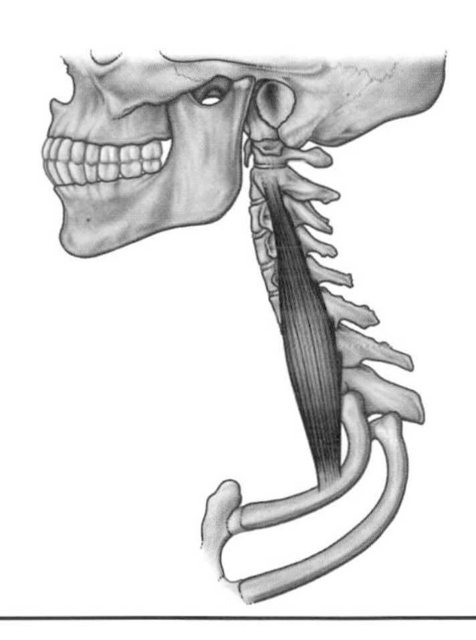

Stretching technique B:

The insertion of *scalenus anterior* may lie beneath the sternocleidomastoideus muscle making direct contact impossible. The therapist presses with the thenar down on the second rib, just below the collarbone. The other hand completes the stretch by bending the head and cervical spine forward combined with rotation and side bending to the contralateral side.

Tension–relaxation technique: Patient attempts to bend head towards the side of the muscle for 5 sec while therapist resists movement or patient takes a deep breath in. Patient then relaxes gradually while therapist performs stretch.

Notice: Considering the origin, it may appear logical to rotate the cervical spine in the ipsilateral direction to produce a stretch. If there is good mobility in the cervical spine stretching may be performed in this way. However, limited mobility due to 'locking' of the vertebral facets during rotation often make this technique less effective. Thus, stretching in the direction of physiologic movement i.e. lateral flexion and rotation towards the same direction is recommended.

Warning ❗ In cases of root canal blockage due to prolapsed disc or spondylosis, rotation and lateral flexion of the cervical spine may reproduce radiating symptoms into the upper extremity and stretching should be stopped. The therapist should be careful while using the body to support the head as this should not place compression on the vertebral discs and cause further stenosis.

Stretching techniques performed by the thumb must be short and near to the muscle insertions, because pressure higher up may affect the carotid artery and cause vascular complications in patients suffering from arteriosclerosis. Compression over carotid sinus should be avoided, because it may cause arrhythmia.

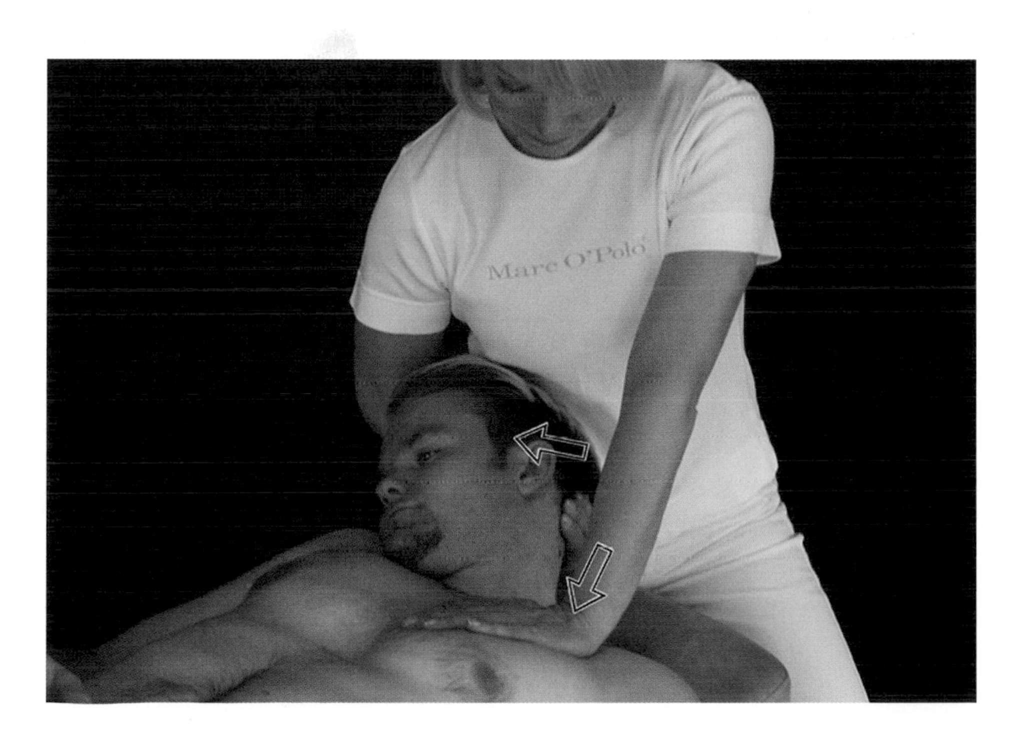

Scalenus minimus

Appears in only one-third of patients with high percentage of atrophy or may present as the transverse copular ligament.

Nerve, supply: Ventral rami of the spinal nerves, C7–8.

Origin: Transverse processes of C6–7.

Insertion: First rib with scalenus medius and the apex of pleural membrane of lungs.

Function: Lifts first rib and pleural membrane, bends cervical spine to same side. Assists in deep inspiration.

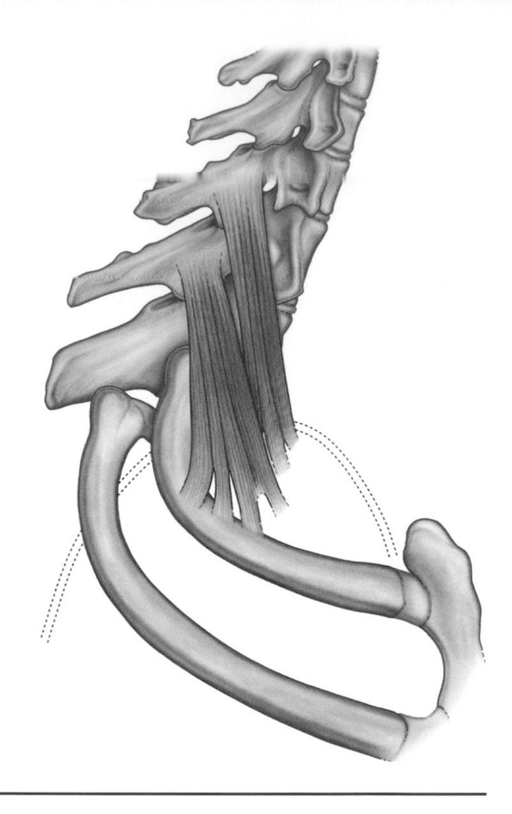

Stretching technique A:

Patient is lying on stomach, head and cervical spine in forward flexion, rotated and bent to contralateral side to expose muscle. Therapist stretches with pressure of hypothenar to the body of the muscle, down towards the first and second rib, while pulling with the other hand placed over the facet joints at the level of C4–7 to increase rotation and later flexion of the cervical spine. Stretch is performed at the end of exhalation.

Tension–relaxation technique: Patient attempts to bend head towards the side of the muscle for 5 sec while therapist resists movement or patient takes a deep breath in. Patient then relaxes gradually while therapist performs stretch.

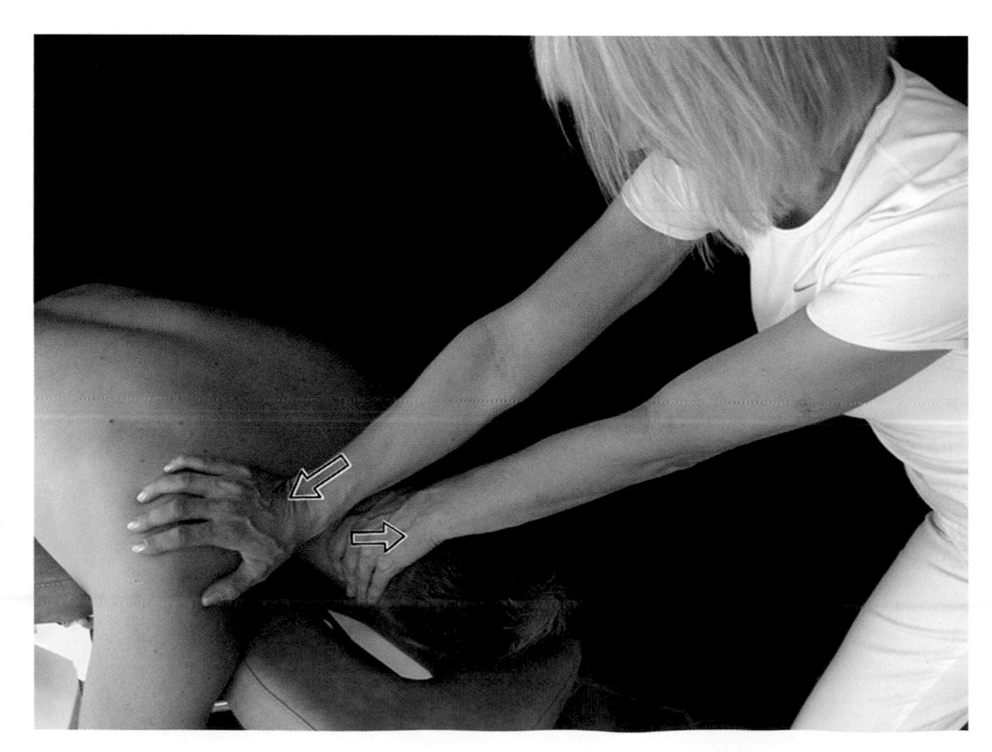

Scalenus posterior

Nerve, supply: Ventral rami of spinal nerves, C6–8.

Origin: Transverse processes of C4–7.

Insertion: Second rib and sometimes the third rib.

Function: Lifts rib and bends cervical spine to same side. Assists in deep inspiration.

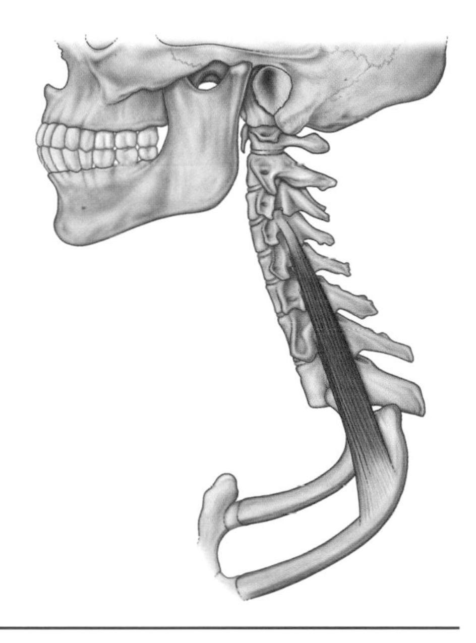

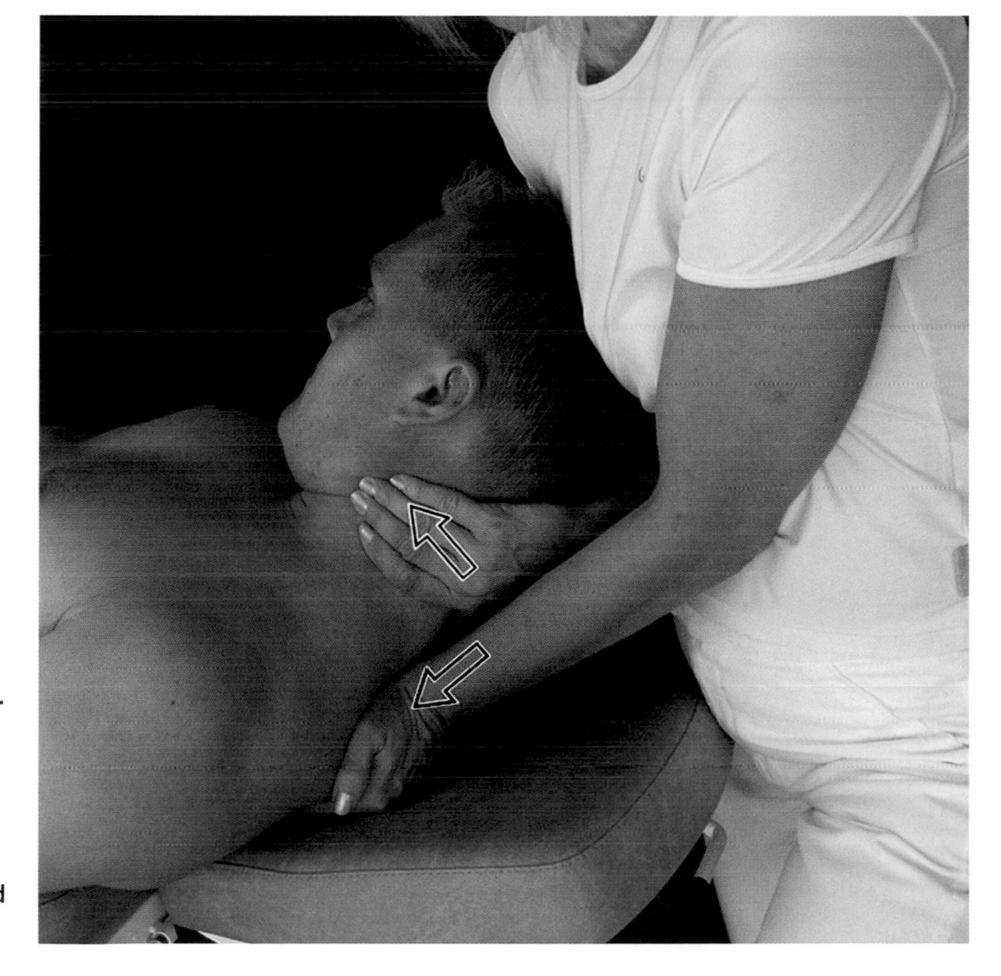

Stretching technique B:

Patient is lying on back, head and cervical spine in forward flexion, slightly rotated and bent to contralateral side to expose muscle. Therapist pulls at level of C4–7 while increasing rotation and lateral flexion. The other hand presses down diagonally and to the side on the second rib. Stretch is performed at the end of exhalation.

Geniohyoid

Nerve, supply: Ventral rami of spinal nerve, C1.

Origin: Middle part of anterior and inner surface of the mandible.

Insertion: Middle of the hyoid bone.

Function: Draws mandible down, lifts and draws hyoid bone forward.

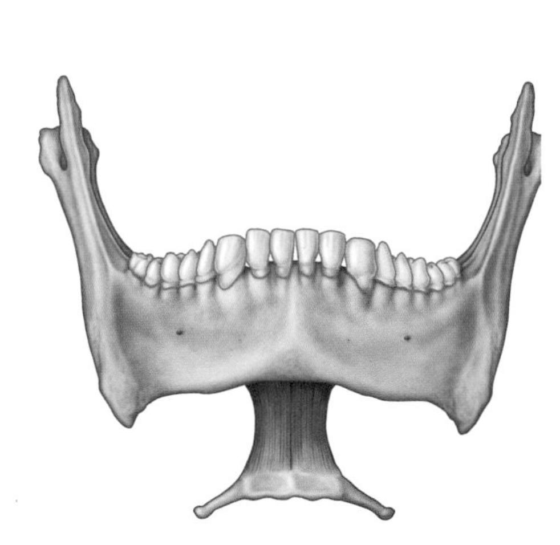

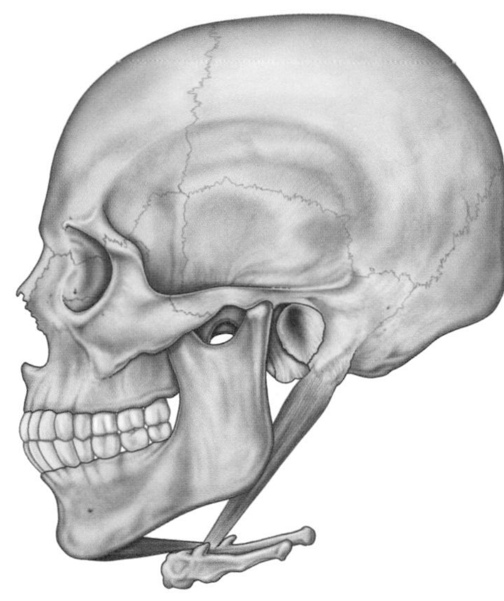

Digatric (anterior belly)

Nerve, supply: Trigeminal nerve (V cranial nerve) divides into the inferior alveolar nerve, and finally the mylohyoid nerve.

Origin: Inner surface of the mandible.

Insertion: Tendon located beneath the lateral transverse ligament of hyoid bone.

Function: Draws mandible down, lifts and draws hyoid bone forward.

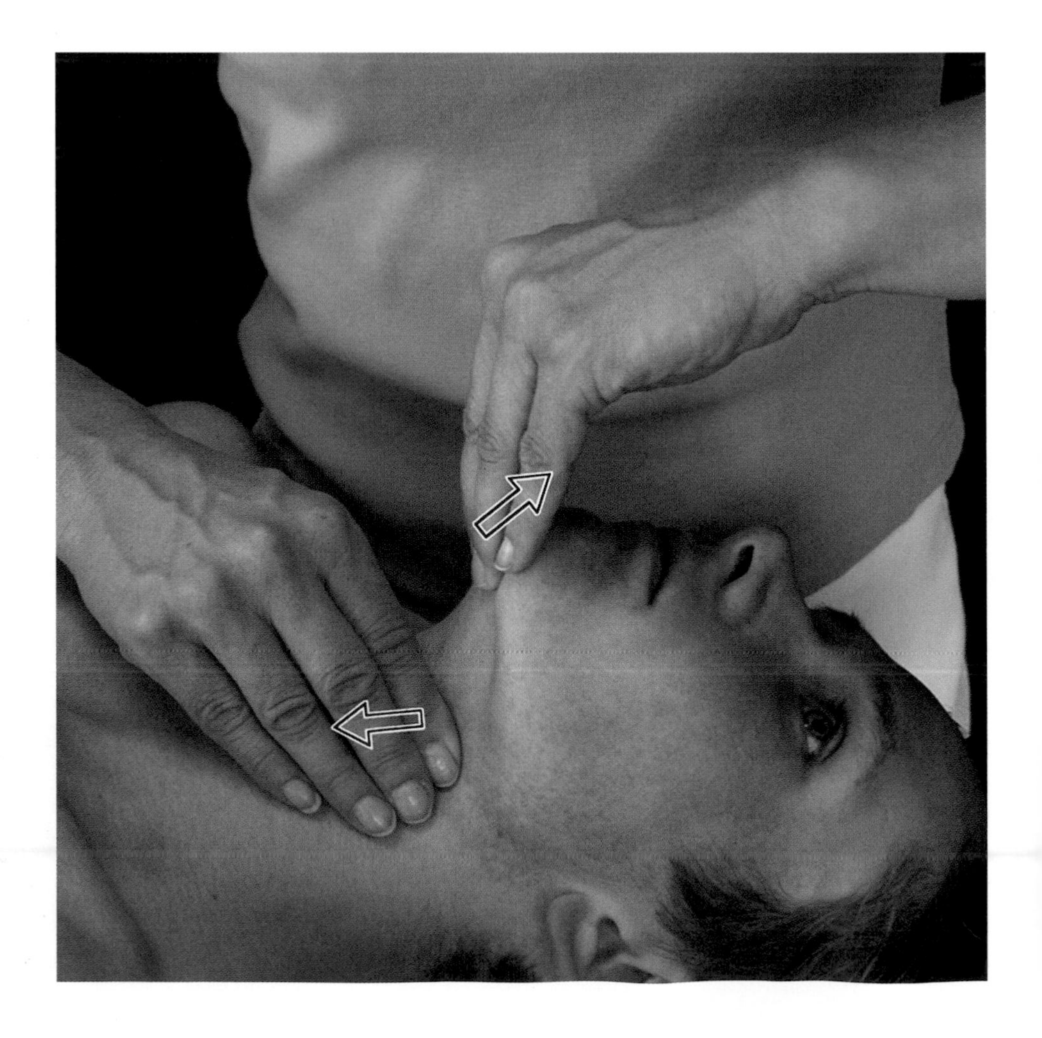

Stretching technique:

Patient is lying on back, neck slightly bent back. Therapist presses with fingers against the base of chin while drawing hyoid bone downwards using the thumb and forefinger of the other hand.

Warning ! Do not place any pressure on the carotid artery. Contact should not be below the hyoid bone.

Mylohyoid

Nerve, supply: Trigeminal nerve (V cranial nerve) divides into the inferior alveolar nerve, and finally the mylohyoid nerve.

Origin: Inner surface of the mandible.

Insertion: Middle of the hyoid bone.

Function: Draws mandible down, lifts and draws hyoid bone forward.

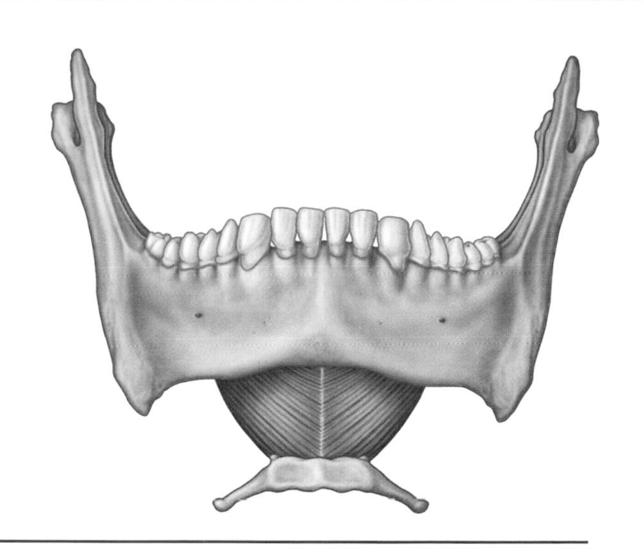

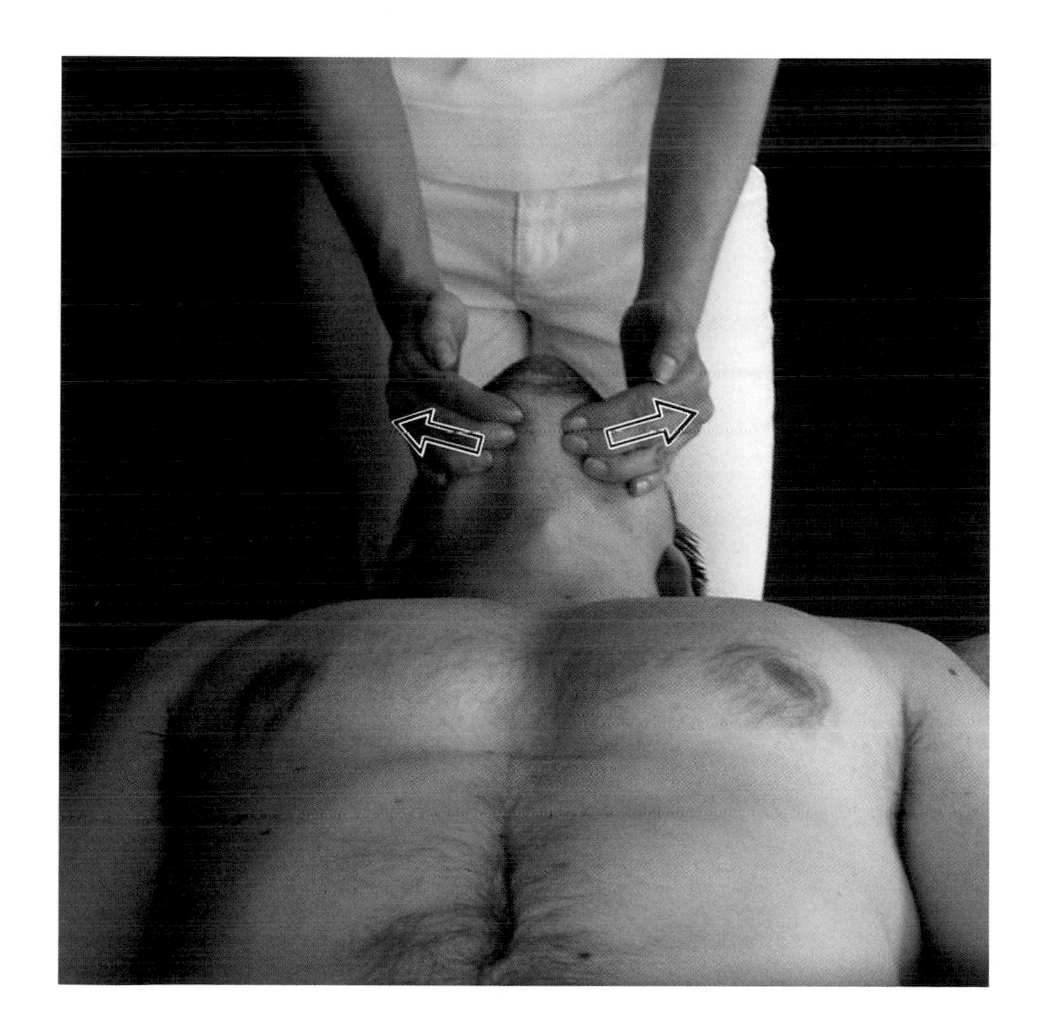

Stretching technique A:

Patient is lying on back, head and cervical spine slightly bent back. Therapist applies pressure at insertion of muscle on mandible and stretches backwards.

Stretching technique B:

Patient is lying on back, head and cervical spine slightly bent back and side bend. Therapist uses fingers of one hand to apply pressure to muscle origin on mandible while using thumb and forefinger of the other hand to stretch muscle tissue down and away from insertion on hyoid bone.

Warning ❗ Do not place pressure on the carotid artery. Contact should not extend below the hyoid bone.

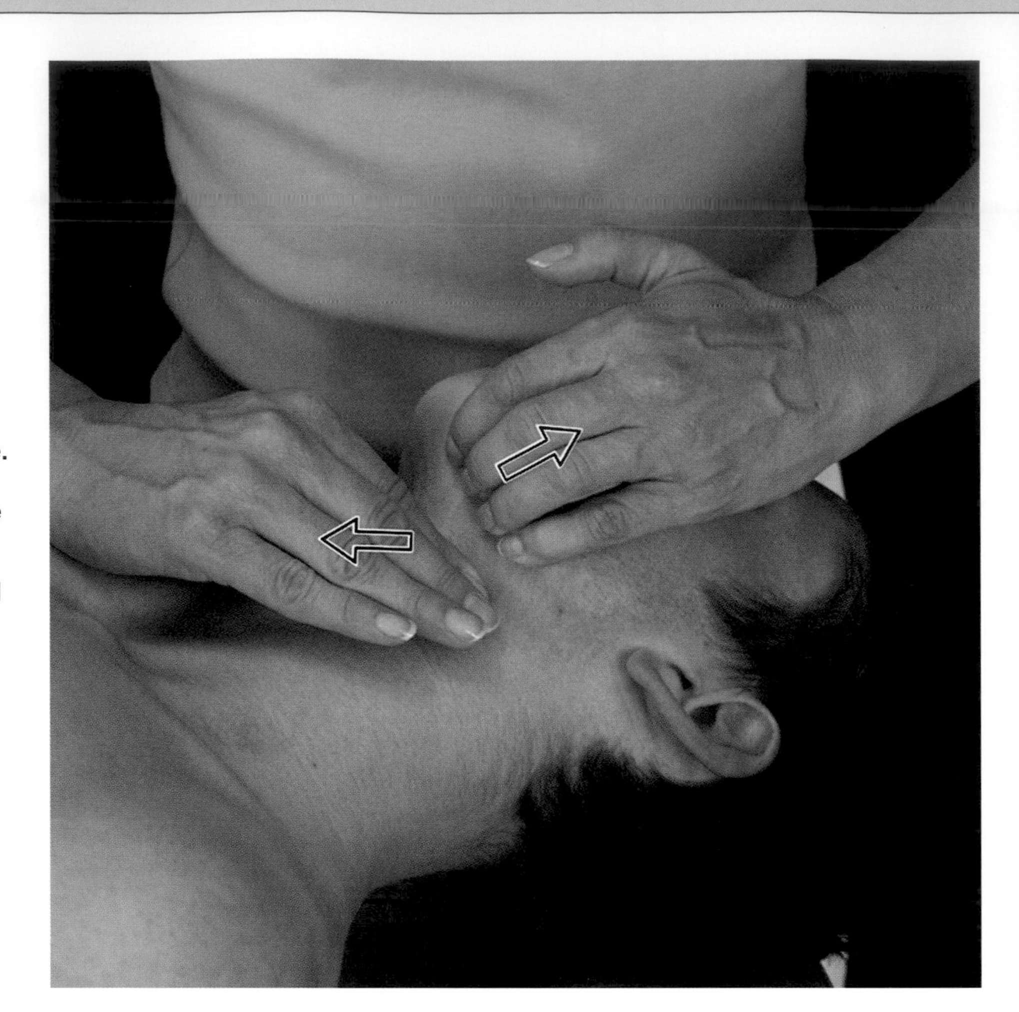

Digastric (posterior belly)

Nerve, supply: Facial nerve (VII cranial nerve).

Origin: Mastoid processes of temporal bone.

Insertion: Tendon of hyoid bone located beneath lateral transverse ligament.

Function: Raises hyoid bone.

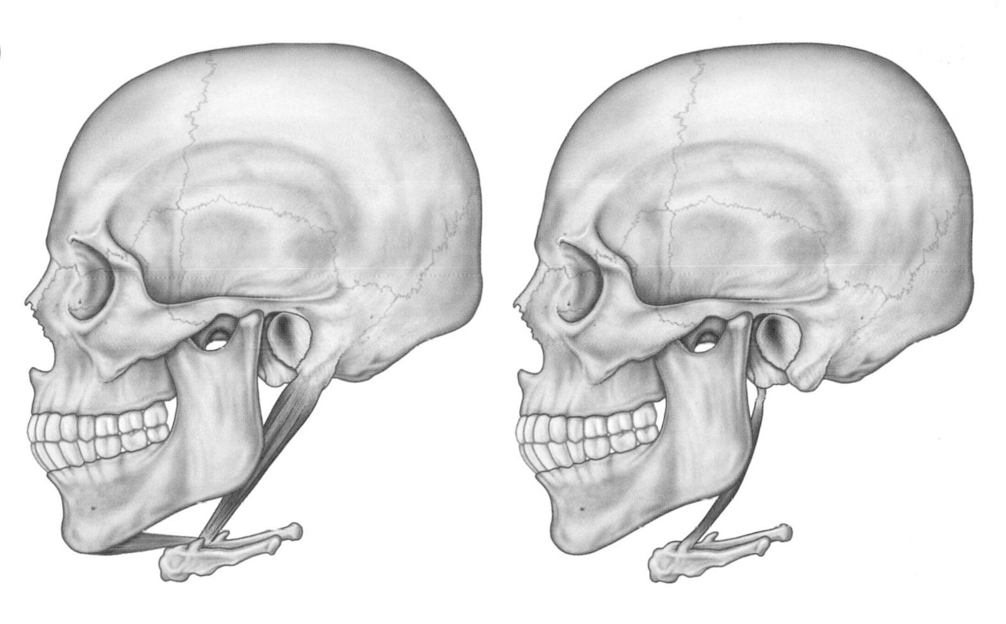

Stylohyoid

Nerve, supply: Facial verve (VII).

Origin: Styloid process at base of skull.

Insertions: Lesser horn of hyoid bone.

Function: Raises hyoid bone and draws backward.

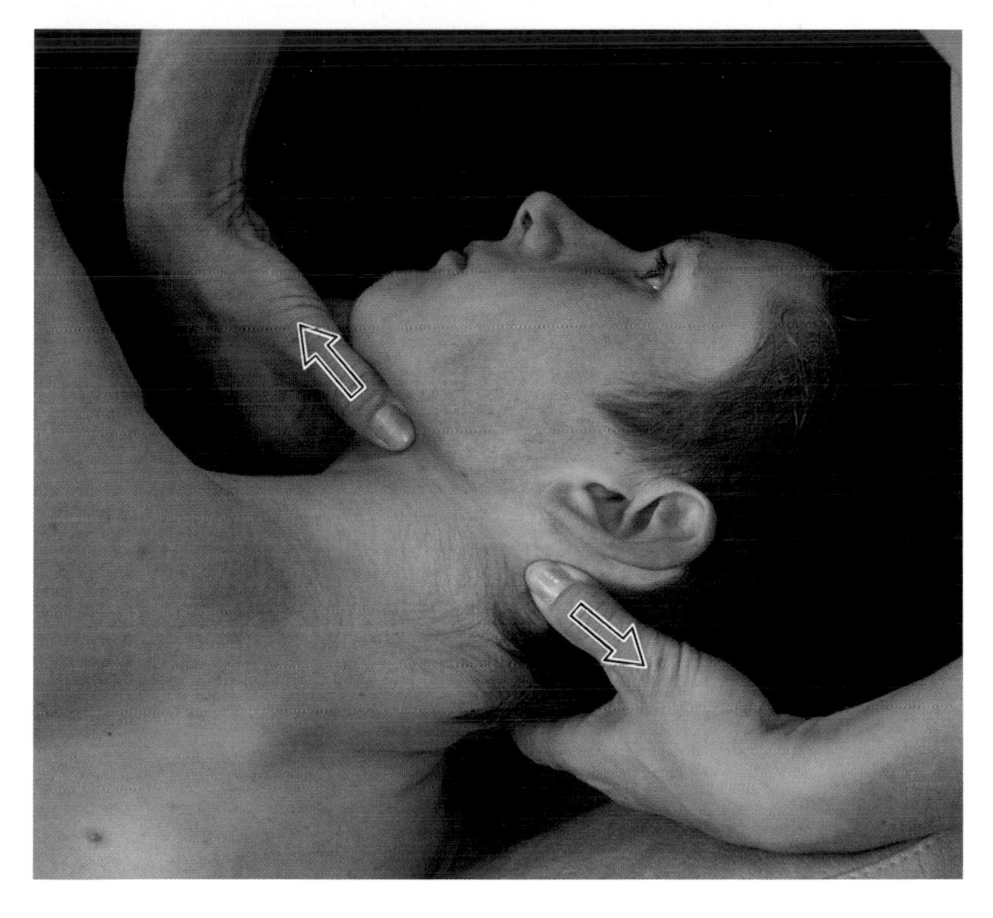

Stretching technique:

Patient is lying on side, head and cervical spine rotated to same side as muscle treated. Therapist takes contact with thumb on the mastoid processes, while using the thumb and forefinger of the other hand to grasp the hyoid bone. Stretching is achieved by pulling hands away from each other.

Warning ❗ Do not place pressure on the carotid artery. Contact should not extend below the hyoid bone.

Omohyoid

Nerve, supply: Ventral rami of spinal nerves, C1–3.

Origin: Medial to scapular notch.

Insertion: Lateral one-third of lower border of the hyoid bone.

Function: Draws hyoid bone downwards.

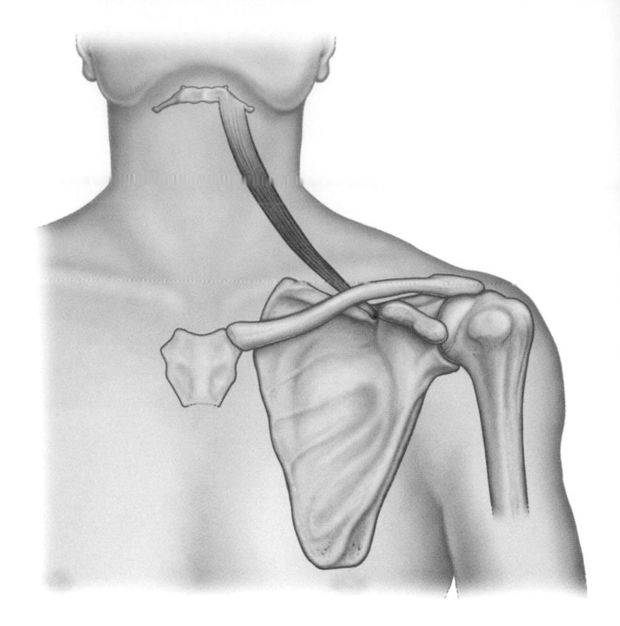

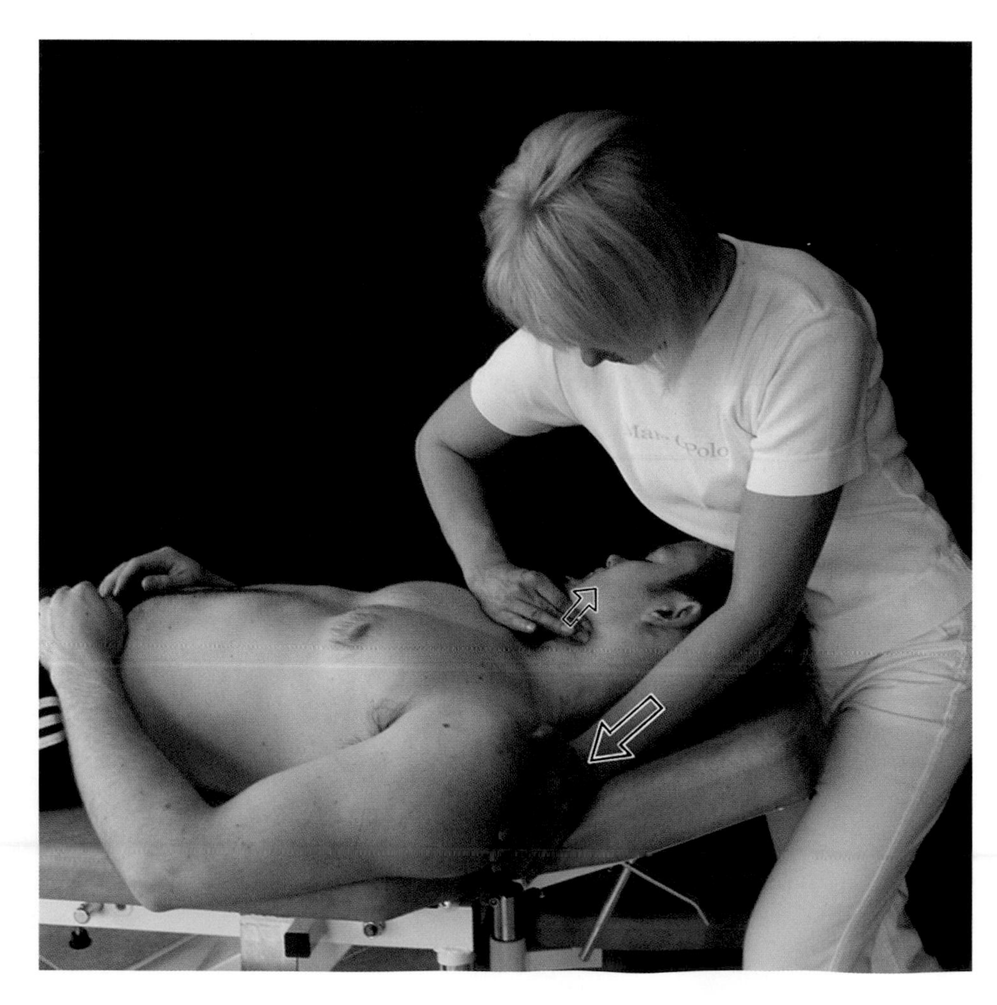

Stretching technique:

Patient is lying on back, head and cervical spine bent forwards, side bent and rotated as far as possible away from the muscle. Therapist presses with the thenar down on the origin of the muscle, located on the scapula. Stretching is achieved by pulling up on the hyoid bone, with fingertips of the other hand, at the point of insertion.

Warning ! Do not place pressure on the carotid artery. Contact should not extend below the hyoid bone.

Sternohyoid

Nerve, supply: Ventral rami of spinal nerves, C1–3 from cervical plexus.

Origin: Upper and posterior surface of manubrium of sternum and the medial end of clavicle.

Insertion: Inner surface of the hyoid bone.

Function: Draws hyoid bone downwards.

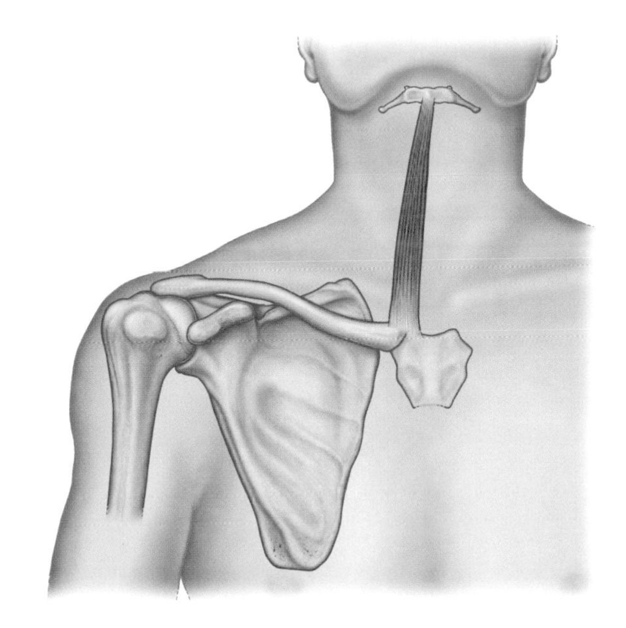

Stretching technique:

Patient is lying on back, head and cervical spine slightly bent back. Therapist presses with the hypothenar down on sternum near the origin of muscle. Therapist uses fingertips of the other hand to push hyoid bone upwards. Forearms will cross over each other as they press in opposite directions.

Warning ! Extreme extension of cervical spine should be avoided as it increases pressure on the vertebral artery. Do not place pressure on the carotid artery. Contact should not extend below the hyoid bone.

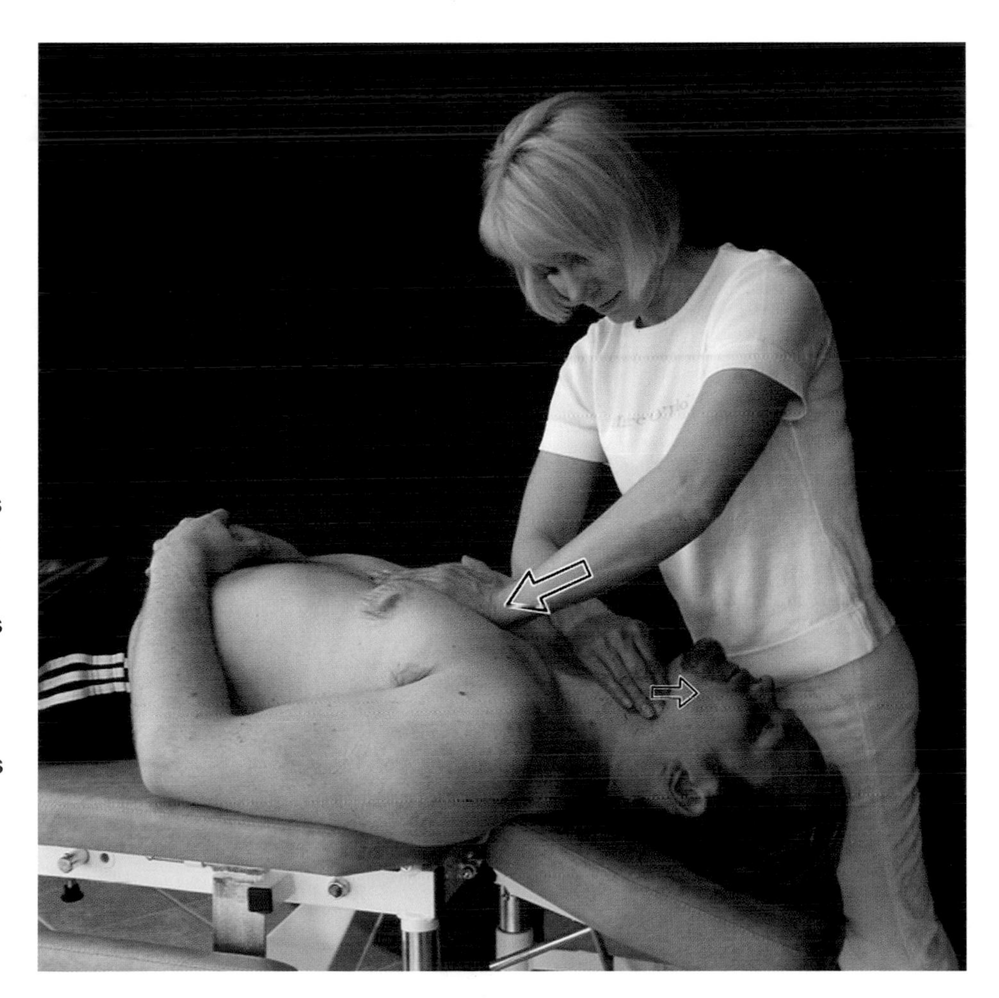

Thyrohyoid

Nerve, supply: Ventral rami of spinal nerve, C1.

Origin: Greater horn of hyoid bone.

Insertion: Thyroid cartilage.

Function: Draws hyoid bone and thyroid cartilage towards each other.

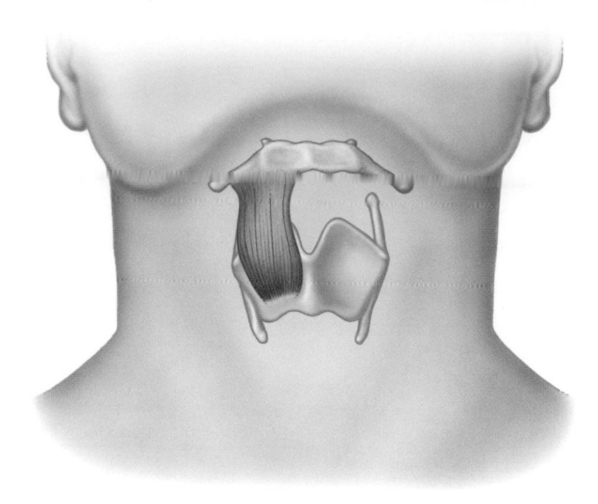

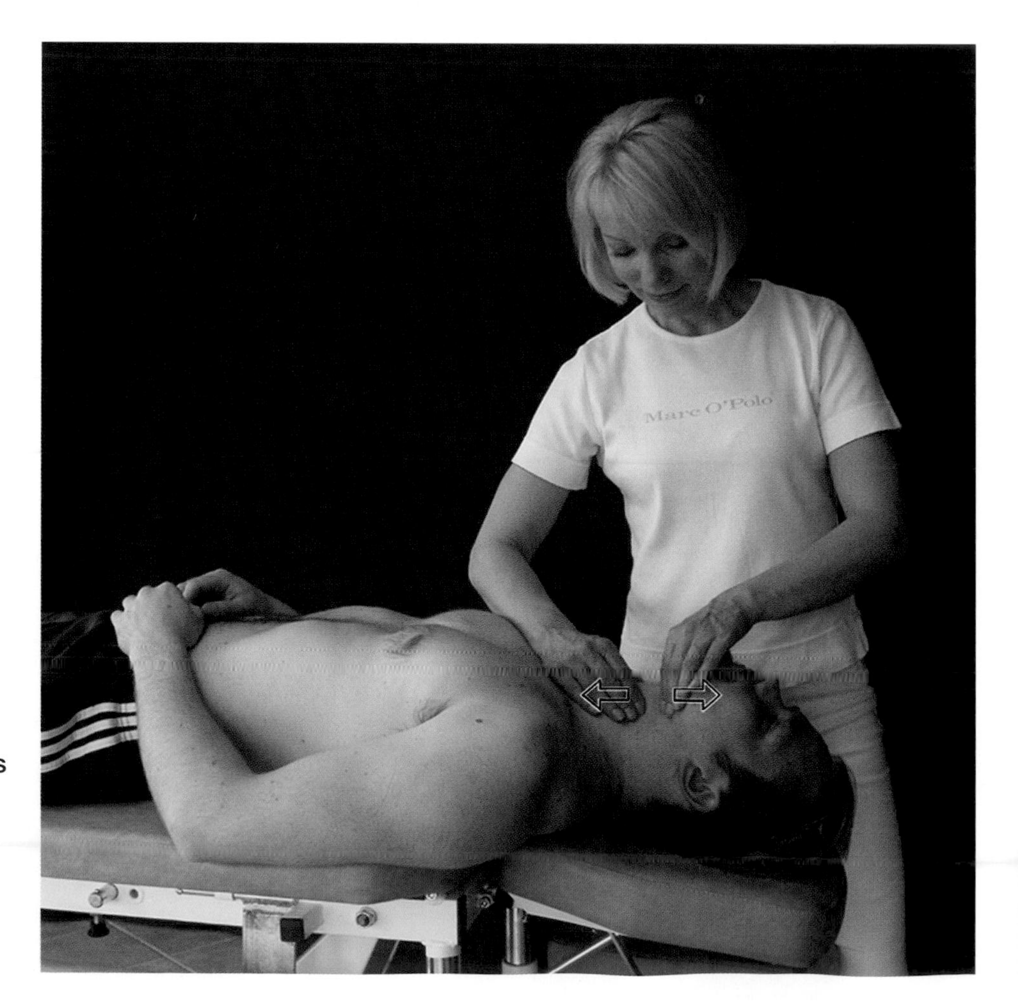

Stretching technique:

Patient is lying on back, head and cervical spine slightly bent back. Using fingertips of both hands, therapist pulls hyoid bone and thyroid cartilage away from each other.

Warning ! Extreme extension of cervical spine should be avoided as it increases pressure on the vertebral artery. Do not place pressure on the carotid artery. Contact should not extend outside the hyoid and thyroid bones.

Sternothyroid

Nerve, supply: Ventral rami of spinal nerves, C1–3.

Origin: Posterior surface of manubrium of sternum and costal cartilage of first rib.

Insertion: Lamina of thyroid cartilage.

Function: Draws thyroid down.

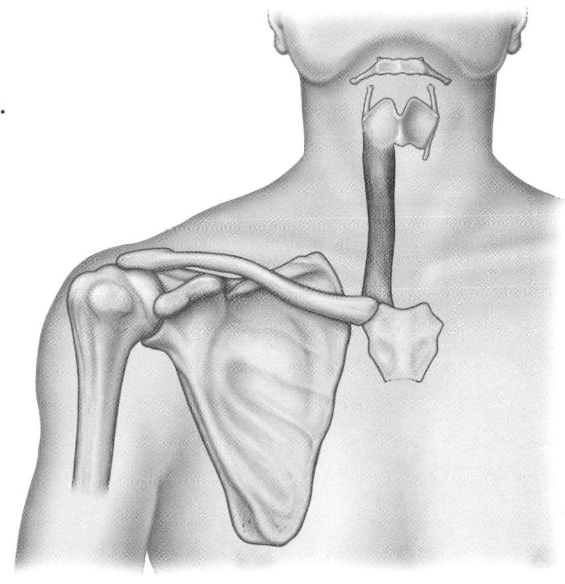

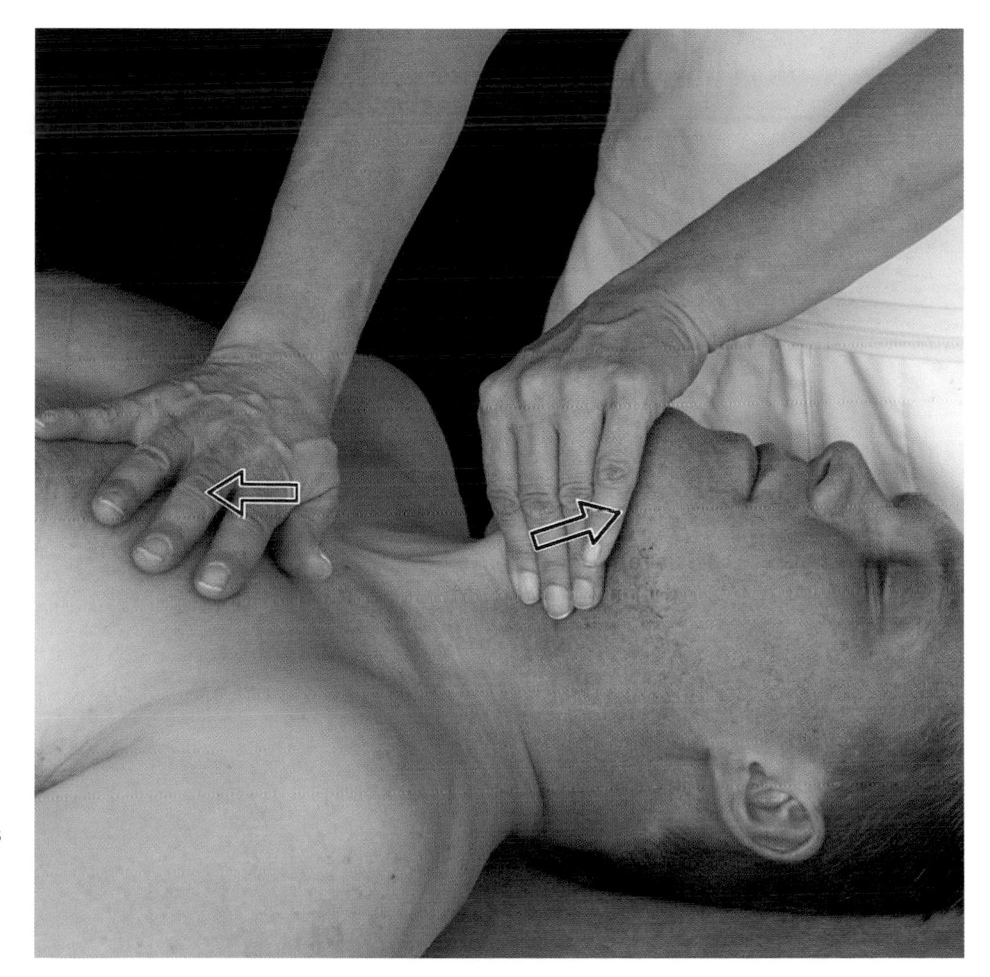

Stretching technique:

Patient is lying on back. Press sternum downward with the thenar. Grasp thyroid cartilage at muscle insertion with fingertips of the other hand, and stretch upwards.

Warning ❗ Pressure on the carotid artery is to be avoided. The grasp is not very wide and should not extend past the edges of the thyroid cartilage.

Longus capitis

Nerve, supply: Ventral rami of spinal nerves, C1–4.

Origin: Anterior tubercles of transverse processes of C3–6.

Insertion: Basal part of occipital bone, anterior to the great foramen.

Function: Forward and lateral flexion of head and cervical spine.

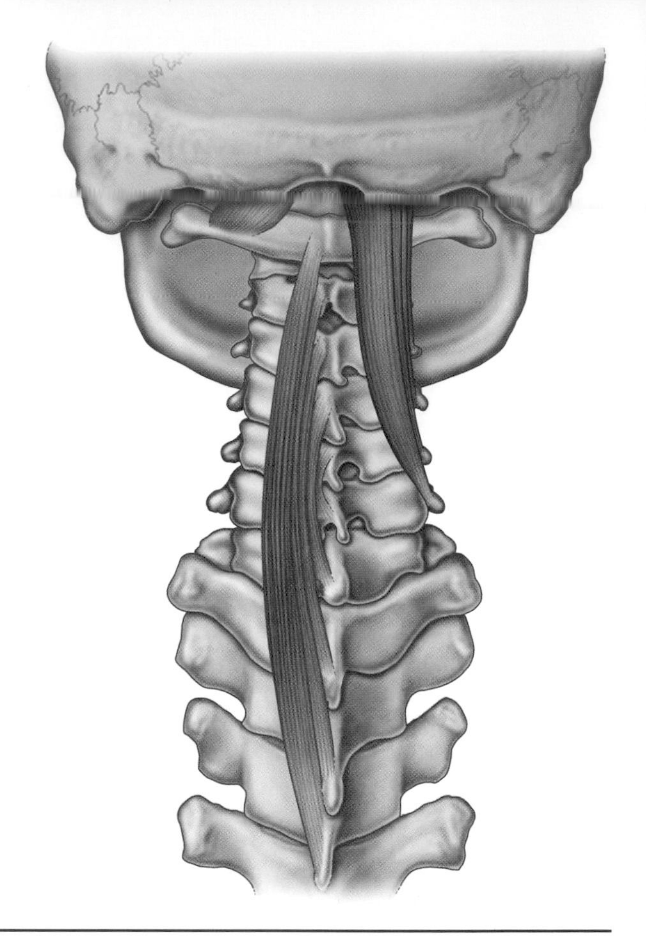

Longus colli

Nerve, supply: Ventral rami of spinal nerves, C2–7.

Origin:

a) Superior oblique fibres from anterior tubercles of transverse processes of C2–5.
b) Medial fibres from bodies of C5–Th3.
c) Inferior oblique fibres from bodies of Th1–3.

Insertion:

a) Anterior tubercle of anterior arch of atlas.
b) Bodies of C2–4.
c) Anterior tubercles of transverse processes of C5–6.

Function: Forward flexion of head and cervical spine, bending to the same side, rotation to the opposite side.

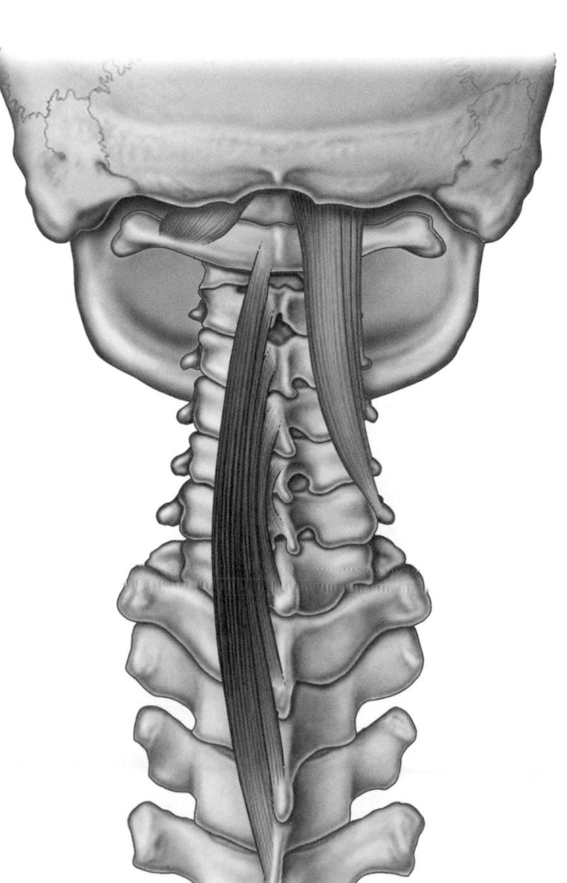

Rectus capitis anterior

Nerve, supply: Ventral rami of spinal nerve, C1–2.

Origin: Lateral mass of atlas.

Insertion: Bassilar process of occipital bone, anterior to the great foramen.

Function: Forward flexion of head.

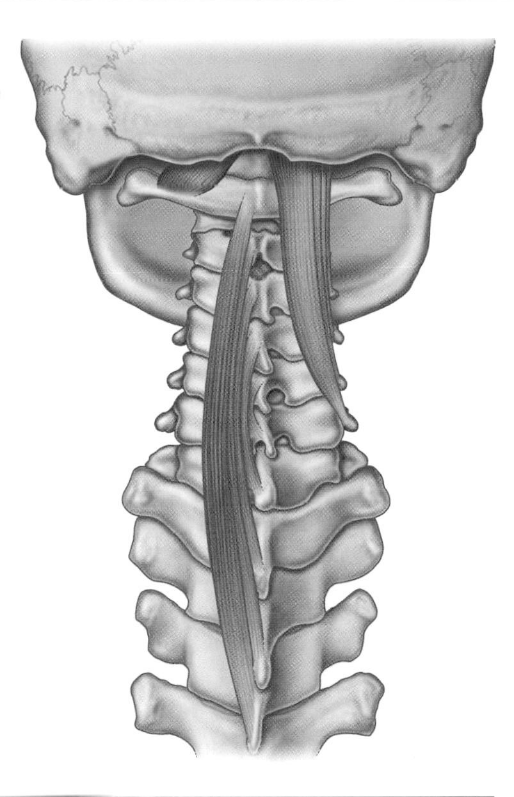

Stretching technique

Patient is lying on back, therapist bends cervical spine back. This technique is not recommended. Fixation and/or direct contact are not possible with these muscles and effective stretching cannot be applied, because of the limitation in the movement of the cervical spine.

Notice: Deep muscles anterior to cervical spine are often weak in painful conditions of the neck and seldom suffer from shortening while anterior superficial muscles are often quite tense.

Warning ! Extreme extension of head may cause blockage in the vertebral artery. Risk increases in the elderly suffering from arteriosclerosis. The risk of aneurysm, more likely in younger patients, should also be noted!

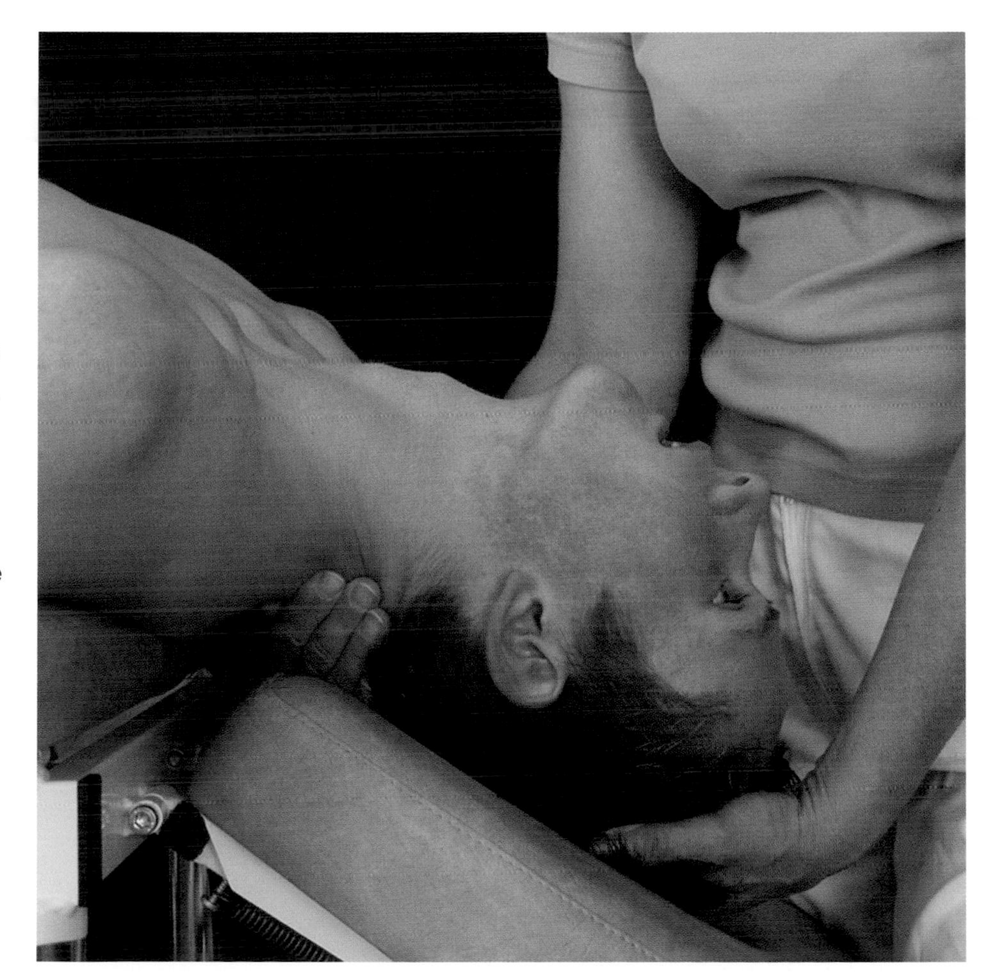

Trapezius (superior descending part)

Nerve, supply: Accessory nerve (XI cranial nerve) and spinal nerves, C2–4.

Origin: Superior nuchal line, the external occipital protuberance and the ligamentum nuchae arising from spinous processes of C1–7.

Insertion: Lateral third of the clavicle and the spine of scapula.

Function: Stabilizes, lifts, adducts and rotates up the scapula. Lateral flexion of the head and cervical spine. Assists in deep inspiration.

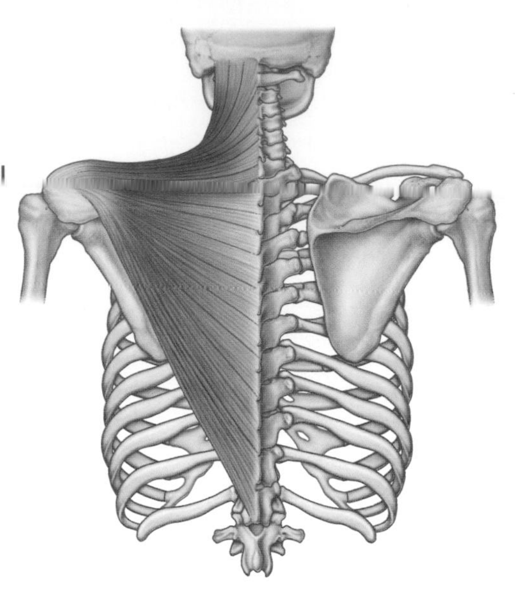

Stretching technique A:

Patient is lying on back, head supported against therapist in slight flexion. Therapist stretches with the thenar of the hand down towards muscle insertion while using the other hand and the body to bend the head and cervical spine to the opposite side.

Tension–relaxation technique: Patient tries to lift shoulder up for 5 sec while therapist actively resists. Patient is then advised to gradually relax as therapist performs stretch.

Notice: Some rotation of the head and cervical spine to the same side as lateral flexion is allowed to avoid locking of the facet joints in the cervical spine.

Notice: Fixation of hands on the origin and insertion of the muscle while using body movement to produce stretch — instead of hands — is more effective and places less stress on the therapist.

Notice: The hand supports the upper cervical spine in order to avoid excessive stress, which may result from flexion of the upper cervical spine. This is important especially in cases of hypermobility.

Warning ! The therapist's body should not lean in axial direction on the patient head to avoid pressure on the cervical discs.

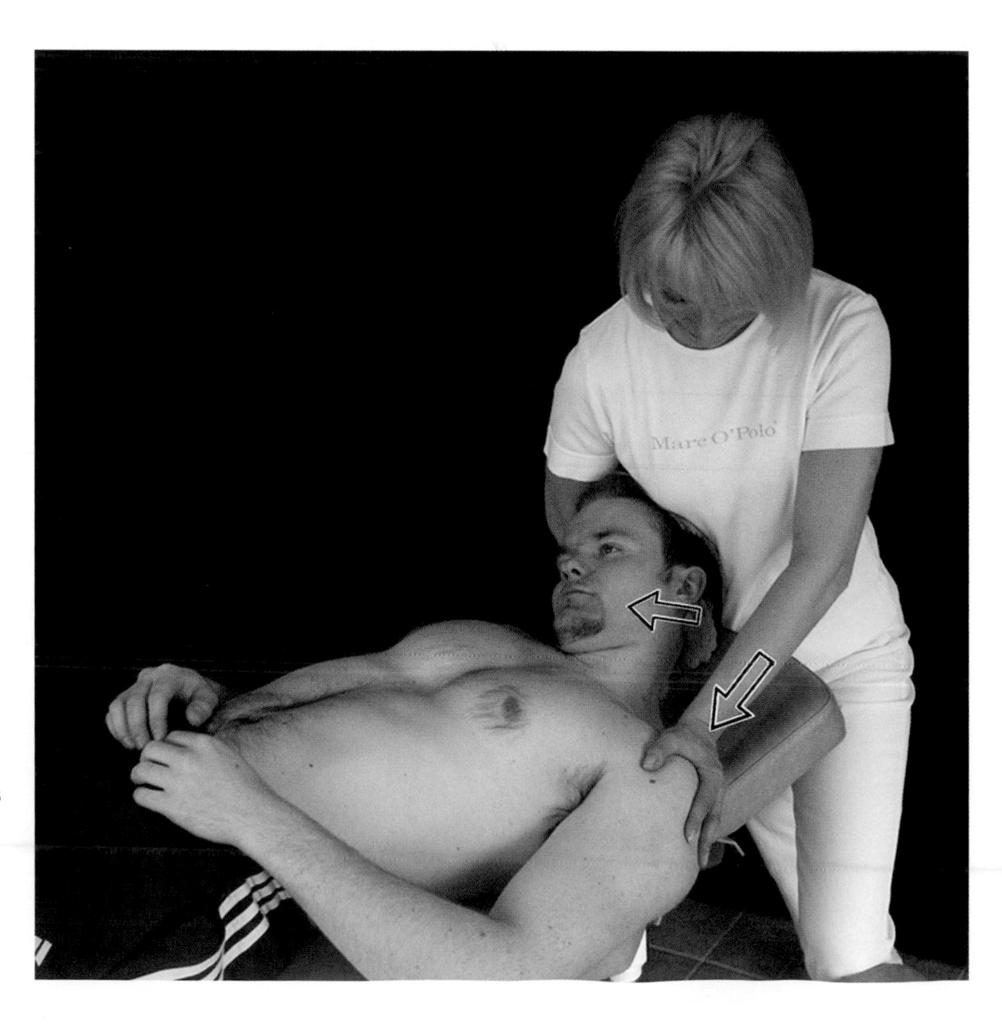

Stretching technique B:

Patient is lying on back, head and cervical spine bent away from muscle to be treated. Therapist's forearm wraps around under patient's upper arm, grasps spine of scapula, and pulls downwards while stretching upwards along muscle fibres with thumb and the first metacarpal bone towards origin.

Notice: Do not press against transverse or spinous processes, which is painful and cause easily muscle damage. Pressure should be directed to the facet joints.

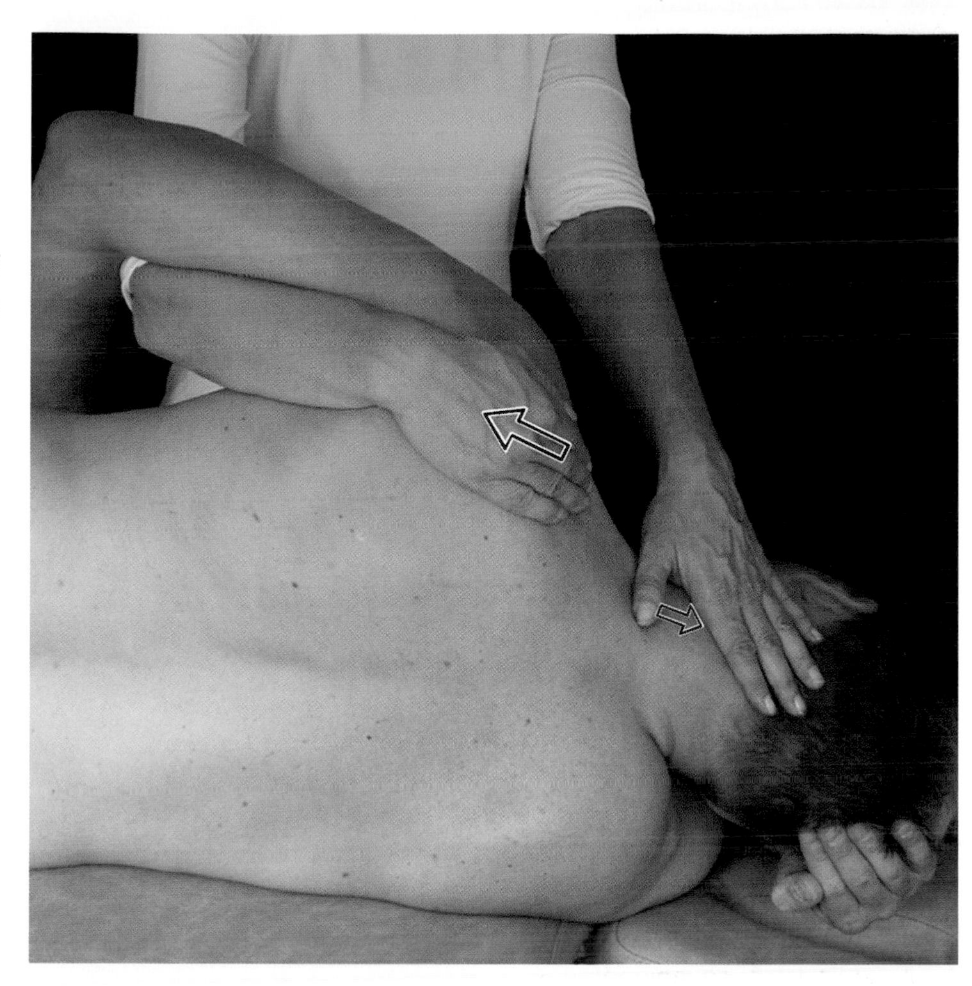

Levator scapulae

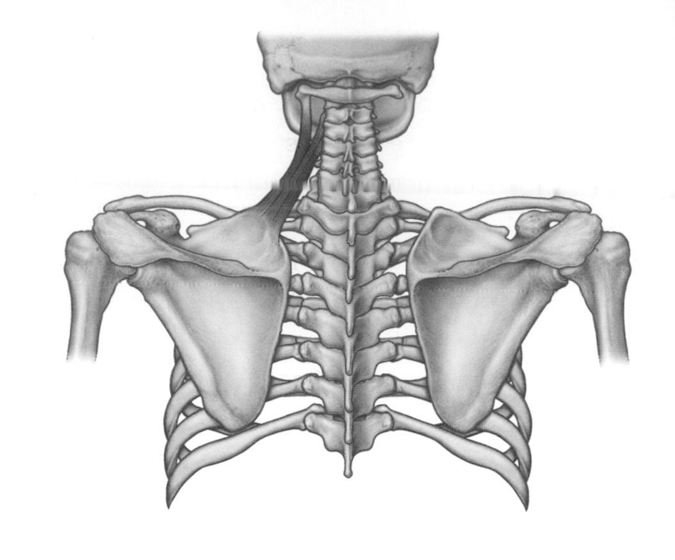

Nerve, supply: Dorsal scapular nerve, C3–5.

Origin: Dorsal tubercles of the transverse processes of C1–4.

Insertion: Superior angle of scapula and the adjacent part of the medial border of the scapula.

Function: Extension and lateral flexion of cervical spine. Raises, abducts and rotates scapula. Assists in deep inspiration.

Stretching technique A:

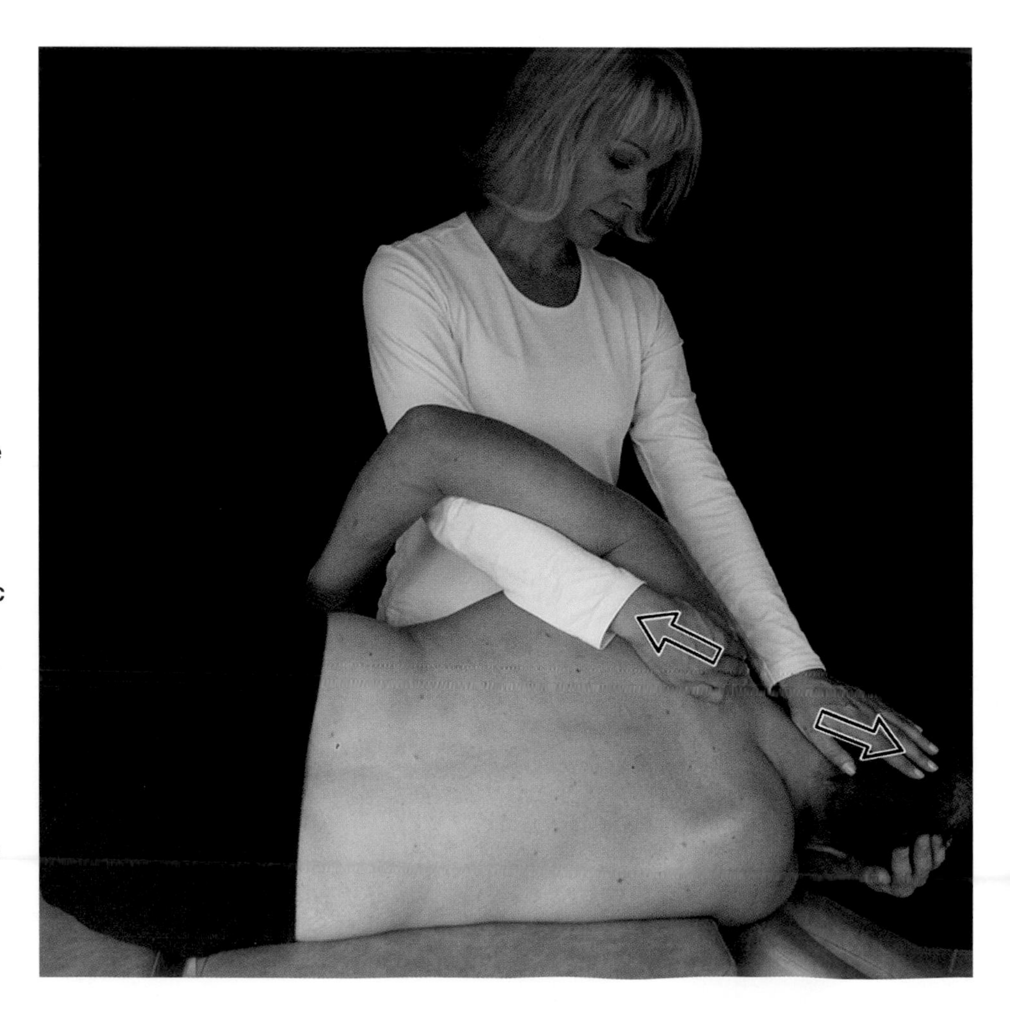

Patient is lying on side with the upper arm over therapist's forearm. Therapist grasps around the superior, medial angle of the scapula and pulls the scapula downwards while using the thenar of other hand to rotate and lateral flex cervical facet joints away in the contralateral direction.

Tension–relaxation technique: Patient tries to lift head up for 5 sec while therapist actively resists. Patient is then advised to gradually relax as therapist performs stretch.

Notice: Side bending and rotation is allowed to happen in the same direction, because rotation towards opposite direction will restrict the side bending and thus stretching will be less effective.

Stretching technique B:

Patient is lying on back with head flexed and supported against therapist's body. Therapist rotates and lateral flexes facet joints at level C1–4 to same side by moving her body forwards while with the thenar of the other hand pressing down on superior angle of scapula at the muscle insertion.

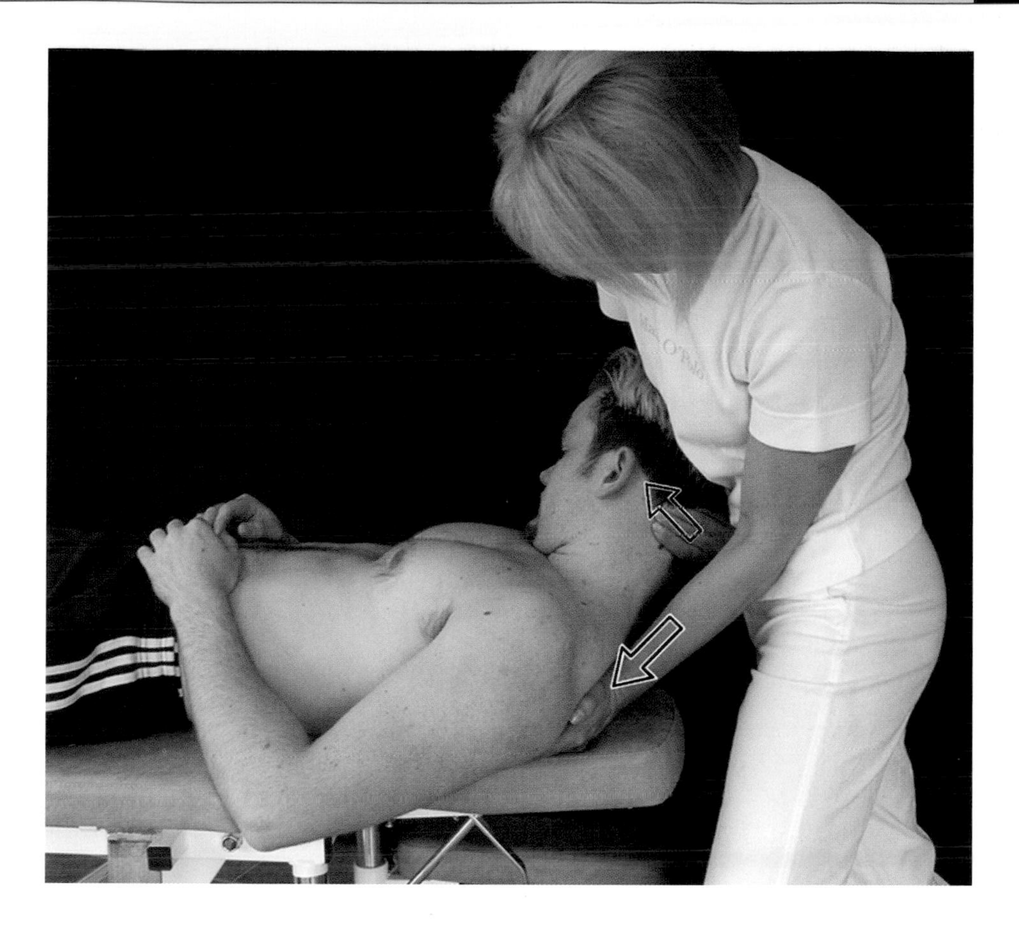

Stretching technique C:

Patient is lying on stomach, arm raised above head so that muscle insertion rotates downwards. Therapist presses with the hypothenar towards insertion on the superior angle of scapula to the side and downwards while using the other hand to press diagonally down on cervical facet joints to rotate and lateral flex them. Forearms cross over each other to produce the stretch.

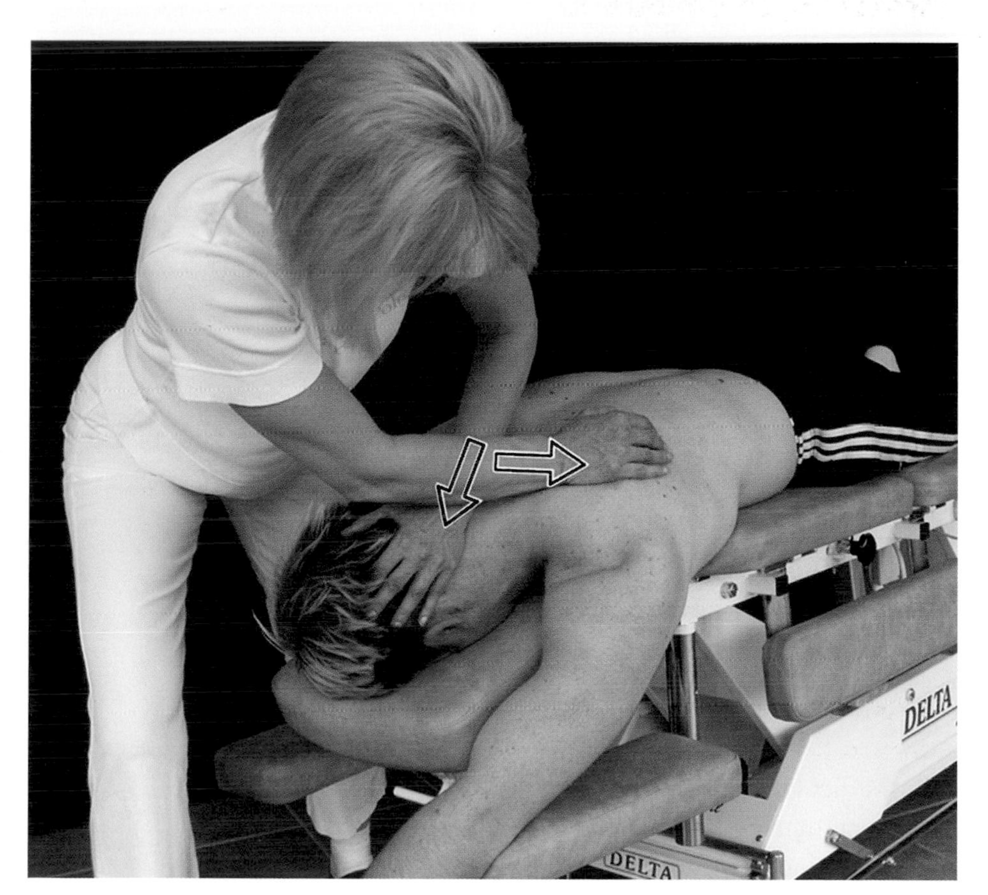

Splenius capitis

Nerve, supply: Posterior rami of spinal nerves, C3–5.

Origin: Inferior half of ligament nuchae and spinous processes of C7–Th3.

Insertion: Mastoid process of temporal bone.

Function: Extension and rotation of the head and cervical spine.

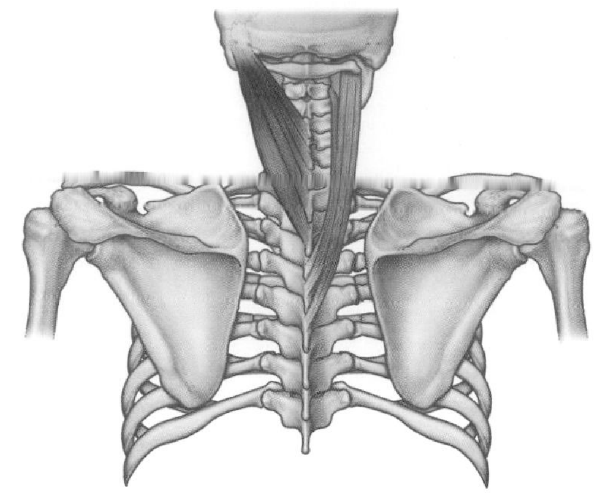

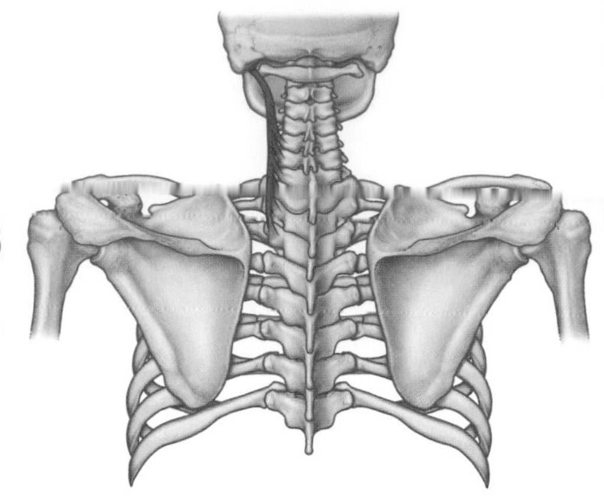

Longissimus capitis

Nerve, supply: Posterior rami of spinal nerves, C2–Th4.

Origin: Transverse processes of C5–7 and Th1–3 (5).

Insertion: Mastoid process.

Function: Extension, lateral flexion and rotation of head and cervical spine.

Stretching technique:

Patient is lying on stomach, head slightly bent forwards and to the side away from muscle to be treated. Therapist applies pressure with the thenar of the hand next to transverse processes on the facet joints at the level of C5–C7 and presses diagonally down and away from the spine and moves then at the level of Th1–3. The other hand, wrapped around the mastoid process and occiput, is used to increase lateral flexion and rotation by pulling from the base of the skull.

Tension–relaxation technique: Patient tries to rotate neck against therapist's forearm for 5 secs while therapist resists. Then the patient is advised to gradually relax muscles while the therapist gently increases stretch.

Notice: Splenius capitis is the strongest rotator muscle in the back of the neck. Thus, it is important to instruct the patient to use only moderate force while trying to rotate the head, e.g. 20% of the maximum force.

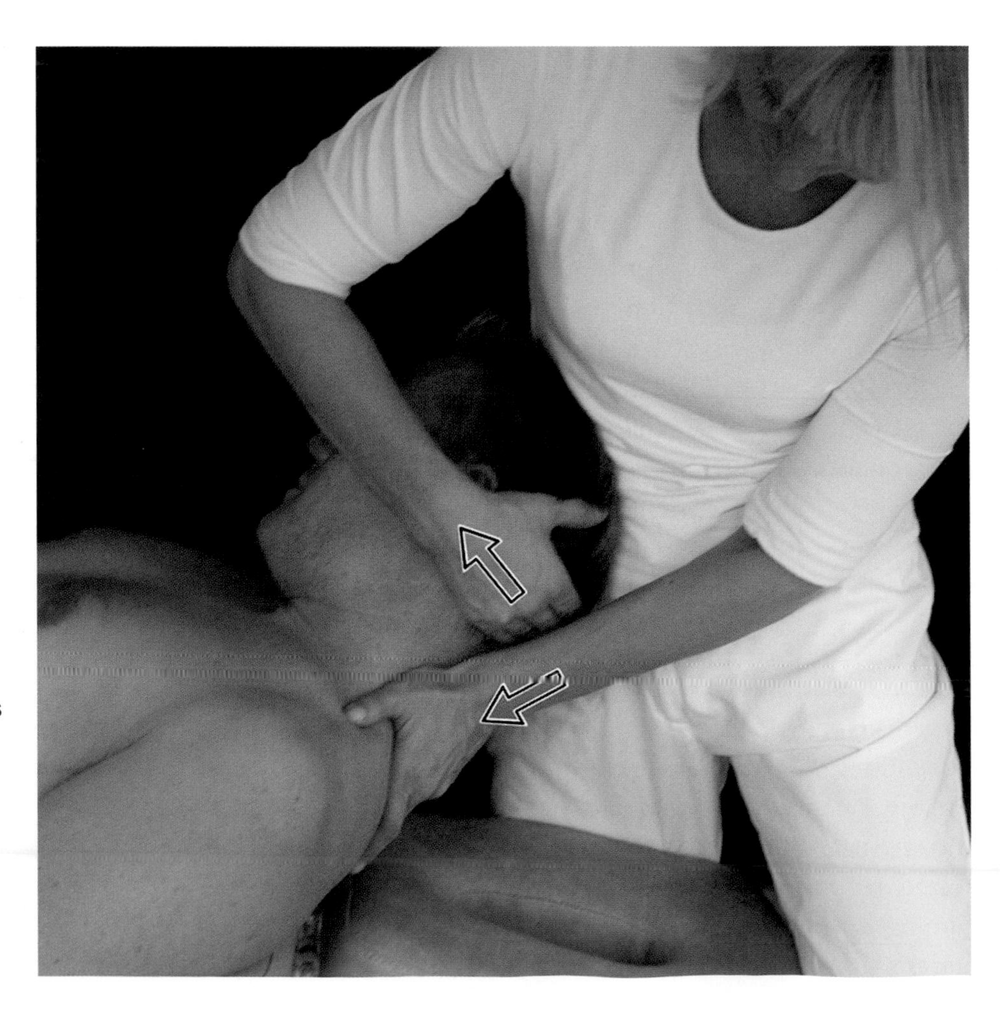

Splenius cervicis

Nerve, supply: Posterior rami of spinal nerve, C5–7.

Origin: Spinous processes of Th3–6.

Insertion: Transverse processes of atlas and axis, C1–2(3).

Function: Extension, lateral flexion and rotation of cervical spine.

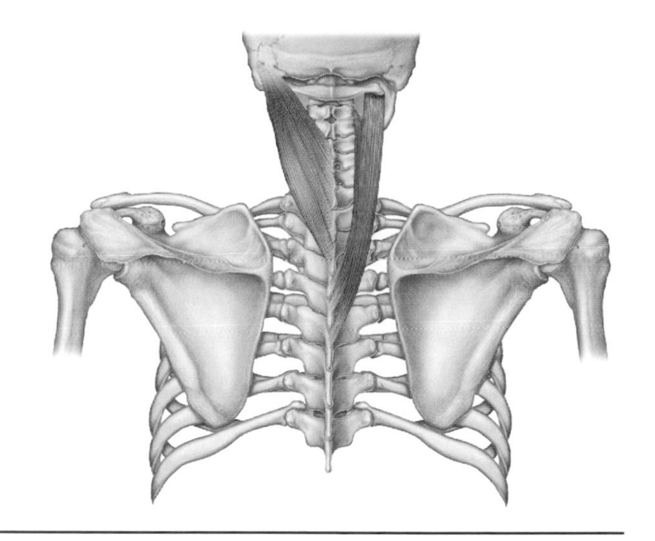

Stretching technique:

Patient is lying on stomach, head slightly in forward flexion and rotated, and bent away from the muscle to be treated. Therapist cups hand around atlas (C1) and axis (C2). Stretching is achieved by gently pulling on the muscle insertions to increase rotation and lateral flexion while using the thenar of the other hand to apply pressure downwards next to the spinous processes of Th3–6 on the facet joints.

Tension–relaxation technique: Patient tries to rotate head against the forearm for 5 sec while therapist resists. Patient is then advised to gradually relax muscles while therapist gently increases stretch.

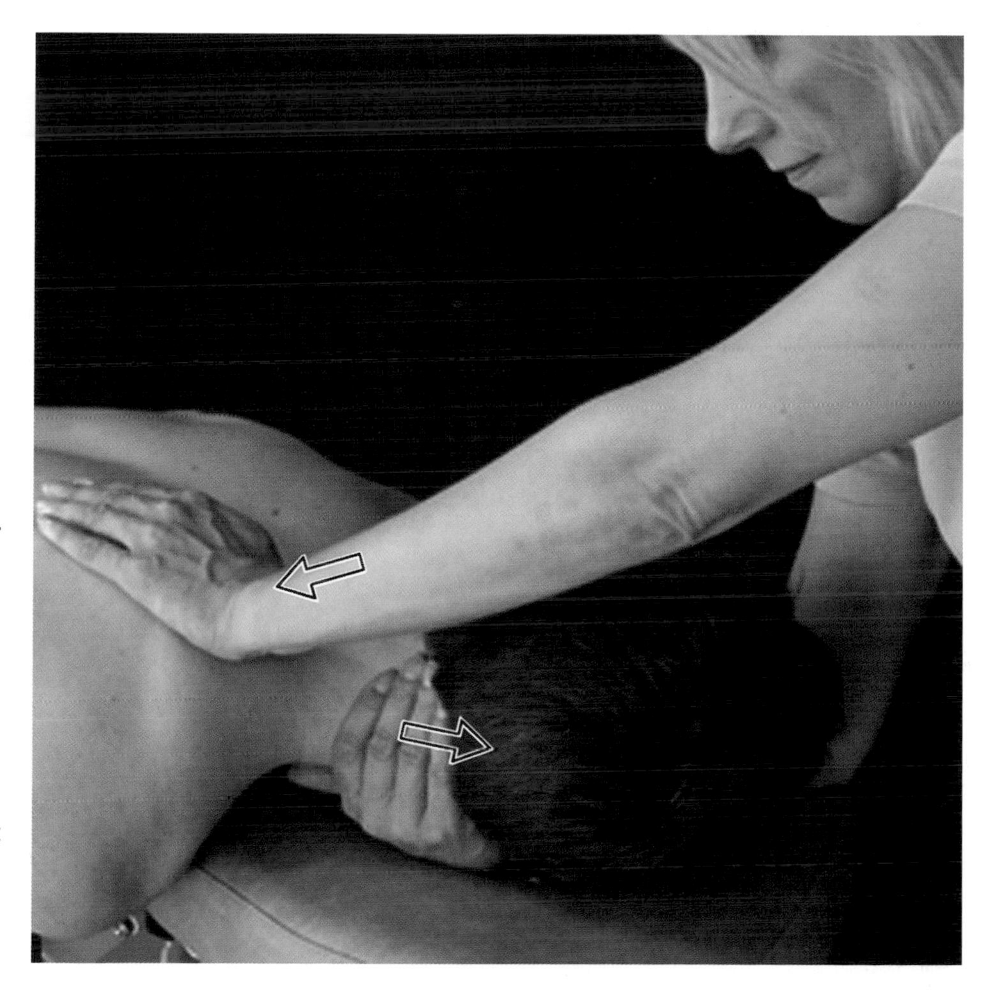

Iliocostalis cervicis

Nerve, supply: Posterior rami on spinal nerves, C4–6.

Origin: Posterior angles of ribs 3–6.

Insertion: Transverse processes of C4–6.

Function: Extension, lateral flexion and rotation of cervical spine.

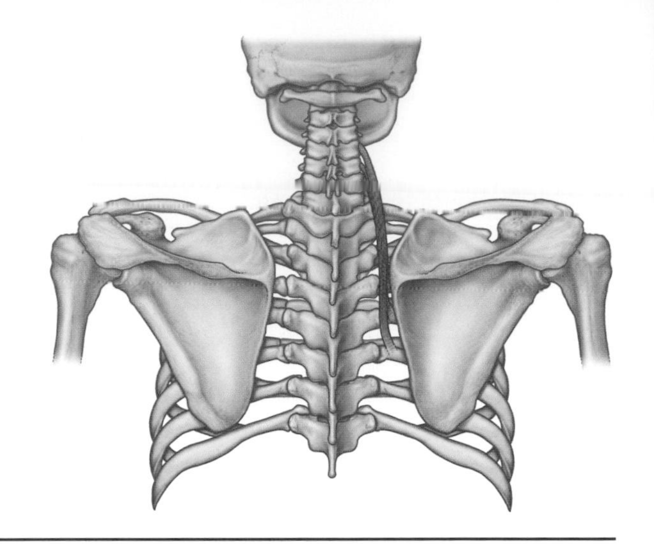

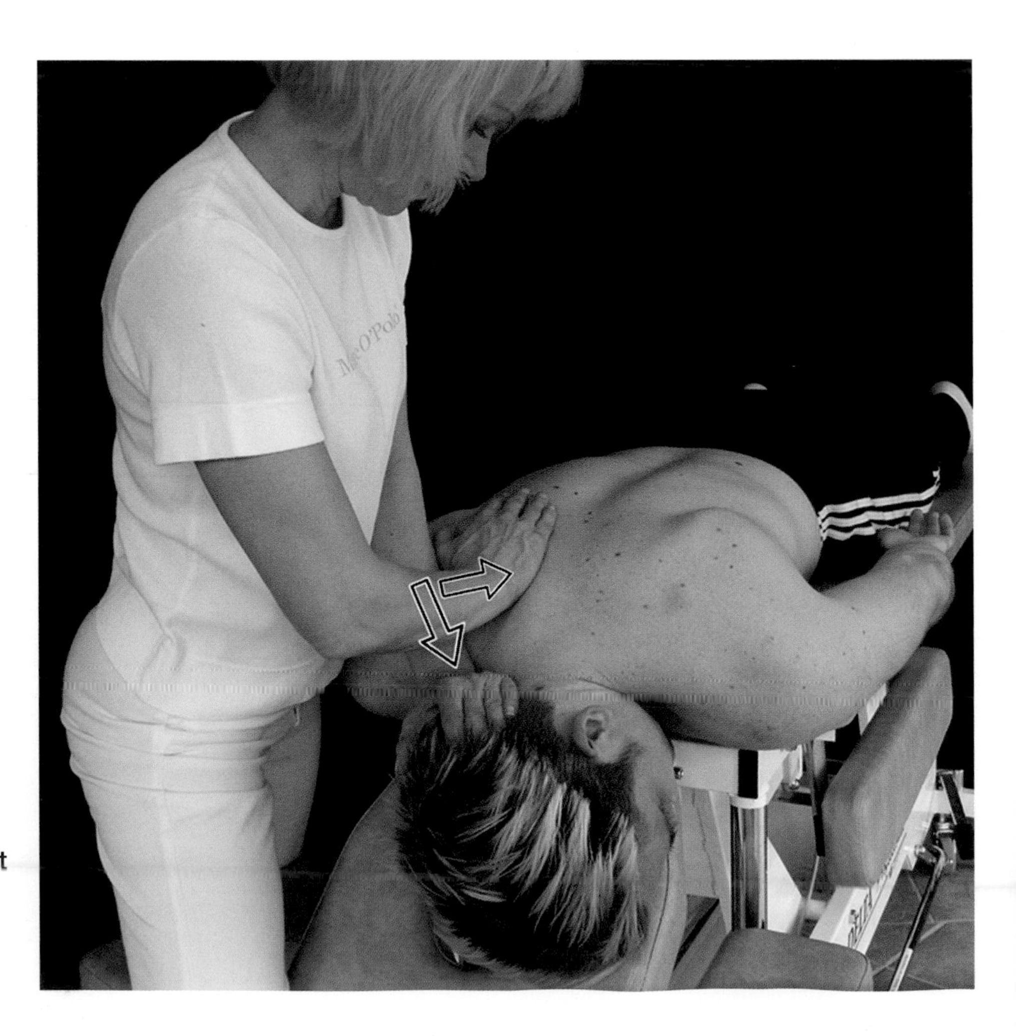

Stretching technique:

Patient is lying on stomach, head bent slightly forward, lateral flexed and rotated away from the muscle to be treated. Therapist presses with the hypothenar next to the spinous processes of C4–6 on the facet joints to increase lateral flexion and rotation. The hypothenar of the other hand presses diagonally away from the cervical spine on ribs 3–6. The forearms of the therapist are crossed.

Tension–relaxation technique: Patient tries to extend neck for 5 sec while therapist resists. Patient is then advised to gradually relax muscles while therapist gently increases stretch.

Longissimus cervicis

Nerve, supply: Posterior rami of spinal nerves, C4–Th5.

Origin: Transverse processes of Th1–5(6).

Insertion: Posterior tubercles of transverse processes of C2–5(6).

Function: Extension, lateral flexion and rotation of cervical spine.

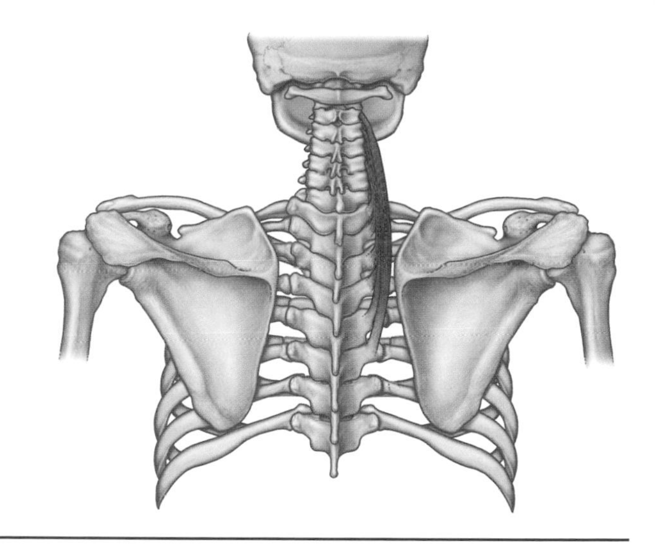

Stretching technique:

Patient is lying on stomach, head bent slightly forward, lateral flexed and rotated away from muscle to be treated. Therapist places thenar of the hand next to spinous processes of C2–5, on the facet joints and applies pressure in a diagonal direction, to the side with rotation. The other hand, placed on the facet joints next to the spinous processes of Th1–6, presses diagonally away from the cervical spine. The therapist's arms are crossed.

Tension–relaxation technique: Patient tries to extend neck for 5 sec while therapist resists. Patient is then advised to gradually relax muscles while therapist gently increases stretch.

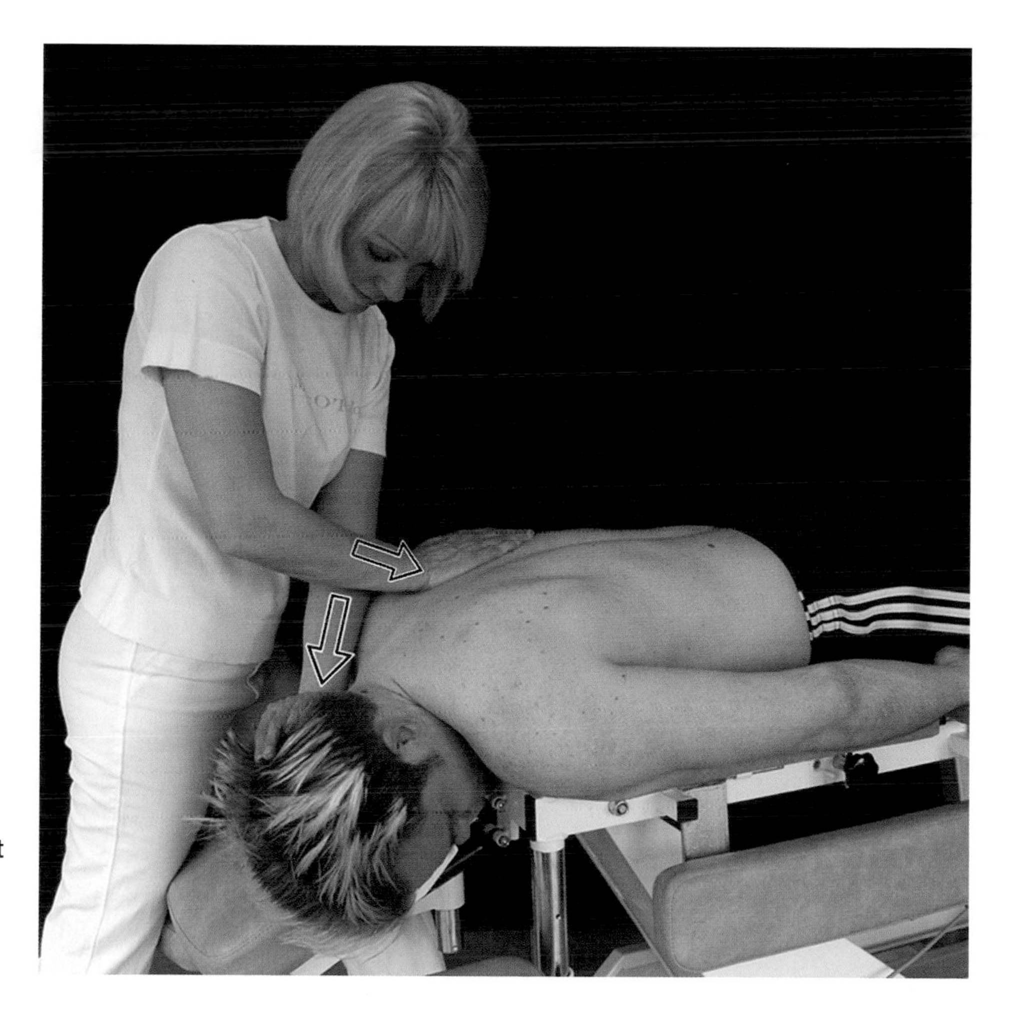

Spinalis capitis

Nerve, supply: Posterior rami of spinal nerves, C2–Th1.

Origin: Spinous processes of C6–Th2.

Insertion: At base of occipital bone.

Function: Extension, lateral flexion and rotation of head and cervical spine.

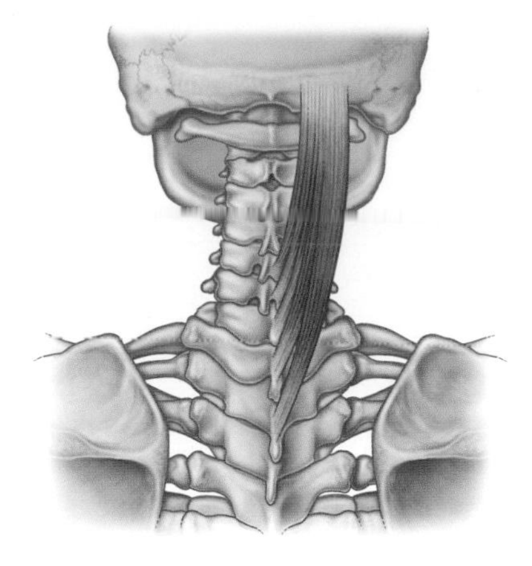

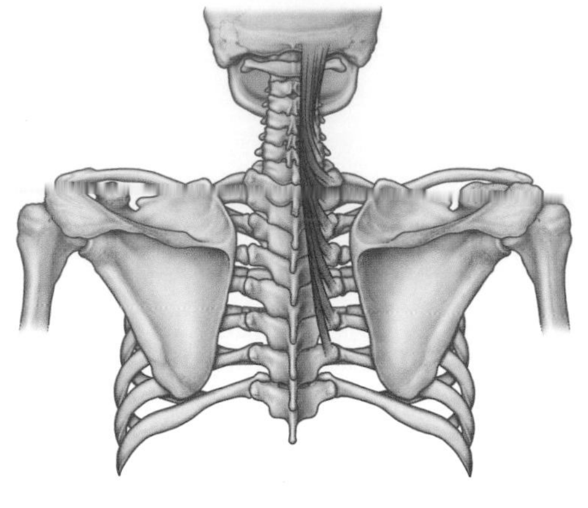

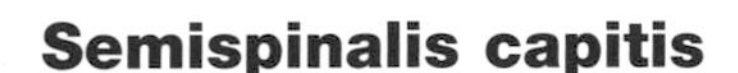

Semispinalis capitis

Nerve, supply: Posterior rami of spinal nerves, C1–Th6.

Origin: Transverse processes of Th1–4 (7) and articular processes of C3–7.

Insertion: Between the superior and inferior nuchal line of skull, occipital bone.

Function: Extension, lateral flexion and rotation of head.

Stretching technique:

Patient is lying on back, head flexed and supported against therapist. Therapist wraps one hand around the occiput to rotate and laterally flex cervical spine away from the muscle. The hypo-thenar of the other hand presses downward and away from the head on the facet joints next to spinous processes at the level of C3–7. Then the hand is moved over the facet joints at the level of Th1–4 and stretching is repeated.

Tension–relaxation technique: Patient tries to extend neck for 5 sec against the forearm while therapist actively resists. Patient is then instructed to gradually relax muscles while therapist performs stretch.

Notice: The semispinalis capitis is one of the strongest extensor muscles of the neck. The head is supported by the body and therapist's elbow by the hip to avoid excessive loading of upper extremities.

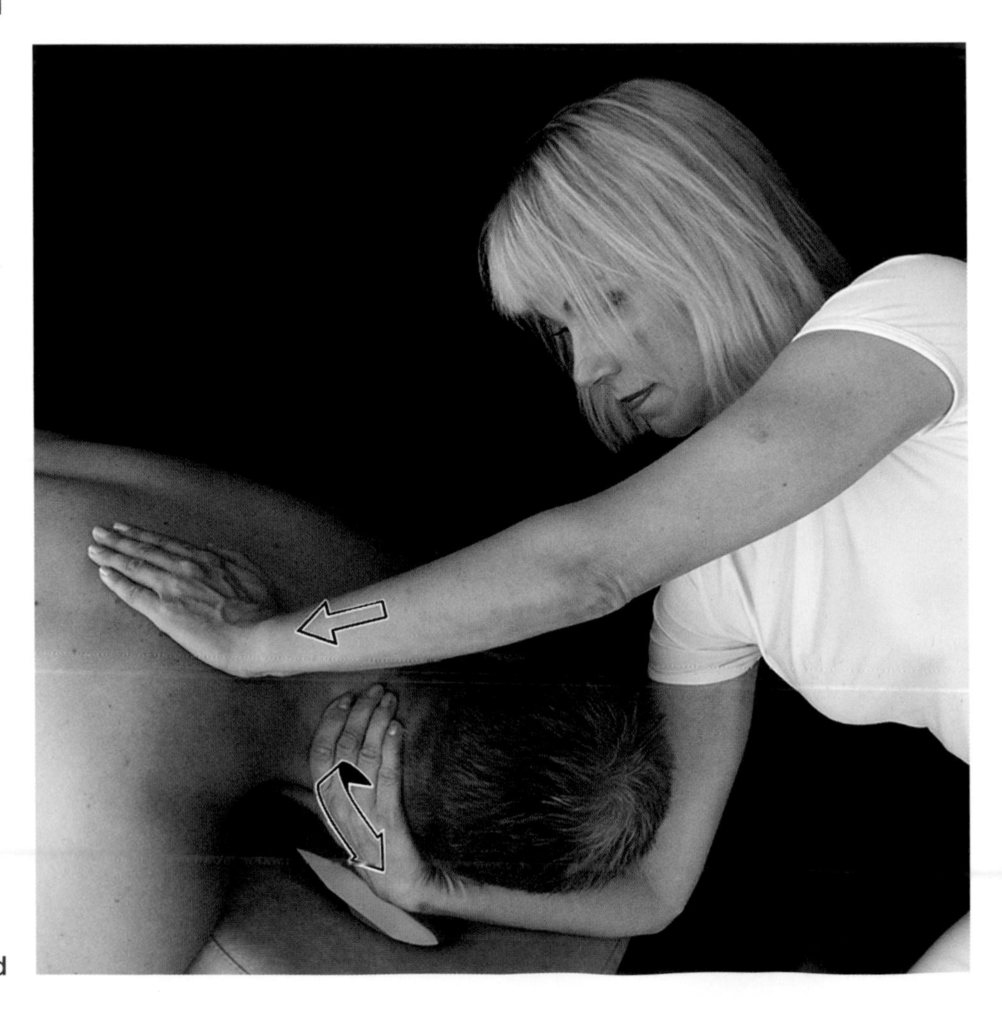

Semispinalis cervicis

Nerve, supply: Posterior rami of spinal nerves, C2–Th6.

Origin: Transverse processes of Th1–6.

Insertion: Cross over at least 4 vertebrae to insert on spinous processes of C2–5.

Function: Rotating lateral flexion and extension of the cervical and thoracic spine.

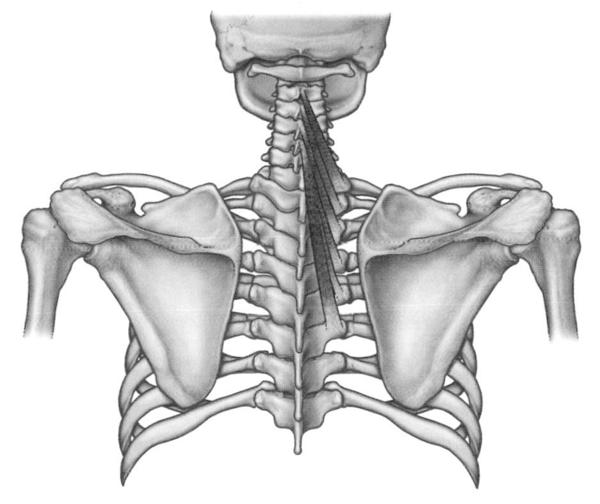

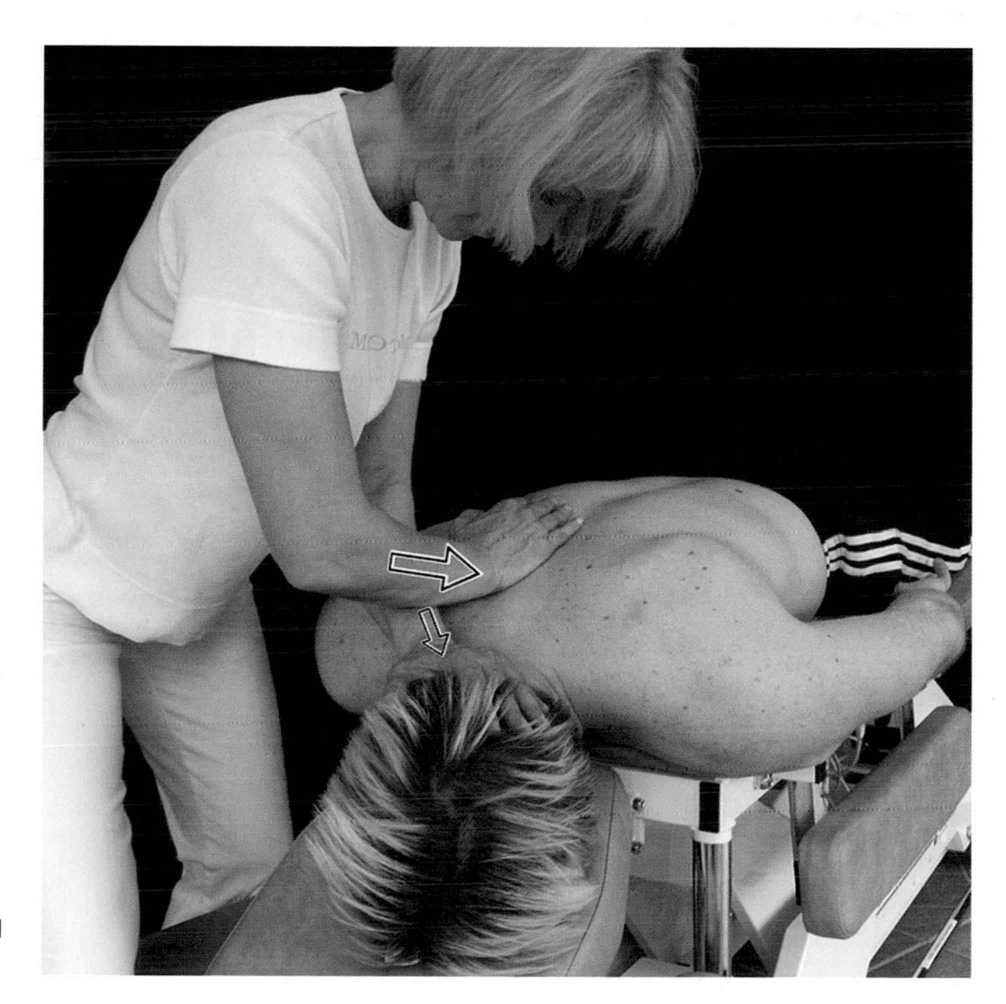

Stretching technique:

Patient is lying on stomach, neck bent slightly away from muscle to be treated without rotation. Therapist presses with the hypothenar next to spinous processes C2–5 on facet joints and applies pressure diagonally up towards the skull. Placing the hypothenar of the other hand next to the spinous processes on the facet joints of Th1–6 of the same side, the therapist presses down diagonally and away from the neck.

Tension–relaxation technique: Patient tries to lift head for 5 sec while therapist resists. Patient is then advised to gradually relax muscles while therapist gently presses cervical spine upwards and thoracic spine downwards.

Semispinalis thoracis

Nerve, supply: Posterior rami of spinal nerves, C1–Th6.

Origin: Transverse processes of Th7–10(12).

Insertion: Cross over at least 5 vertebrae to insert on the spinous processes of C6–Th6.

Function: Rotation lateral flexion and extension of cervical and thoracic spine.

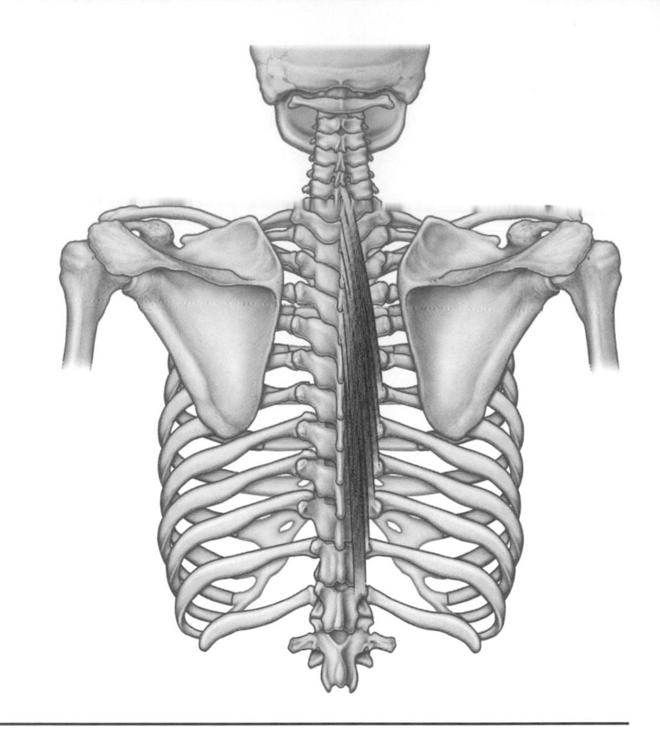

Stretching technique:

Patient is lying on stomach, inferior part of cervical spine rotated and bent to side to expose muscle to be treated. Therapist presses with the hypothenar diagonally upward towards head on the facet joints next to the spinous processes of C2–5. The hypothenar of the other hand presses diagonally down and away from the neck on the facet joints next to the spinous processes of Th1–6 on the same side.

Tension–relaxation technique: Patient tries to extend upper thoracic spine for 5 sec while therapist resists. Patient is then advised to gradually relax muscles while therapist increases stretch.

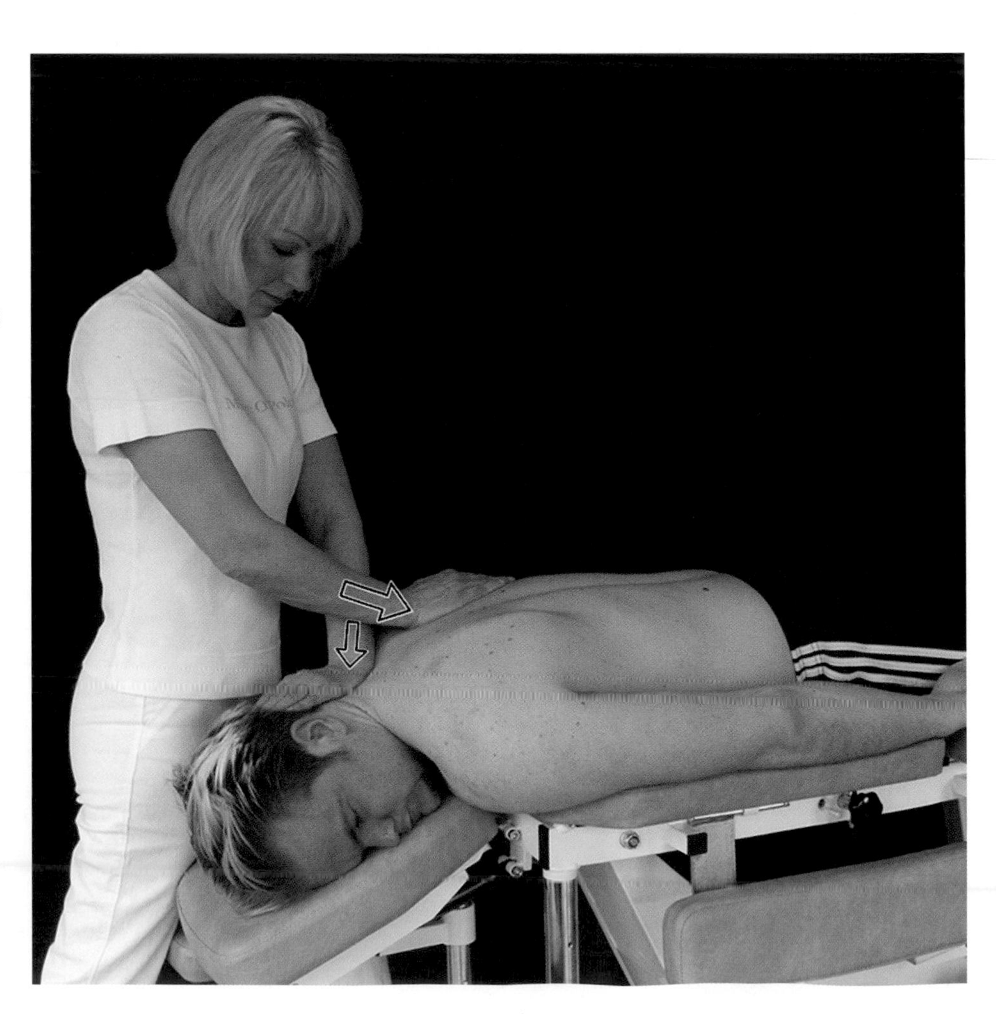

Spinalis cervicis

Nerve, supply: Posterior rami of spinal nerves, C2–Th1.

Origin: Spinous processes of C6–Th2.

Insertion: Spinous processes of C2–4.

Function: Extension of cervical spine.

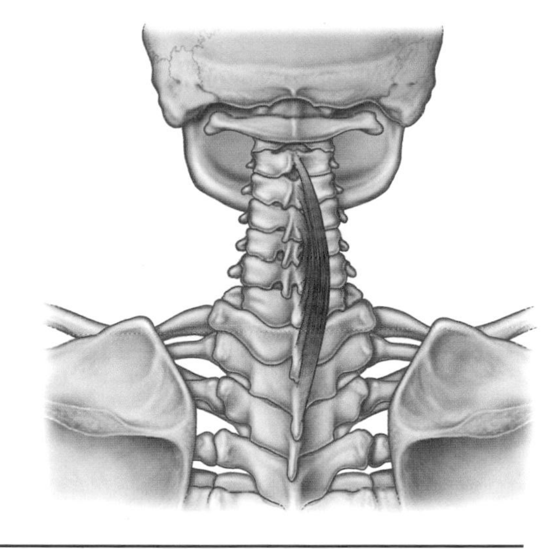

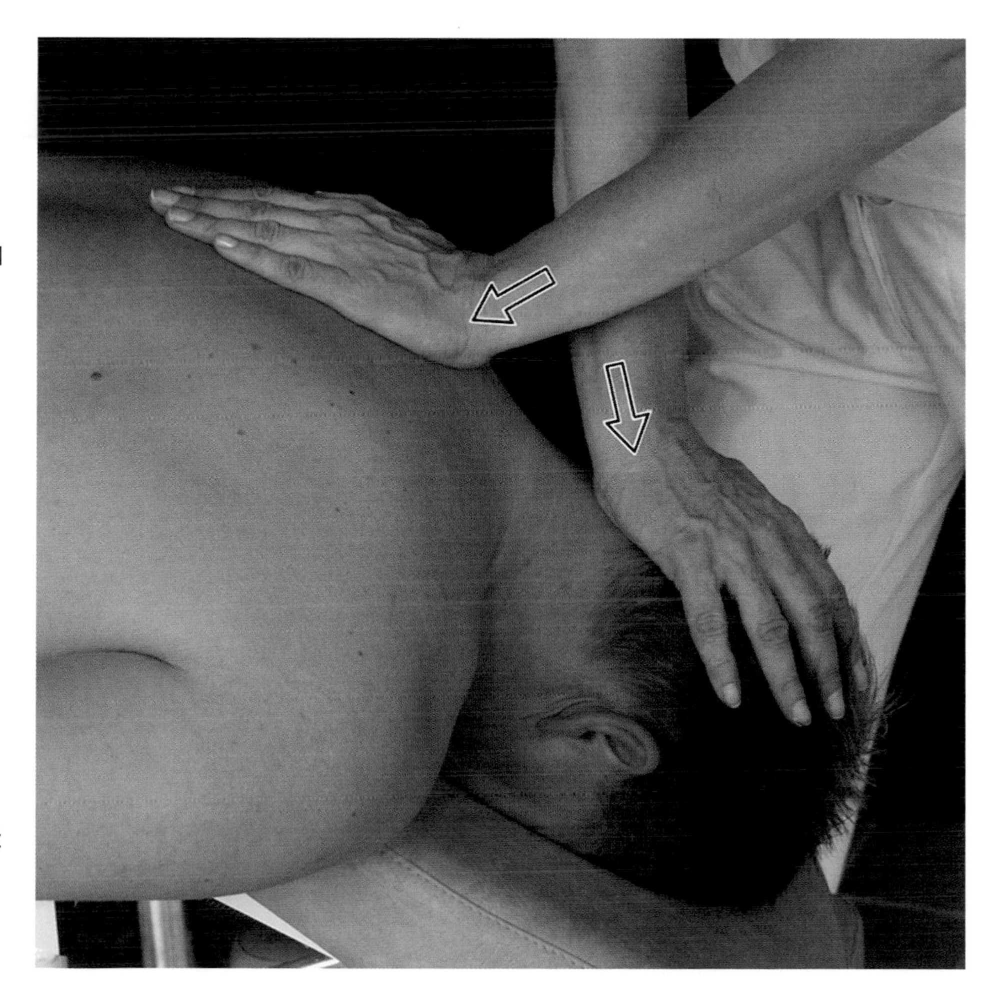

Stretching technique:

Patient is lying on stomach, cervical spine bent noticeably forward. Therapist presses with the hypothenar diagonally upward towards head on the facet joints next to the spinous processes of C2–4. The hypothenar of the other hand presses diagonally down and away from the neck on the facet joints next to the spinous processes of C6–Th2 on the same side.

Tension–relaxation technique: Patient tries to extend neck for 5 sec while therapist resists. Patient is then advised to gradually relax muscles while therapist increases pressure to increase stretch effect.

Posterior superior serratus

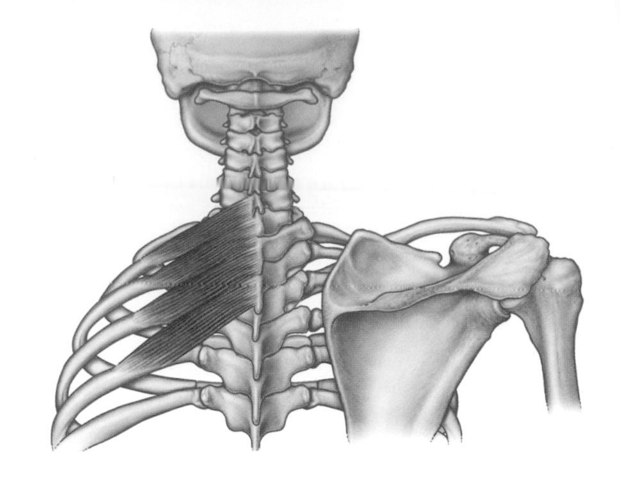

Nerve, supply: Intercostal nerves, Th1–4.

Origin: Ligamentum nuchae, Spinous processes C6–Th2.

Insertion: Ribs 2–5.

Function: Raise ribs. Assist in deep inspiration.

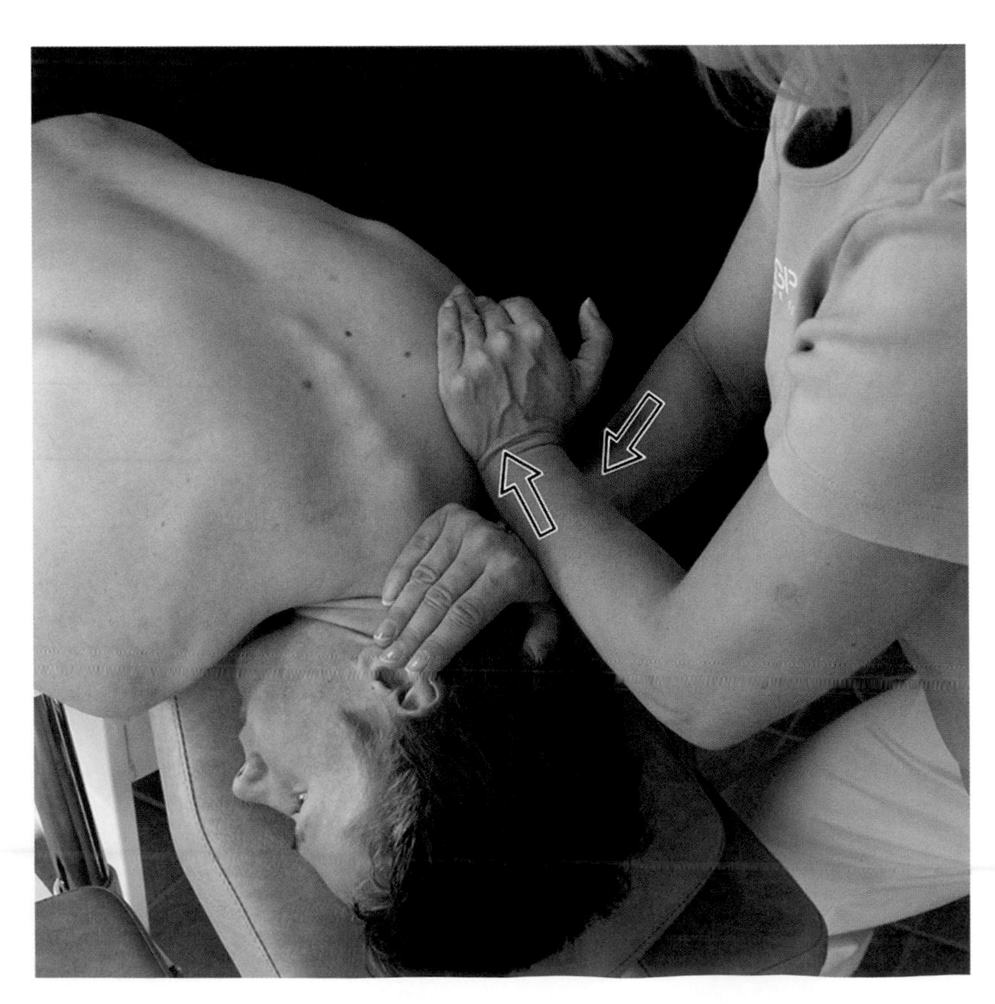

Stretching technique:

Patient is lying on stomach, lower cervical spine flexed forward and head rotated away from muscle to be treated. Therapist presses the hypothenar on the facet joints next to the spinous processes of C6–Th2 towards the head. The hypothenar of the other hand applies pressure diagonally down and to the side on ribs 2–5. The forearms of the therapist are crossed.

Patient takes a deep breath in. Patient is then advised to gradually relax muscles while therapist increases pressure to increase stretch effect.

Interspinales cervicis

(Six pairs of muscles)

Nerve, supply: Posterior rami of spinal nerves, C2–6.

Origin: Spinous processes of C2–7.

Insertion: Spinous processes of next vertebrae below.

Function: Extension of cervical spine.

Interspinalis thoracis

(Upper part; two pairs of muscles)

Nerve, supply: Posterior rami of spinal nerves, Th1–2.

Origin: Spinous processes Th1–2.

Insertion: Spinous processes of next vertebrae below.

Function: Extension of upper thoracic spine.

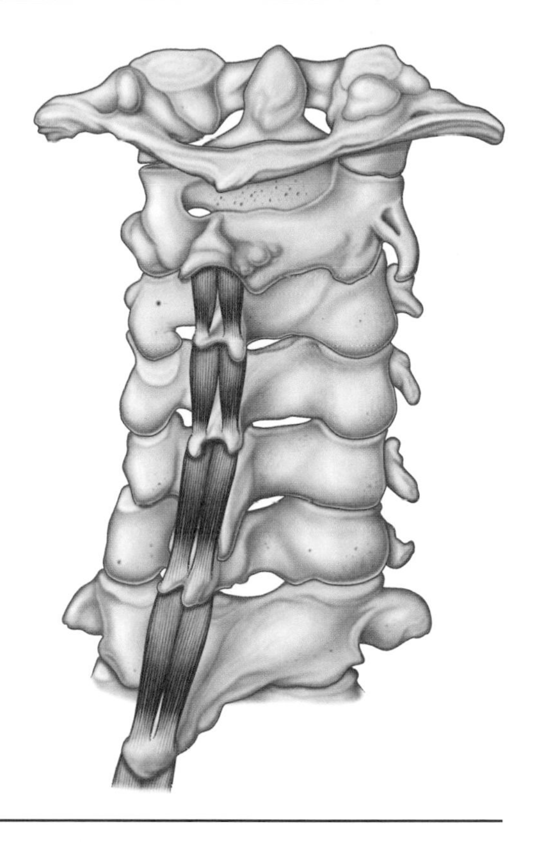

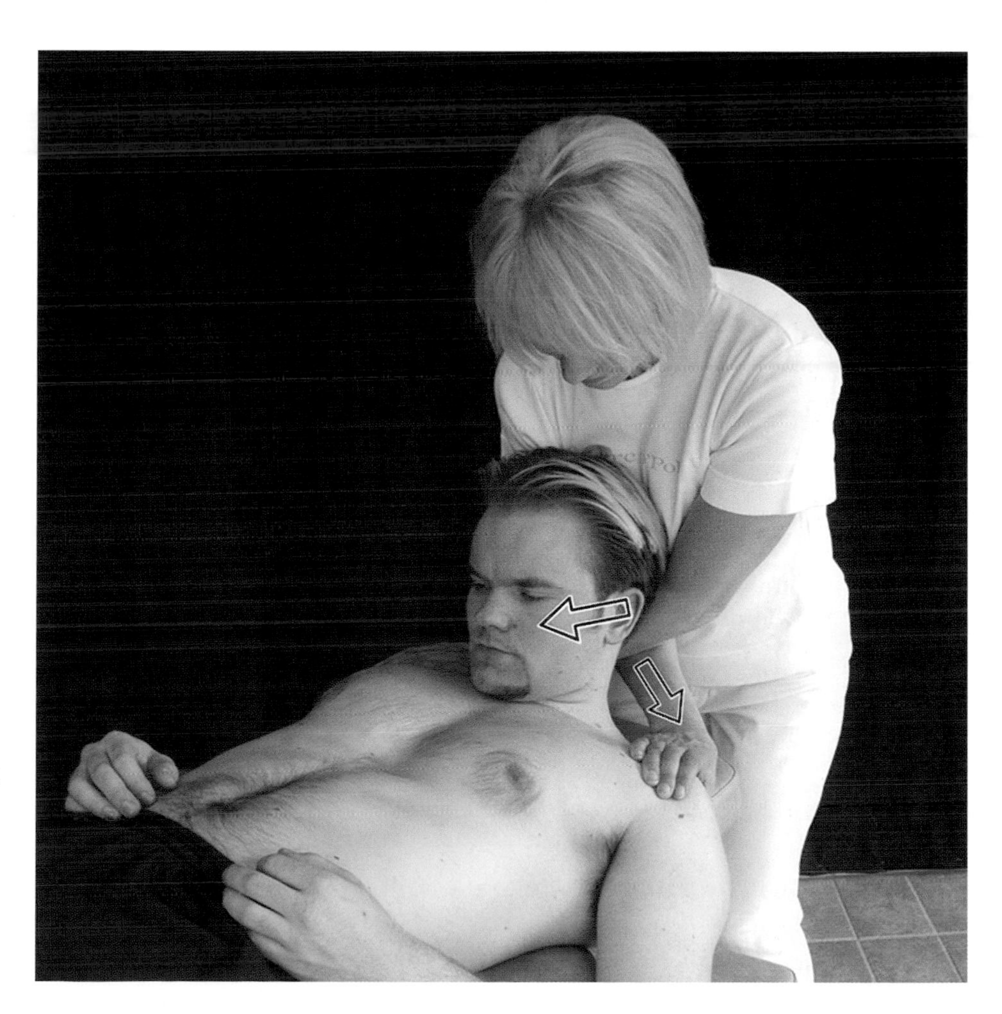

Stretching technique:

Patient is lying on back, head flexed forward. Therapist presses down on shoulders with both hands and with forearms crossed, leans forward and presses the head forward as far as possible.

Tension–relaxation technique: Patient tries to press the head backwards for 5 sec while therapist resists. Patient is then advised to gradually relax muscles while therapist increases stretch by pressing forward with forearms and upper body.

Rectus capitis posterior major

Nerve, supply: Suboccipital nerve, C1.

Origin: Spinous process of axis, C2.

Insertion: Inferior nuchal line at base of occipital bone.

Function: Extension, lateral flexion and rotation of head.

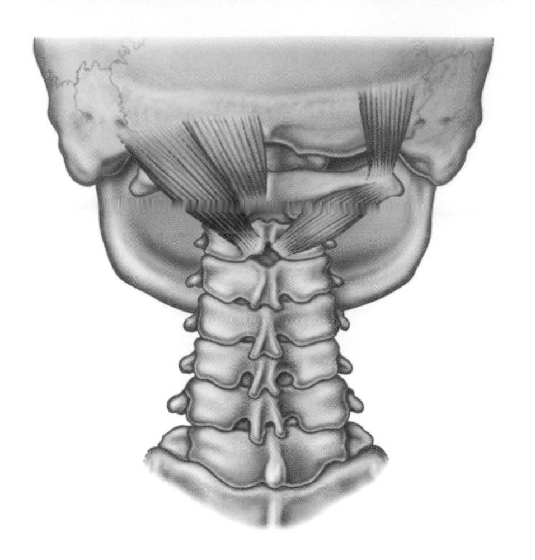

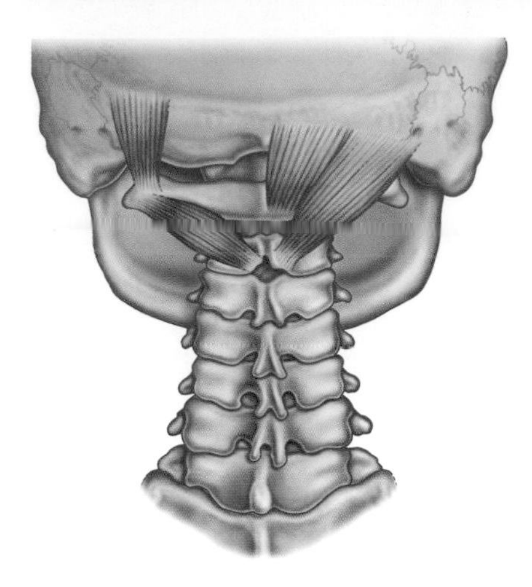

Obliquus capitis inferior

Nerve, supply: Suboccipital nerve, C1.

Origin: Spinous process of axis, C2.

Insertion: Transverse process of atlas, C1.

Function: Rotation of atlas.

Stretching technique:

Patient is lying on back, cervical spine straight, head bent slightly away from muscle to be treated. Therapist cups hand under the cervical spine so that the spinous process of axis rests firmly at the base of the forefinger. Therapist applies pressure with the other hand on the chin to rotate the head towards the side of the muscles to be stretched, while increasing lateral flexion to the contralateral side, and pulls diagonally back at about a 45° angle.

Tension–relaxation technique: Patient tries to extend neck for 5 sec while therapist resists. Patient is then advised to gradually relax muscles while therapist presses chin diagonally back to increase stretch further.

Notice: This technique should not be applied in cases of instability at the atlanto axial joint in rheumatoid arthritis or after high energy cervical trauma.

Warning ! The head is bent to the side so much that movement occurs only in the superior cervical spine and the same applies to rotation. There should not be extension of the cervical spine but slight forward flexion instead.

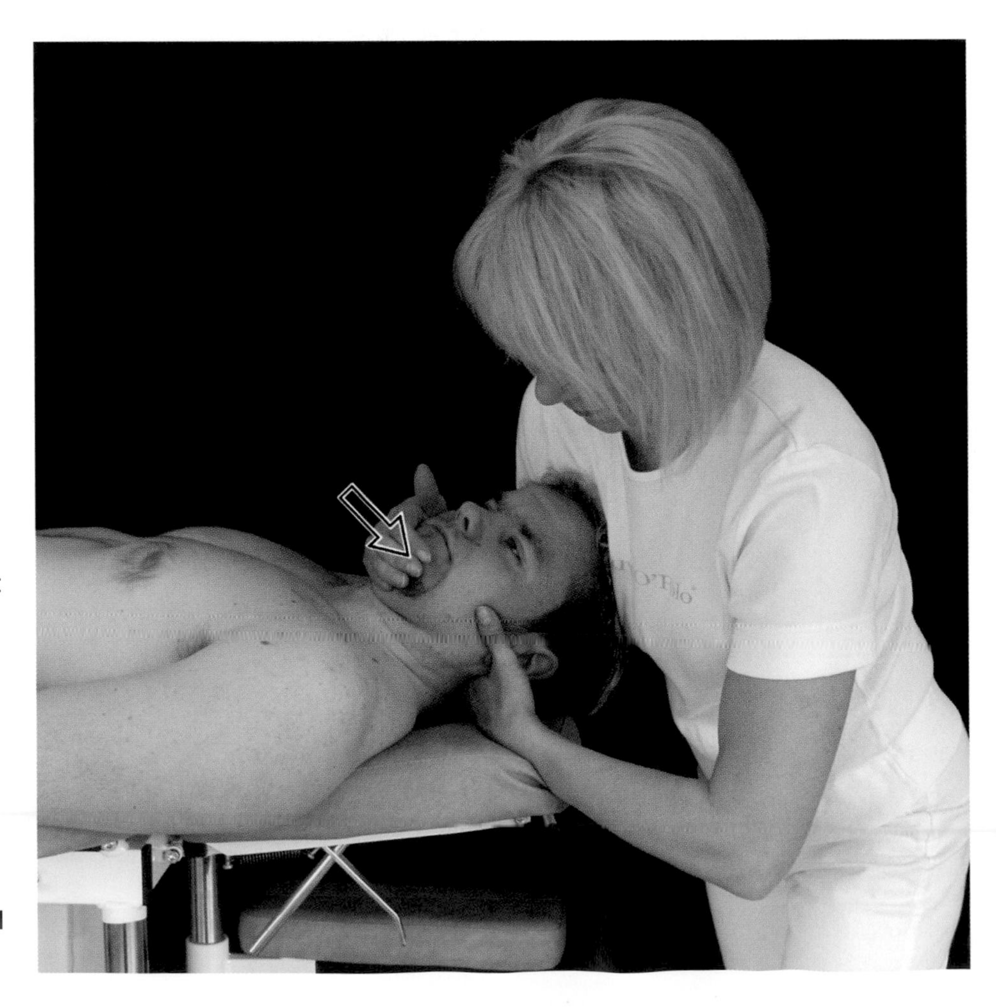

Rectus capitis posterior minor

Nerve, supply: Suboccipital nerve, C1.

Origin: Posterior arch of atlas, C1.

Insertion: Inferior nuchal line at base of skull.

Function: Rotation, lateral flexion and extension of head.

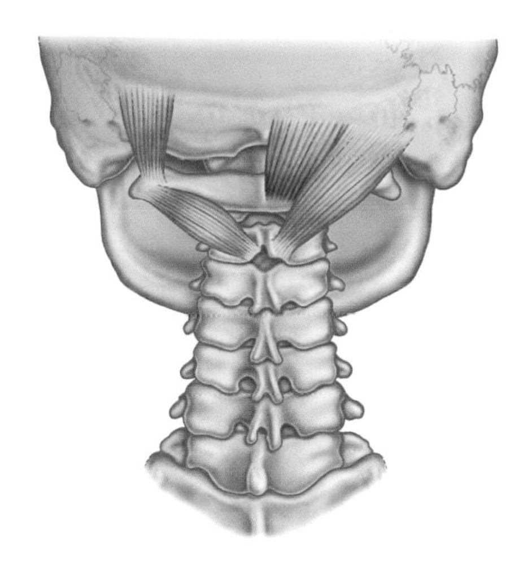

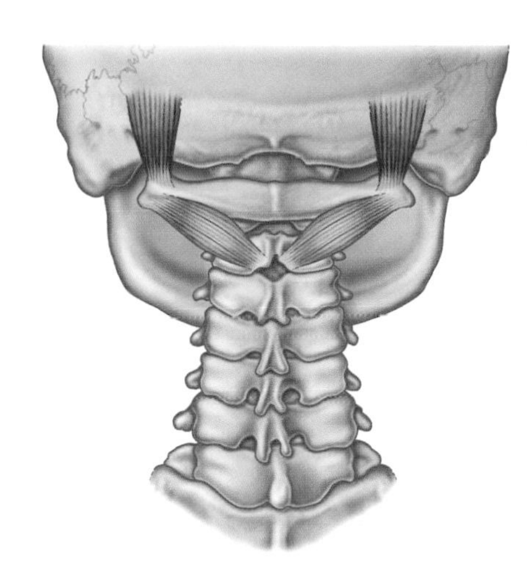

Obliquus capitis superior

Nerve, supply: Suboccipital nerve, C1.

Origin: Transverse process of atlas, C1.

Insertion: Occipital bone at base of skull.

Function: Rotation, lateral flexion and extension of head.

Stretching technique:

Patient is lying on back, cervical spine straight. Therapist cups hand under the cervical spine so that the posterior arch of atlas rests firmly at the base of the forefinger. Therapist applies pressure with the other hand on the chin and pulls back at about a 45° angle.

Tension–relaxation technique: Patient tries to extend head for 5 sec while therapist resists. Patient is then instructed to gradually release tension while therapist pulls chin to improve stretch effect.

Notice: This technique should not be applied in cases of instability at the atlanto axial joint in rheumatoid arthritis or after high energy cervical trauma.

Warning ❗ Upper cervical spine should not be extended. It should be in slight forward flexion during stretch.

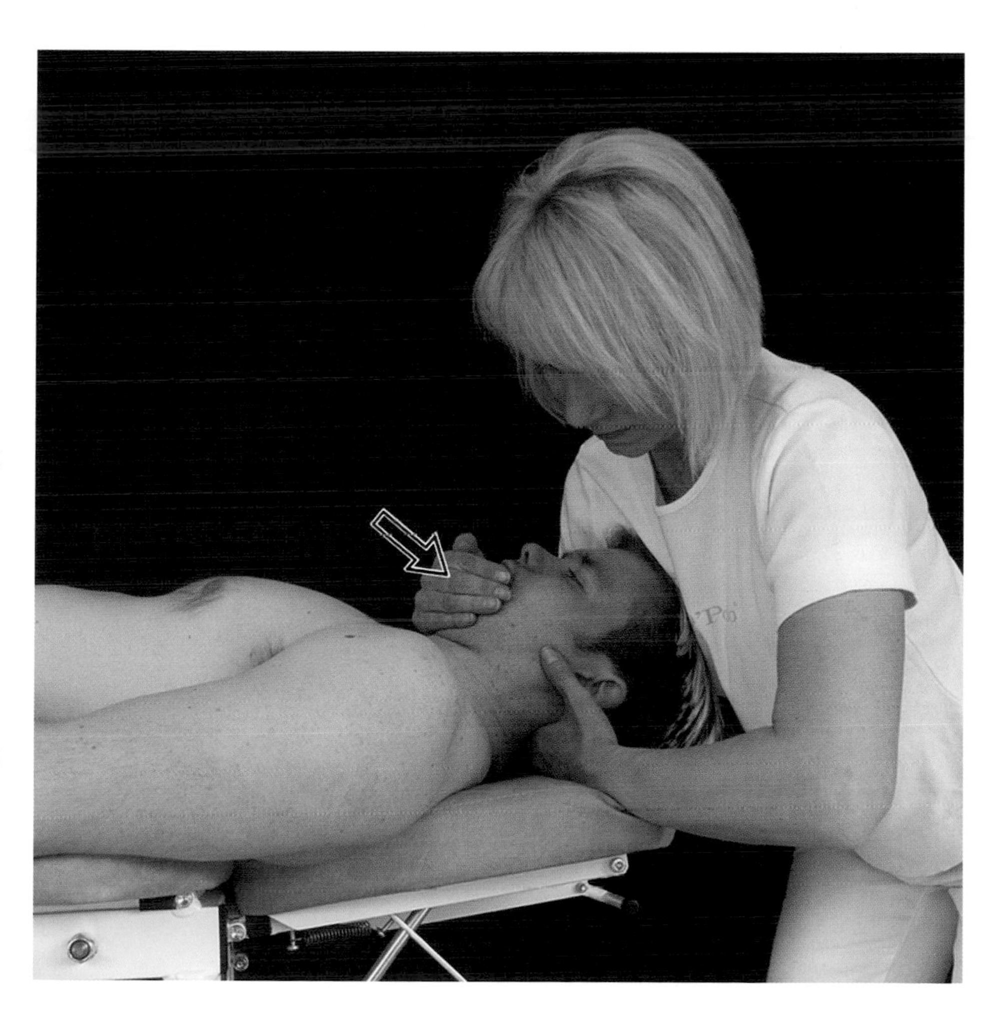

Rectus capitis lateralis

Nerve, supply: Ventral rami of spinal nerves, C1–2.

Origin: Transverse process of atlas, C1.

Insertion: Jugular process of the occipital bone at base of skull.

Function: Stabilization and lateral flexion of head.

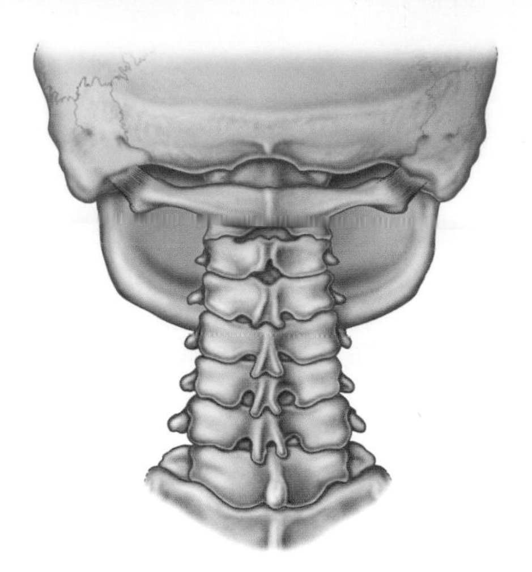

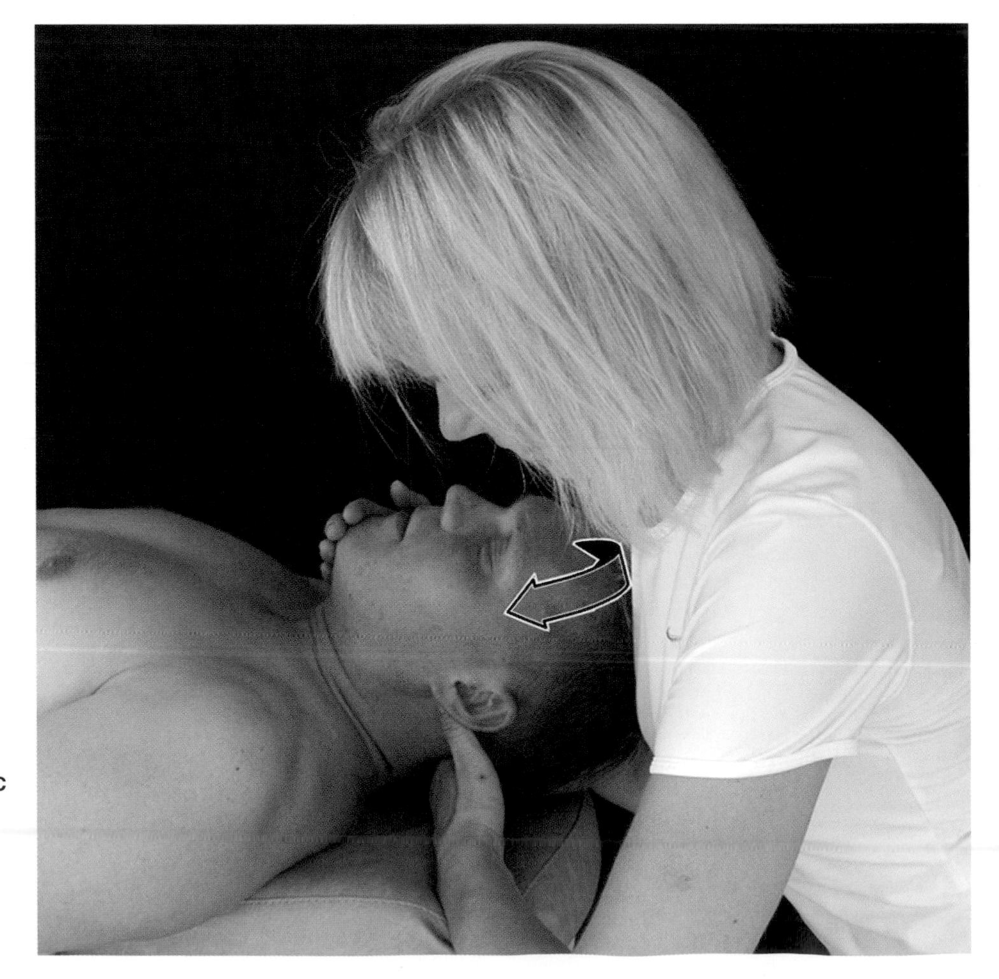

Stretching technique:

Patient is lying on back, cervical spine straight. Therapist cups hand under the head so that the occiput rests on the base of the forefinger. Therapist grasps under the chin and applies pressure with the forearm of the other hand on the side of the head and sidebends only the upper cervical joints.

Tension–relaxation technique: Patient tries to sidebend the head towards opposite direction for 5 sec while therapist resists. Patient is then instructed to gradually release tension while therapist increases stretch effect.

Intertransversarii muscles

Nerve, supply: posterior rami of spinal nerves, C2–C7.

Anterior intertransversarii muscles

Origin: anterior tubercles of transverse processes of C2–6.

Insertion: Transverse processes of next vertebrae below.

Posterior intertransversarii muscles

Origin: Posterior tubercles of transverse processes of C2–6.

Insertion: Transverse processes of next vertebrae below.

Function: Stabilization and lateral flexion of vertebrae.

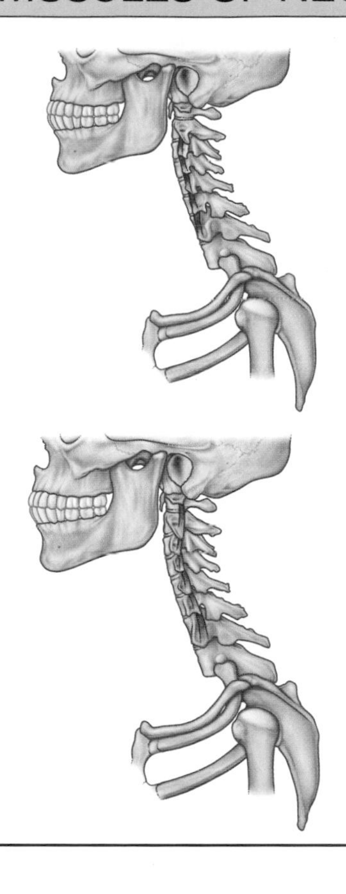

Stretching technique:

Patient is lying on back and therapist holds the head with both hands with index finger just under the occiput. The head is bent to the side from just below the grip. The stretch effect is strongest between the joints immediately inferior to the position of the therapist's hands. By replacing hands and progressing down the cervical spine from joint to joint, stretching can be intensified with each muscle the head and neck are straightened each time as the place of grip is moved.

Tension–relaxation technique: Patient attempts to extend head for 5 sec while therapist resists. Patient is then instructed to gradually relax muscles while the therapist increases the stretch further.

Notice: This technique is very specific. There should not be pressure down on the shoulder. It would result in stretching of only the trapezius muscle.

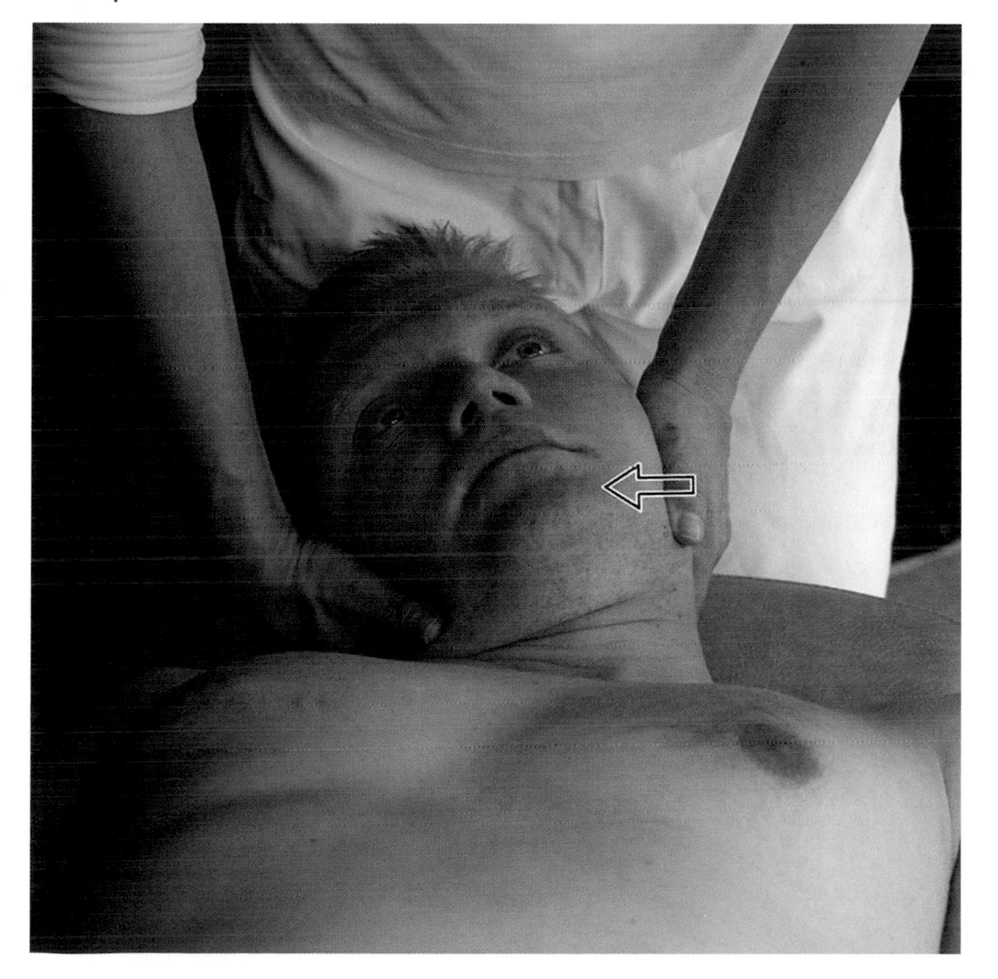

Multifidus cervicis

Nerve, supply: Posterior rami of spinal nerves, C3–4.

Origin: Articular processes of C5–7.

Insertion: Cross over two or three vertebrae to insert at spinous processes of C2–4.

Function: Stabilization extension, rotation and lateral flexion of cervical spine.

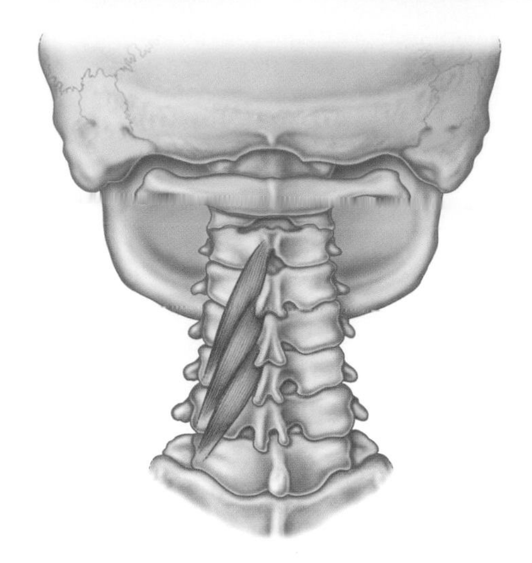

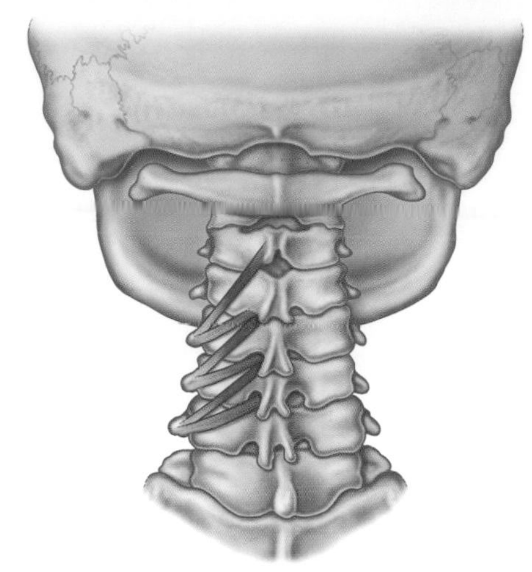

Rotator cervicis

Nerve, supply: Posterior rami of spinal nerves, C3–7.

Origin: Transverse processes of cervical vertebrae.

Insertion of short muscles: Lamina at base of the spinous process of the next higher vertebrae.

Insertion of long muscles: Lamina at base of the spinous process of the second higher vertebrae.

Function: Stabilization extension, rotation and lateral flexion of cervical spine.

Stretching technique:

Patient is lying on back and therapist holds the head and neck with both hands so that fingers overlay each other fully. Therapist supports the head and neck in slightly flexed position and rotates and lateral flexes the cervical spine to the same side. The stretch effect is most intense on the deep muscles of the vertebral joint immediately inferior to area of contact. Muscles of each joint can be individually treated by moving hands on the facet joints of the adjacent vertebrae, working down the spine.

Tension–relaxation technique: Patient attempts to rotate head for 5 sec while therapist resists. Patient is then instructed to gradually relax muscles while the therapist increases the stretch further.

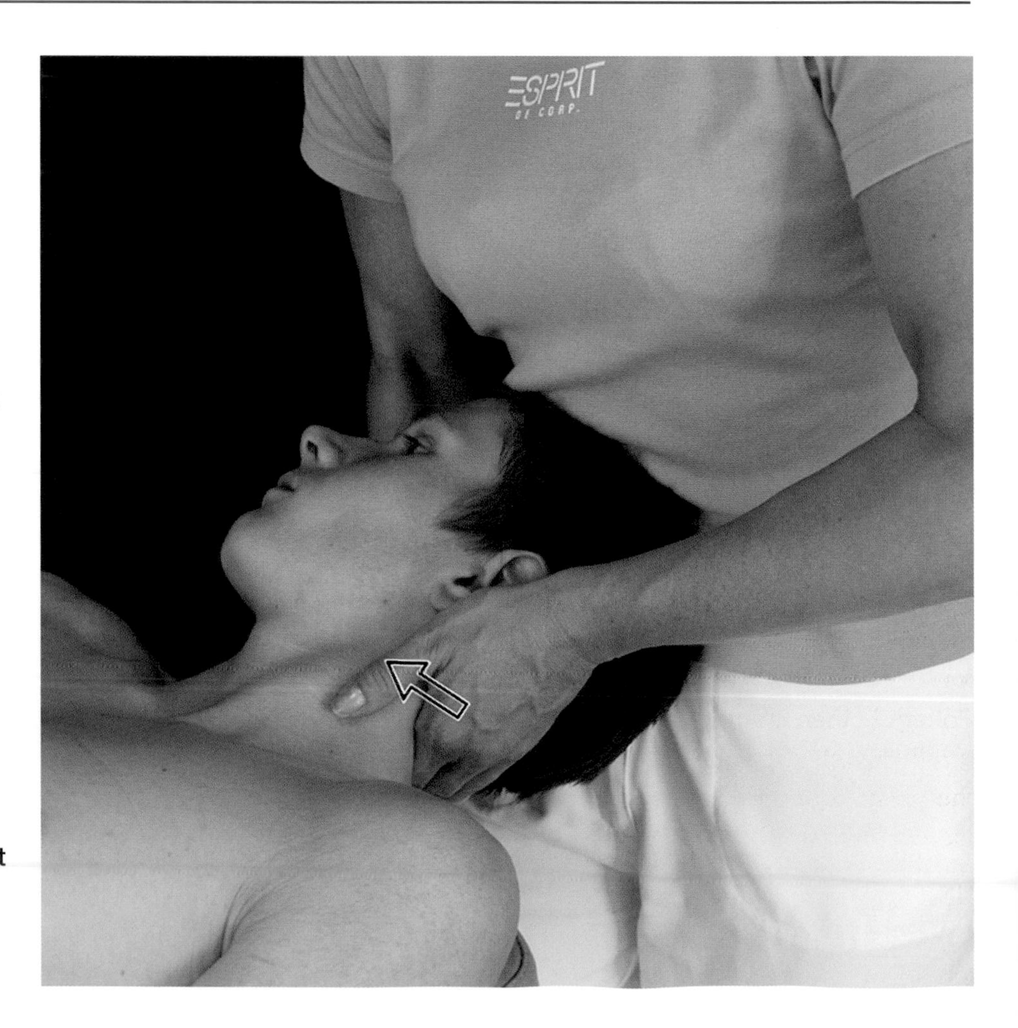

Deltoid anterior part of the deltoid muscle

Nerve, supply: Axillary nerve, C4–6.

Origin: Lateral third of the clavicle, the acromion, and the lower border of the spine of the scapula.

Insertion: Deltoid tuberosity on the humerus.

Function: Flexion and internal rotation of the shoulder joint.

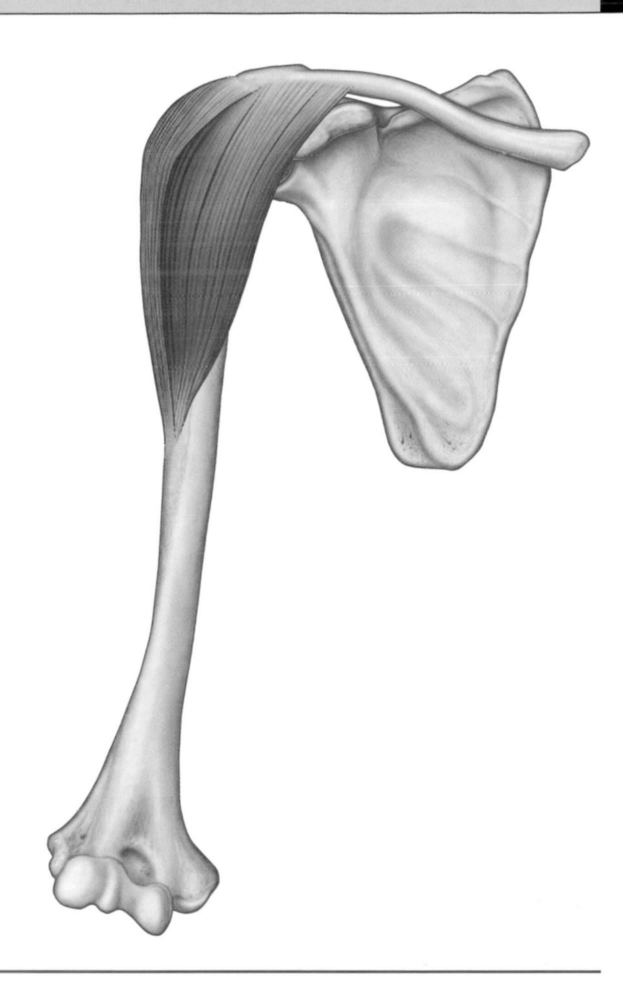

Stretching technique (extension):

Patient is lying on back and therapist uses the thenar of hand to press up, away from muscle insertion. Stretch is improved by pressing down on upper arm with other hand.

Tension–relaxation technique: Patient tries to flex shoulder joint for 5 sec while therapist resists. Patient is then instructed to gradually relax muscles while therapist extends shoulder joint to increase stretch.

Notice: Patient's elbow is slightly flexed to avoid stretching of the long head of the biceps.

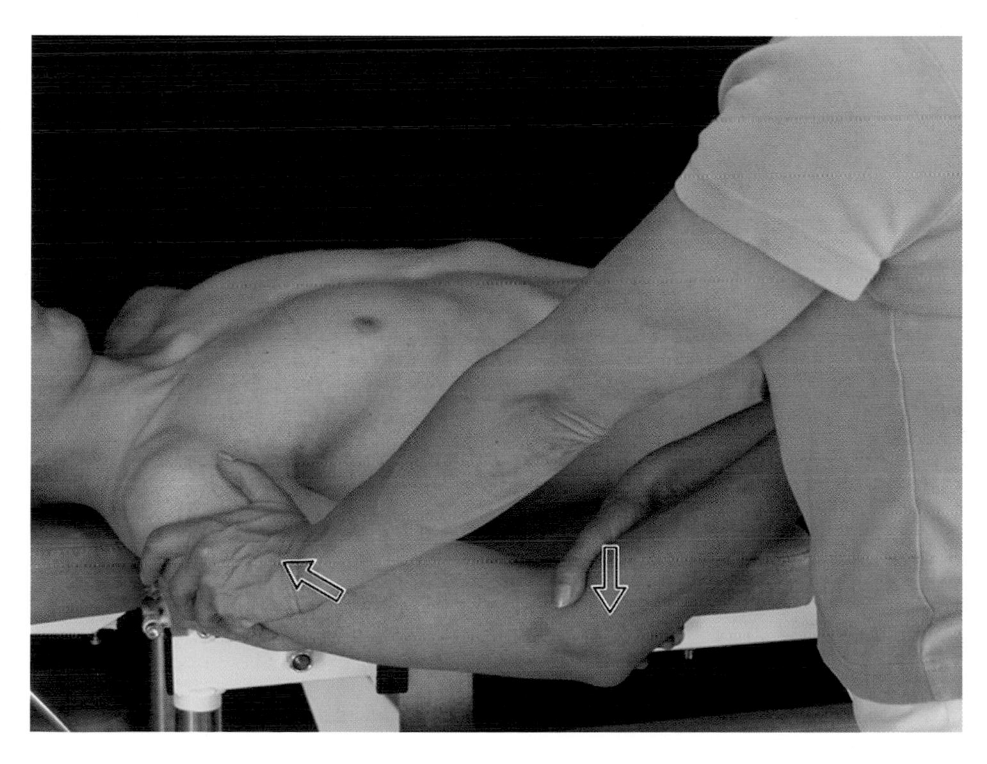

Deltoid

(Medial part of the deltoid muscle)

Function: Abduction.

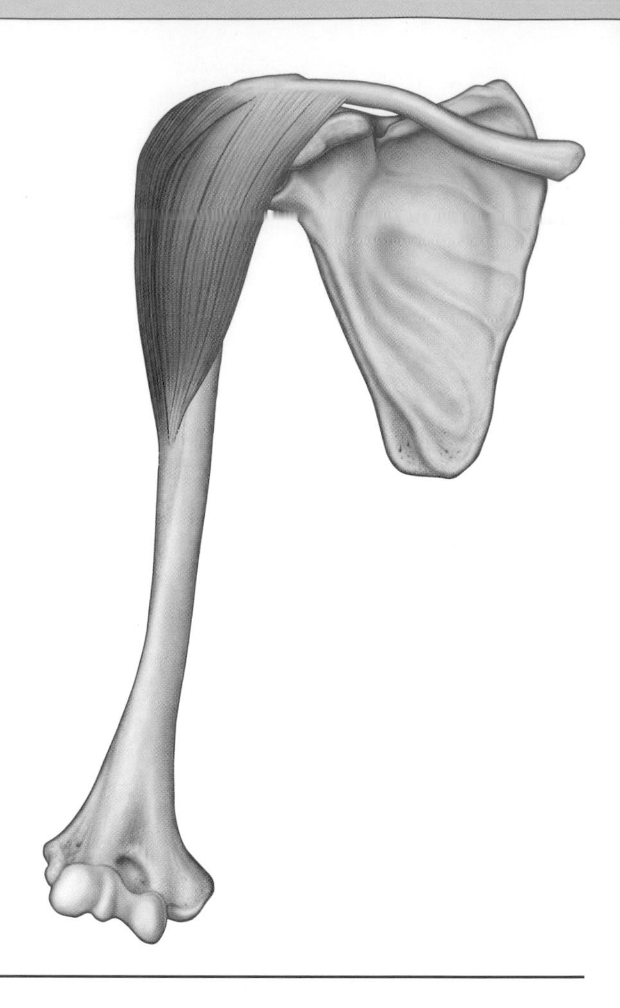

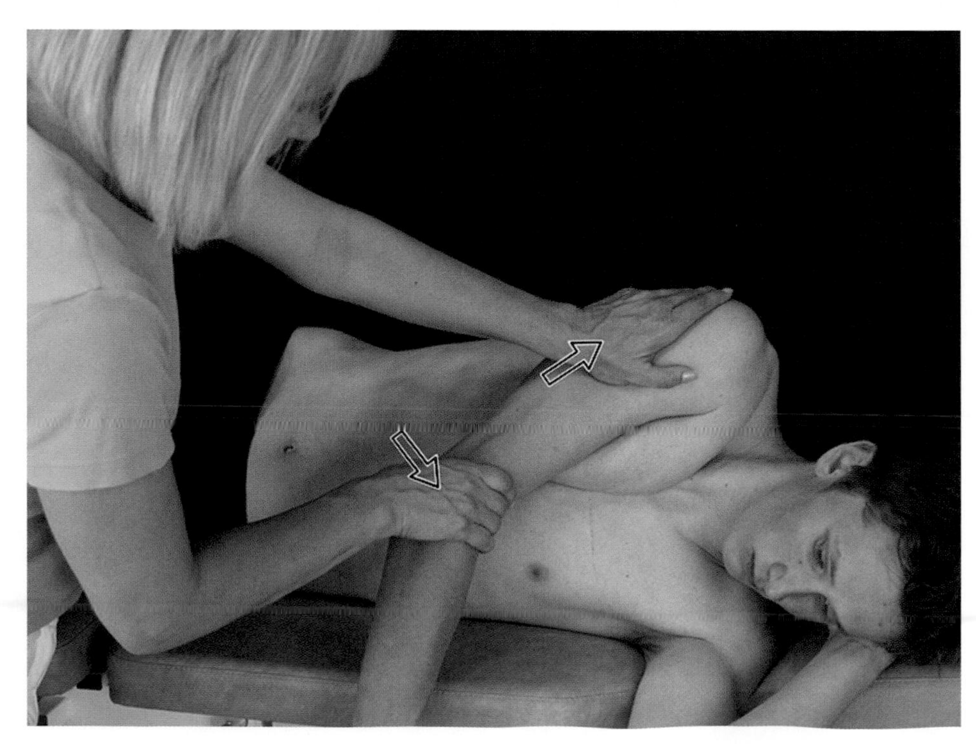

Stretching technique (adduction):

Patient is lying on side and therapist uses the thenar of hand to press immediately above insertion towards the body of muscle. The stretch effect is improved by pressing upper arm down in front of chest.

Tension–relaxation technique: Patient tries to abduct shoulder joint for 5 sec while therapist resists. The patient is then instructed to gradually relax muscle while therapist increases stretch.

Deltoid

(Posterior part of the deltoid muscle)

Function: Extension and external rotation of the shoulder joint.

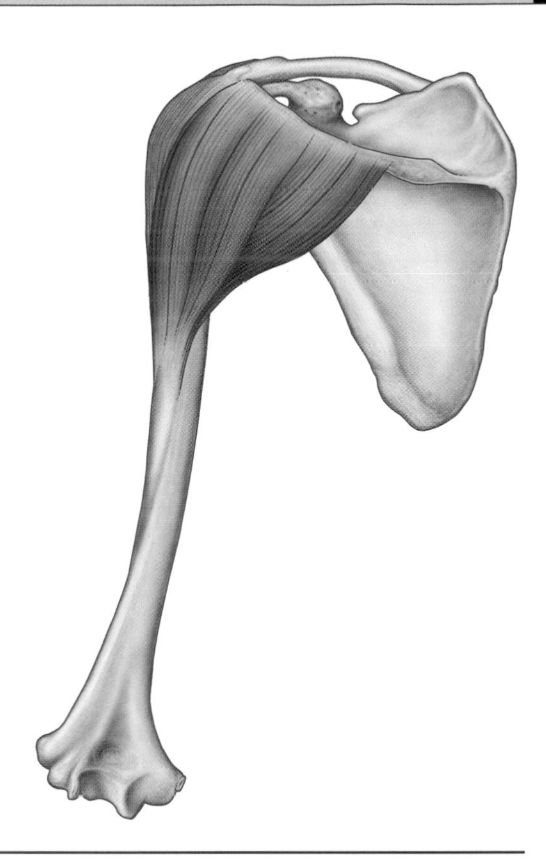

Stretching technique:

Patient is lying on back with arm raised up beside head and shoulder joint flexed to approximately 135°. The therapist, using the thenar of one hand, stretches the muscle beginning proximal to the insertion and pressing along the body of the deltoid. The stretch will be more effective if the arm is pressed downward on the elbow using the other hand.

Tension–relaxation technique: Patient tries to extend shoulder for 5 sec while therapist resists. Patient is then instructed to gradually relax while therapist increases pressure to further stretch muscle.

Notice: Elbow joint should be kept slightly flexed to avoid stretching process to prevent the long head of triceps.

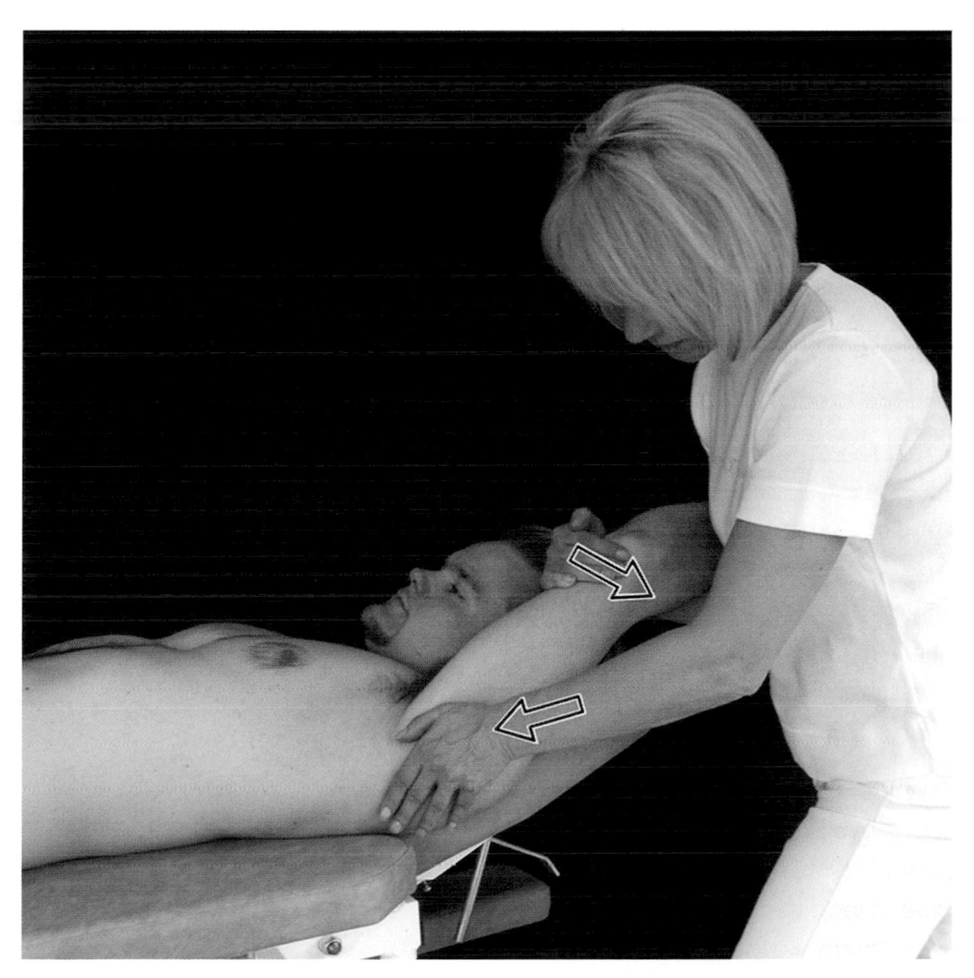

Supraspinatus

Nerve, supply: Suprascapular nerve, C4–6.

Origin: Supraspinous fossa on the posterior surface of the scapula.

Insertion: Joint capsule and greater tubercle of the humerus.

Function: Abduction and external rotation of the shoulder joint.

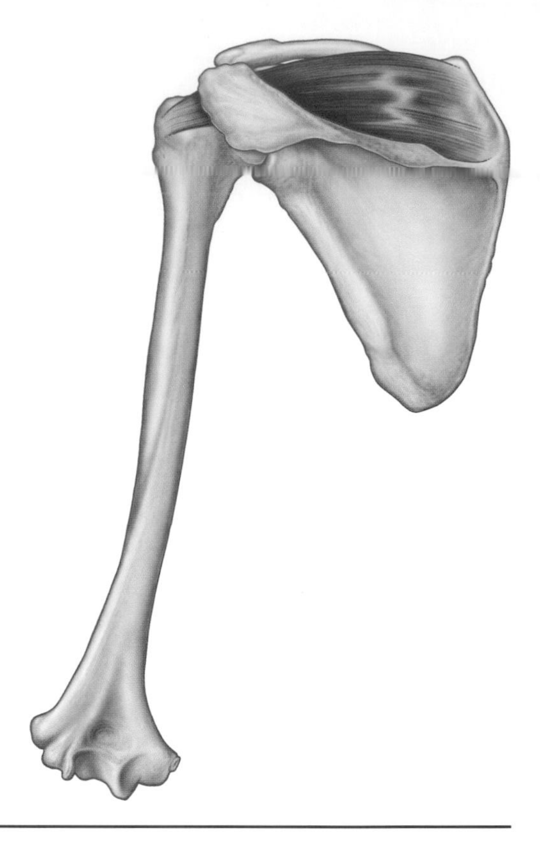

Stretching technique (extension + adduction + internal rotation):

Patient is lying on side with arm drawn behind back and internally rotated. Therapist further extends and adducts arm by applying pressure at elbow while the other hand presses upon the body of the muscle towards the origin.

Tension–relaxation technique: Patient tries to abduct arm for 5 sec while the therapist resists. Patient is then instructed to gradually relax muscles while the therapist increases the stretch.

Notice: This stretch can be made more effective by placing a flexible round object in the armpit to act as a lever and expose the head of the humerus from the joint socket.

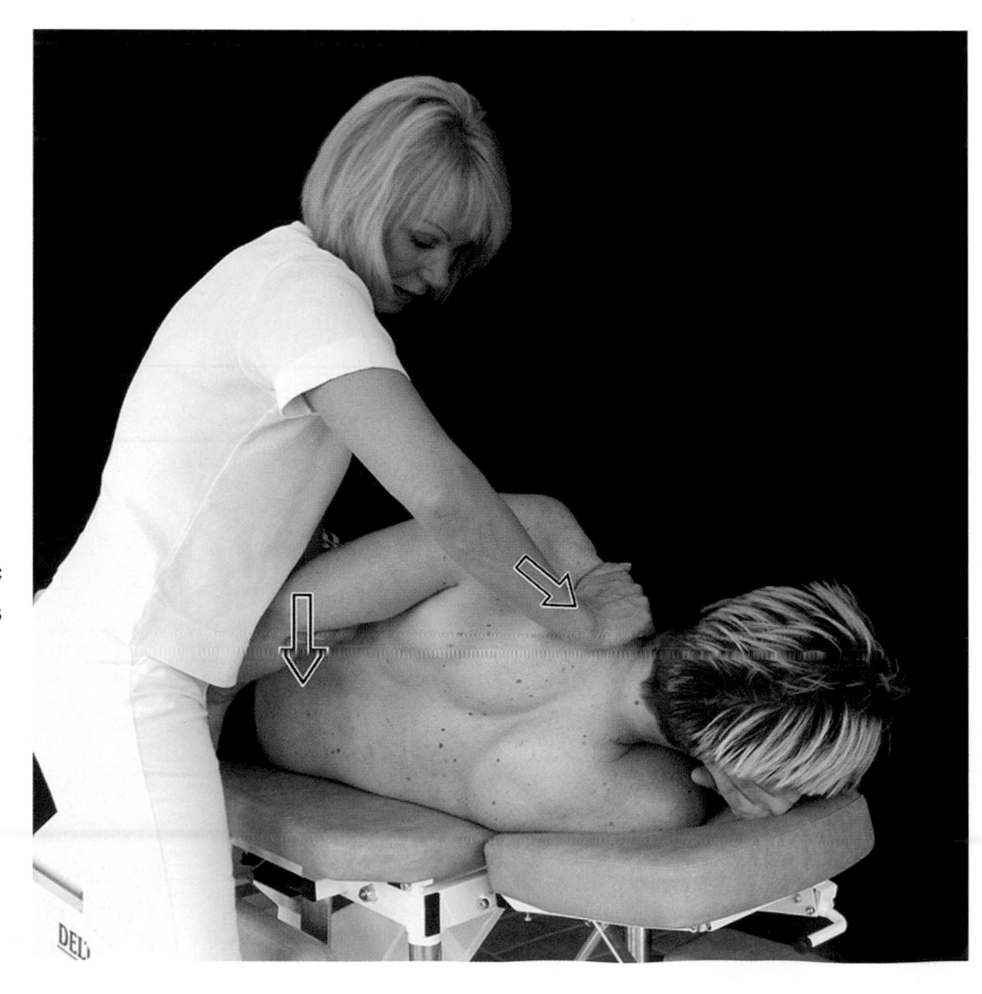

Infraspinatus

Nerve, supply: Suprascapular nerve, C4–6.

Origin: Infraspinatus fossa and the spine of scapula.

Insertion: Joint capsule and greater tubercle of the humerus.

Function: External rotation and abduction of the shoulder joint.

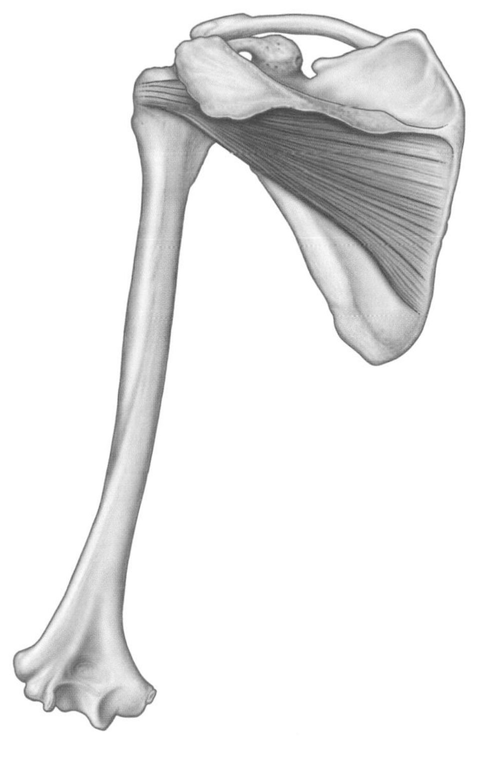

Stretching technique A (flexion + abduction + internal rotation):

Patient is lying on side with shoulder joint abducted to 135° and elbow flexed about 90°. Therapist uses the thenar of the hand to stretch along the body of the muscle away from the insertion while internally rotating and pulling down on the elbow with the other hand.

Tension–relaxation technique: Patient tries to externally rotate upper arm while therapist resists. Patient is then instructed to gradually relax muscles while therapist gently increases abduction and internal rotation.

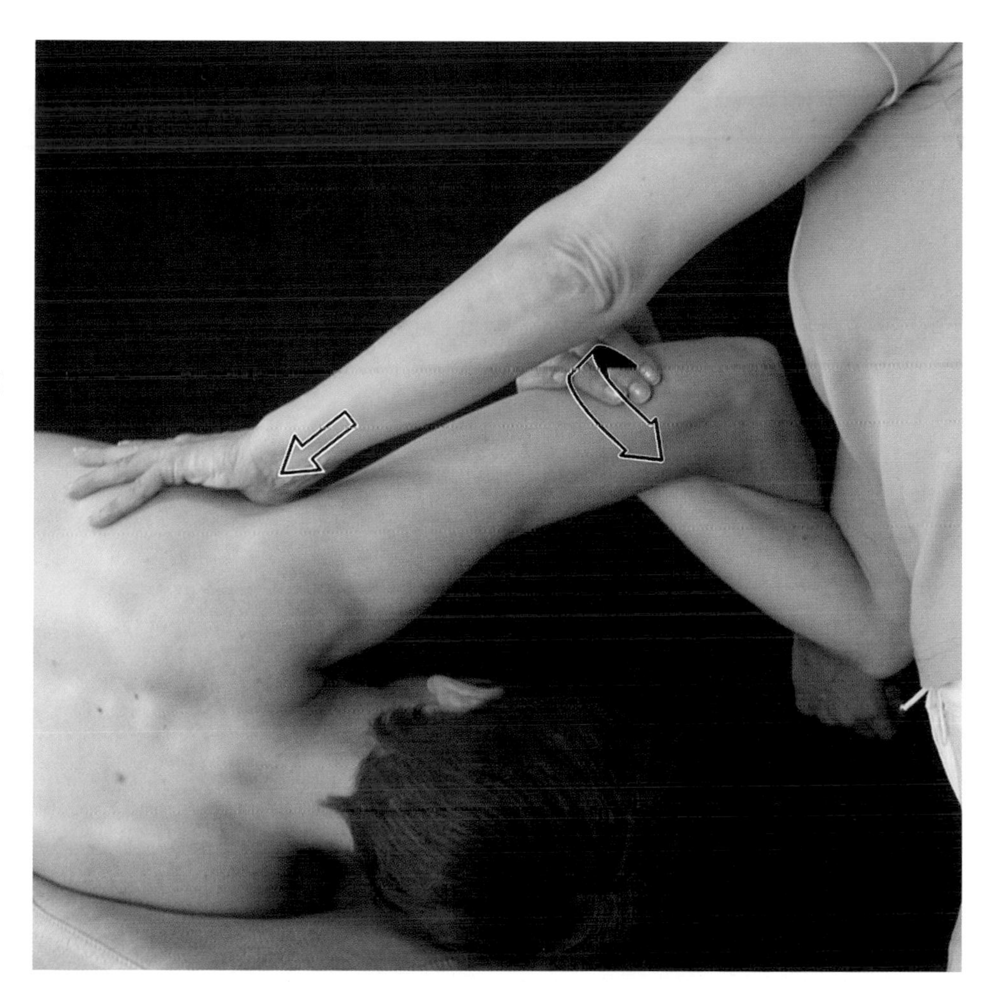

Teres minor

Nerve, supply: Axillary Nerve, C5–6.

Origin: Posterior, lateral border of the scapula.

Insertion: Joint capsule and lower facet of the greater tubercle of the humerus.

Function: External rotation of the shoulder joint.

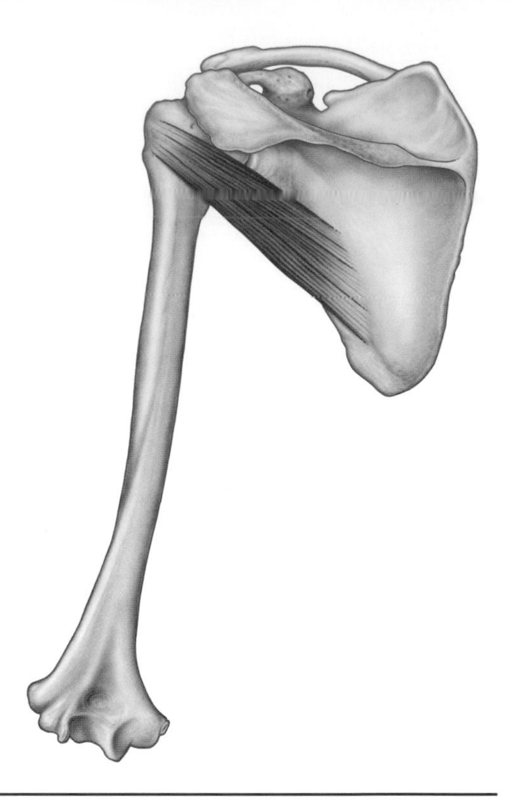

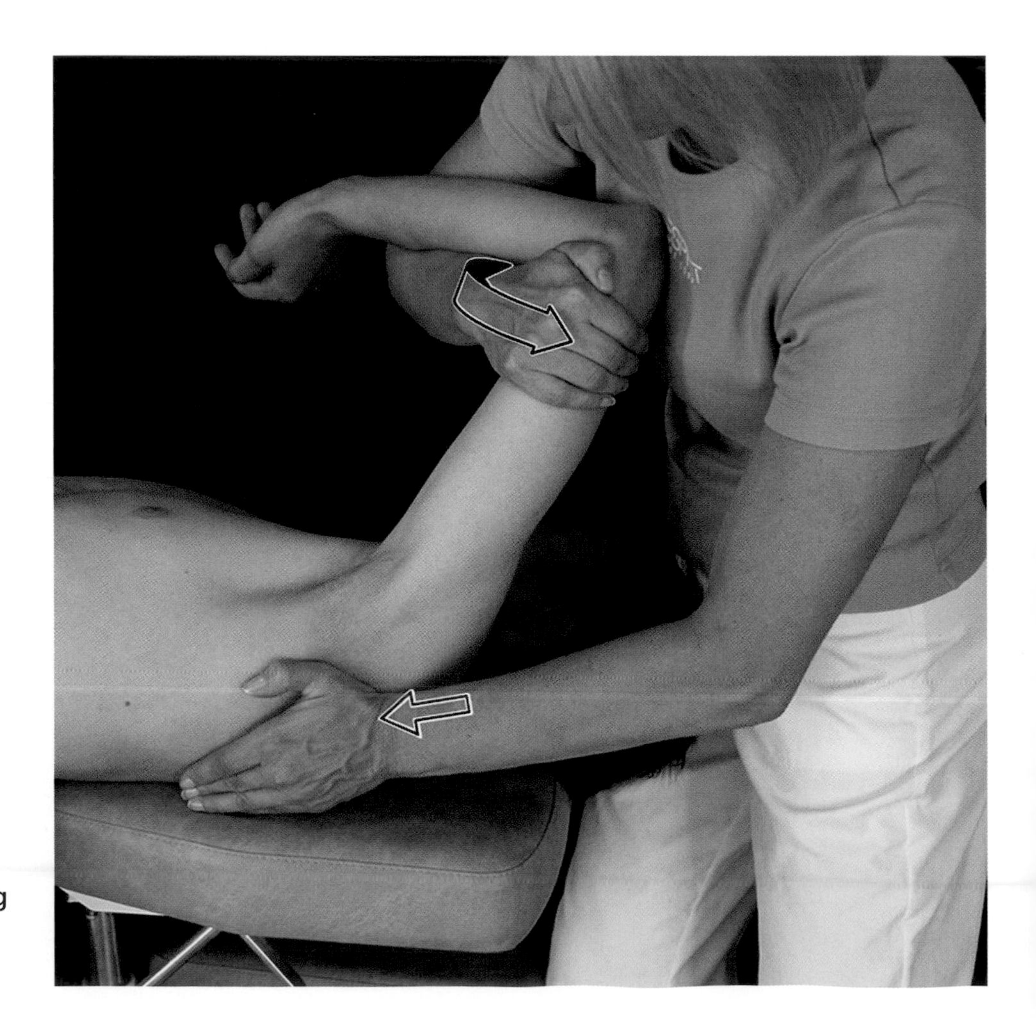

Stretching technique B (flexion + abduction + internal rotation):

Patient is lying on back with shoulder joint flexed about 120° and elbow flexed 90°. Therapist uses the thenar of the hand to stretch along the body of the muscle away from the insertion while internally rotating and pulling down on the elbow with the other hand.

Teres major

Nerve, supply: Subscapular nerve, C6–7.

Origin: Posterior, inferior border of the scapula.

Insertion: Crest of lesser tubercle of the humerus.

Teres major may join with the latissimus dorsi muscle or not exist at all.

Function: Internal rotation, extension and adduction of the shoulder joint.

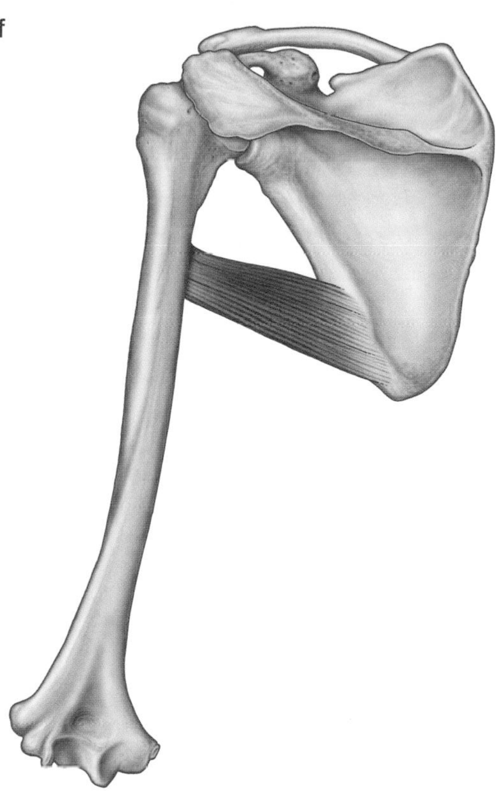

Stretching technique (external rotation + flexion + abduction):

Patient is lying on side with the shoulder joint flexed to 135° and elbow to 90°. Therapist presses along body of muscle with the thenar of the hand, while pulling down and rotating outwards on the elbow with the other hand.

Tension–relaxation technique: Patient tries to internally rotate shoulder joint while therapist resists. Patient is then instructed to relax while therapist repeats stretch.

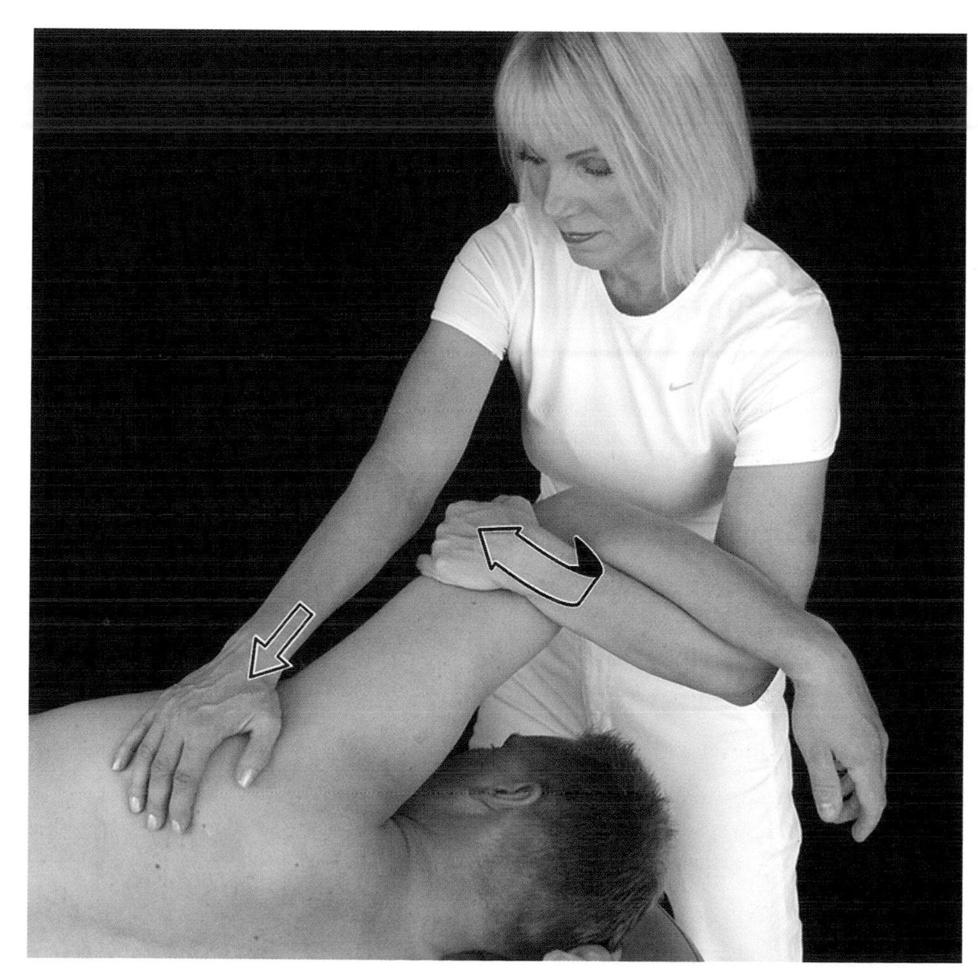

Latissimus dorsi

Nerve, supply: Thoracodorsal nerve, C6–8.

Origin: Inferior angle of the scapula, back of the 10–12th ribs, spinous processes of Th7–12, thoracolumbar fascia arising from spinous processes of L1–5, sacrum and iliac crest.

Insertion: Crest of the lesser tubercle of the humerus.

Function: Extension, adduction and internal rotation of the shoulder joint. Assist in deep exhalation.

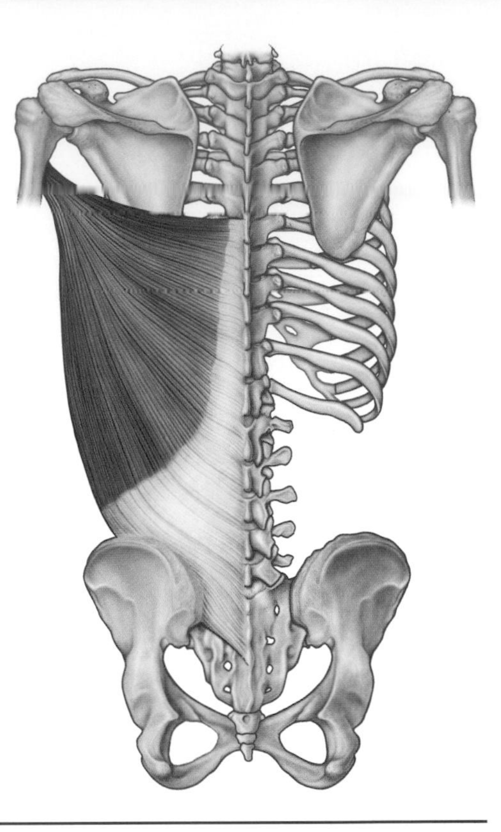

Stretching technique (flexion + abduction + external rotation):

Patient is lying on side with shoulder joint abducted 135° and elbow flexed about 90°. Therapist presses against the body of the muscle with the thenar of the hand while pulling on the elbow gradually down and towards external rotation with the other hand.

Tension–relaxation technique: Patient tries to pull upper arm down while therapist resists for 5 sec. Patient is then instructed to relax while therapist increases stretch.

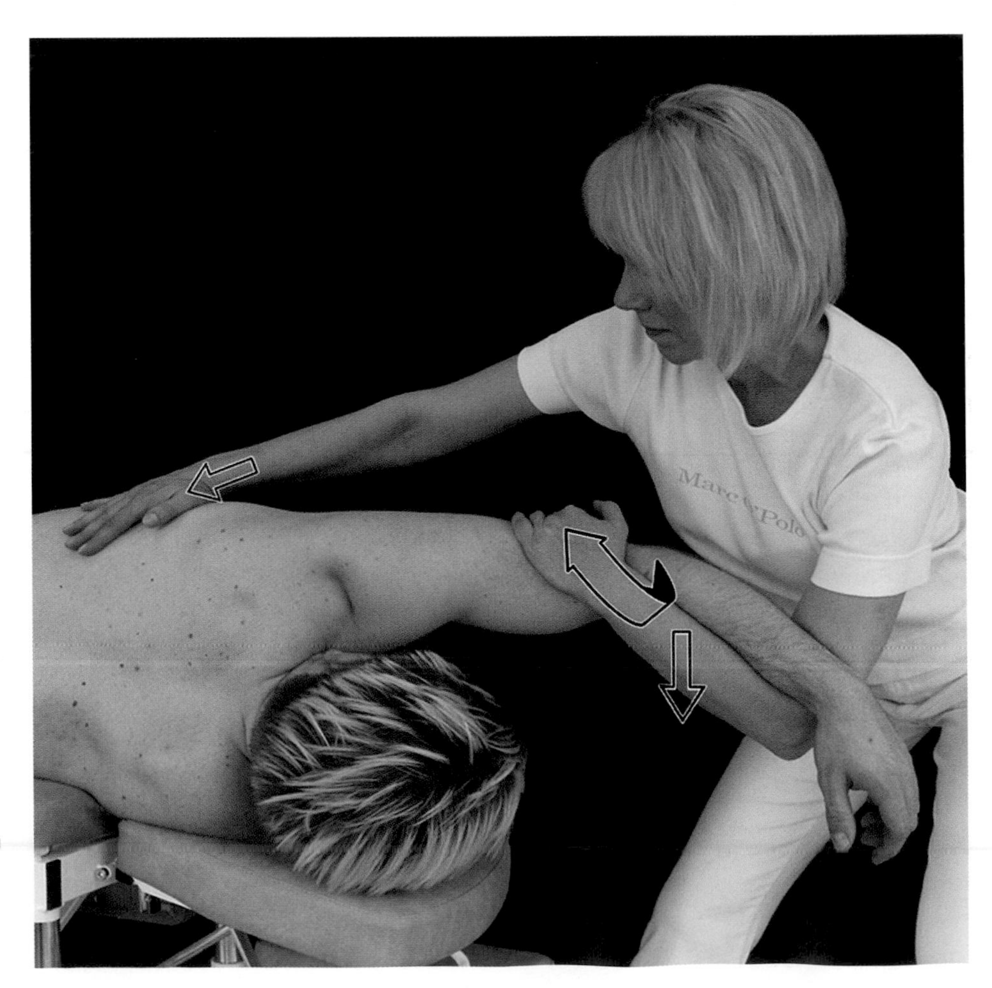

Subscapularis

Nerve, supply: Subscapular nerve, C5–8.

Origin: Subscapular fossa in the anterior surface of the scapula.

Insertion: Lesser tubercle of the humerus and capsule of shoulder joint.

Function: Internal rotation of the shoulder.

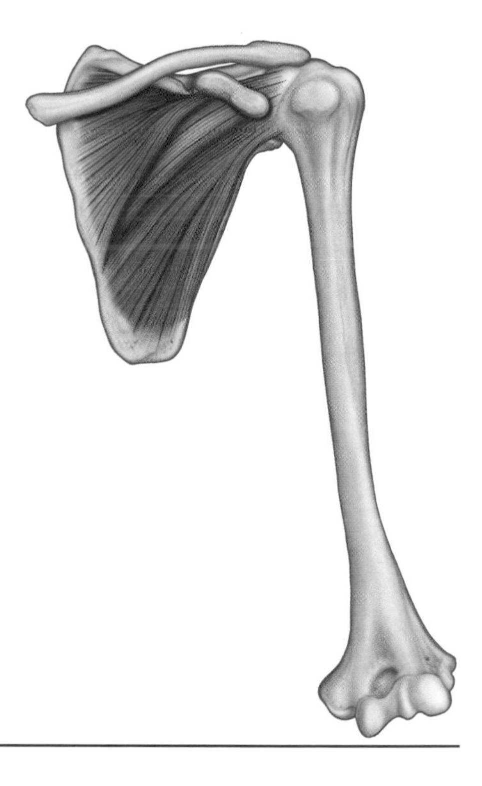

Stretching technique (external rotation):

Patient is lying on back with upper arm next to body and the elbow flexed about 90°. Therapist puts the hypothenar of the hand next to the lesser tubercle and below the coracoid process and pushes towards the body of the muscle while the other hand grasps the elbow and with forearm and externally rotates patient's upper arm.

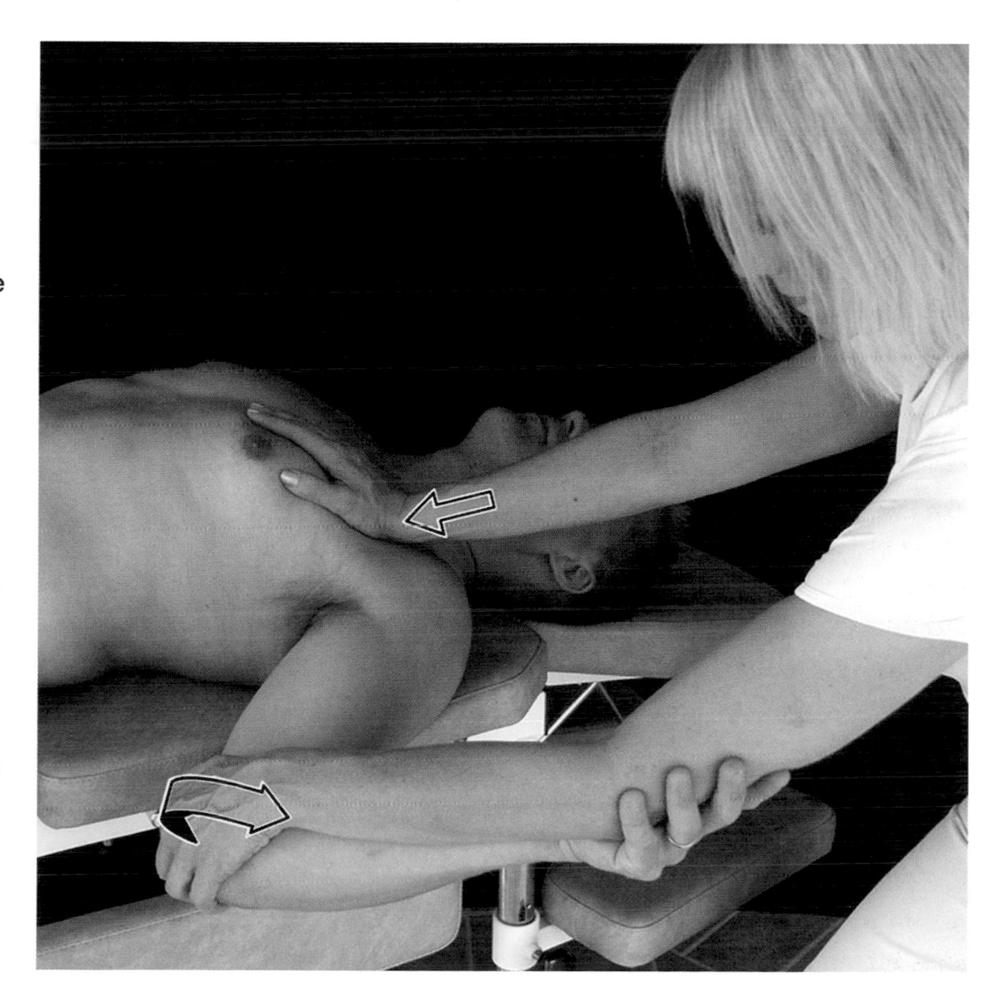

Tension–relaxation technique: Patient tries to internally rotate the shoulder for 5 sec while therapist resists. Patient is then instructed to gradually relax muscles while therapist applies stretching technique.

Notice: There should be only slight abduction of the arm, because abduction will cause the pectorals major to tense preventing the manual stretch from reaching the subscapular muscle.

Long head of the biceps brachii

Nerve, supply: Musculocutaneous nerve, C5–6.

Origin: Supraglenoid tubercle of the scapula.

Insertion: Radial tuberosity and with bicipital aponeurosis into the antebrachial fascia on the ulnar side of the forearm.

Function: Flexion and adduction of the shoulder joint and flexion and external rotation of the elbow joint. Stabilizes shoulder joint.

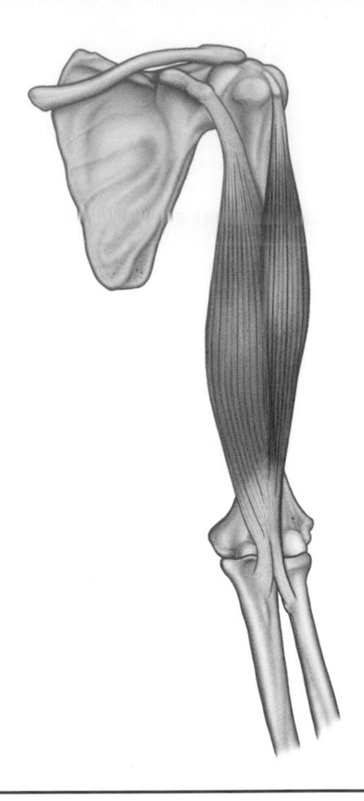

Stretching technique A (extension + abduction + internal rotation):

Patient is lying on back with arm abducted about 45° and elbow straight. Therapist applies pressure at the lower muscle–tendon junction towards the body of the muscle with the hypothenar of the hand while keeping the arm internally rotated.

Notice: This is a forceful technique due to long lever arm. Excessive extension of shoulder joint should be avoided.

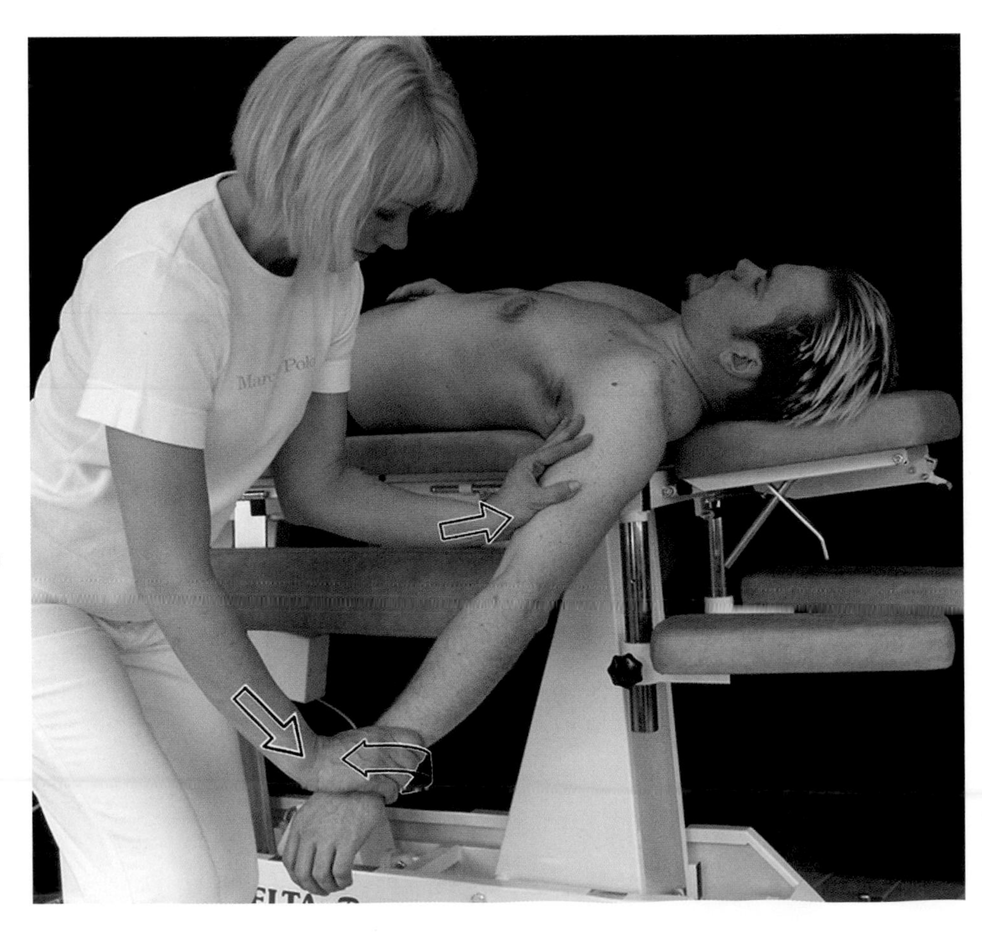

Stretching technique B (extension + abduction + internal rotation):

Patient is lying on back with arm abducted about 45°. Therapist applies pressure from the upper muscle–tendon junction towards the body of the muscle with the thumb of the hand and then gradually lets it slide downwards while keeping the arm internally rotated with the other hand.

Tension–relaxation technique: Patient tries to flex shoulder joint for 5 sec while therapist resists. Patient is then instructed to gradually relax muscles while therapist applies stretching technique.

Warning ❗ Excessive pressure to the upper arm should be avoided as it can cause damage to the shoulder joint ligaments. Intense wrenching of the shoulder joint can cause rupture of the long head.

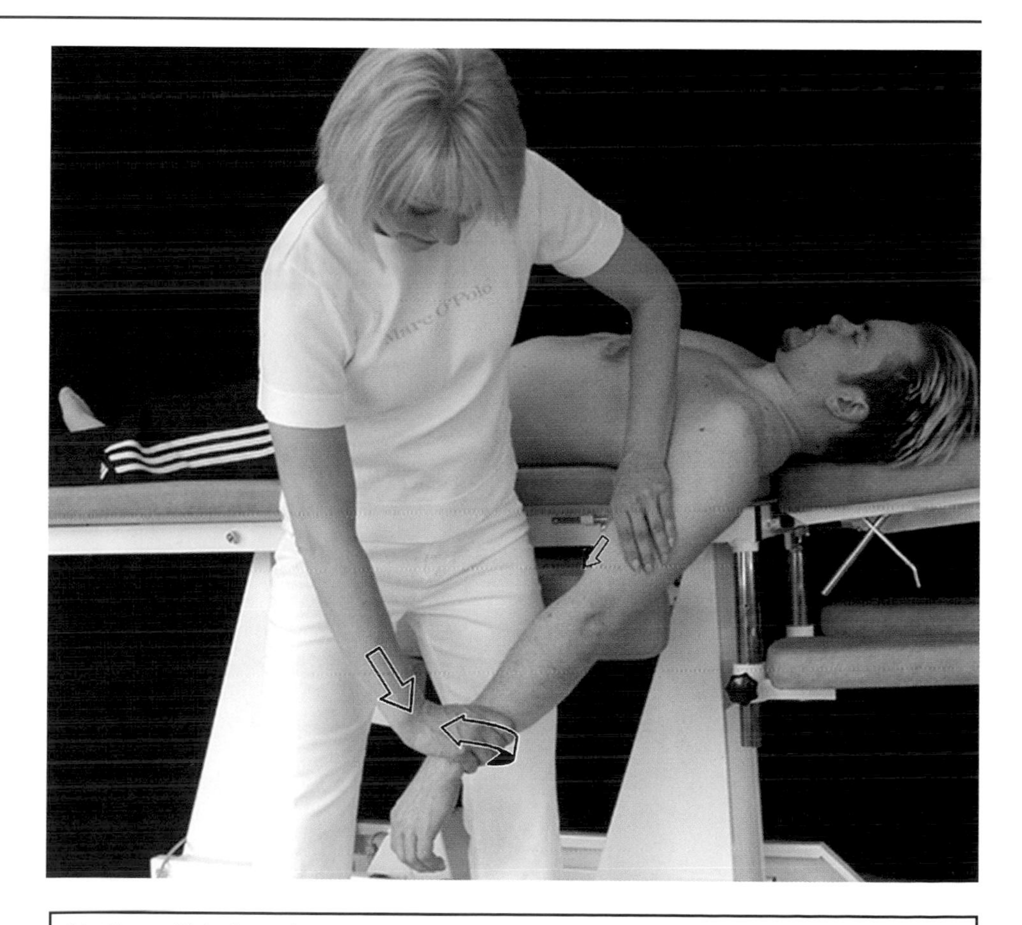

Notice: This is only an example to avoid unnecessary repeat. The manual stretching towards belly of the muscle can be performed starting from the proximal musculotendinous junction to distal direction or distal musculotendinous junction to proximal direction also with other muscles.

Coracobrachialis

Nerve, supply: Musculocutaneous nerve, C6–7.

Origin: Coracoid process.

Insertion: Middle of anteromedial surface of the humerus.

Function: Flexion and adduction of the shoulder joint.

Short head of the biceps brachii

Nerve, supply: Musculocutaneous nerve, C5–6.

Origin: Coracoid process.

Insertion: Radial tuberosity and with bicipital aponeurosis into the antebrachial fascia on the ulnar side.

Function: Flexion and adduction of the shoulder joint and flexion and external rotation of the elbow joint.

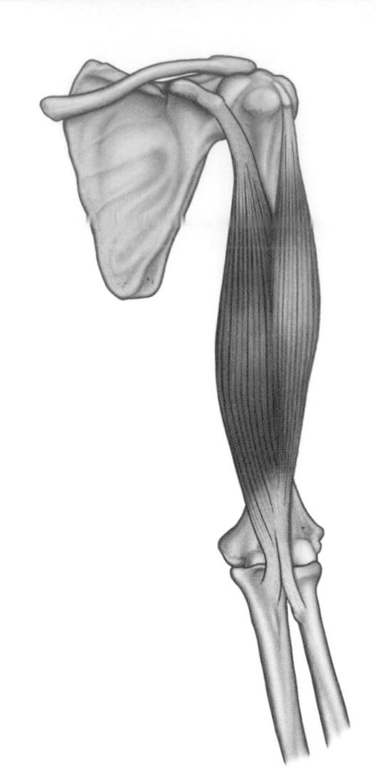

Stretching technique:

Patient is lying on back with upper arm abducted approximately 45°. Therapist applies pressure at the muscle–tendon junction towards the body of the coracobrachialis muscle with the hypothenar of the hand while using other hand to press down on the upper arm.

Tension–relaxation technique: Patient tries to flex shoulder joint for 5 sec while therapist resists. Patient is then instructed to gradually relax muscles while therapist applies stretching technique.

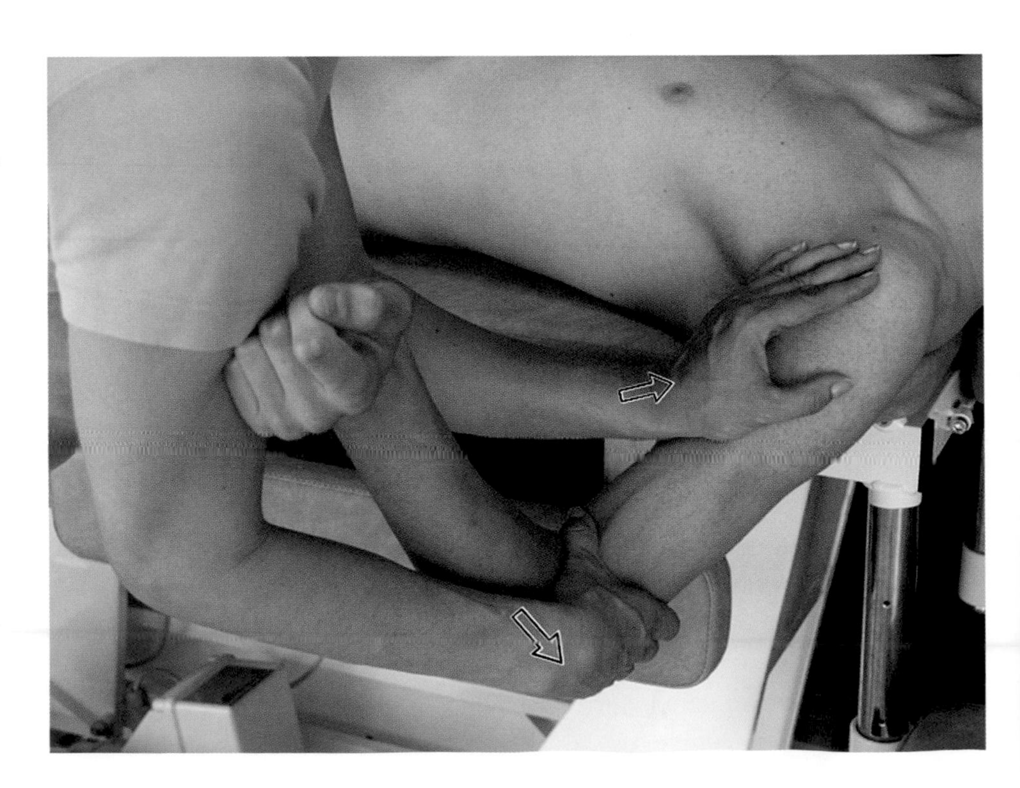

Brachialis

Nerve, supply: Musculocutaneous nerve, C5–6.

Origin: Distal half of the anterior surface of the humerus.

Insertion: Ulnar tuberosity, coronoid process, the joint capsule and intermuscular septa.

Function: Flexion of the elbow joint.

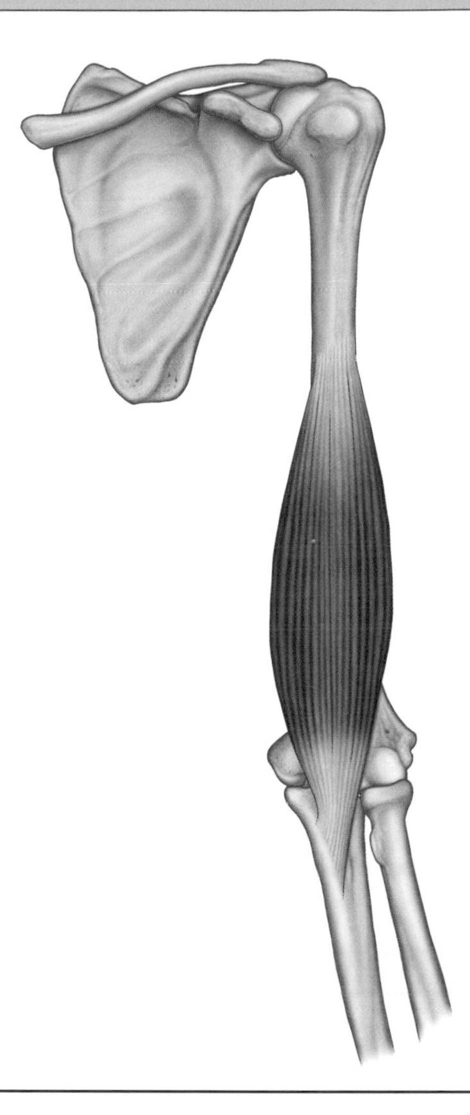

Stretching technique:

Patient is lying on back; arm resting at side with elbow flexed about 45°. Therapist presses with the thenar of the hand above muscle–tendon junction into body of muscle while gradually pulling the forearm down.

Tension–relaxation technique: Patient tries to flex elbow joint for 5 sec while therapist resists. Patient is then instructed to gradually relax muscles while therapist applies stretching technique.

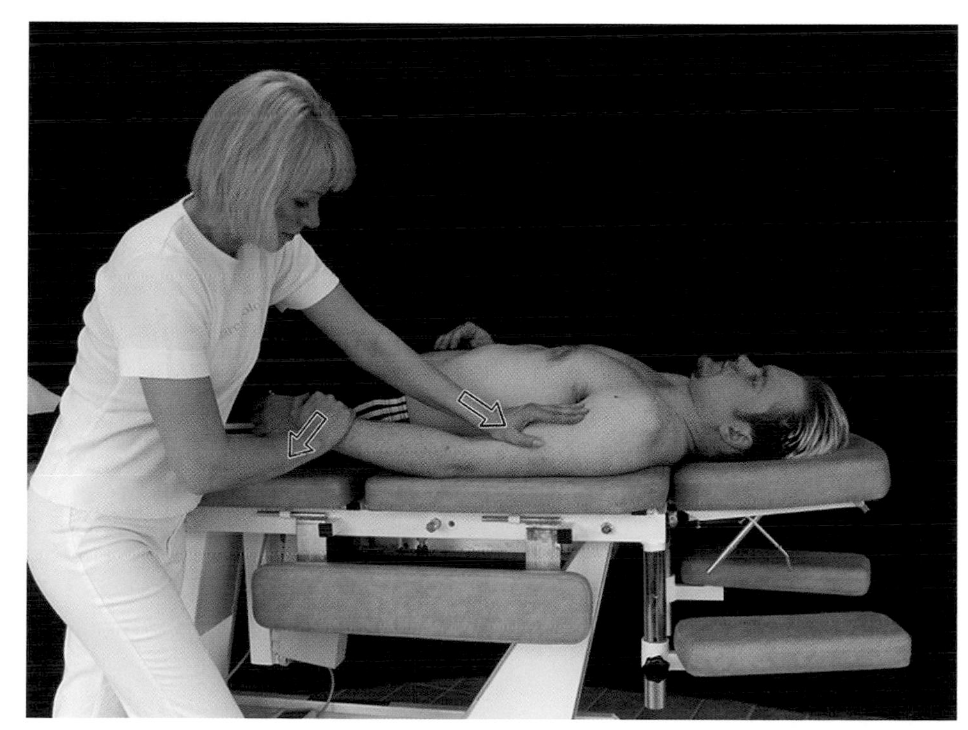

Long head of the triceps brachii

Nerve, supply: Radial nerve, C6–8.

Origin: Infraglenoid tubercle of the scapula and in some cases from the outer edge of the scapula and shoulder joint capsule.

Insertion: Olecranon of the ulna.

Function: Extension of the elbow joint; extension and adduction of the shoulder joint.

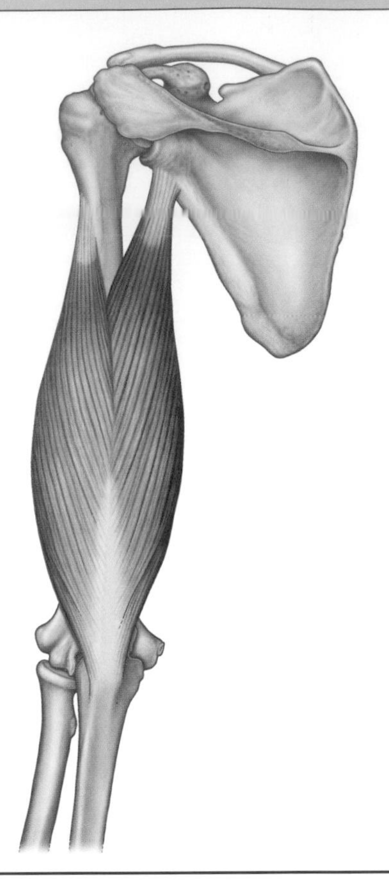

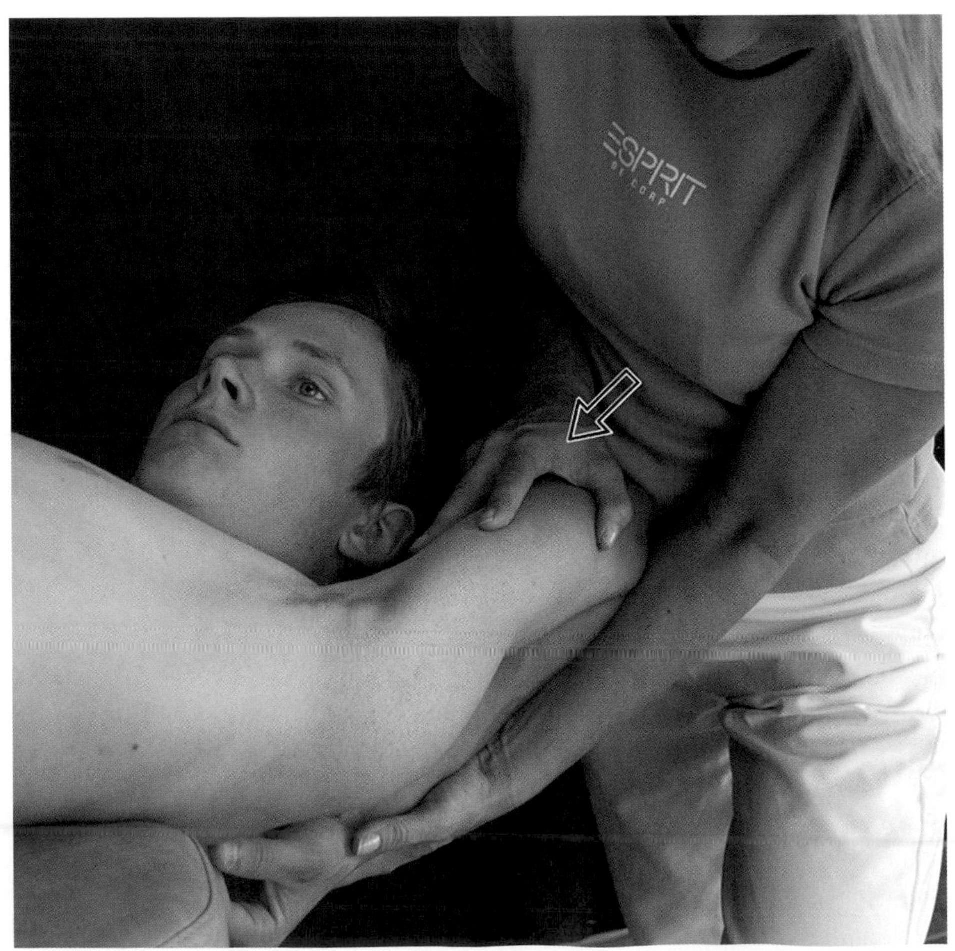

Stretching technique:

Patient is lying on back with shoulder raised up beside head to about 135°. Therapist presses with the hand above muscle–tendon junction into body of muscle while pressing gradually down the arm and holds the elbow in full flexion with the other hand.

Tension–relaxation technique: Patient tries to extend shoulder joint for 5 sec while therapist resists. Patient is then instructed to gradually relax muscles while therapist applies stretching technique.

Medial head of the triceps brachii

Nerve, supply: Radial nerve, C6–8.

Origin: Dorsal surface of the middle and lower third of the humerus.

Insertion: Olecranon of the ulna.

Function: Extension of the elbow joint.

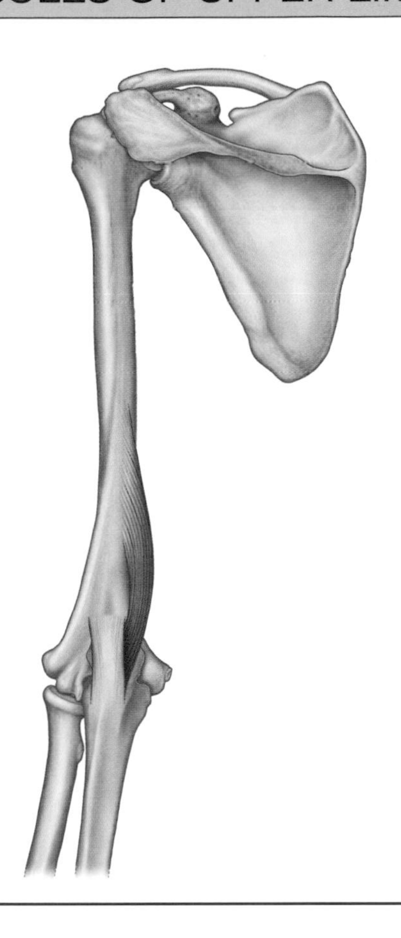

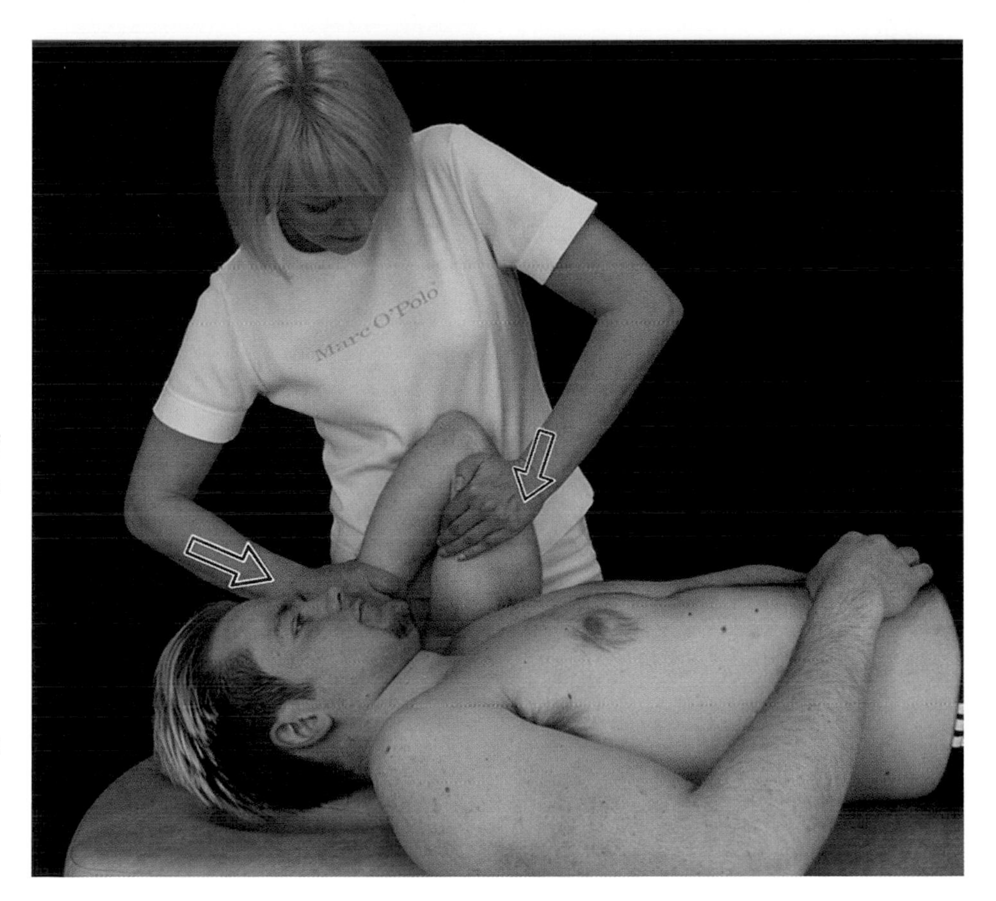

Stretching technique:

Patient is lying on back and shoulder flexed to about 90°. Therapist presses along the body of muscle away from insertion with the thenar of the hand while pressing elbow into flexion with the other hand.

Tension–relaxation technique: Patient tries to extend elbow for 5 sec while therapist resists. Patient is then instructed to gradually relax muscles while therapist applies stretching technique.

Lateral head of the triceps brachii

Nerve, supply: Radial nerve, C6–8.

Origin: Lateral and dorsal surface of the upper half of the humerus.

Insertion: Olecranon of the ulna.

Function: Extension of the elbow joint.

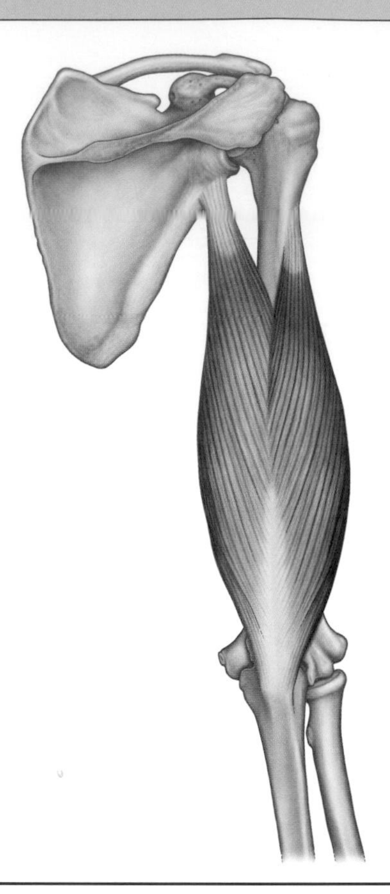

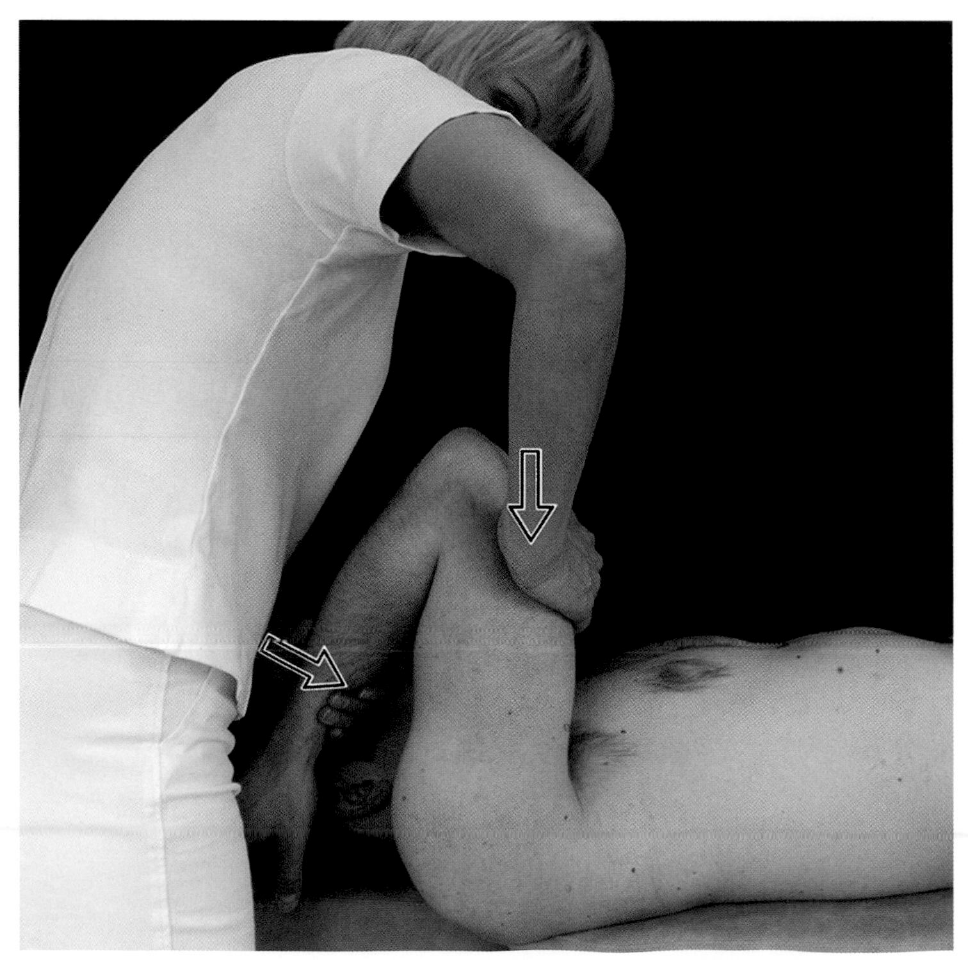

Stretching technique:

Patient is lying on back and shoulder flexed to about 90°. Therapist presses along the body of muscle away from insertion with the thenar of the hand while pressing elbow into flexion with the other hand.

Tension–relaxation technique: Patient tries to extend elbow for 5 sec while therapist resists. Patient is then instructed to gradually relax muscles while therapist applies stretching technique.

Articularis cubiti (subanconeus)

Nerve, supply: Radial nerve, C6–8.

Origin: Lower dorsal surface of the humerus (deep fibres from the medial head of the triceps brachii).

Insertion: Joint capsule of the elbow.

Function: Tightens joint capsule.

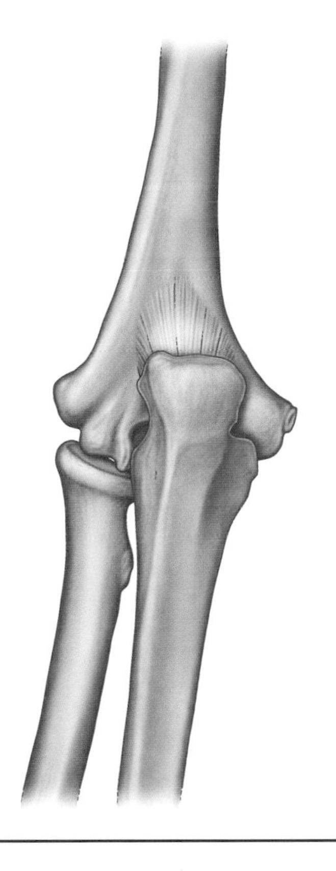

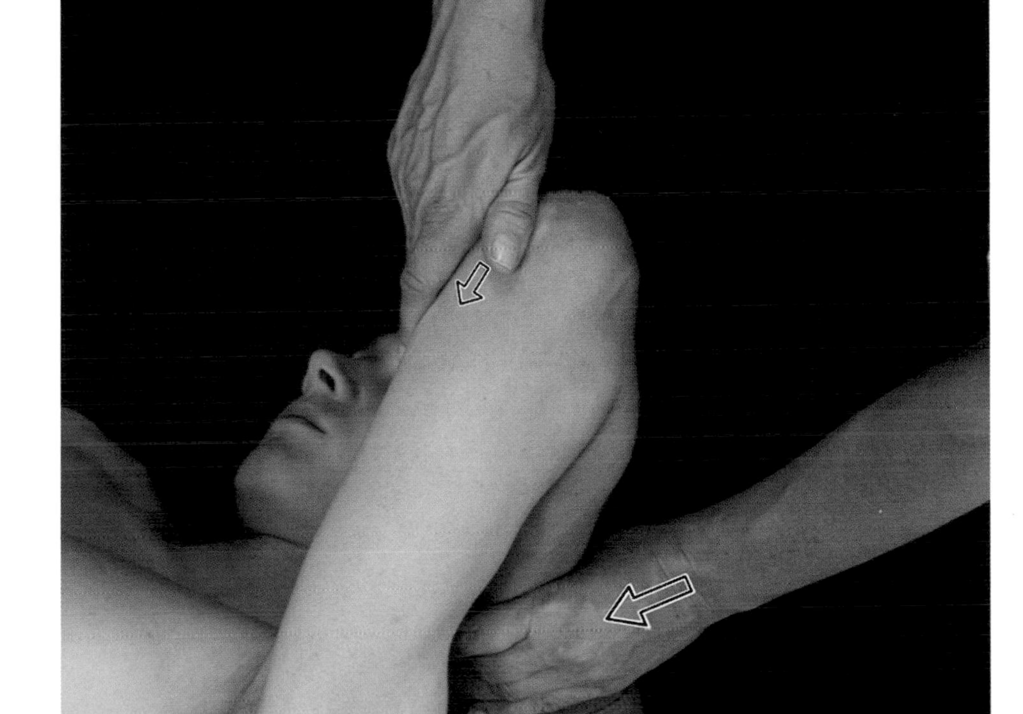

Stretching technique:

Patient is lying on back, shoulder and elbow joints flexed to about 90°. Therapist presses with the thumb of the hand down to the body of muscle while increasing elbow flexion with the other hand.

Anconeus

Nerve, supply: Radial nerve, C7–8.

Origin: Lateral epicondyle of the humerus and the radial collateral ligament.

Insertion: Proximal one fourth of dorsal surface of ulna.

Function: Extension of the elbow joint.

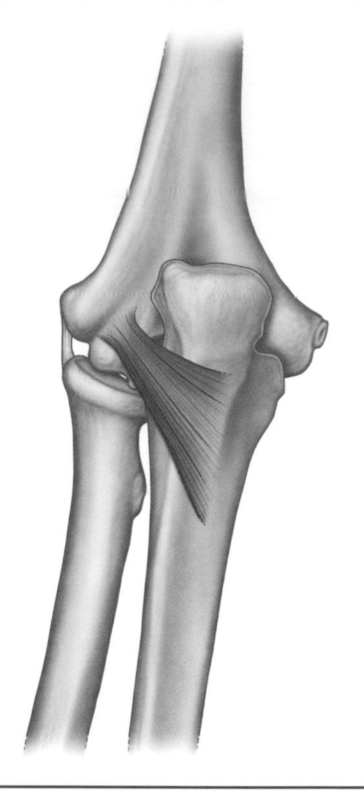

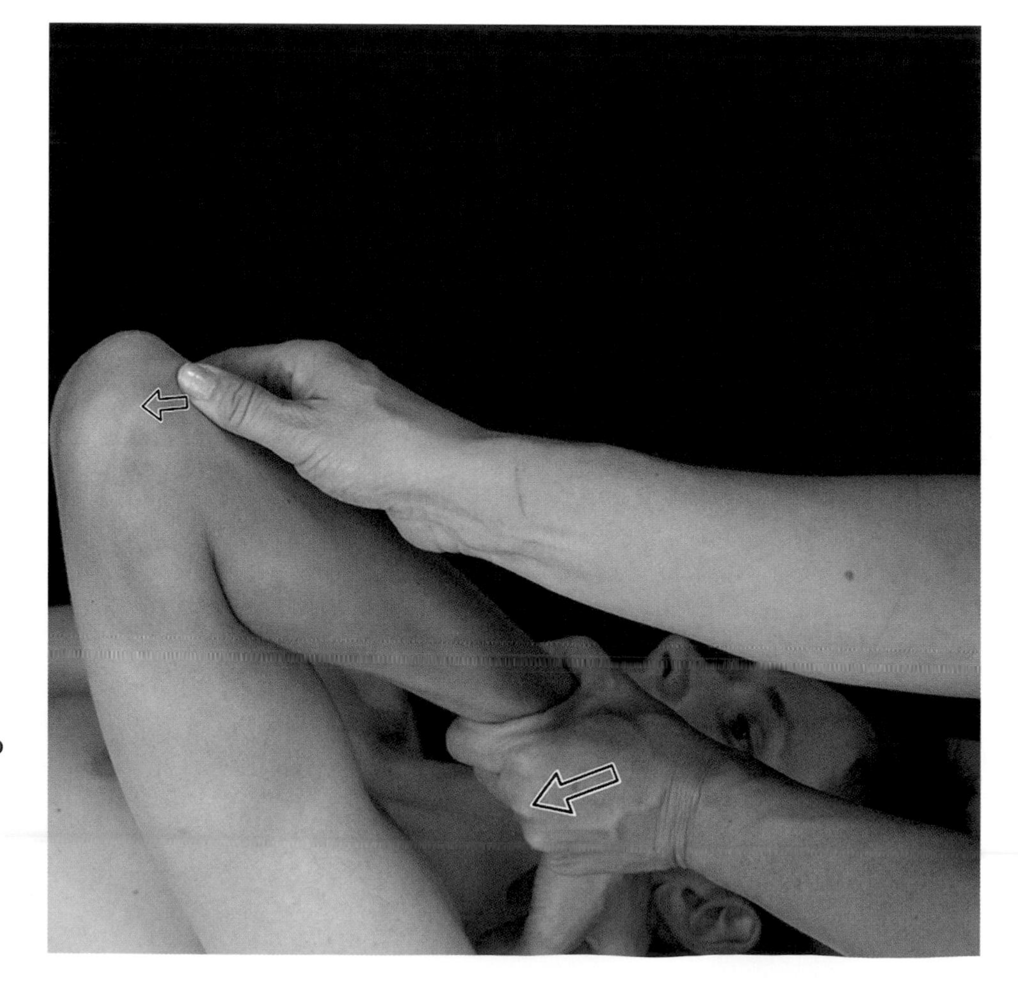

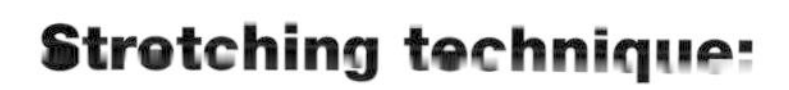

Stretching technique:

Patient is lying on back with shoulder and elbow joints flexed to 90°. Therapist presses with the thumb of the hand the body of muscle away from insertion while increasing elbow flexion with the other hand.

Brachioradialis

Nerve, supply: Radial nerve, C5–6.

Origin: Supracondylar crest of the humerus and the intermuscular septum.

Insertion: Styloid process of the radius.

Function: Brings forearm into the mid-position between pronation and supination and flexion of the elbow joint.

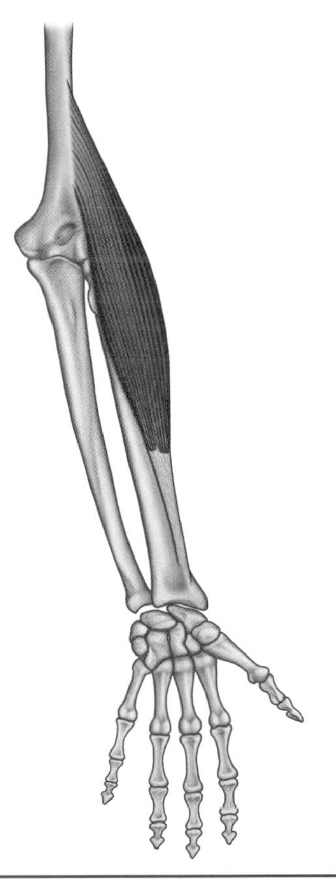

Stretching technique: (pronation + extension)

Patient is lying on back and elbow flexed 45°. Therapist presses with the thenar of the hand along body of muscle while using the other hand to internally rotate and extend the elbow joint.

Tension–relaxation technique: Patient tries to flex elbow for 5 sec while therapist resists. Patient is then instructed to gradually relax muscles while therapist applies stretching technique.

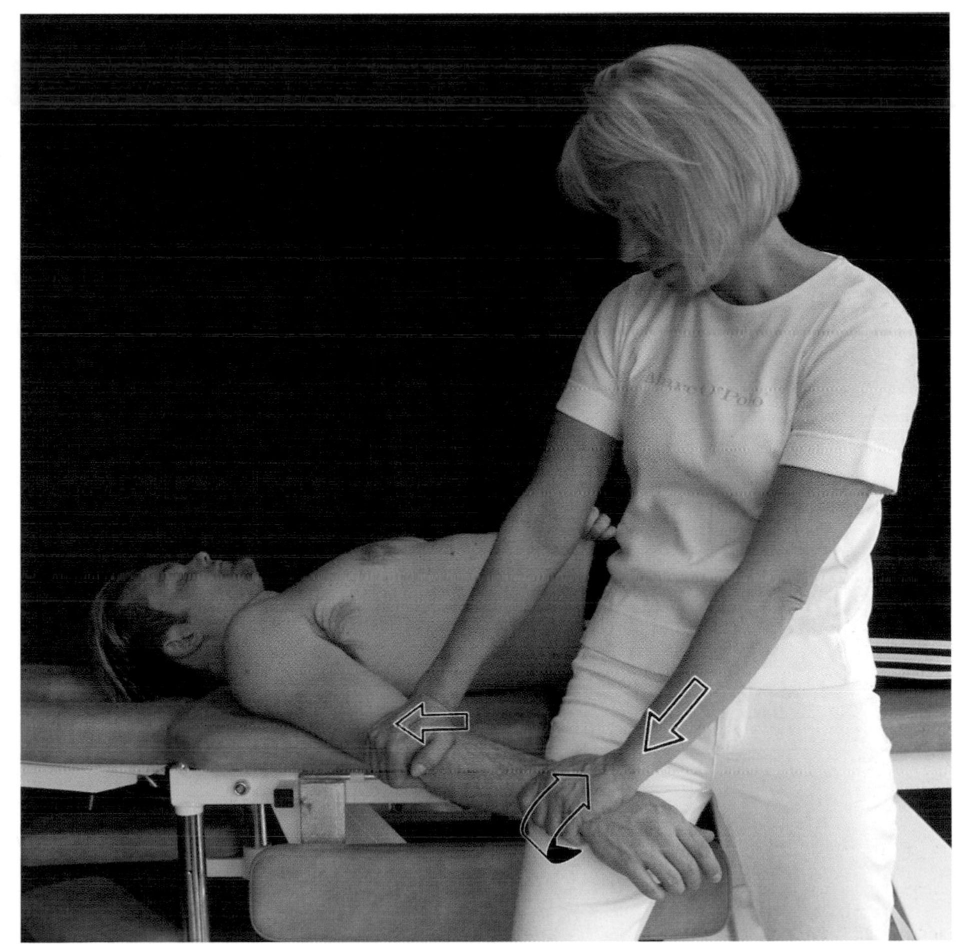

Pronator teres

Nerve, supply: Median nerve, C6–7.

Origin: Medial epicondyle, the intermuscular septum and the coronoid process of the ulna.

Insertion: Pronator tuberosity of the radius.

Function: Internal rotation of forearm and flexion of the elbow joint.

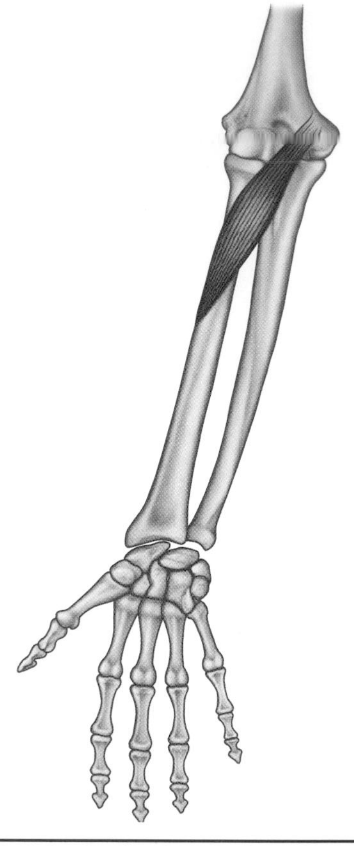

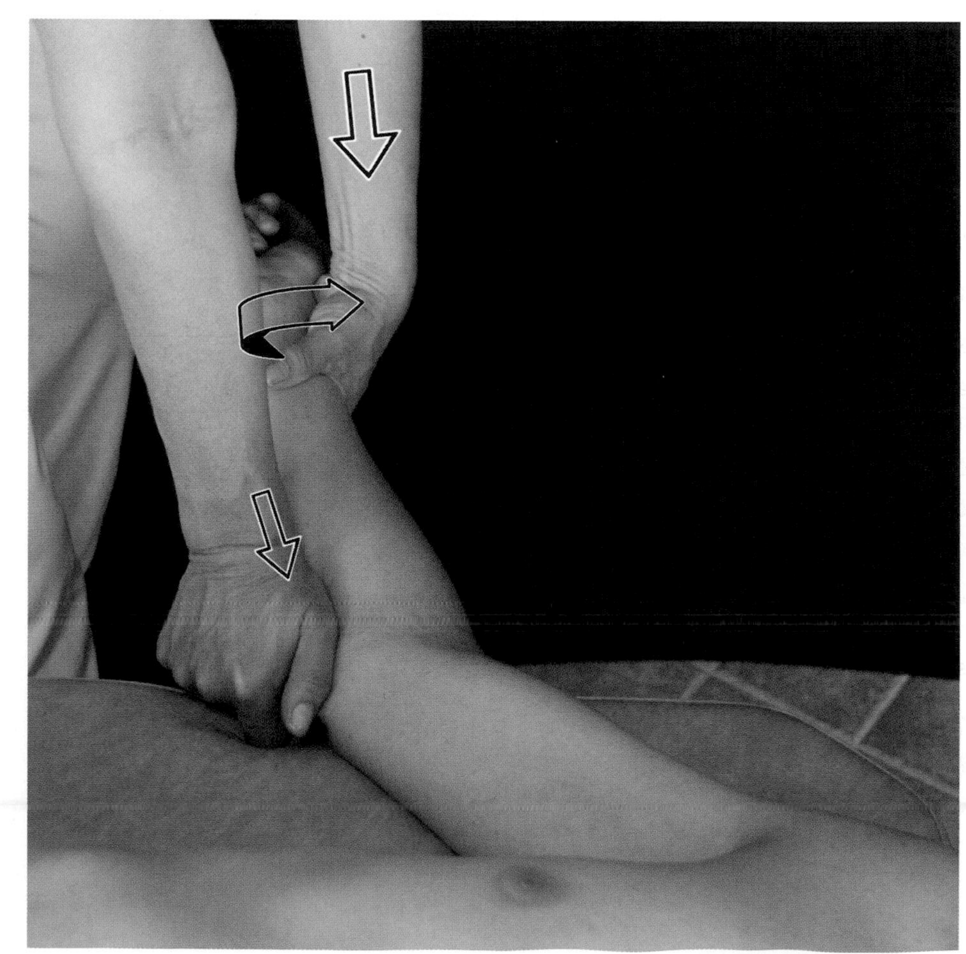

Stretching technique (supination + extension):

Patient is lying on back and elbow flexed to 45°. Therapist uses the thenar of the hand to press immediately above insertion across or towards the body of muscle while using other hand to extend the elbow joint and externally rotate forearm.

Tension–relaxation technique: Patient tries to internally rotate forearm for 5 sec while therapist resists. Patient is then instructed to gradually relax muscles while therapist applies stretching technique.

Flexor carpi radialis

Nerve, supply: Median nerve, C6–7.

Origin: Medial epicondyle of the humerus and from the superficial fascia of the forearm.

Insertion: Palmar surface at base of second metacarpal and in some cases on third metacarpal.

Function: Flexion and radial abduction of wrist. Flexion and pronation of the elbow joint.

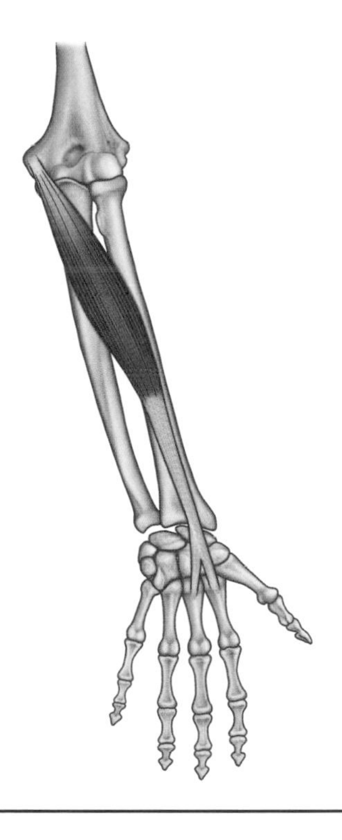

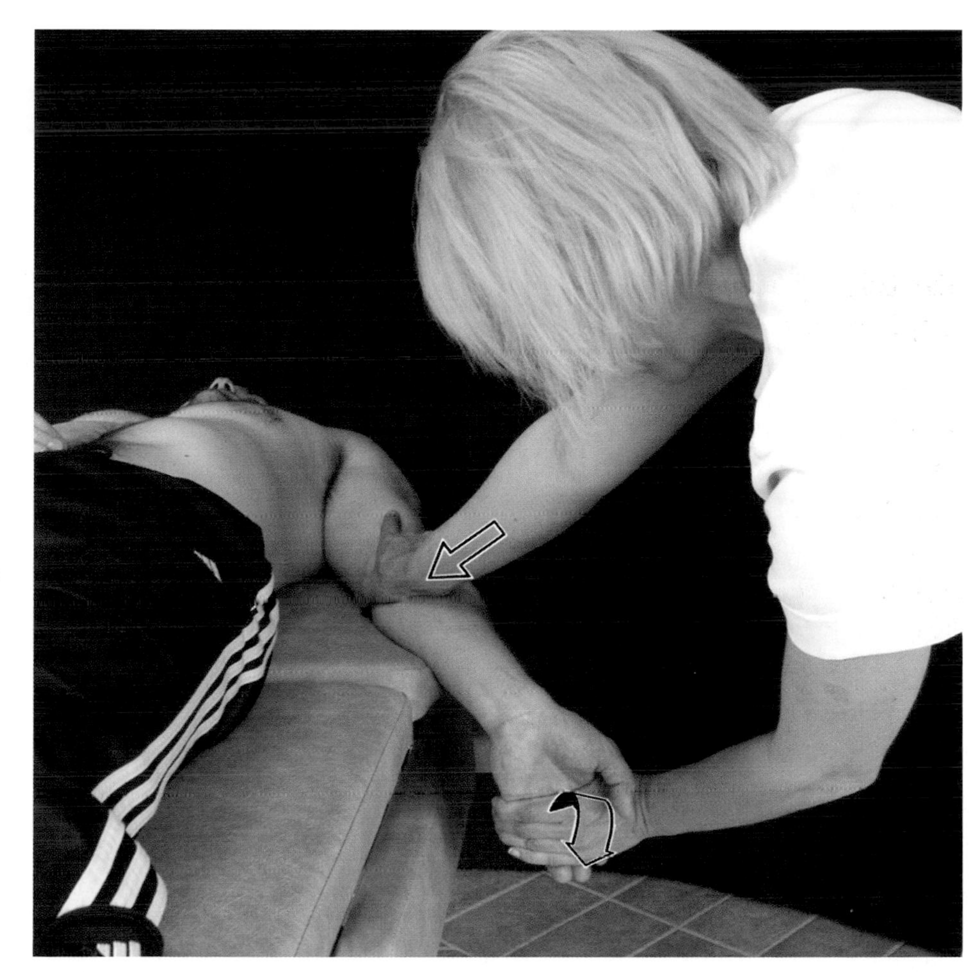

Stretching technique (supination + extension):

Patient is lying on back with the arm straight and beside the body. Therapist uses the hypothenar of the hand to press from muscle tendon junction towards the body of muscle while using other hand to press down on palm and externally rotate the forearm starting from the second metacarpal bone.

Tension–relaxation technique: Patient tries to flex wrist for 5 sec while therapist resists. Patient is then instructed to gradually relax muscles while therapist applies stretching technique.

Flexor carpi ulnaris

Nerve, supply: Ulnar nerve, C7–8.

Origin: Medial epicondyle of the humerus, olecranon of ulna and the upper two-thirds of the posterior margin of the ulna.

Insertion: Pisiform, hamate and fifth metacarpal bones and the pisohamate and pisometacarpal ligaments.

Function: Flexion and ulnar adduction of the wrist.

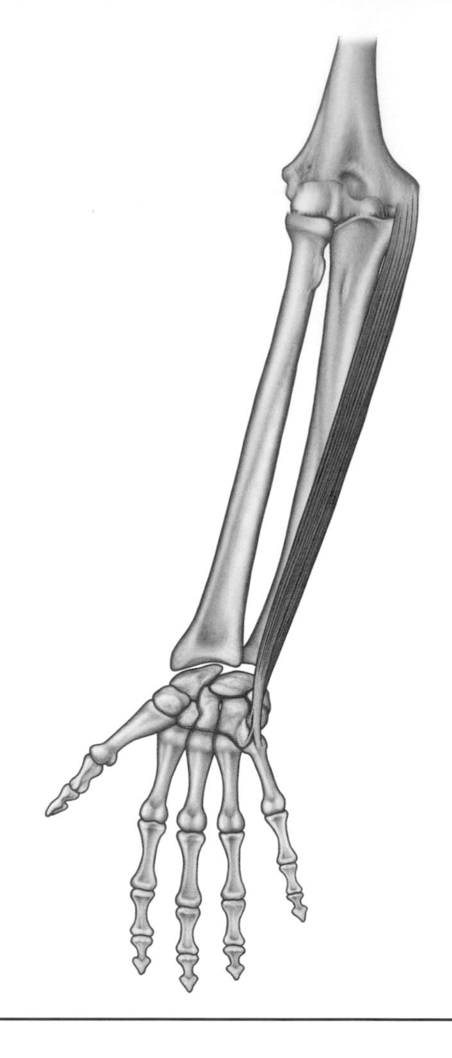

Stretching technique (pronation + extension):

Patient lies on stomach with the arm straight and beside the body. Therapist applies pressure with thenar of the hand towards the body of muscle away from insertion while using the other hand to extend wrist and internally rotate the forearm starting from the fifth metacarpal bone.

Tension–relaxation technique: Patient tries to flex wrist for 5 sec while therapist resists. Patient is then instructed to gradually relax muscles while therapist applies stretching technique.

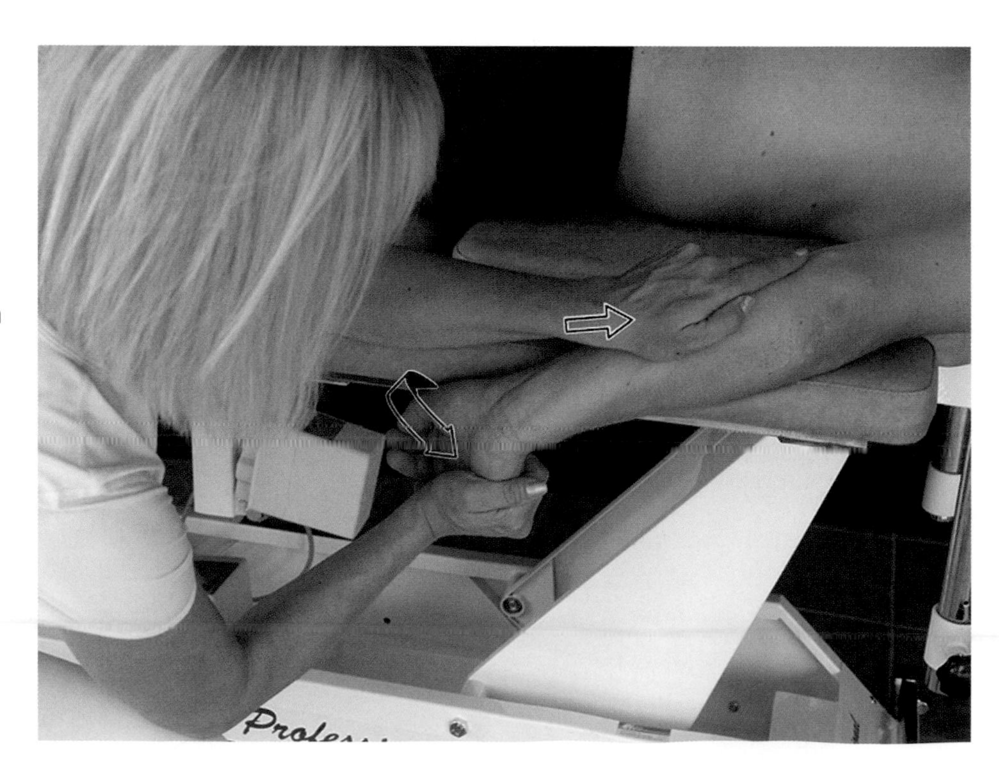

Palmaris longus

Nerve, supply: Median nerve, C7–Th1.

Origin: Medial epicondyle of the humerus.

Insertion: Palmar aponeurosis joins to the tendon sheaths of the flexor tendons, the transverse metacarpal and metacarpophalangeal ligaments, the corium of the palm and the deep palmar fascia by nine septa, which border both sides of the tendons of the superficial and deep flexors of the fingers and the radial side of the first lumbrical muscle.

It may be absent (10 per cent) of peope, although palmar aponeurosis is present.

Function: Flexion of wrist and tensing palmar aponeurosis.

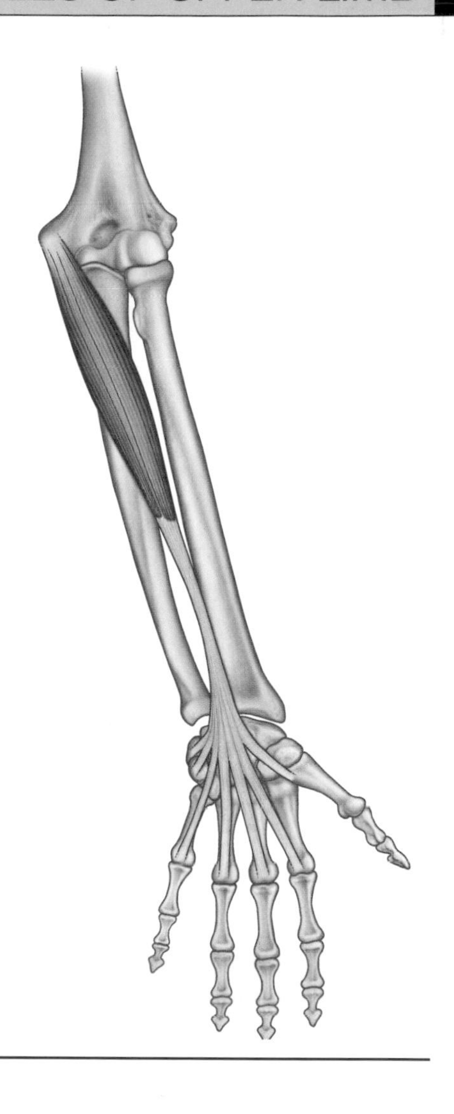

Stretching technique (supination + extension):

Patient lies on back with forearm extended at side. Therapist applies pressure with thenar of the hand towards the body of muscle away from insertion while using the other hand to extend wrist and 2–5 metacarpophalangeal joints and externally rotate the forearm.

Tension–relaxation technique: Patient tries to flex wrist for 5 sec while therapist resists. Patient is then instructed to gradually relax muscles while therapist applies stretching technique.

Notice: The muscle may be absent.

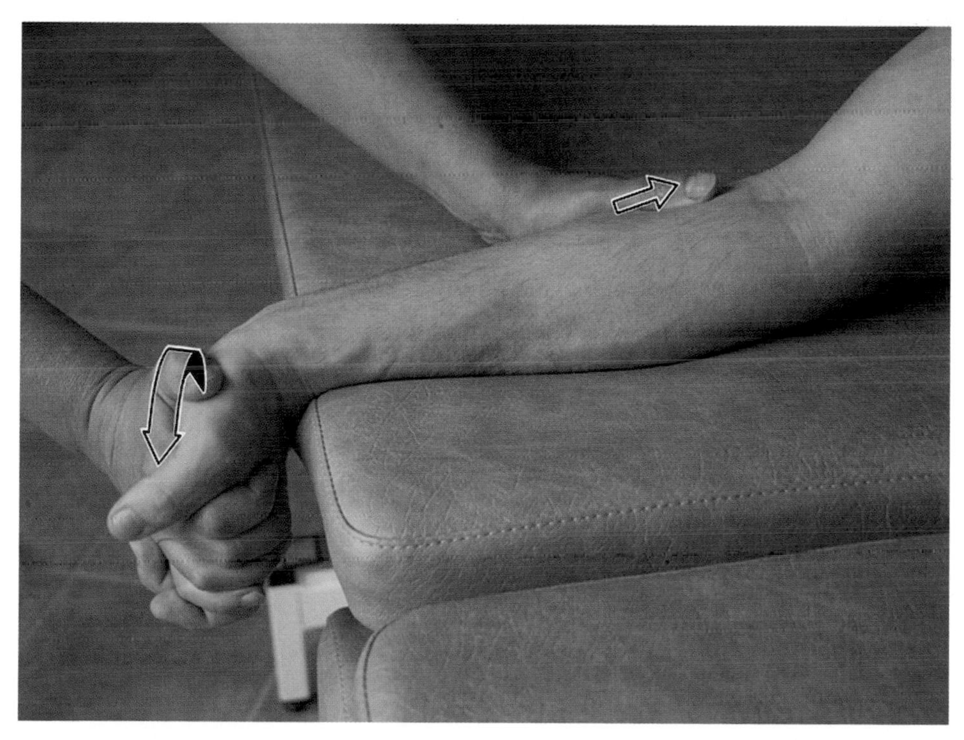

Flexor digitorum superficialis

Nerve, supply: Median nerve, C7–Th1.

Origin: Medial epicondyle of the humerus, coronoid process of the ulna and anterior surface of the radius.

Insertion: Centre of the middle phalanges of fingers 2–5.

Function: Flexion of wrist, 2–5 metacarpophalangeal and proximal finger joints.

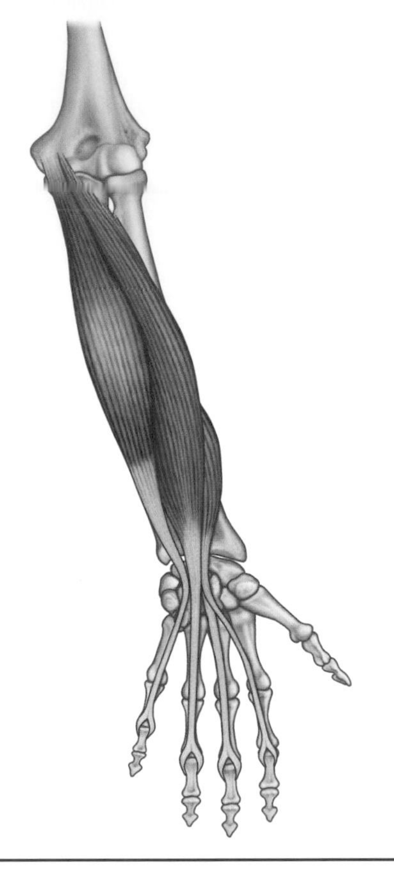

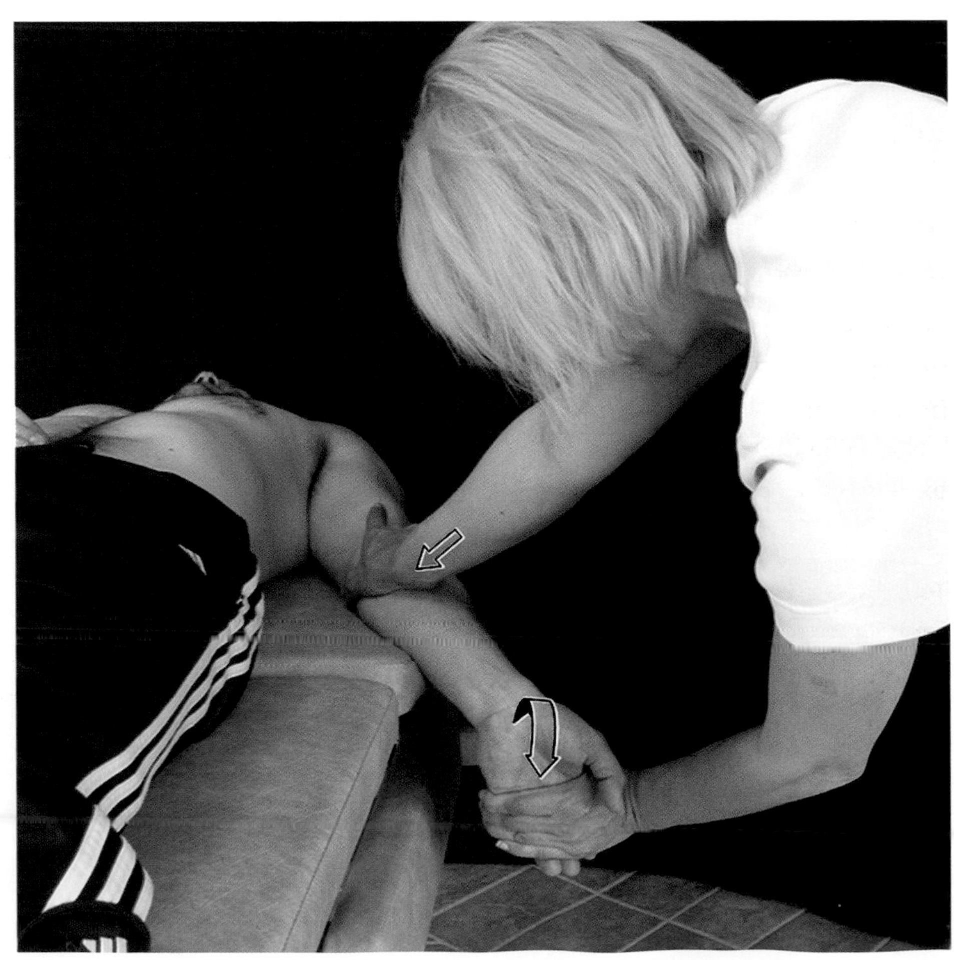

Stretching technique (supination + extension):

Patient is lying on back with the elbow extended at side. Therapist applies pressure with the thenar of the hand towards the body of muscle away from insertion while using the other hand to extend the wrist, 2–5 metacarpophalangeal and proximal phalangeal joints, allowing the distal joints to remain flexed, and externally rotates the forearm.

Tension–relaxation technique: Patient tries to make a fist for 5 sec while therapist resists. Patient is then instructed to gradually relax muscles while therapist applies stretching technique.

Flexor digitorum profundus (perforatus)

Nerve, supply: Median and ulnar nerve, C7–Th1.

Origin: Proximal two-thirds of the anterior surface of the ulna and the interosseus membrane.

Insertion: Base of distal phalanges of fingers 2–5.

Function: Flexion of wrist and finger joints.

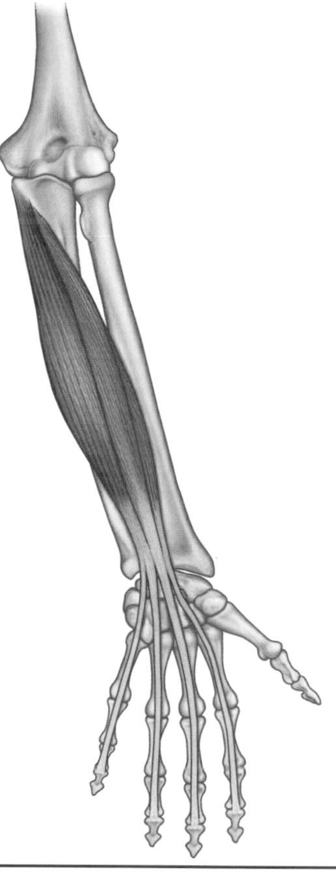

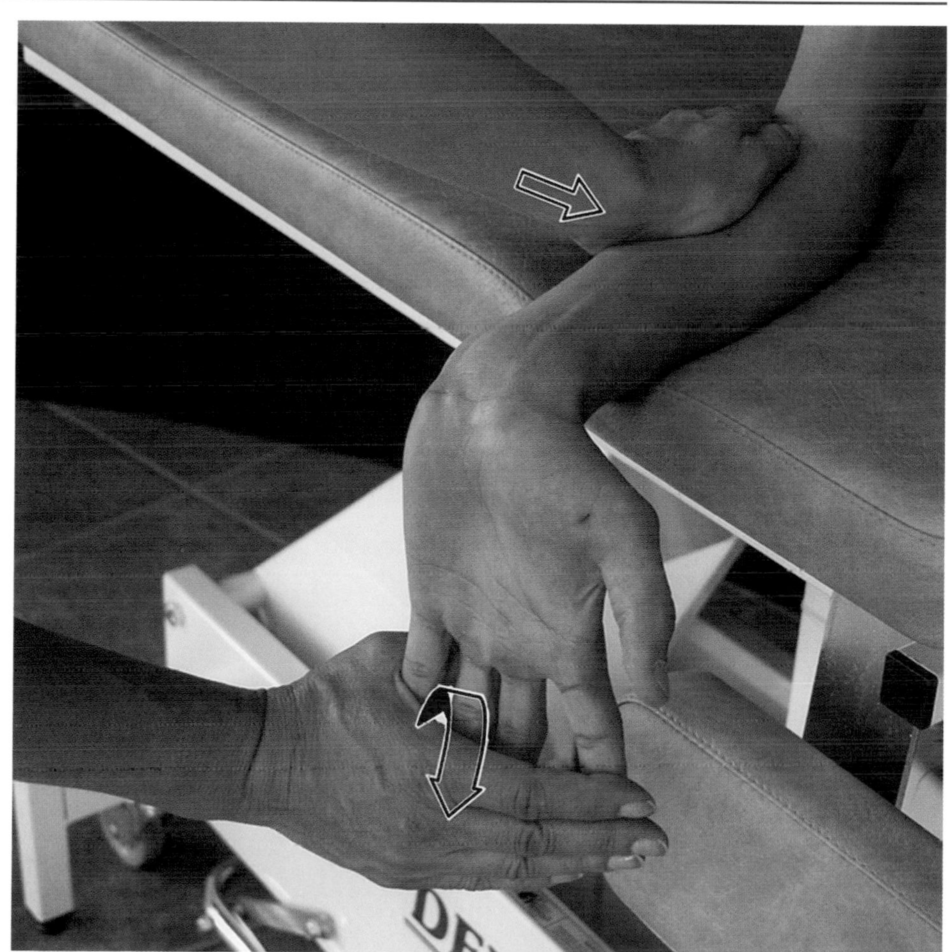

Stretching technique (supination + extension):

Therapist applies pressure with the thenar of the hand towards the body of muscle away from insertion while using the other hand to extend the wrist and fingers 2–5 and externally rotate the forearm.

Tension–relaxation technique: Patient tries to flex fingers 2–5 for 5 sec while therapist resists. Patient is then instructed to gradually relax muscles while therapist applies stretching technique.

Notice: Elbow joint is kept flexed to avoid stretching flexor muscles attaching to the medial epicondyle.

Flexor pollicis longus

Nerve, supply: Median nerve, C7–8.

Origin: Mid third of anterior surface of radius, interosseus membrane and in some people also from the medial epicondyle (40%).

Insertion: Distal phalange of thumb and often connects with the tendon of flexor digitorum superficialis.

Function: Thumb and wrist flexion and assists with radial abduction.

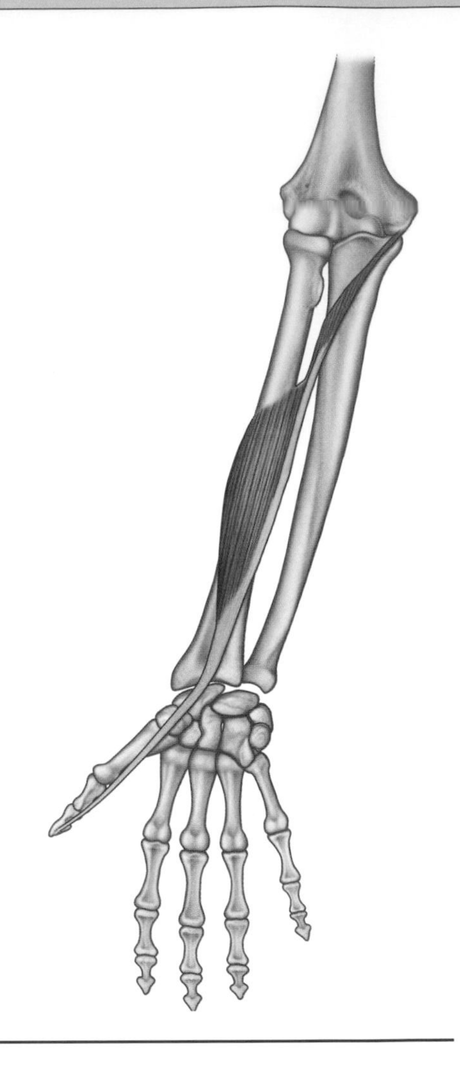

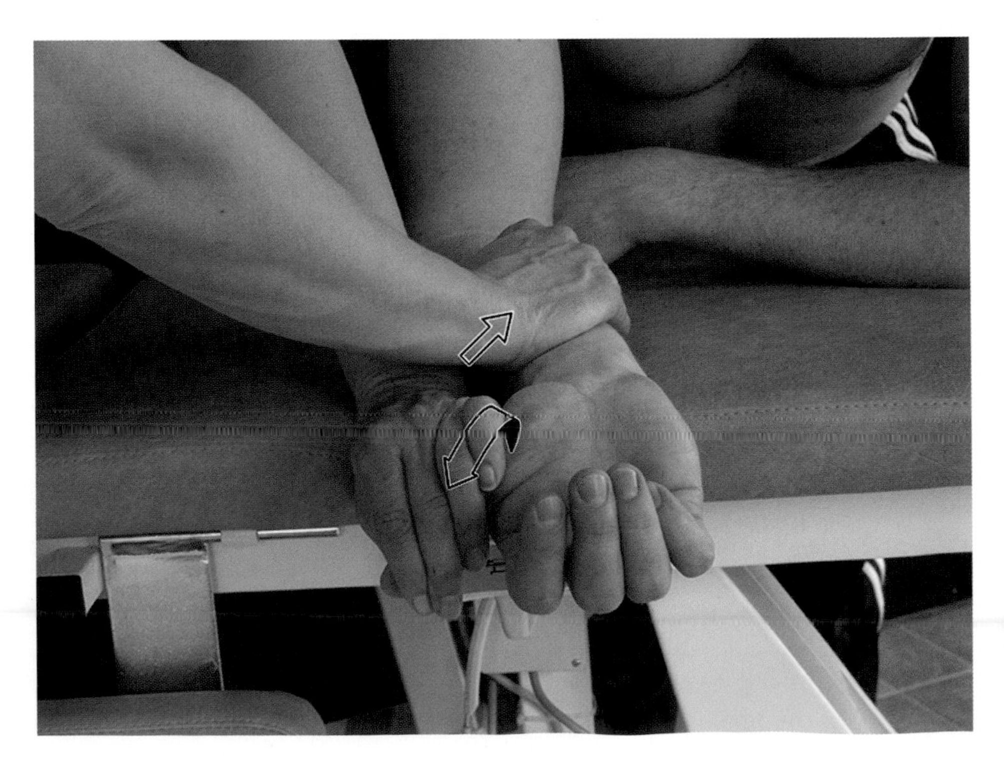

Stretching technique (supination + extension):

Therapist applies pressure with the thenar of the hand towards the body of muscle away from insertion while using the other hand to extend the thumb and wrist and externally rotate the forearm.

Tension–relaxation technique: Patient tries to flex thumb for 5 sec while therapist resists. Patient is then instructed to gradually relax muscles while therapist applies stretching technique.

Pronator quadratus

Nerve, supply: Anterior interosseus nerve, of median nerve, C8–Th1.

Origin: Distal fourth of anterior surface of ulna.

Insertion: Distal fourth of anterior surface of radius.

Function: Internal rotation of forearm.

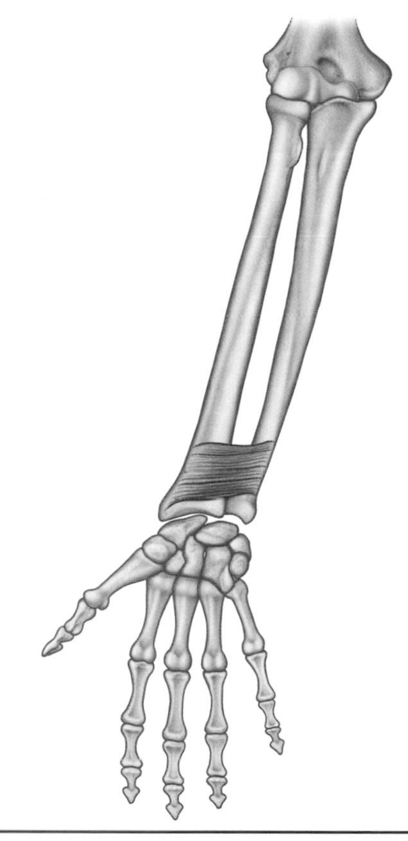

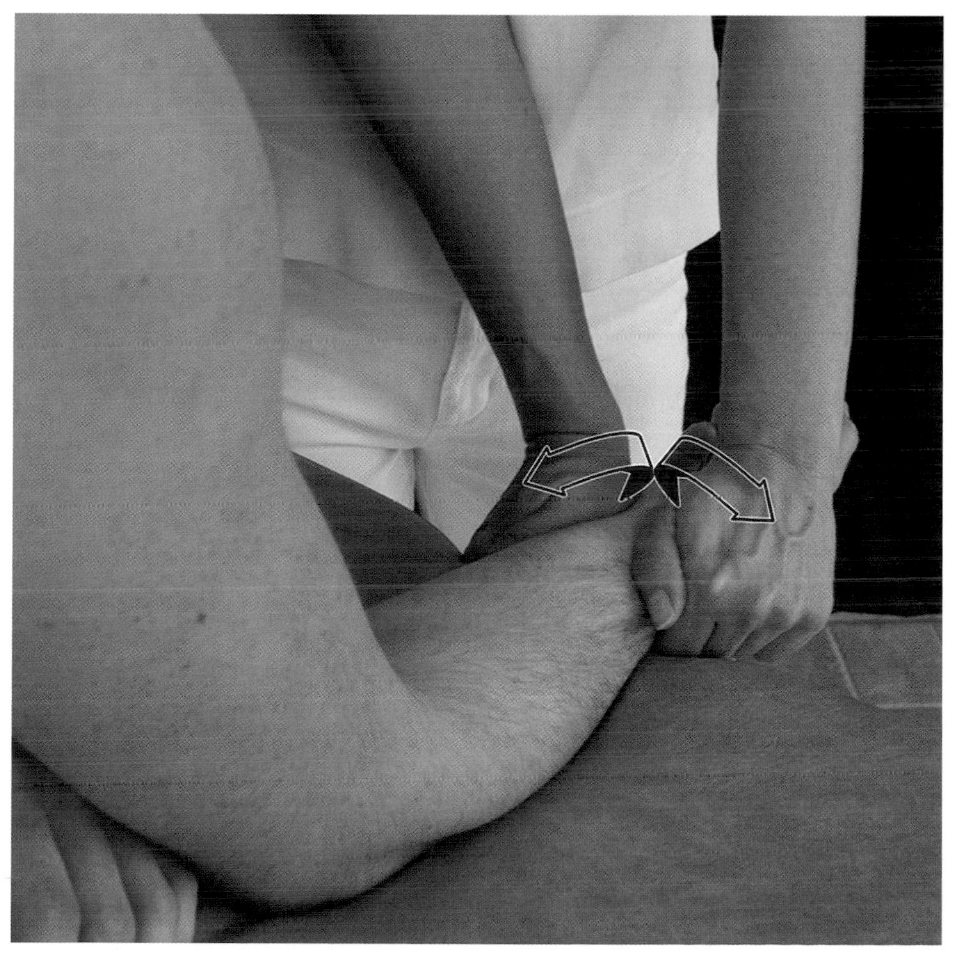

Stretching technique (supination):

Therapist grasps the thumb and radius with thumb and thenar of one hand and the little finger and styloid process of ulna with the other hand respectively bones and rotates hands away from each other.

Tension–relaxation technique: Patient tries to rotate wrist internally while therapist resists. Patient is then instructed to gradually relax muscles while therapist applies stretching technique.

Notice: The muscle may be absent.

Supinator

Nerve, supply: Posterior interosseus nerve, of radial nerve, C5–6.

Origin: Supinator crest of the ulna, lateral epicondyle of the humerus, the radial collateral ligament and the annular ligament of the radioulnar joint.

Insertion: Between the radial tuberosity and insertion of pronator teres muscle on the radius.

Function: External rotation of forearm.

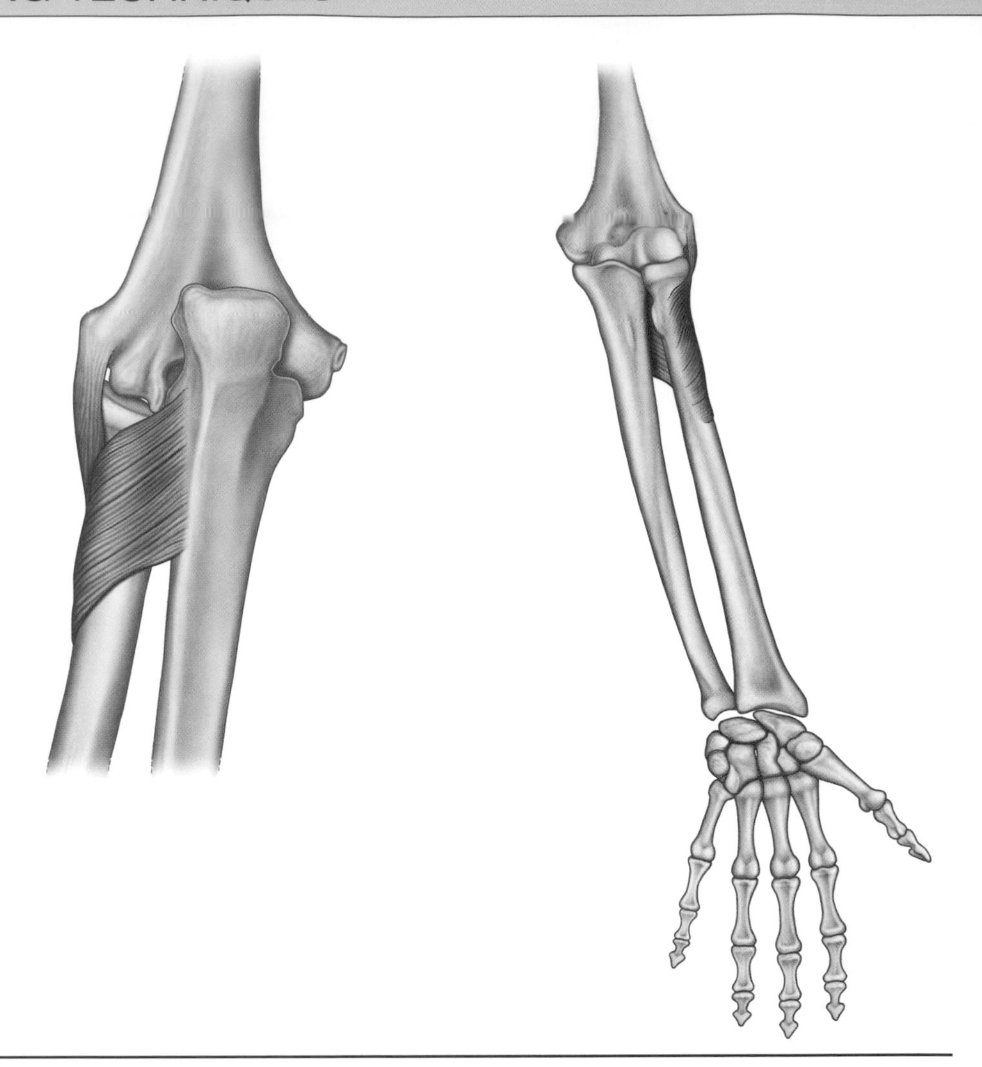

Stretching technique: (pronation + extension)

Patient is lying on back with the elbow flexed about 45°. Therapist applies pressure with the thenar of the hand across the body of muscle while using the other hand to internally rotate and extend the forearm.

Tension–relaxation technique: Patient tries to externally rotate forearm for 5 sec while therapist resists. Patient is then instructed to gradually relax muscles while therapist applies stretching technique.

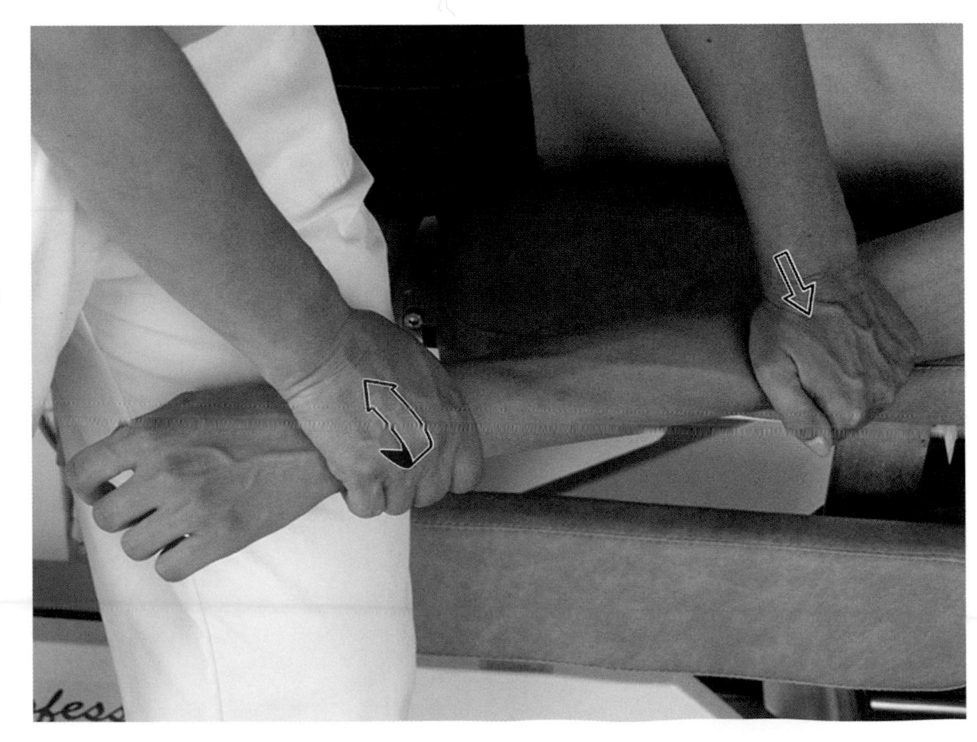

Extensor carpi radialis longus

Nerve, supply: Radial nerve, C6–8.

Origin: Lateral epicondyle and lateral supracondylar crest of the humerus.

Insertion: Base of the second metacarpal.

Function: Extension and radial abduction of wrist, weak flexor of the elbow and brings forearm into the mid-position between pronation and supination.

Extensor carpi radialis brevis

Nerve, supply: Posteror interosseus nerve of radial nerves C6–8.

Origin: Lateral epicondyle, radial collateral ligament and annular radial ligament.

Insertion: Base of the third metacarpal.

Function: Extension and radial abduction of wrist, weak flexor of the elbow and brings forearm into the mid-position between pronation and supination.

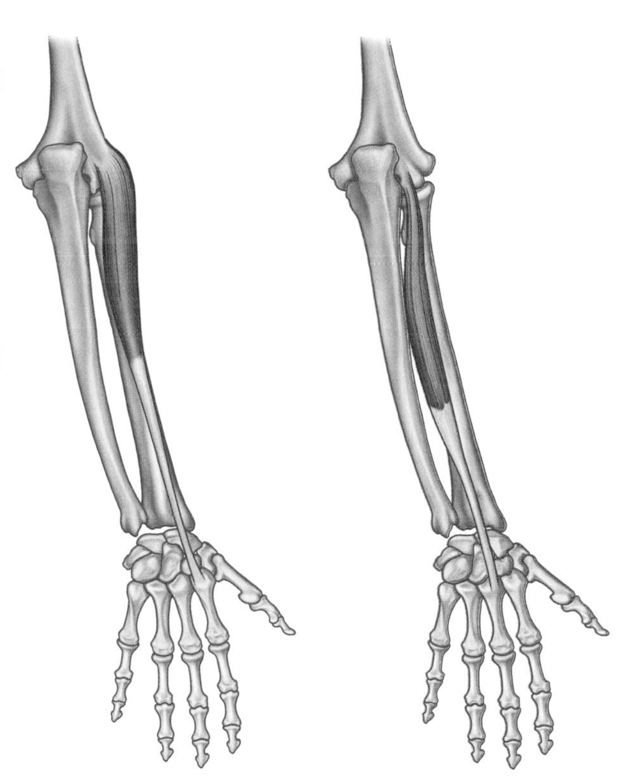

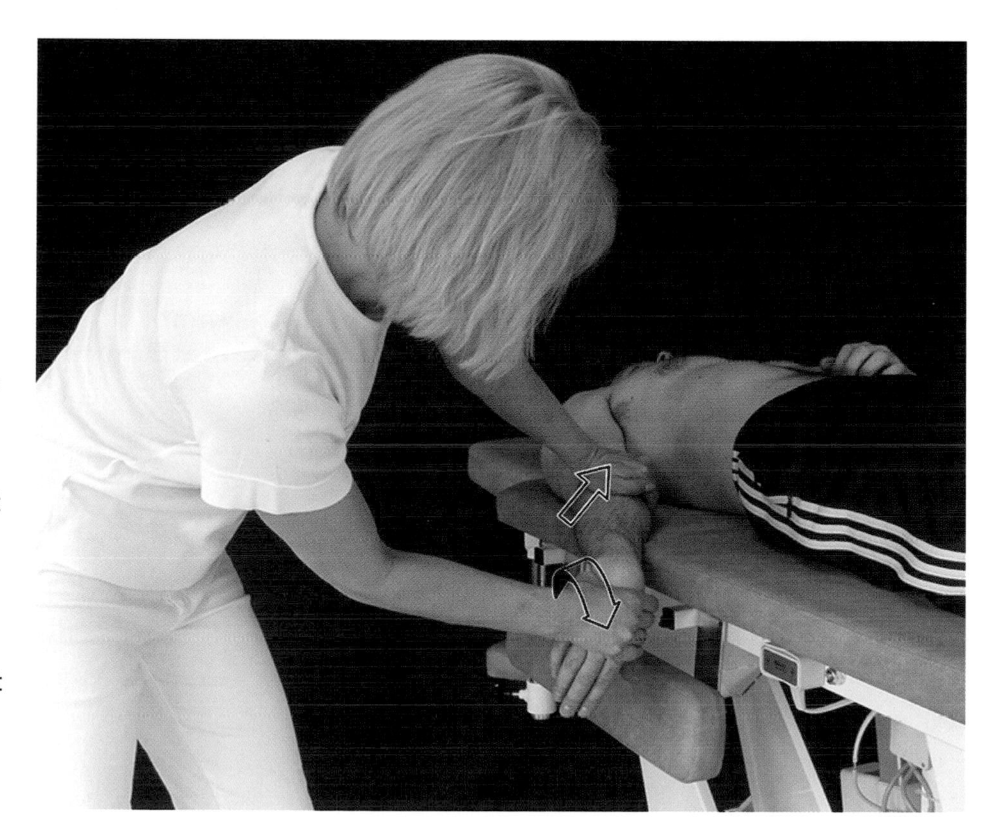

Stretching technique (pronation + flexion):

Patient lies on back with the arm straight and beside the body. Therapist applies pressure with the thenar of the hand towards the body of muscle away from insertion while the other hand is used to grasp the second and third metacarpal bones and flex the wrist and internally rotate the forearm.

Tension–relaxation technique: Patient tries to extend the wrist for 5 sec while therapist resists. Patient is then instructed to gradually relax muscles while therapist applies stretching technique.

Extensor carpi ulnaris

Nerve, supply: Posterior interosseus nerve, of radial nerve, C6–8.

Origin: Medial epicondyle, radial collateral ligament and middle third of posterior surface of ulna.

Insertion: Base of fifth metacarpal.

Function: Extension and ulnar abduction of the wrist.

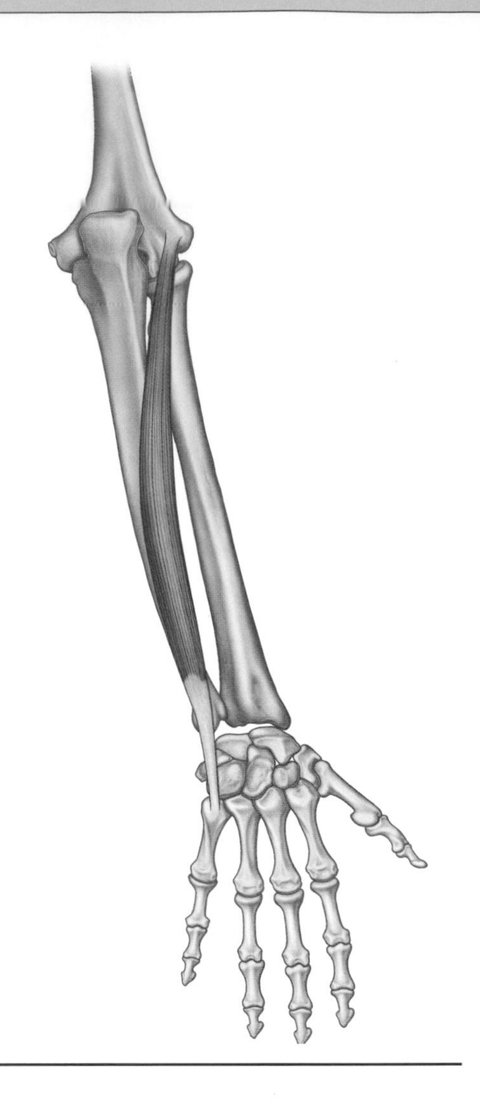

Stretching technique (supination + flexion):

Patient is lying on stomach and arm extended at side. Therapist applies pressure towards the body of muscle from the tendon–muscular junction with the thenar of the hand while using the other hand to grasp the fifth metacarpal and flex the wrist and externally rotate the forearm.

Tension–relaxation technique: Patient tries to extend wrist for 5 sec while therapist resists. Patient is then instructed to gradually relax muscles while therapist applies stretching technique.

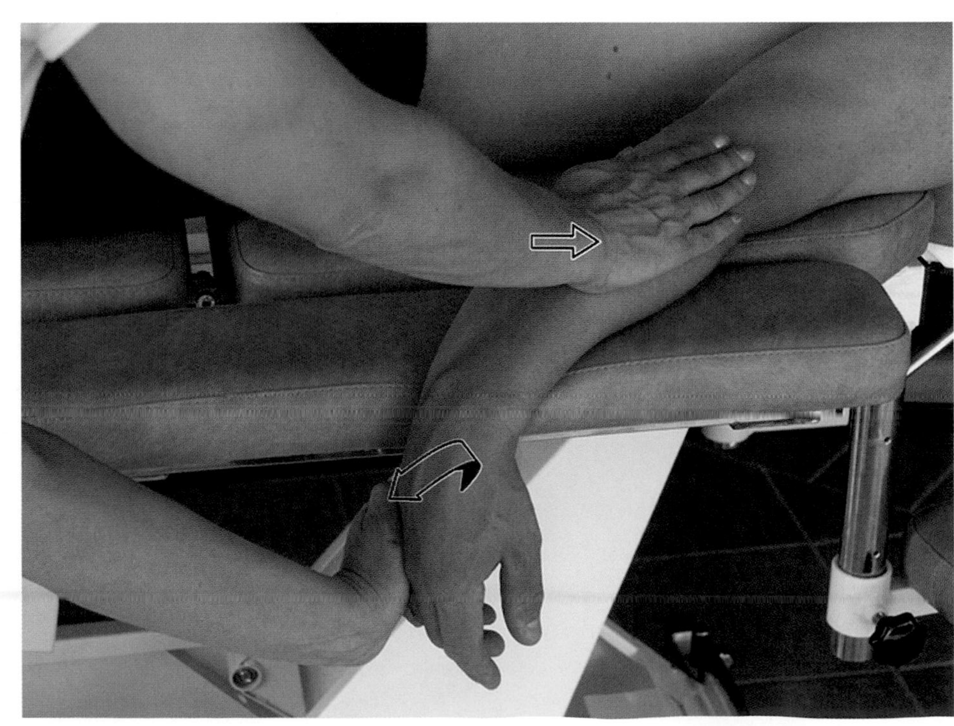

Extensor digitorum

Nerve, supply: Posterior interosseus nerve of radial nerve, C6–8.

Origin: Lateral epicondyle, radial collateral ligament, annular radial ligament and antebrachial fascia.

Insertion: Via the dorsal aponeurosis to the capsules of the metacarpophalangeal joints, bases of proximal and distal phalanges of fingers 2–5.

The tendon to the fifth finger may be absent.

Function: Extension and separation of fingers, and extension and ulnar abduction of wrist.

Extensor digitorum is the strongest extensor of wrist and fingers.

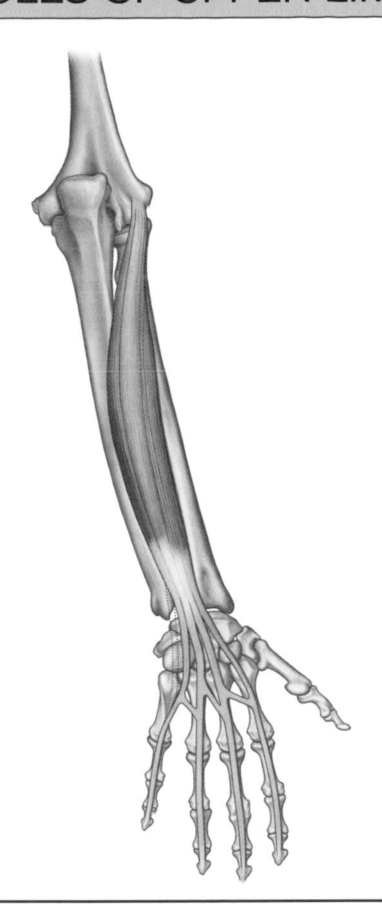

Stretching technique (pronation + flexion):

Patient is lying on back with the elbow extended at side and fingers in tight fist. Therapist applies pressure with the thenar of the hand towards the body of muscle away from insertion while using the other hand to grasp the fist, flex the wrist and internally rotate forearm.

Tension–relaxation technique: Patient tries to extend wrist for 5 sec while therapist resists. Patient is then instructed to gradually relax muscles while therapist applies stretching technique.

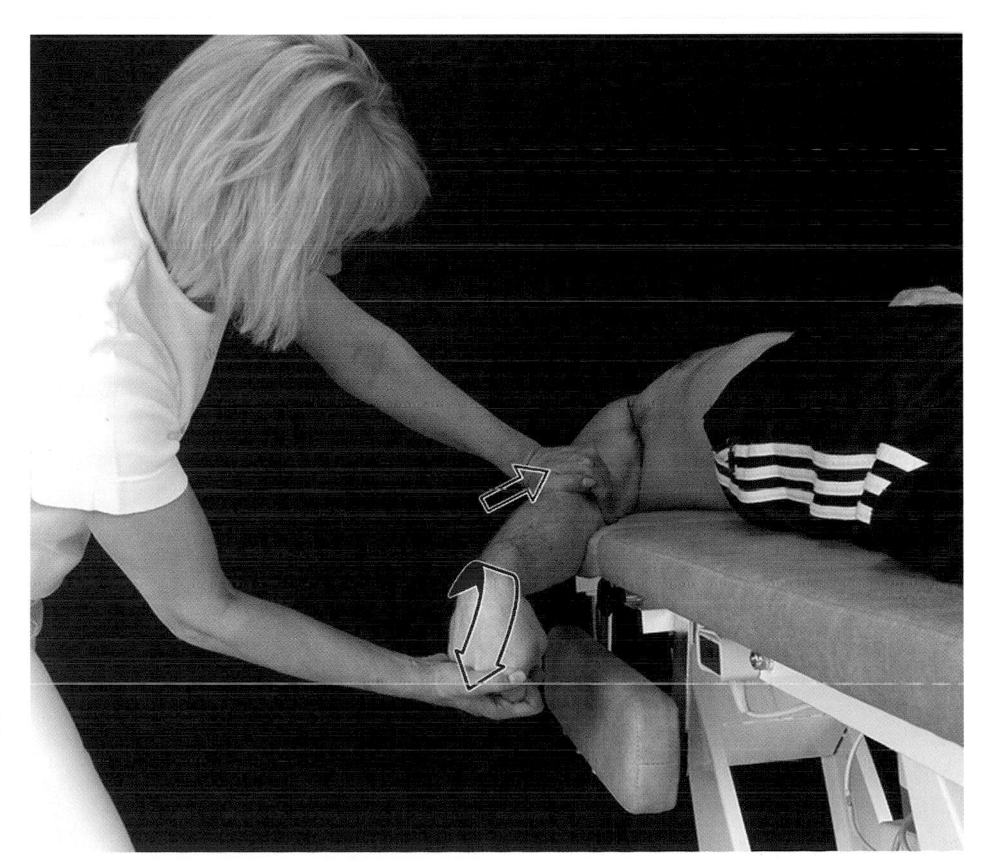

Extensor digiti minimi

Nerve, supply: Posterior interosseus nerve, of radial nerve, C6–8.

Origin: Lateral epicondyle.

Insertion: Dorsal aponeurosis of fifth finger.

The muscle may be absent and the function is fulfilled by the extensor digitorum.

Function: Extension of little finger and extension and ulnar abduction of wrist.

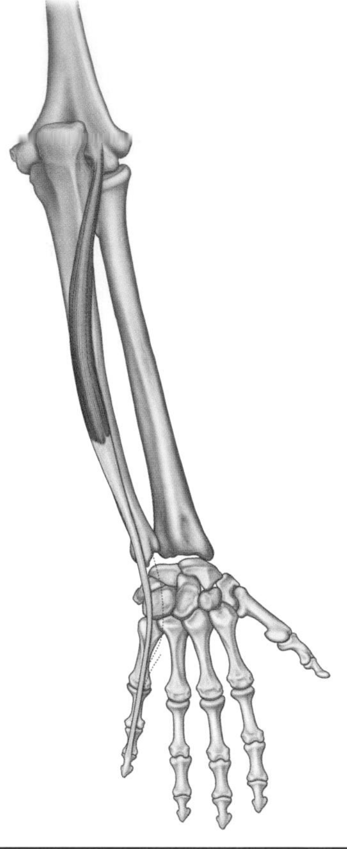

Stretching technique (supination + flexion):

Patient is lying on stomach with the elbow extended at side and the little finger flexed. Therapist applies pressure with the thenar of the hand towards the body of muscle away from insertion while using the other hand to grasp the flexed little finger, flex the wrist and externally rotate forearm.

Tension–relaxation technique: Patient tries to extend the wrist for 5 sec while therapist resists. Patient is then instructed to gradually relax muscles while therapist applies stretching technique.

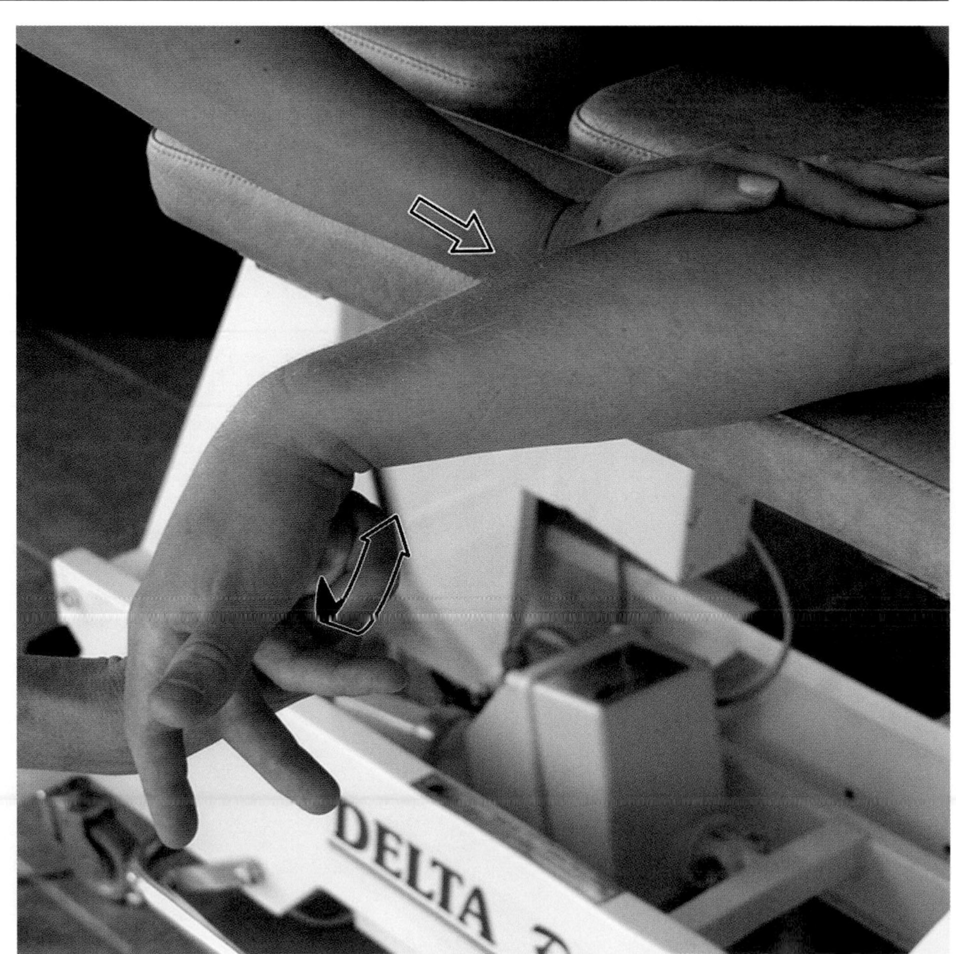

Abductor pollicis longus

Nerve, supply: Posterior interosseus nerve, of radial nerve, C7–8.

Origin: Dorsal surfaces of ulna and radius, and interosseus membrane.

Insertion: Base of first metacarpal, trapezium bone of wrist, and tendons of the extensor pollicis brevis and abductor pollicis brevis.

Function: Extension and abduction of thumb and radial abduction of wrist.

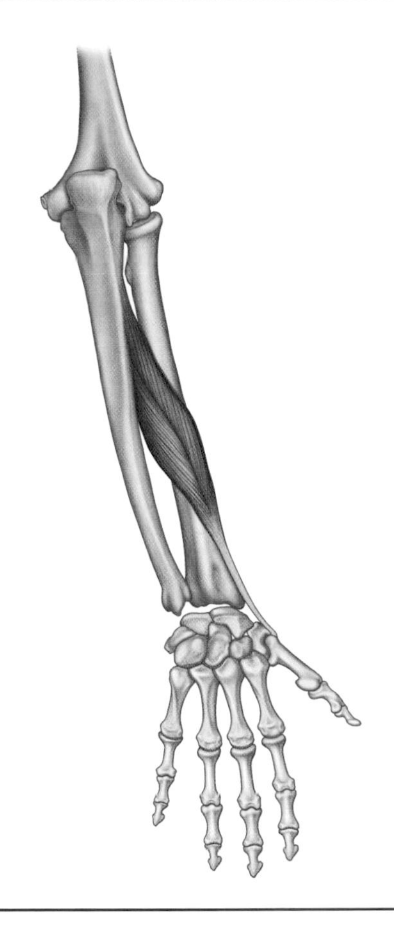

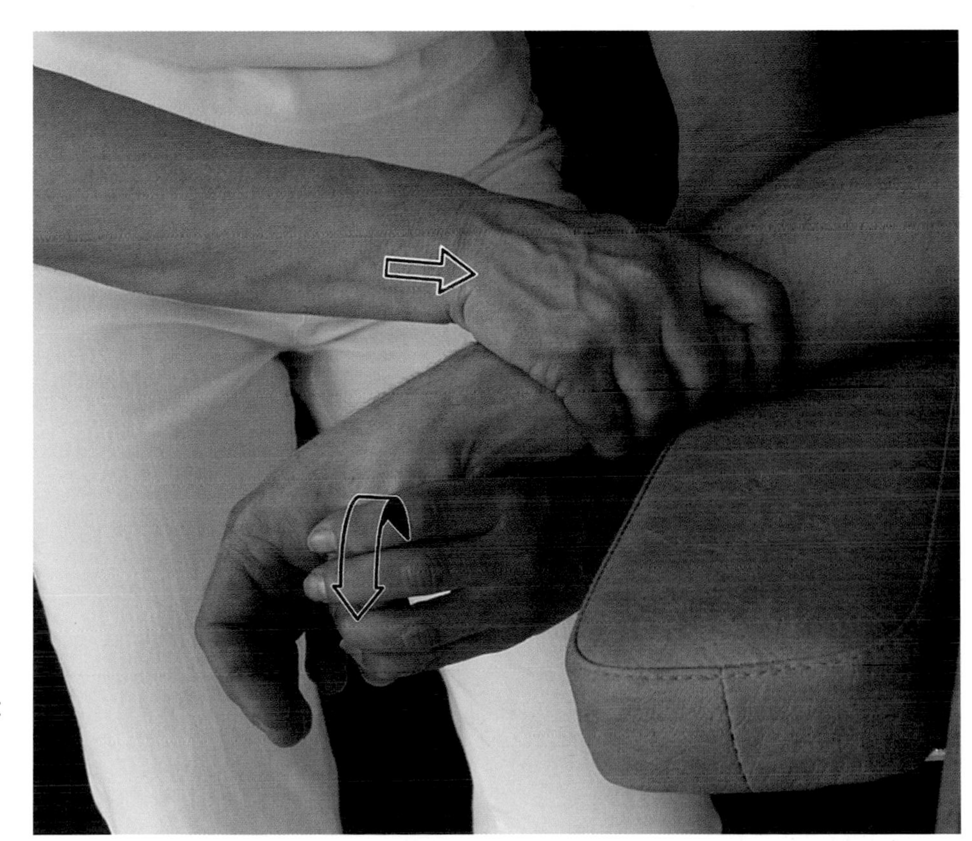

Stretching technique (ulnar deviation + flexion + pronation):

Therapist applies pressure with the thenar of the hand towards the body of muscle away from insertion while using the other hand to grasp the thumb, flex the metacarpophalangeal and wrist joints and internally rotate the forearm.

Tension–relaxation technique: Patient tries to extend the wrist for 5 sec while therapist resists. Patient is then instructed to gradually relax muscles while therapist applies stretching technique.

Extensor pollicis longus

Nerve, supply: Posterior interosseus nerve, of radial nerve, C7–8.

Origin: Dorsal surface of ulna and interosseus membrane.

Insertion: Base of distal phalanx of thumb.

Function: Extends thumb and extension and radial abduction of wrist.

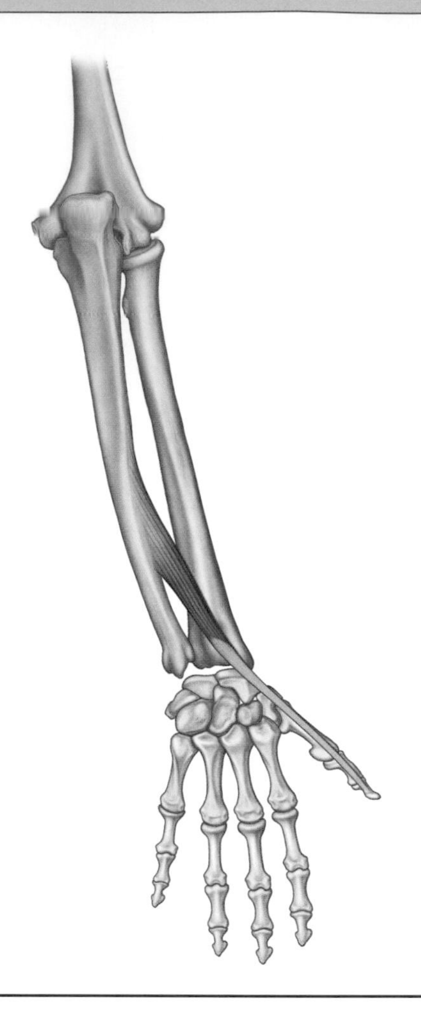

Stretching technique (flexion + ulnar deviation + pronation):

Therapist applies pressure with the thenar of the hand towards the body of muscle away from insertion while using the other hand to flex the thumb, flex the wrist and internally rotate the forearm.

Tension–relaxation technique: Patient tries to extend the wrist for 5 sec while therapist resists. Patient is then instructed to gradually relax muscles while therapist applies stretching technique.

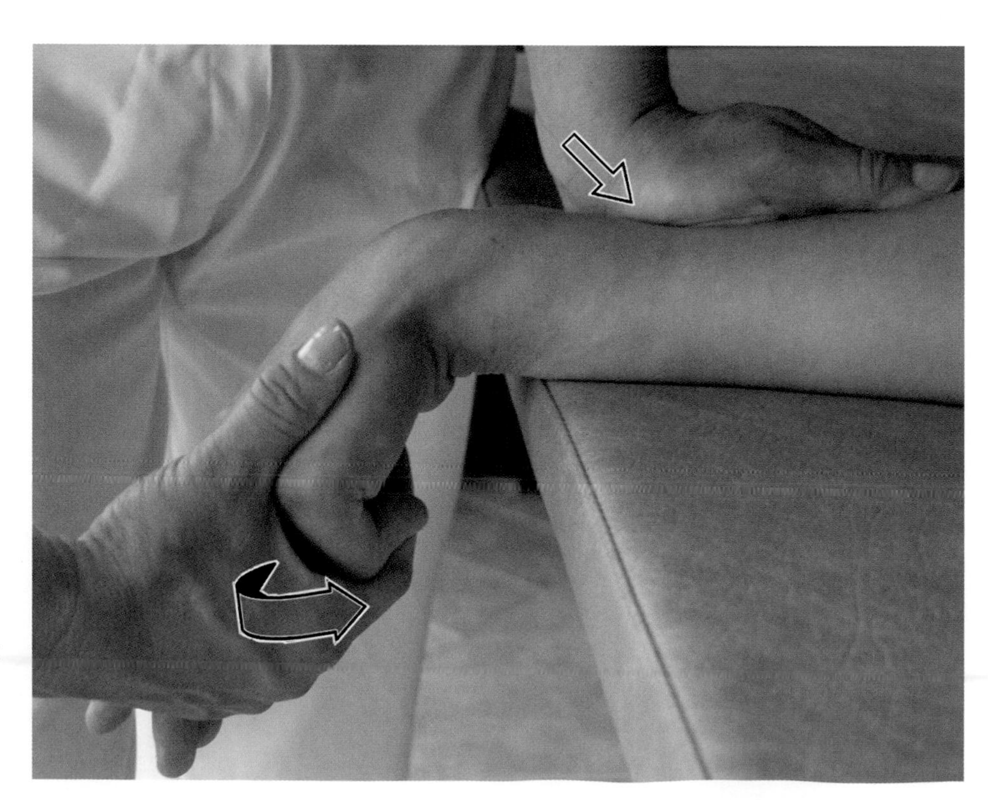

Extensor pollicis brevis

Nerve, supply: Radial nerve, C7–Th1.

Origin: Distal posterior surfaces of radius and ulna and interosseus membrane.

Insertion: Base of the proximal phalanx of thumb.

The muscle may be absent or have two tendons.

Function: Extension and abduction of thumb.

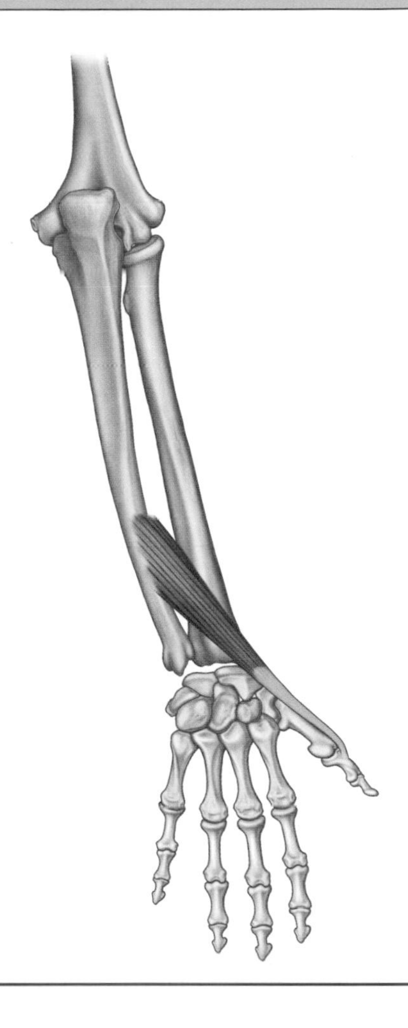

Stretching technique (flexion + ulnar deviation + pronation):

Therapist applies pressure with the thenar of the hand towards the body of muscle away from insertion while using the other hand to flex the metacarpophalangeal joint of the thumb to bend the wrist towards the ulnar side, flex wrist and rotate forearm internally.

Tension–relaxation technique: Patient tries to extend the thumb for 5 sec while therapist resists. Patient is then instructed to gradually relax muscles while therapist applies stretching technique.

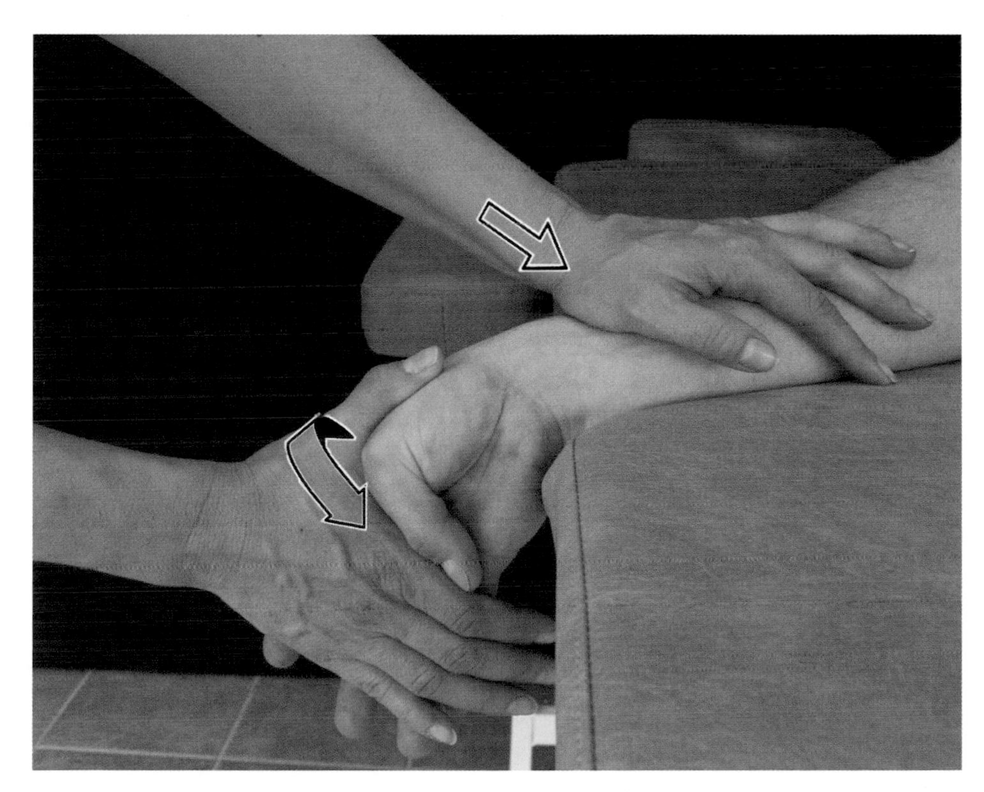

Extensor indicis

Nerve, supply: Posterior interosseus nerve, of radial nerve, C6–8.

Origin: Distal third of posterior ulna and interosseus membrane.

Insertion: Via dorsal aponeurosis to the distal phalan of index finger.

Function: Extension of index finger and assists in wrist extension.

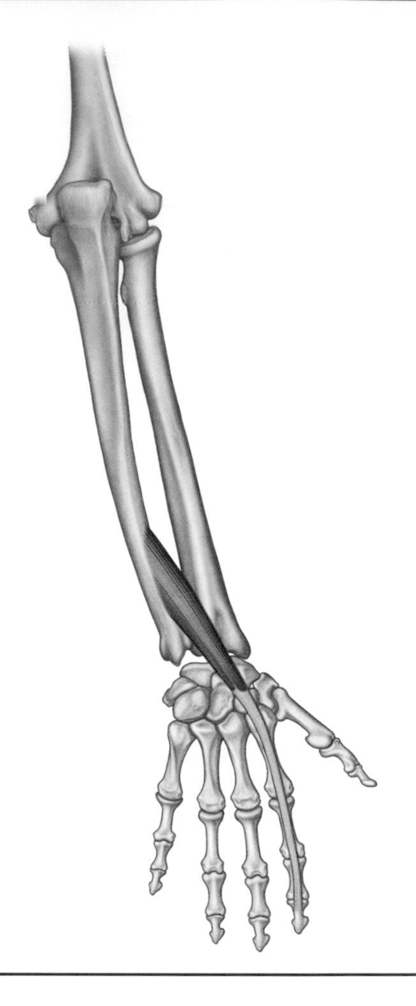

Stretching technique (flexion + ulnar deviation + pronation):

Therapist applies pressure with the thenar of the hand towards the body of muscle away from insertion while using the other hand to flex the index finger, bend the wrist towards the ulnar side, flex the wrist and internally rotate the forearm.

Tension–relaxation technique: Patient tries to extend the index finger for 5 sec while therapist resists. Patient is then instructed to gradually relax muscles while therapist applies stretching technique.

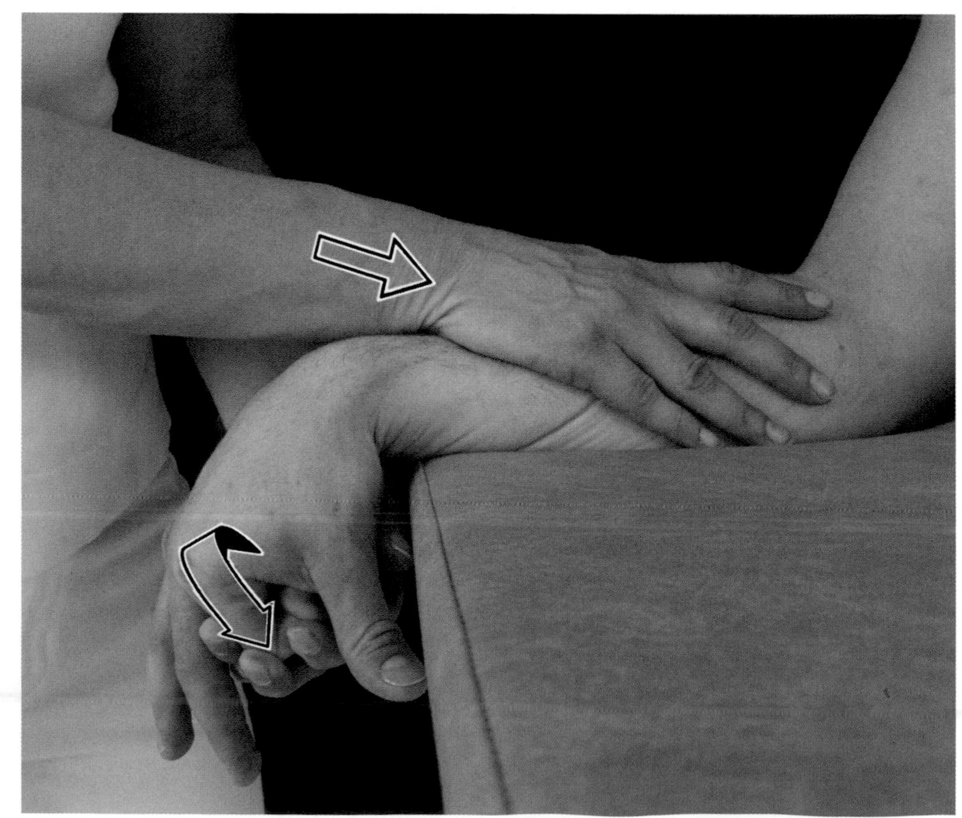

Abductor pollicis brevis

Nerve, supply: Median nerve, C8–Th1.

Origin: Scaphoid bone and flexor retinaculum.

Insertion: Radial sesamoid bone and radially surface of proximal phalanx of the thumb.

Function: Flexion and abduction of thumb.

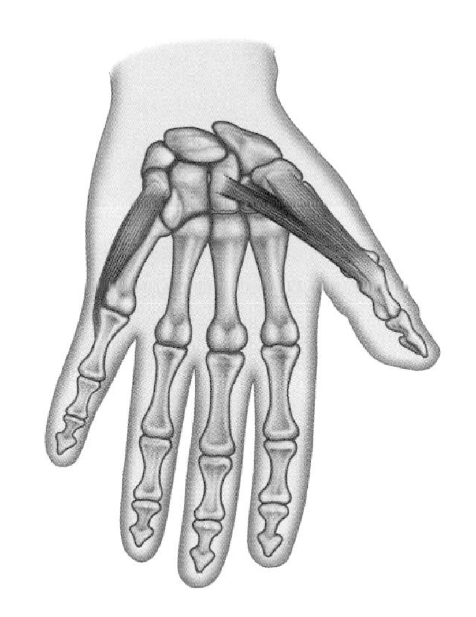

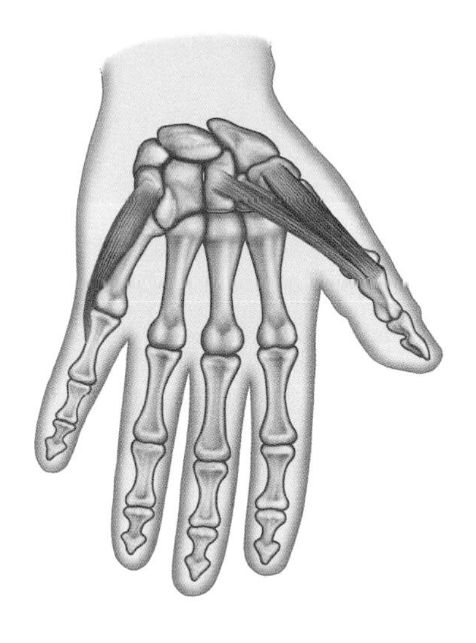

Flexor pollicis brevis

Nerve, supply: Superficially by median nerve, and to deeper layers by ulnar nerve, C8–Th1.

Origin: Superficial head at the flexor retinaculum and the deep head from the trapezium, trapezoid and capitate bones.

Insertion: Radial sesamoid bone and radially surface of proximal phalanx of the thumb.

Function: Thumb flexion, abduction and adduction.

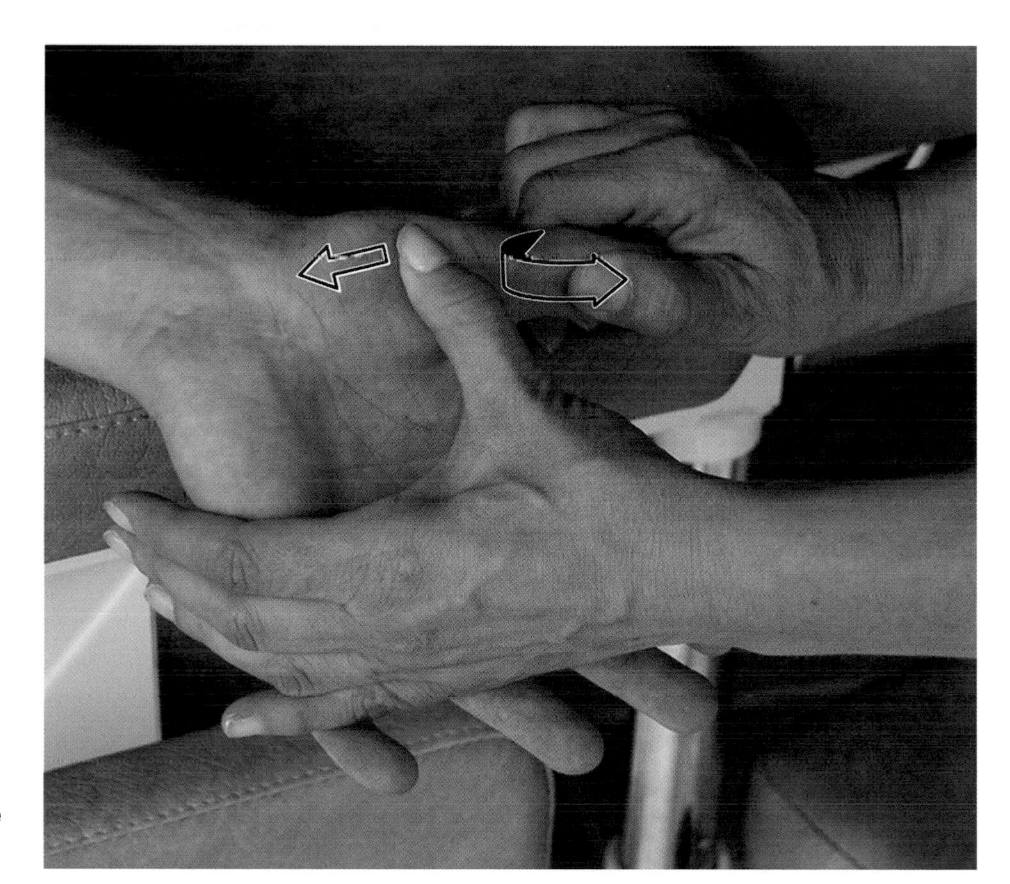

Stretching technique:

Therapist applies pressure with the thumb towards the body of muscle away from insertion while using the other hand to extend the thumb.

Opponens pollicis

Nerve, supply: Median nerve, C6–7.

Origin: Flexor retinaculum and trapezium.

Insertion: Radial surface of the first metacarpal.

Function: Opposition of thumb and assists in adduction.

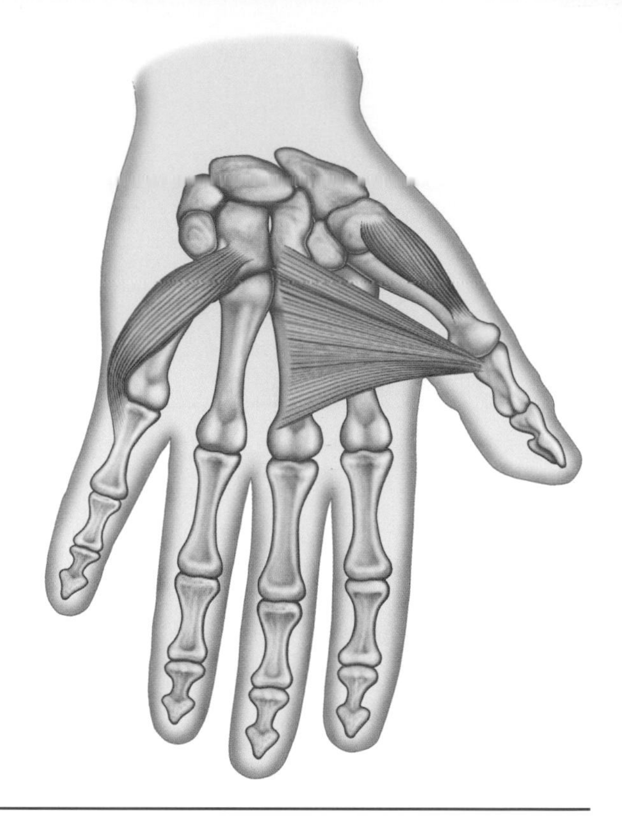

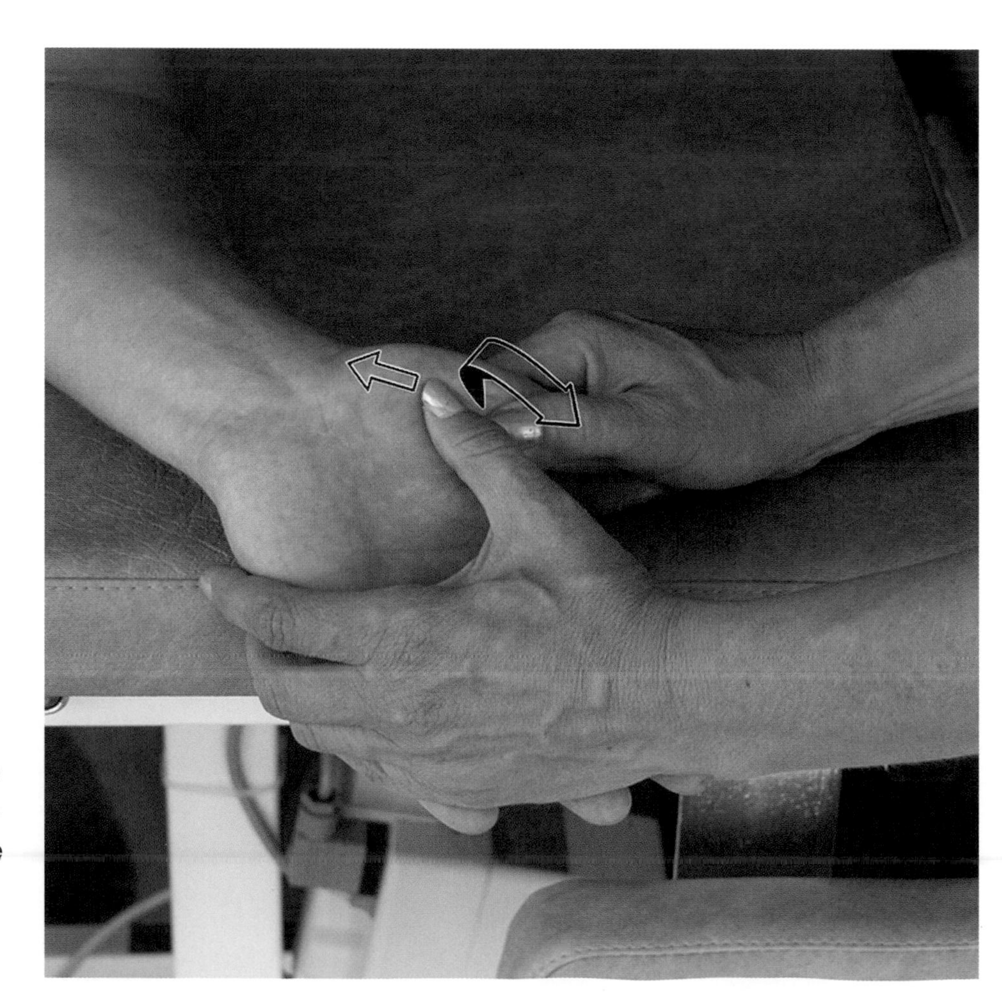

Stretching technique:

Therapist applies pressure with the thumb towards the body of muscle away from insertion while using the other hand to abduct and extend the metacarpophalangeal joint of the thumb.

Adductor pollicis

Nerve, supply: Ulnar nerve, C8–Th1.

Origin: Capitate, trapezoid and the entire length of the third metacarpal.

Insertion: Medial sesamoid bone of the metacarpophalangeal joint of the thumb and ulnar aspect of base of proximal phalanx of thumb.

Function: Adduction and assists in opposition and flexion of thumb.

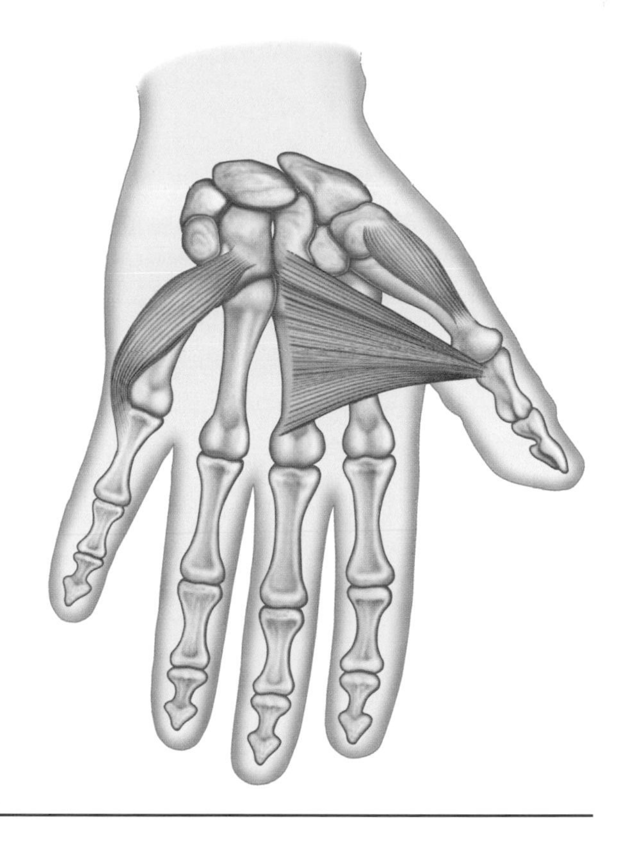

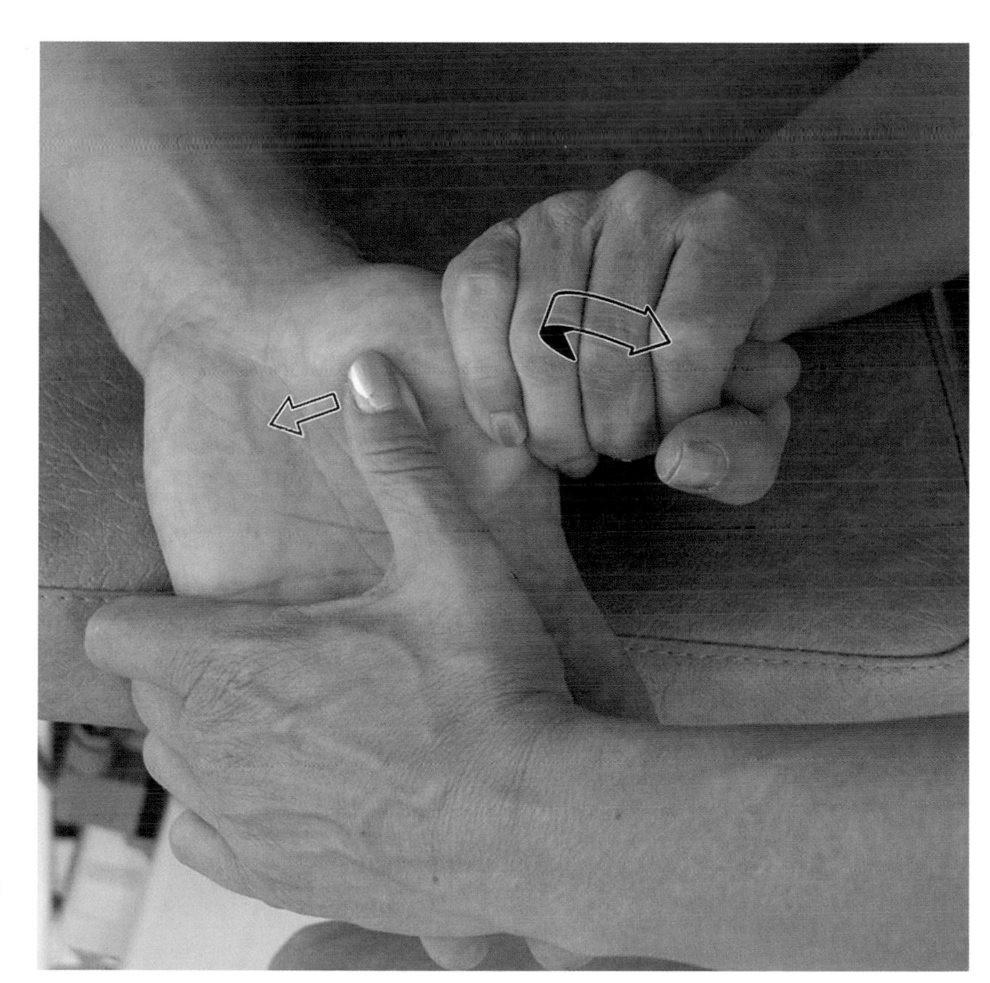

Stretching technique:

Therapist applies pressure with the thumb of the hand towards the body of muscle away from insertion while using the other hand to abduct and extend the thumb.

Abductor digiti minimi

Nerve, supply: Ulnar nerve, C8–Th1.

Origin: Pisiform bone, pisohamate ligament, and flexor retinaculum.

Insertion: Ulnar surface of base of proximal phalanx of the little finger.

Function: Abduction of little finger.

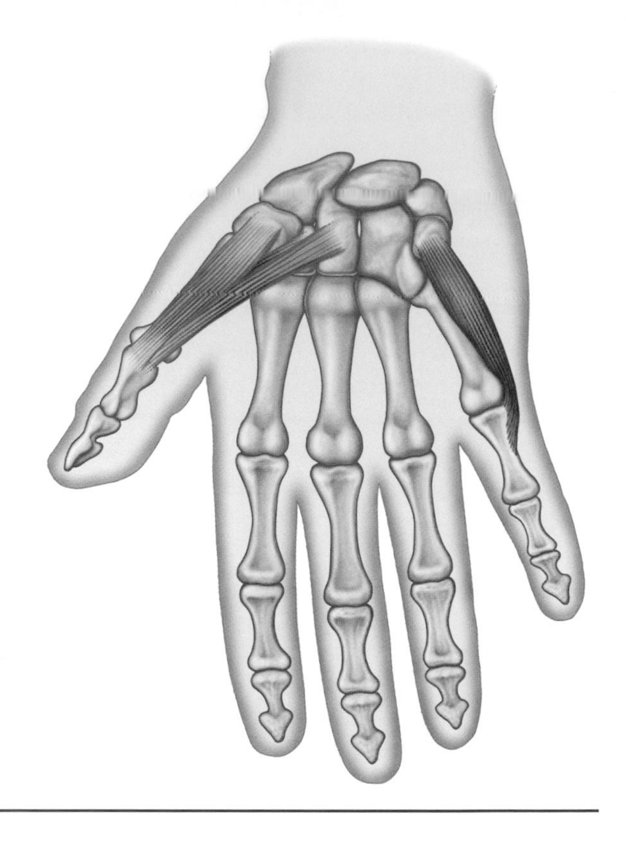

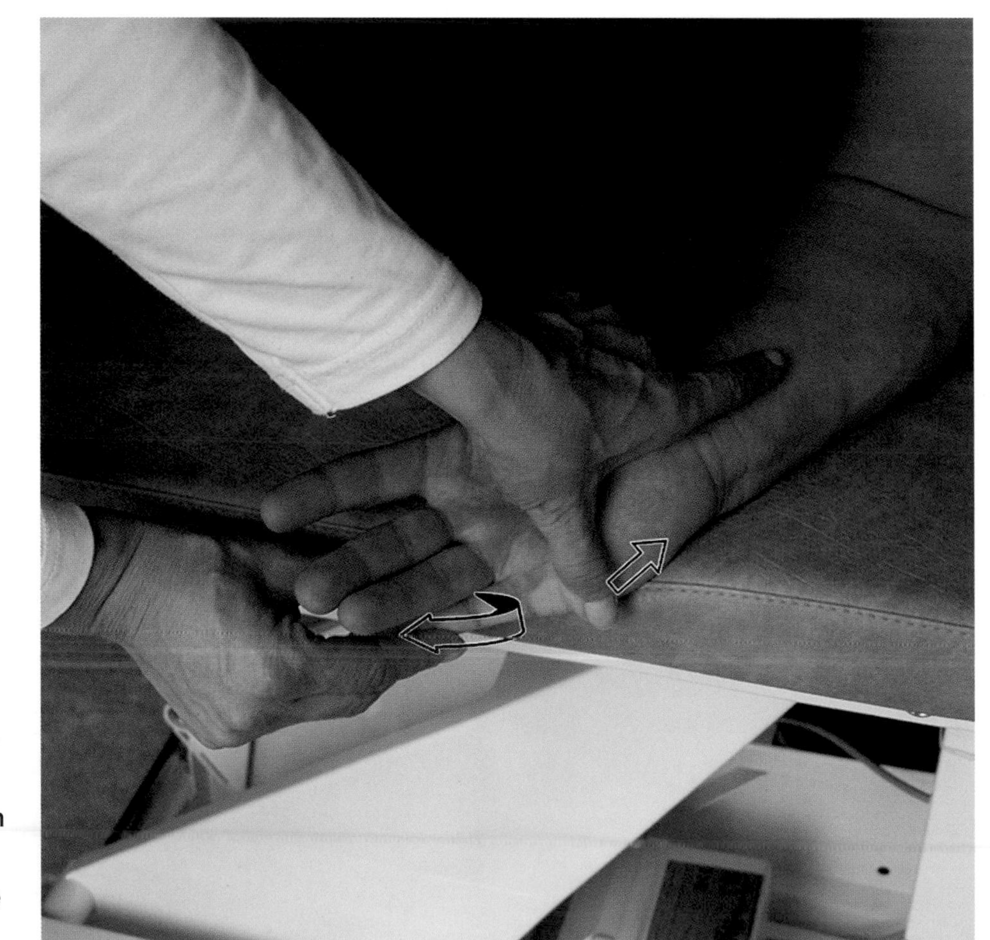

Stretching technique:

Therapist applies pressure with the thumb of the hand towards the body of muscle away from insertion while using the other hand to slightly extend and then adduct the little finger.

Flexor digiti minimi brevis

Nerve, supply: Ulnar nerve, C8–Th1.

Origin: Flexor retinaculum and hamulus of hamate.

Insertion: Tendon of abductor digiti minimi to insert ulnar surface of base of proximal phalanx of little finger.

Function: Flexion of the metacarpophalangeal joint of the little finger.

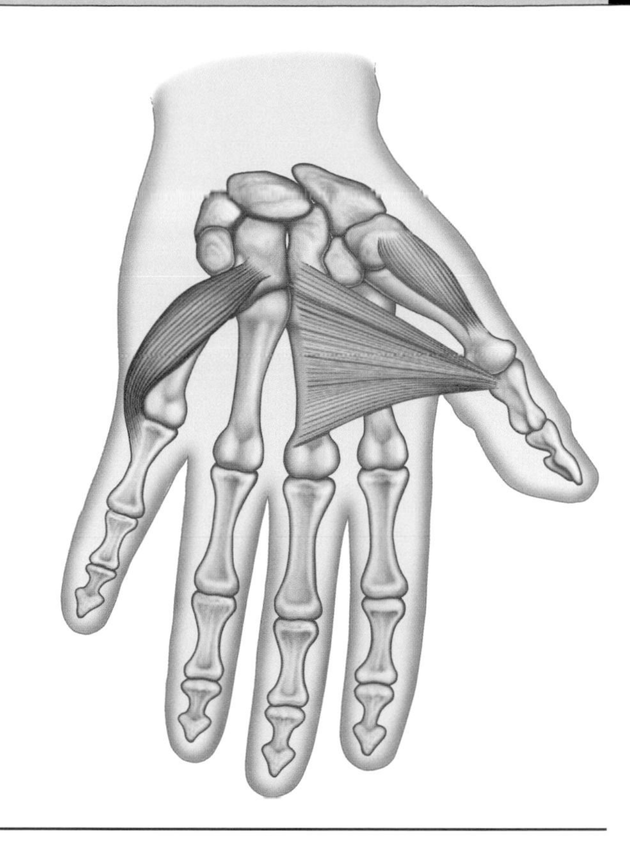

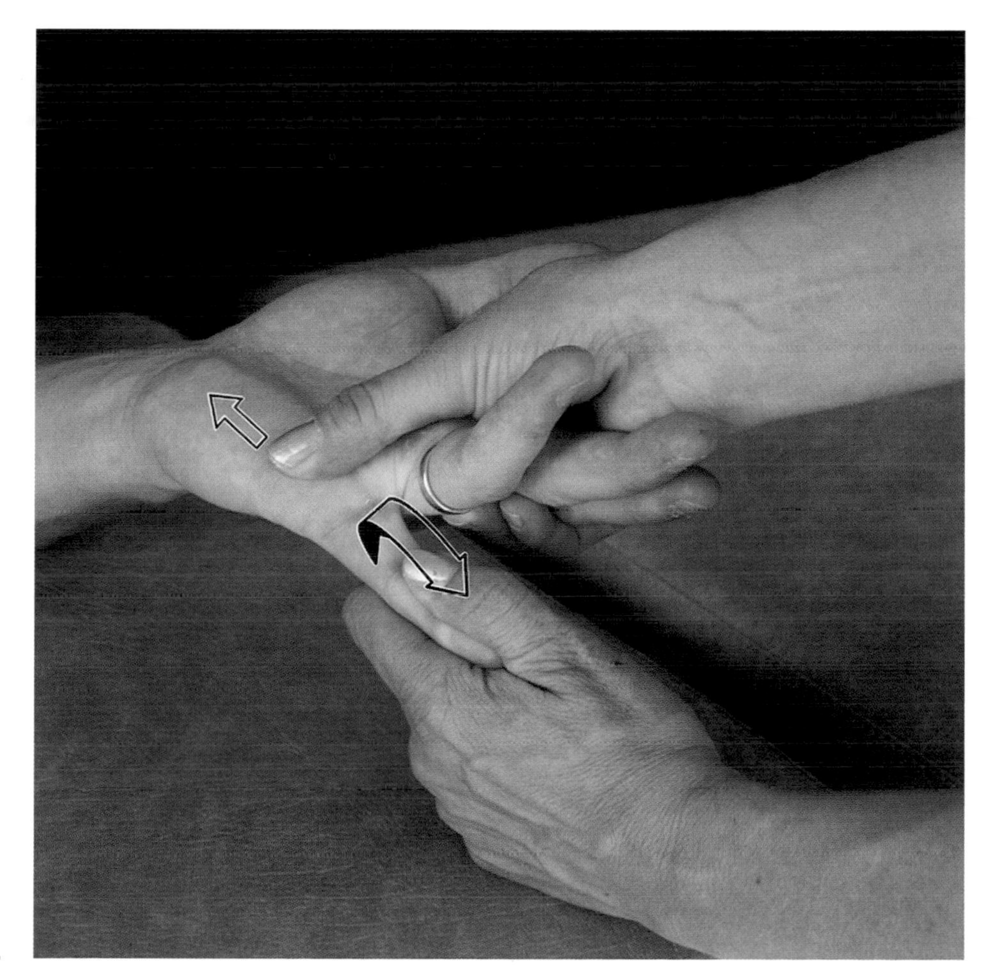

Stretching technique:

Therapist applies pressure with the thumb of the hand towards the body of muscle away from insertion while using the other hand to extend the little finger.

Notice: The muscle may be absent.

Opponens digiti minimi

Nerve, supply: Ulnar nerve, C8–Th1.

Origin: Hamulus of hamate bone and from the flexor retinaculum.

Insertion: Ulnar surface of the fifth metacarpal.

Function: Brings little finger into position for opposition.

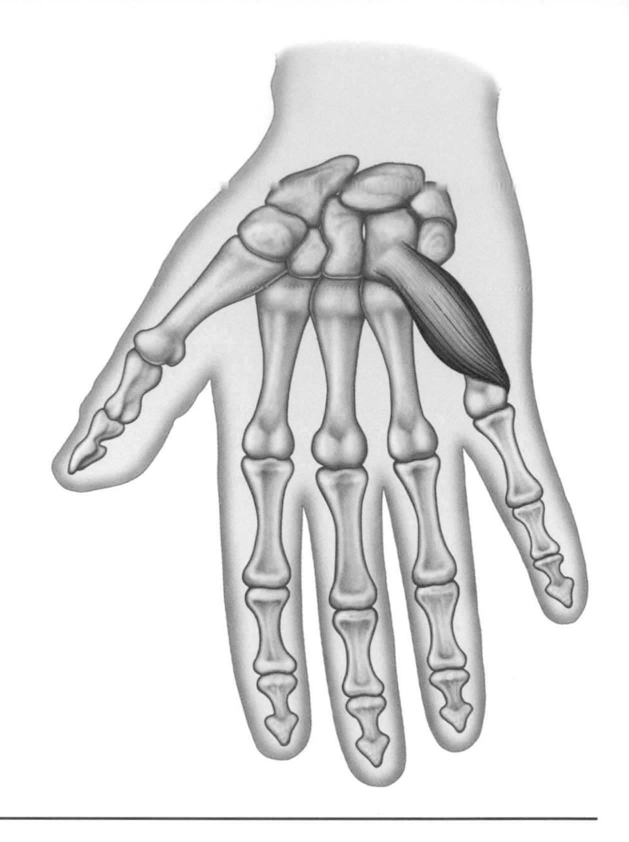

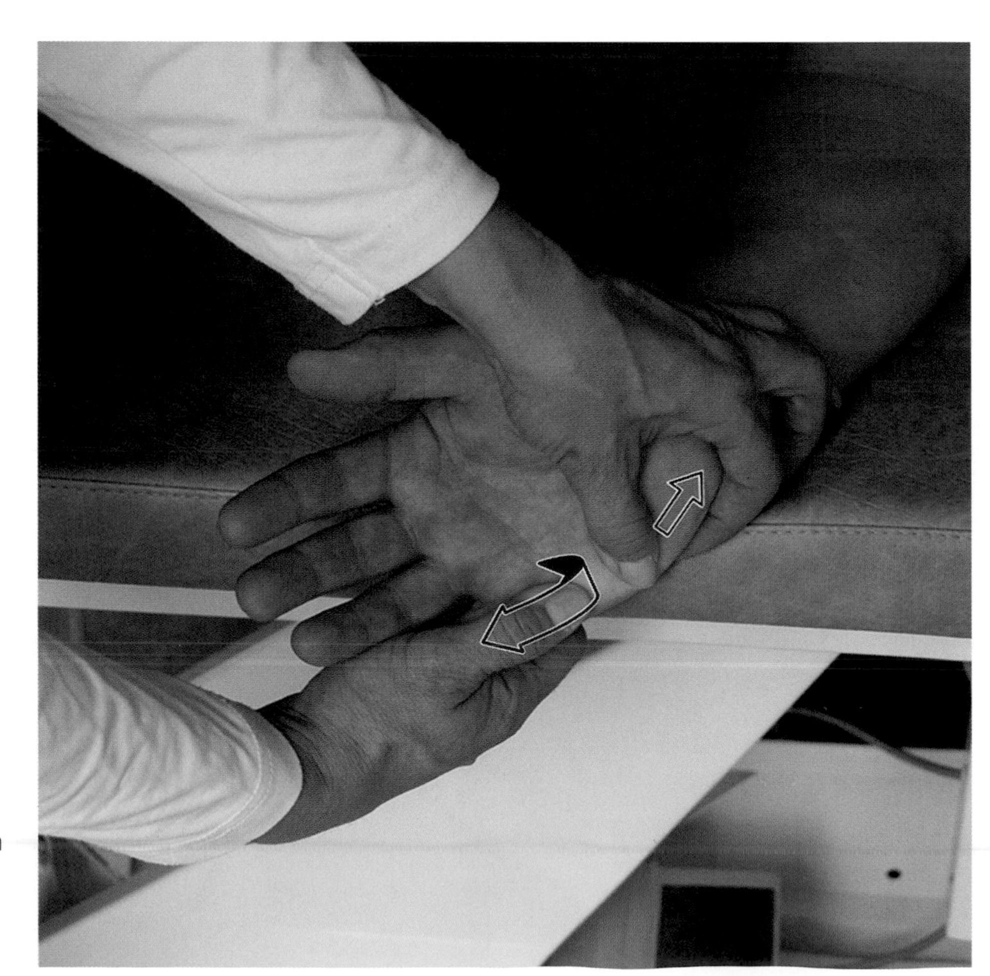

Stretching technique:

Therapist applies pressure with the thumb of the hand towards the body of muscle away from insertion while using the other hand to extend the metacarpophalangeal joint of the little finger.

Palmaris brevis

Nerve, supply: Ulnar nerve, C8–Th1.

Origin: Palmar aponeurosis and flexor retinaculum.

Insertion: Skin of ulnar border of hand.

Function: Thickens palm.

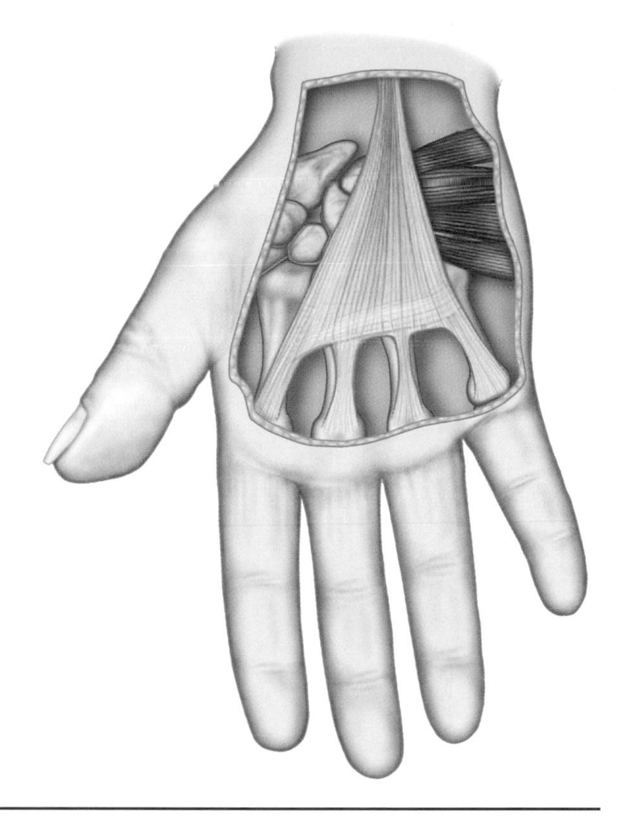

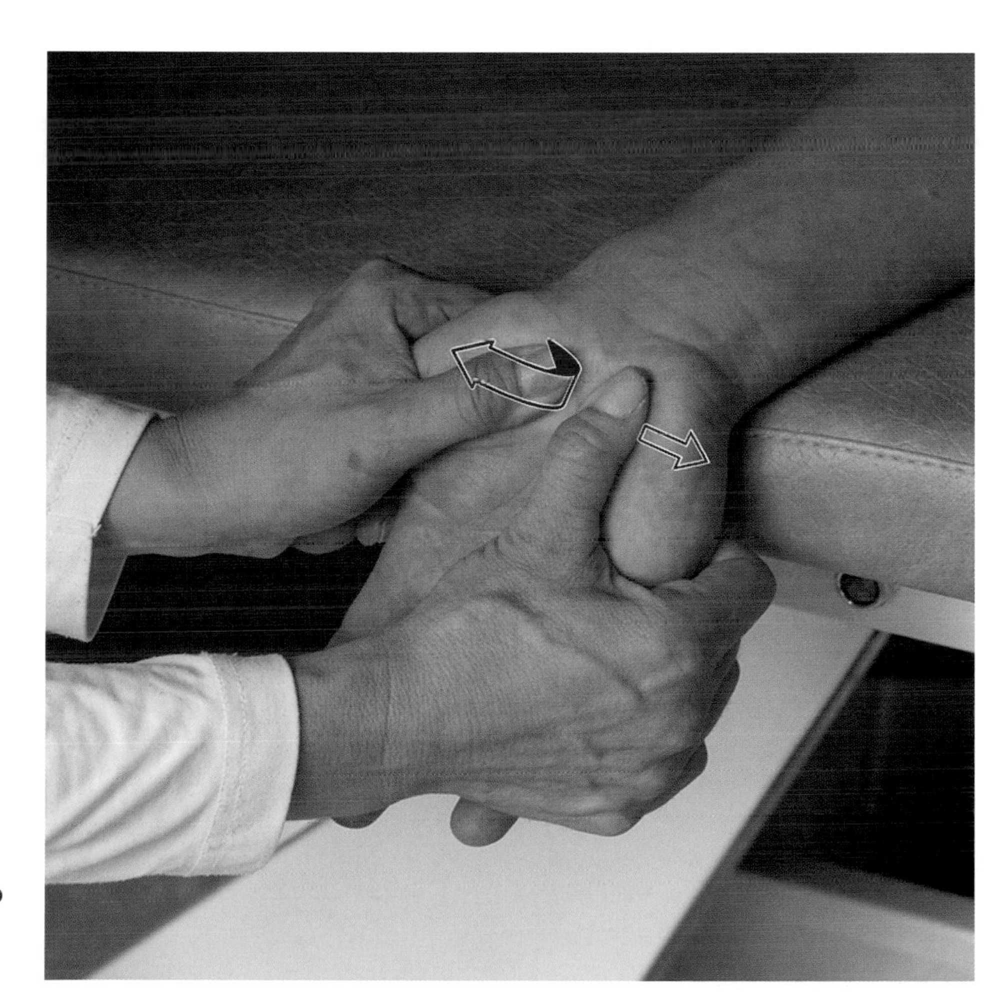

Stretching technique:

Therapist grasps patient's hand at the side of thumb producing counterforce while using the thumb of the other hand to stretch along body of muscle away from origin.

Lumbricales

Nerve, supply: Two radial muscles are supplied by median nerve and two ulnar ones by ulnar nerve, C8–Th1.

Origin: Radial sides of four tendons of flexor digitorum profundus.

Insertion: Radial sides of extensor aponeurosis and joint capsules of metacarpophalangeal joints 2–5.

Function: Flexion of metacarpophalangeal joints and extension of interphalangeal joints.

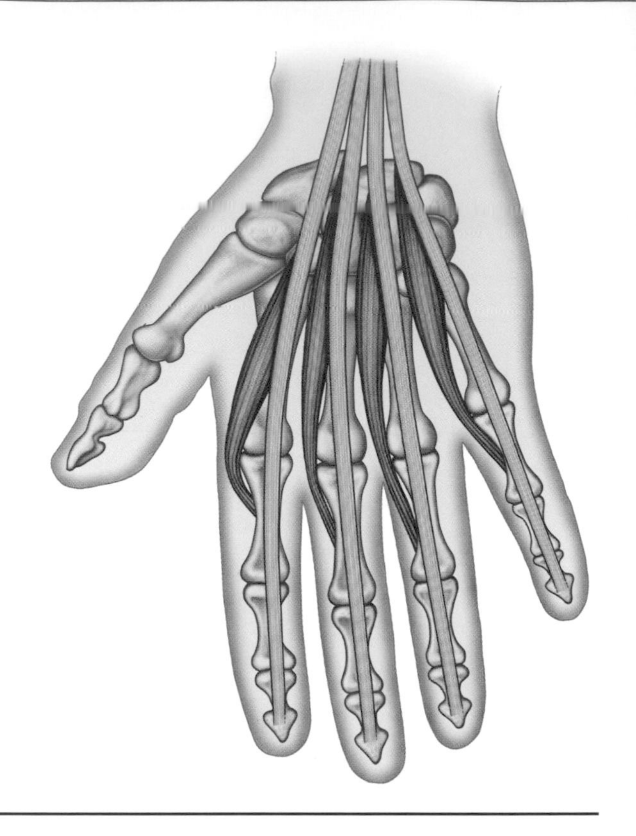

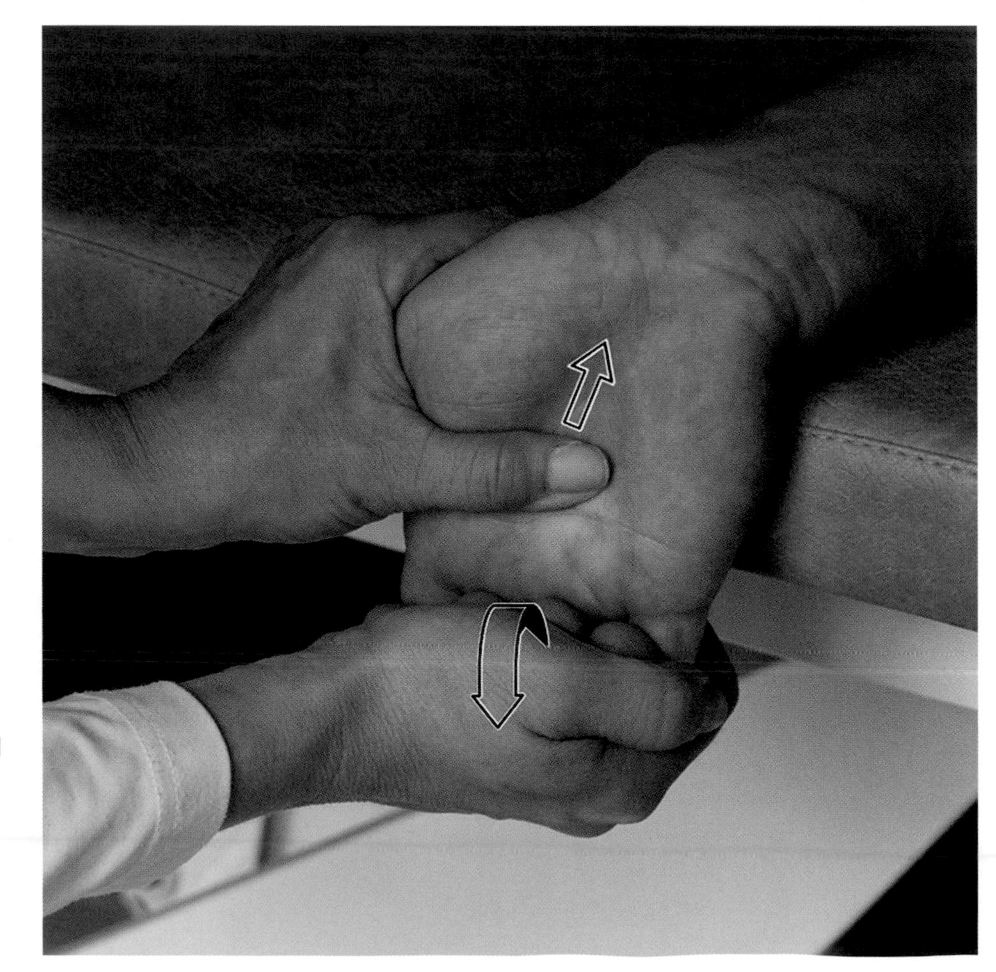

Stretching technique:

Therapist grasps flexed fingers and extends metacarpophalangeal and wrist joints. The thumb of the other hand is used to stretch along bodies of muscles away from insertions.

Palmar interossei

(Three muscles between metacarpal bones)

Nerve, supply: Ulnar nerve, C8–Th1.

Origin: Ulnar side of the second and radial side of the fourth and fifth metacarpals.

Insertion: Bases of proximal phalanges and via extensor aponeuroses to middle and distal phalanges of the corresponding fingers.

Function: Flexion of metacapophalangeal joints, extension of interphalangeal joints and draws fingers together.

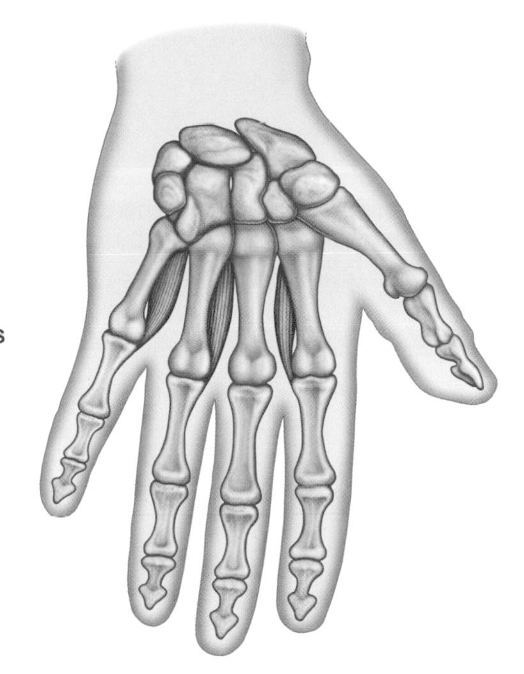

Stretching technique:

Therapist interlocks own fingers with that of patient's, which are in flexion, and extends metacarpophalangeal joints. Therapist uses other hand to stretch along bodies of muscles away from insertions.

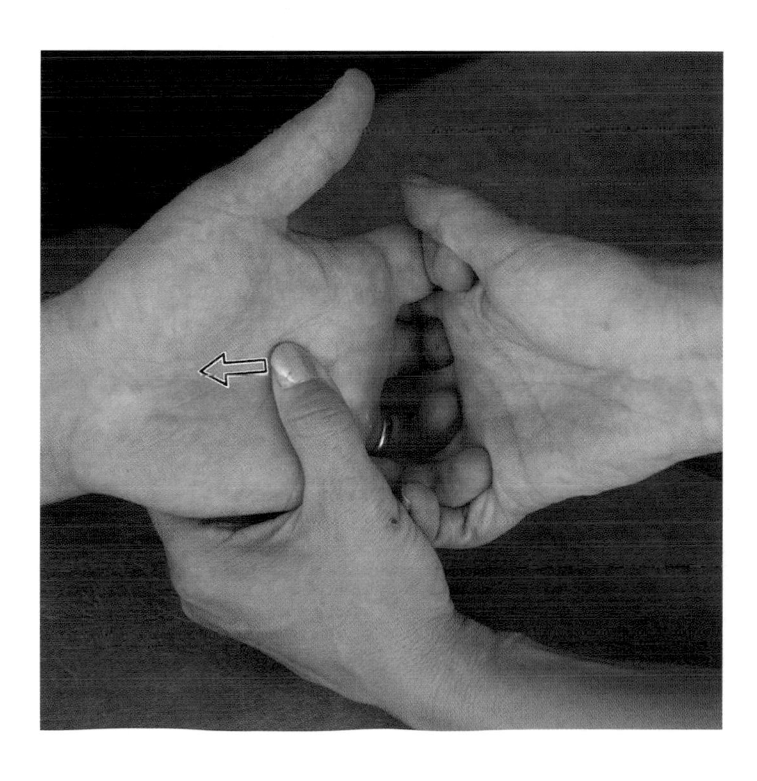

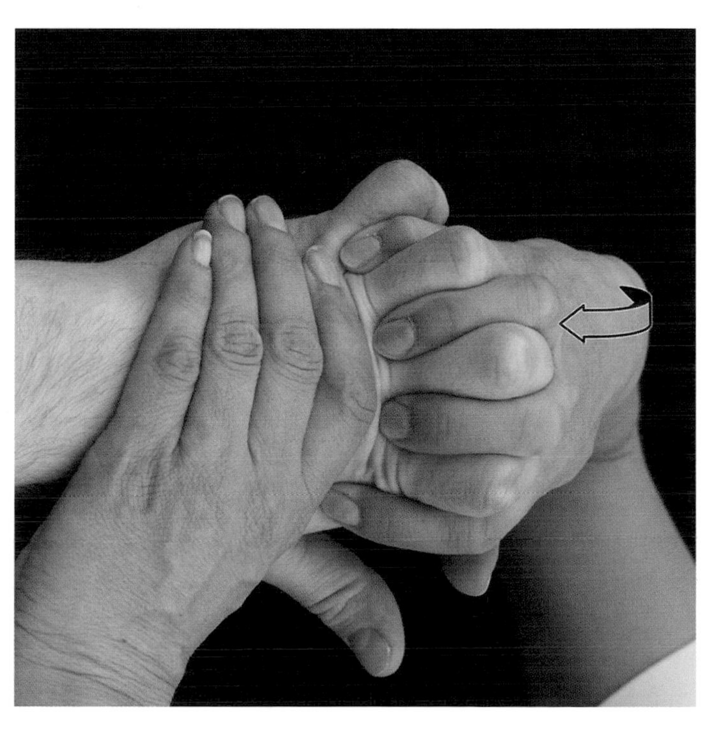

Dorsal interossei

(Four muscles between metacarpals)

Nerve, supply: Ulnar nerve, C8–Th1.

Origin: Each arising from two metacarpal bones from the adjacent sides.

Insertion: Bases of the proximal phalanges and dorsal aponeurosis at the same level of the second and third finger on the radial side and the third finger and fourth finger on the ulnar side.

Function: Flexion of metacarpophalangeal joints, extension of interphalangeal joints and separation of fingers.

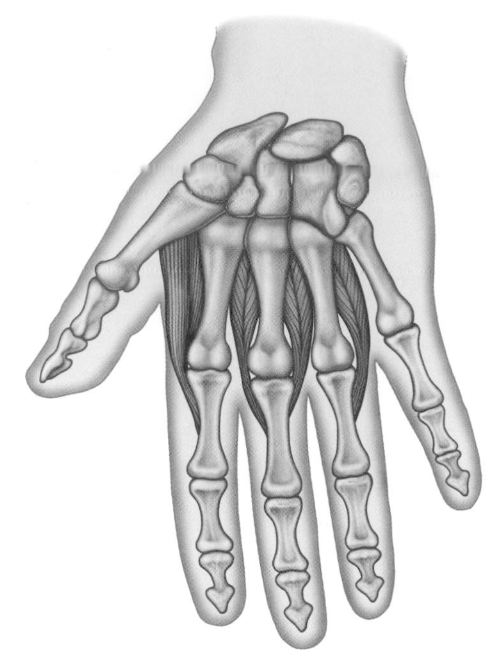

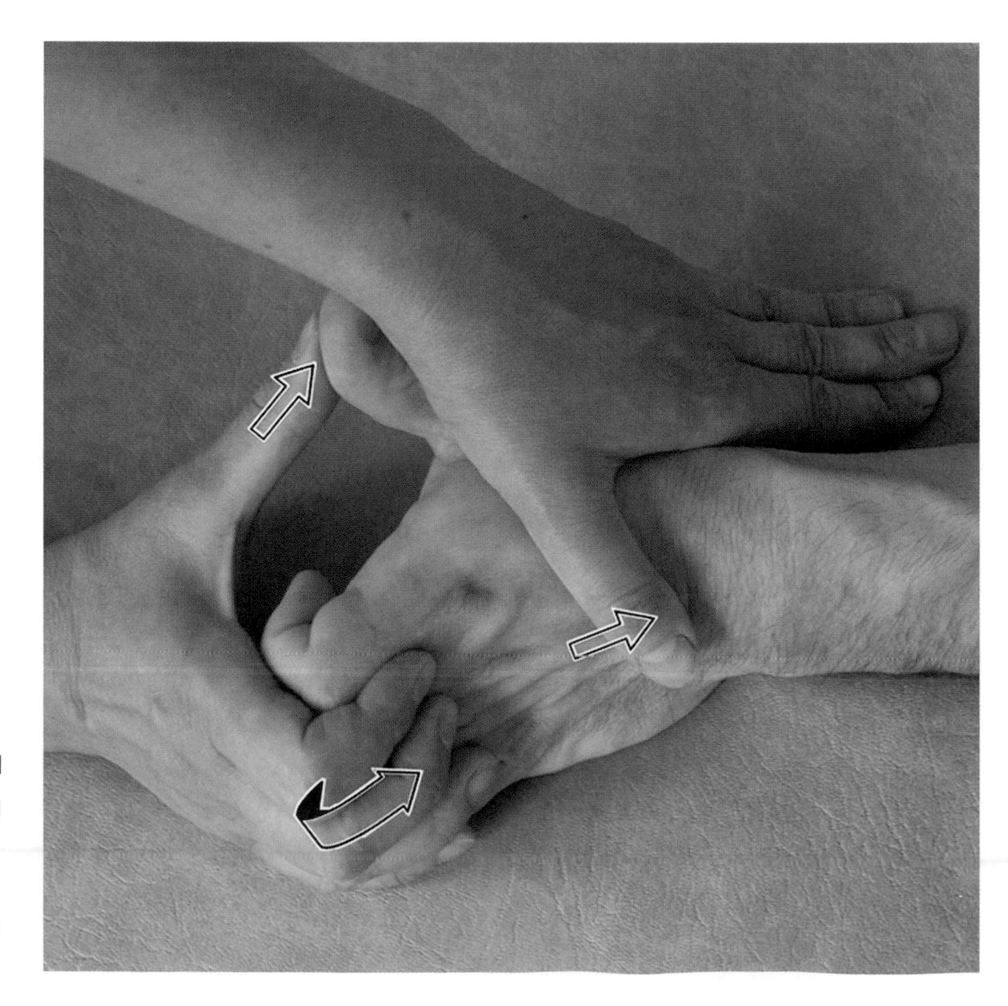

Stretching technique:

Therapist grasps flexed fingers and extends metacarpals while keeping the thumb abducted. Therapist uses the other hand to press along the bodies of the muscles between metacarpals.

Pectoralis major

Nerve, supply: Medial and lateral pectoral nerves, C5–Th1.

Origin: Medial half of anterior surface of clavicle, sternum and cartilages of second–sixth ribs and rectus sheath.

Insertion: Crest of great tubercle of the humerus.

Function: Adduction and internal rotation of the shoulder joint and draws shoulder forward. Superior part flexes shoulder joint and inferior part pulls down the flexed arm. Stabilizes shoulder joint. Assists in deep inhalation, if the arms are fixed in flexed position. Assist in deep exhalation in the neutral position.

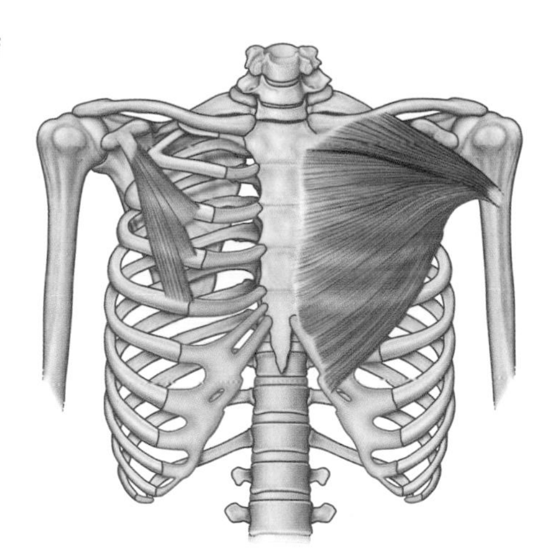

Clavicular part of pectoralis major

Stretching technique:

Patient is lying on back with elbow flexed 90° and shoulder abducted 45°. Therapist applies pressure with the hypothenar of the hand towards the body of muscle away from insertion while using the other hand to grasp the elbow and forearm to press arm down.

Tension–relaxation technique: Patient tries to lift arm for 5 sec while therapist resists. Patient is then instructed to gradually relax muscles while therapist applies stretching technique.

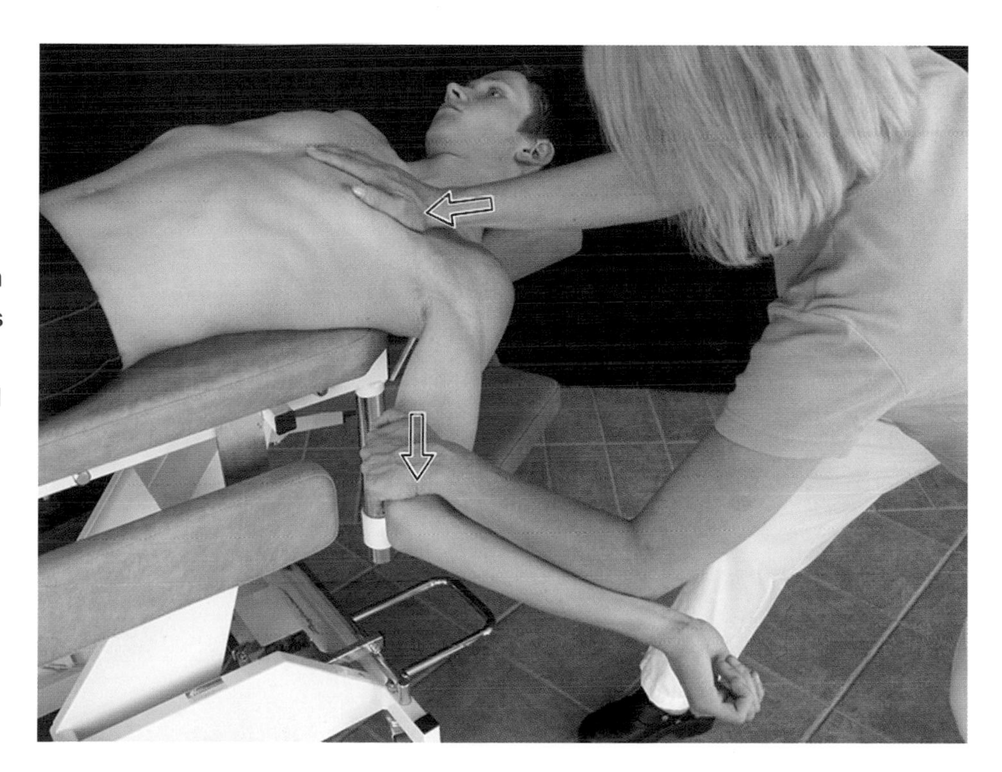

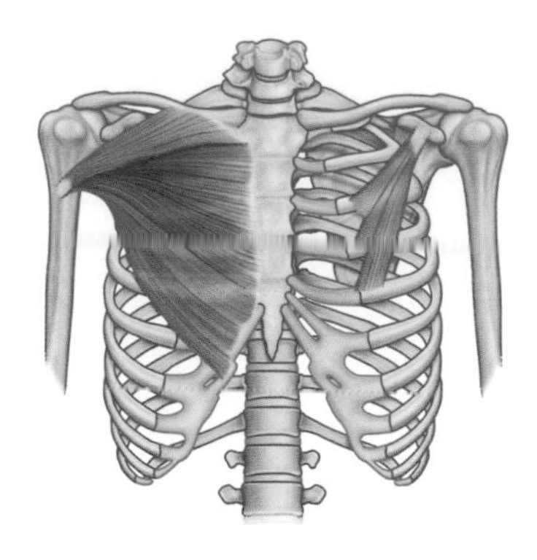

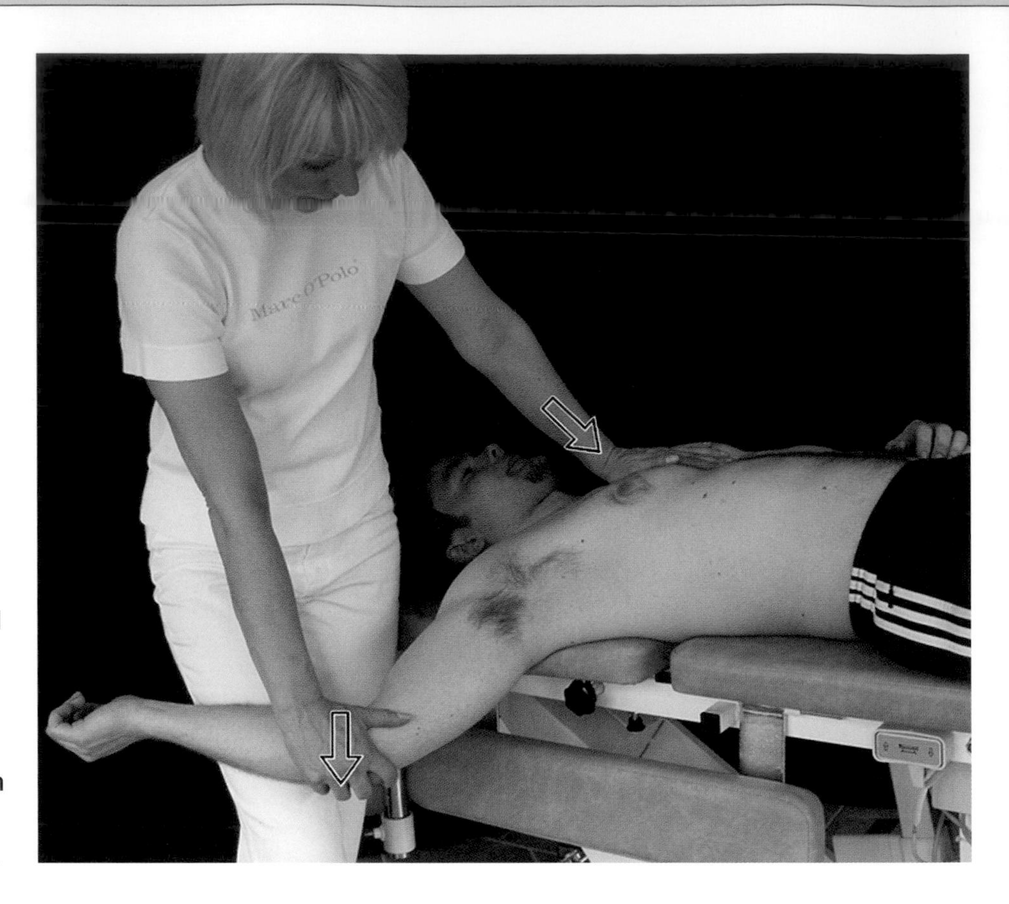

Stern part of pectoralis major

Stretching technique:

Patient is lying on back with elbow flexed 90° and upper arm abducted 90° and externally rotated. Therapist applies pressure with the thenar of the hand towards the body of muscle away from insertion and lets it slide medially in stretching massage while using the other hand to press arm down to horizontal abduction.

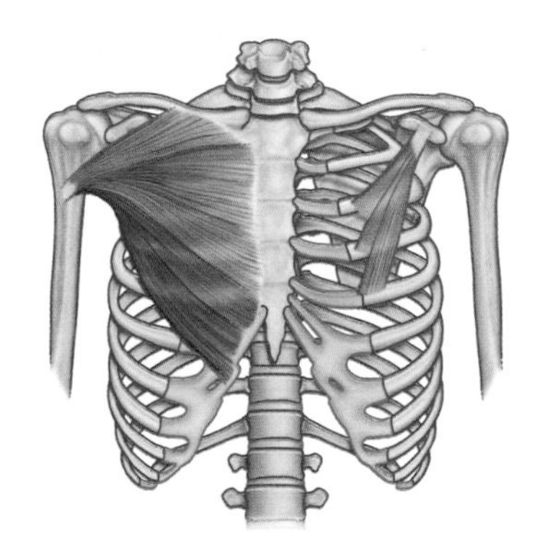

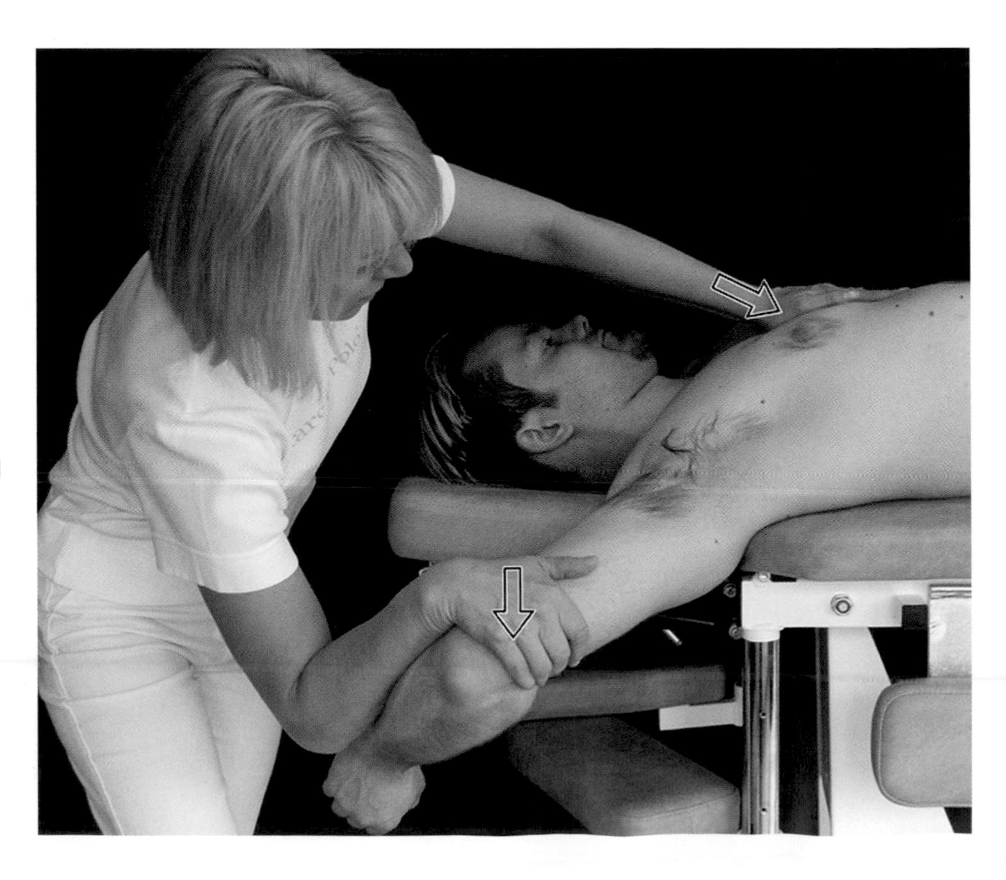

Abdominal part of pectoralis major

Stretching technique:

Patient is lying on back, elbow flexed 90°, upper arm abducted 135°, and externally rotated. Therapist applies pressure with the thenar of the hand towards the body of muscle away from insertion and lets it slide medially in stretching massage while using the other hand to grasp the elbow and forearm to press arm down.

Pectoralis minor

Nerve, supply: Medial pectoral nerve, C5–8.

Origin: Ribs 3–5.

Insertion: Coracoid process.

Function: Draws scapula forward and down. Stabilizes scapula and upper rib cage in lifting. Assists in deep inhalation.

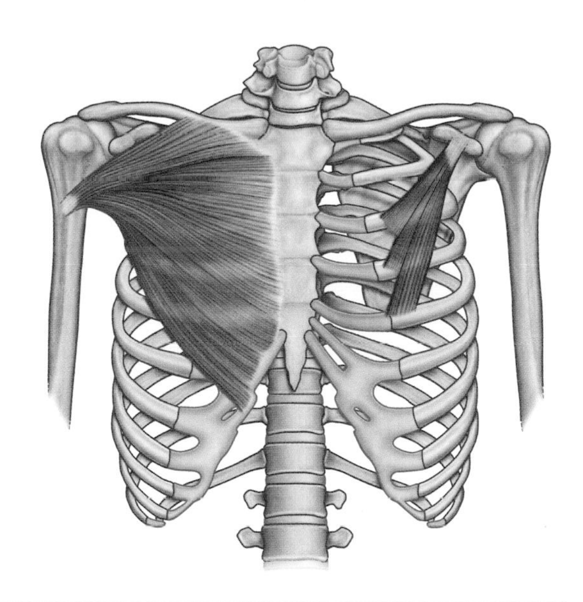

Stretching technique A:

Patient is lying on back with shoulder flexed 90° and elbow in free flexion. Therapist applies pressure with the hypothenar of the hand towards the body of muscle away from insertion while using the other hand to press the elbow downwards.

Tension–relaxation technique: Patient tries to extend shoulder joint for 5 sec while therapist resists. Patient is then instructed to gradually relax muscles while therapist applies stretching technique.

Notice: This stretch often fails by applying pressure either too low or too far towards the middle of the chest. The pressure with the hypothenar should start just below the coracoid process and not reach lower than fifth rib or level of mammary papilla in men. The angle of the therapist's forearm should be about 30–45° depending on patient's chest size. The greater the chest, the smaller the angle should be.

Warning ! Care should be taken not to cause pain in shoulder joint with twisting forces. This stretch is contraindicated if the ROM is restricted due to diseases or trauma of the shoulder joint.

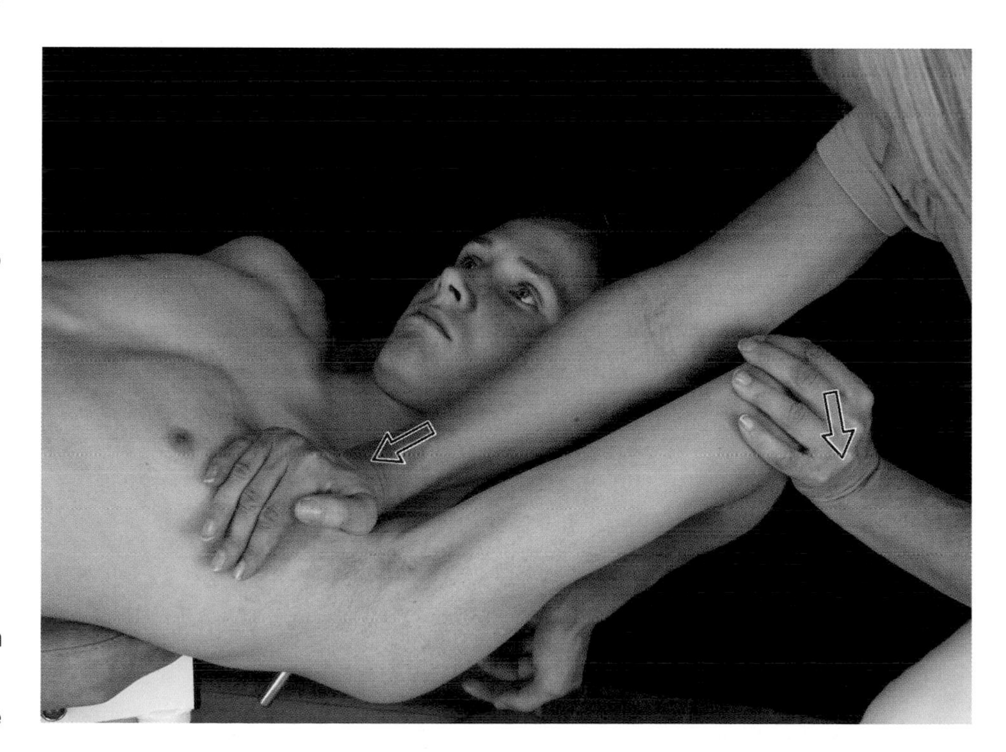

Stretching technique B:

Patient is lying on back with shoulder joint flexed 30° and elbow in complete flexion. Therapist applies pressure below the coracoid process with the hypothenar of the hand towards the body of muscle away from insertion, while using the other hand to push upper arm up, diagonally, in opposite direction.

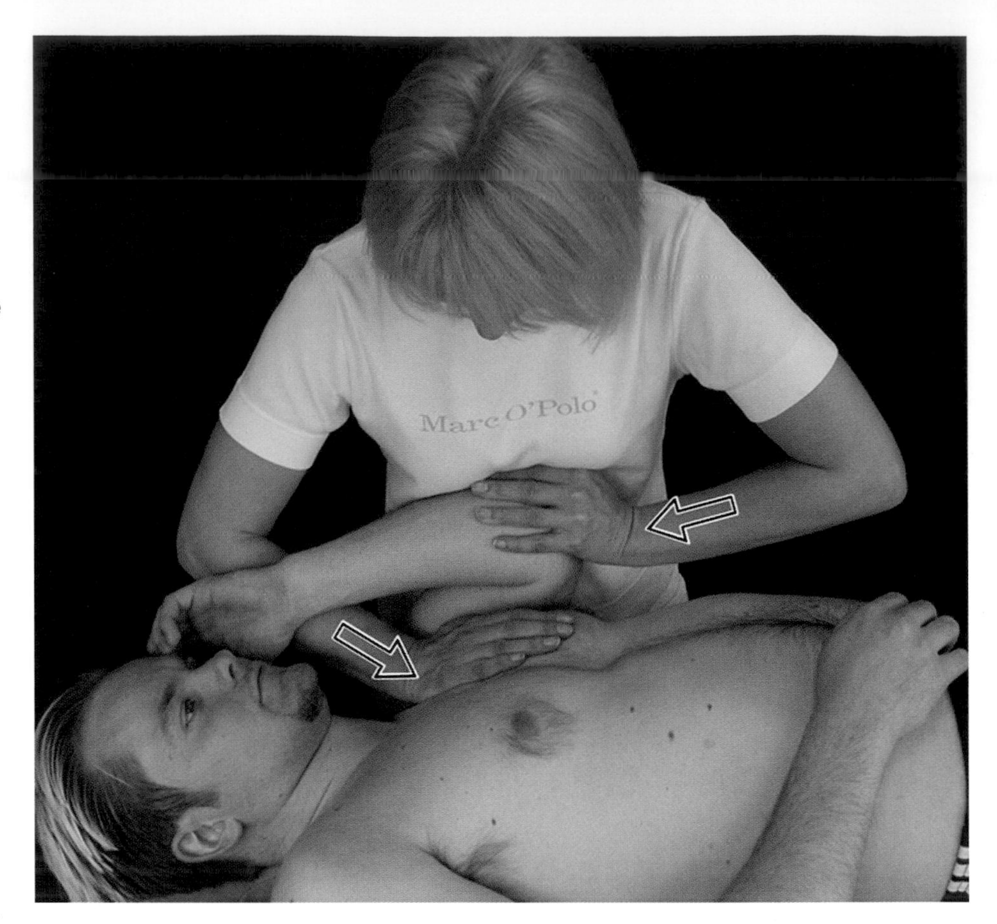

Tension–relaxation technique: Patient tries to push upper arm towards leg for 5 sec while therapist resists. Patient is then instructed to gradually relax muscles while therapist applies stretching technique.

Notice: Pressure must be applied in the same direction as the upper arm of the patient. Thus, therapist's forearm and patient's arm have to be almost in the same line so as to allow pressure in the right direction. This second technique is more difficult, because the therapist cannot use the weight of the body.

It is important to apply pressure on the muscle before pushing the elbow.

Subclavius

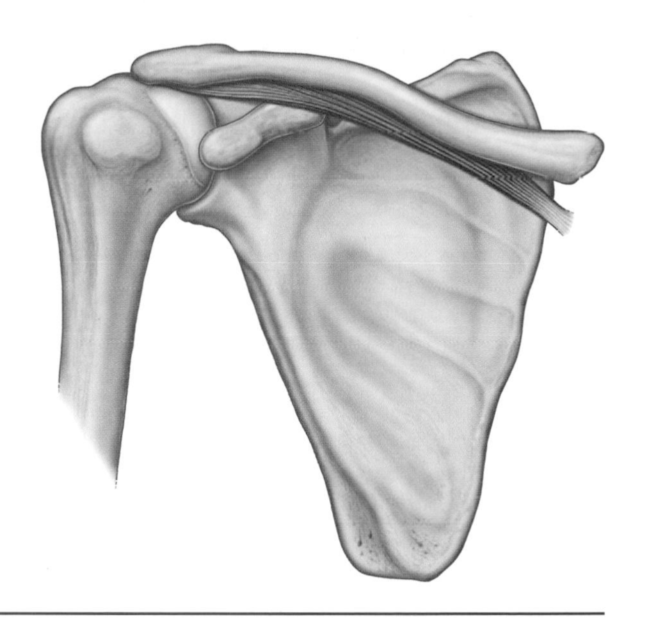

Nerve, supply: Subclavian nerve, C5–6.

Origin: Superior, proximal surface of the first rib.

Insertion: Inferior, distal surface of clavicle.

Function: Draws distal end of clavicle downwards stabilizing the sternoclavicular joint.

Stretching technique A:

Patient is lying on back with shoulder flexed to 45°. Therapist applies pressure with the hypothenar of the hand towards the body of muscle away from insertion while the other hand, presses at the elbow to push the shoulder and distal part of the clavicle upwards.

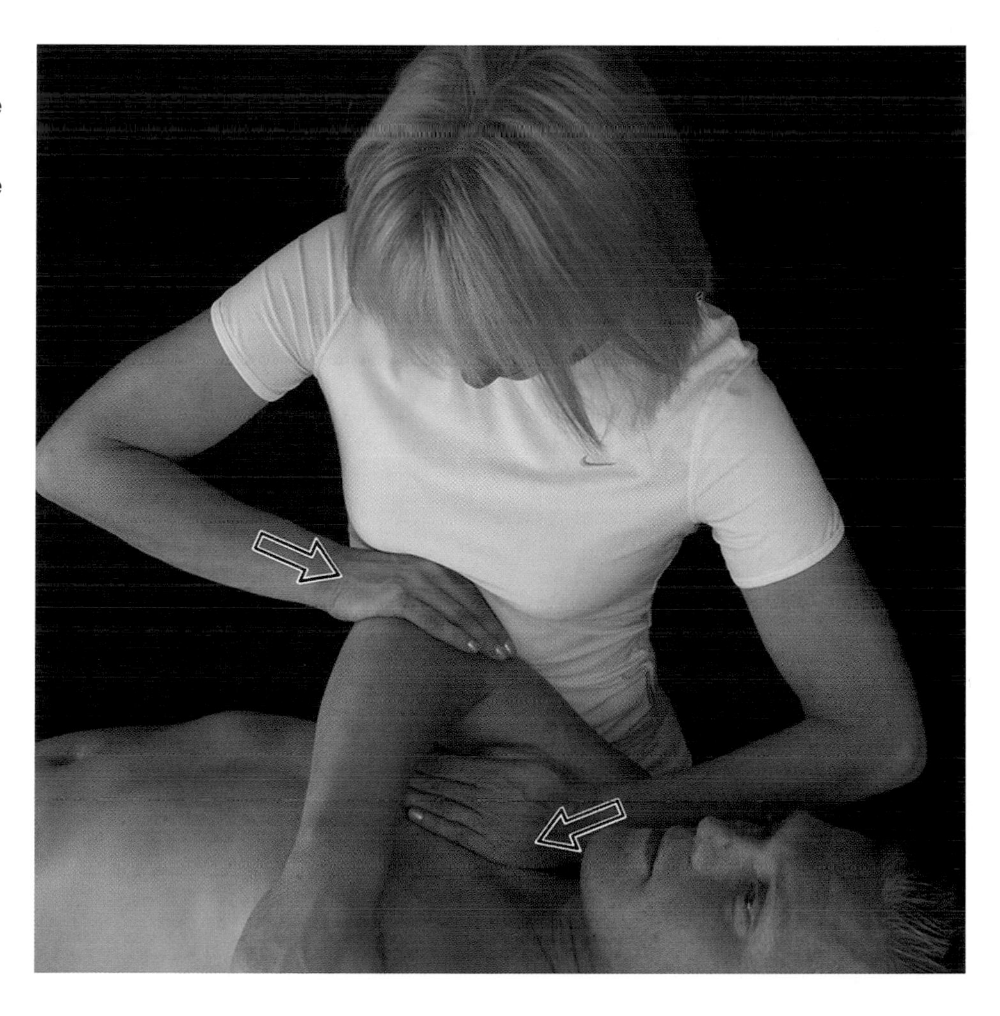

Tension–relaxation technique: Patient tries to push upper arm down for 5 sec while the therapist resists. Patient is then instructed to gradually relax muscles while therapist applies stretching technique.

Notice: Pressure must be applied in the same direction as the upper arm of the patient. Thus, therapist's forearm and patient's arm have to be almost in the same line so as to allow pressure in the right direction.

It is important to apply pressure on the muscle before pushing the elbow.

Stretching technique B:

Patient is lying on back with shoulders on the narrow head rest. Therapist applies pressure with the thenar of both hands towards the bodies of muscles away from insertions while pressing shoulders backwards.

Notice: This stretches pectoralis muscles also.

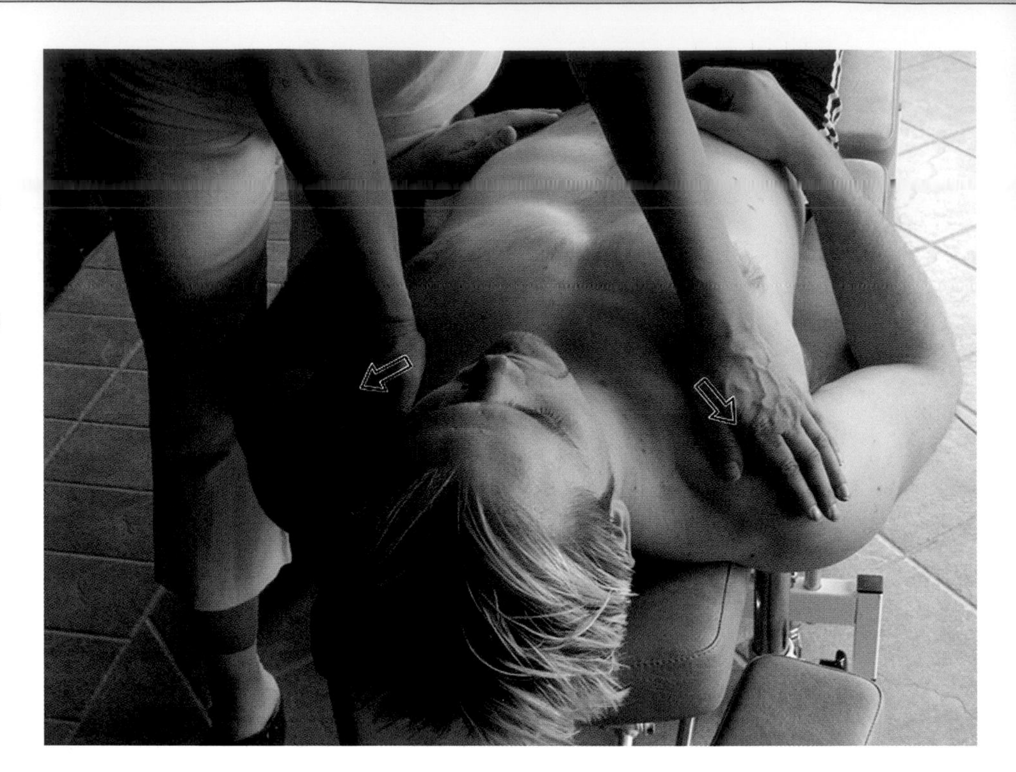

Serratus anterior

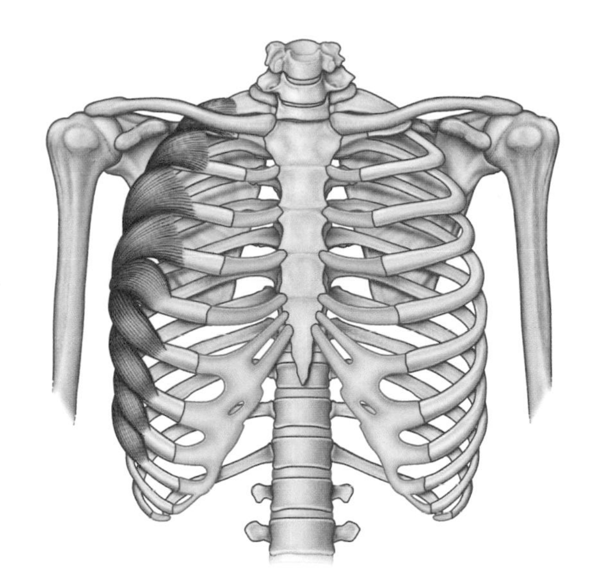

Nerve, supply: Long thoracic nerve, C5–7.

Origin: Ribs 1–9.

Insertion: Medial border of scapula.

Function: Stabilizes and abducts scapula. Rotates inferior part of scapula laterally. Lifts ribs when the shoulder is fixed and assists in deep inhalation.

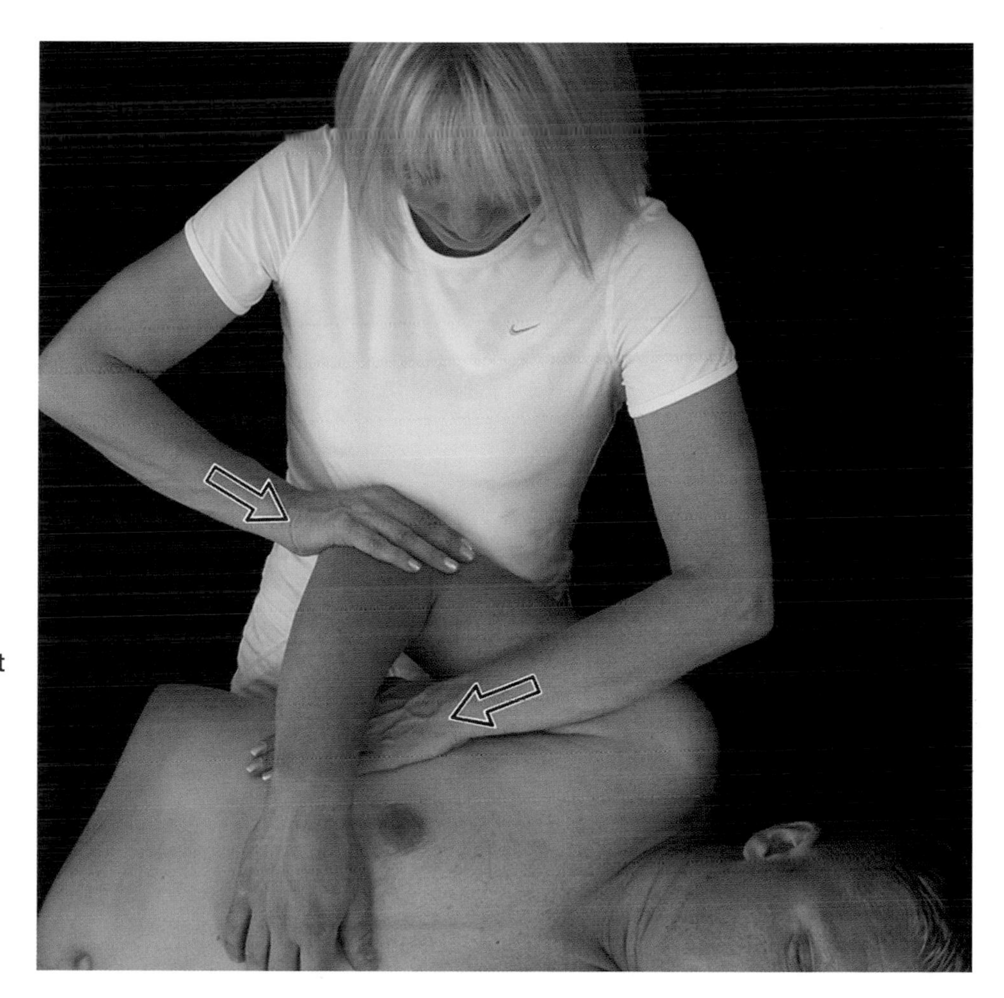

Stretching technique A:

(Lower part)

Patient is lying on side with the shoulder abducted 45°. Therapist applies pressure with the thenar of the hand towards the body of muscle while the other hand presses at the elbow to push the shoulder towards the head.

Tension–relaxation technique: Patient tries to push upper arm in an upward diagonal direction for 5 sec while therapist resists. Patient is then instructed to gradually relax muscles while therapist applies stretching technique.

Notice: It is important to apply pressure on the muscle before pushing the elbow. The forearm must be in-line with patient's arm.

Stretching technique B:

(Middle part)

Patient is lying on back with the shoulder joint abducted 90°. Therapist applies pressure with the thenar of the hand towards the body of muscle away from insertion while the other hand pushes the arm downwards. The thigh pushes the scapula in further adduction and arm towards abduction.

Tension–relaxation technique: Patient tries to abduct scapula for 5 sec while therapist resists. Patient is then instructed to gradually relax muscles while therapist applies stretching technique.

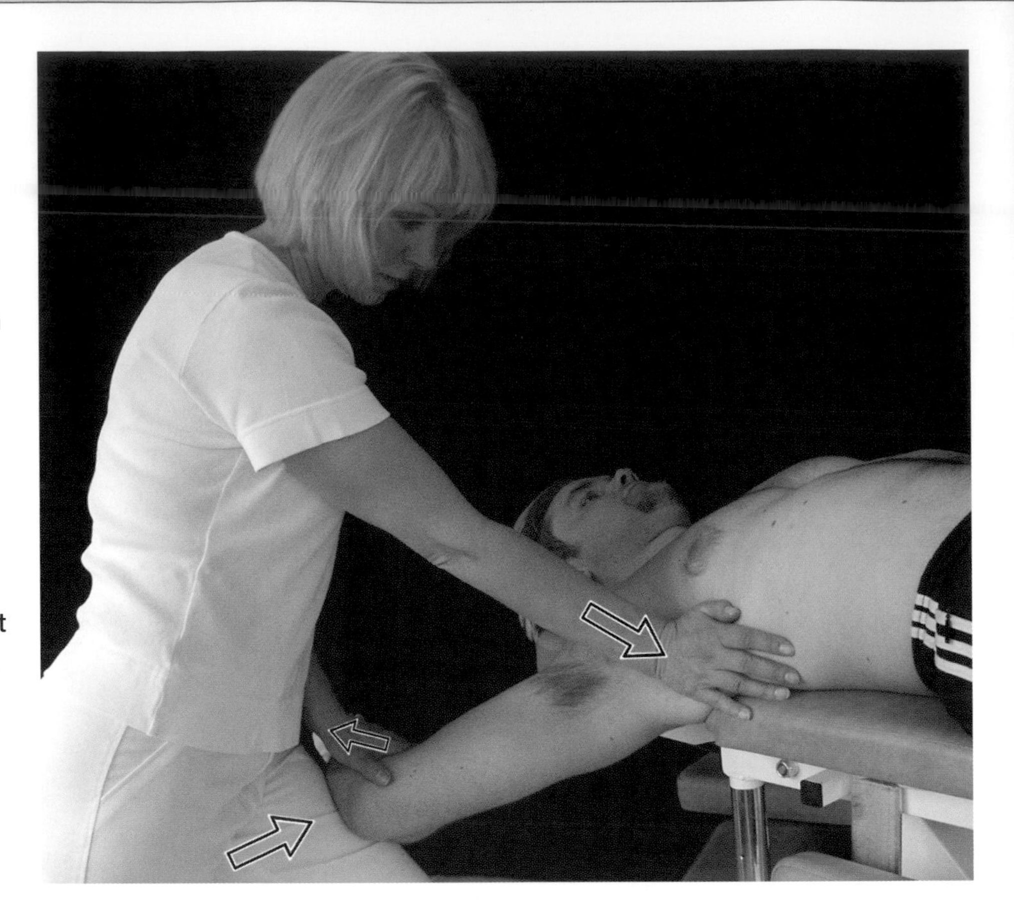

Stretching technique C:

(Upper part)

Patient is lying on back with the shoulder joint abducted to 45°. Therapist applies pressure with the hypothenar of the hand towards the body of muscle away from insertion while the other hand presses at the elbow to raise the and shoulder blade towards the head.

Notice: Pressure must be applied in the same direction as the upper arm of the patient. Thus, therapist's forearm and patient's arm have to be almost in the same line so as to allow pressure in the right direction.

It is important to apply pressure on the muscle before pushing the elbow.

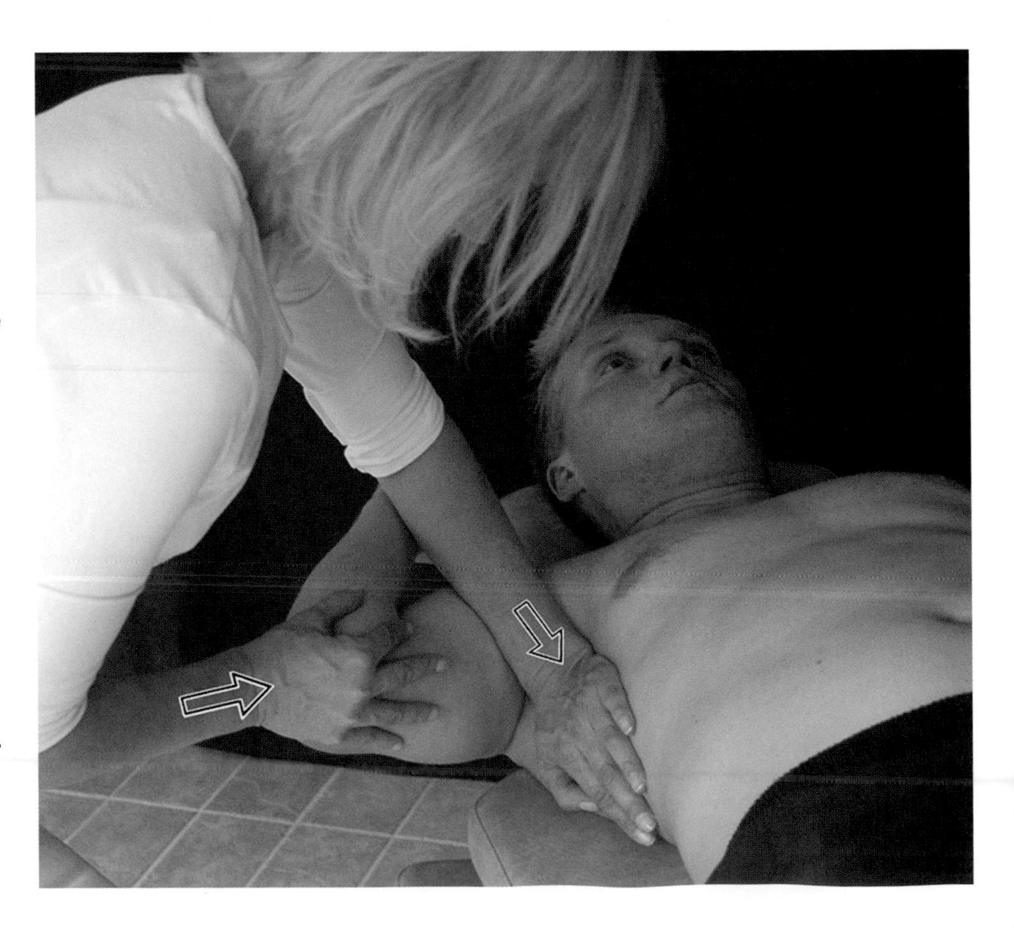

Stretching technique D:

Patient is lying on side with the arm behind the back. Therapist presses with thumbs under the medial edge of the scapula to separate the scapula from the rib cage.

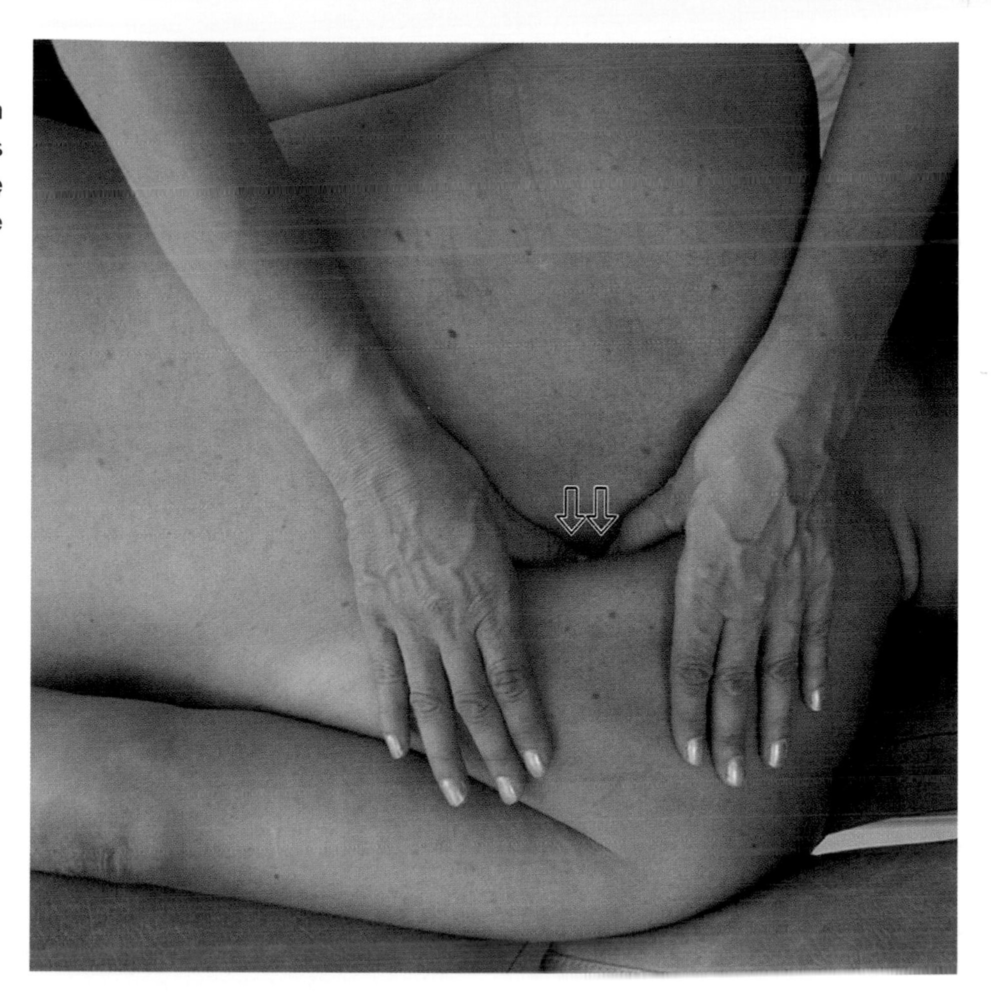

Stretching technique E:

Patient is lying on stomach. Therapist places thigh under shoulder to make a fulcrum under the lateral side of the scapula. Therapist raises the scapula by grasping the medial edge and pulling upwards.

Notice: The knee should not be placed under the shoulder, because the patella is too hard and may place too much pressure on tender structures of the shoulder.

Warning ❗ The scapula should not be pulled down forcefully towards the lower extremities as this may stretch and damage the long thoracic nerve, resulting in winged scapula.

Warning ❗ The forearm may be lifted behind the back in order to raise the medial edge of the scapula, but it has to be done gently. Rapid forceful movement may cause tear in the rotator cuff and in the acromioclavicular joint.

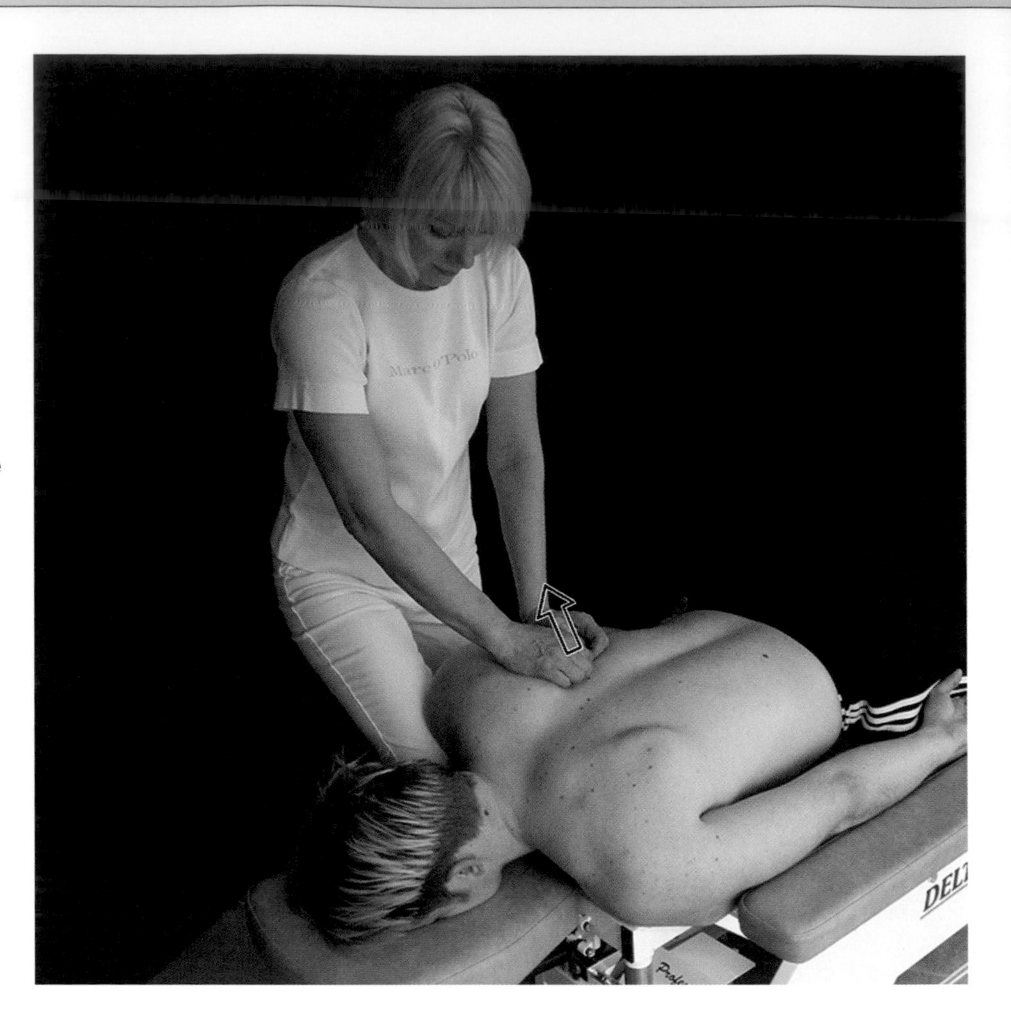

Trapezius

(Middle transverse part)

Nerve, supply: Accessory nerve (XI cranial nerve) and trapezius branch, C2–4.

Origin: Spinous processes Th1–Th5.

Insertion: Lateral end of clavicle, acromion and spine of scapula.

Function: Adducts and stabilizes scapula.

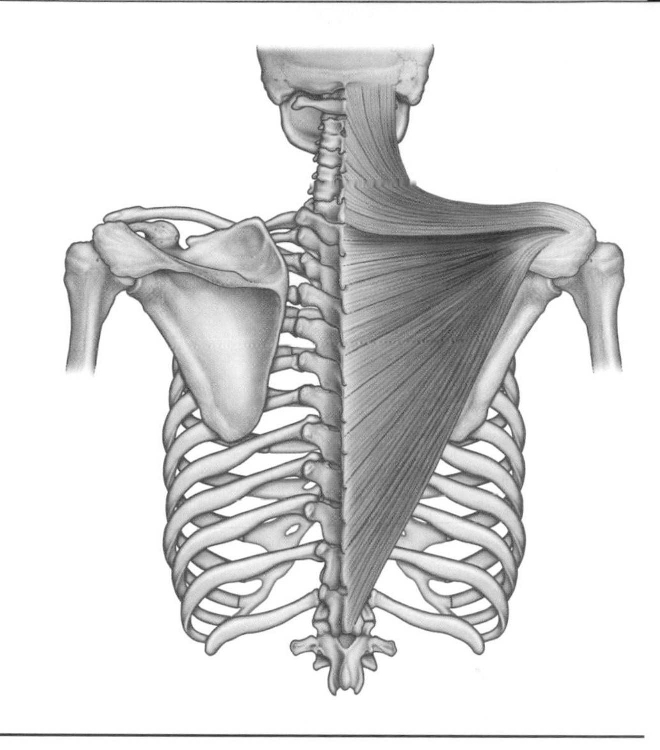

Stretching technique A:

Patient is lying on back with arms hanging down over the sides of the table. Therapist crosses arms and places hands on the spine of each scapula. Stretching is achieved by leaning forward to apply pressure on scapula, forcing them away from each other.

Tension–relaxation technique: Patient tries to adduct shoulder blades for 5 sec while therapist resists. Patient is then instructed to gradually relax muscles while therapist applies stretching technique.

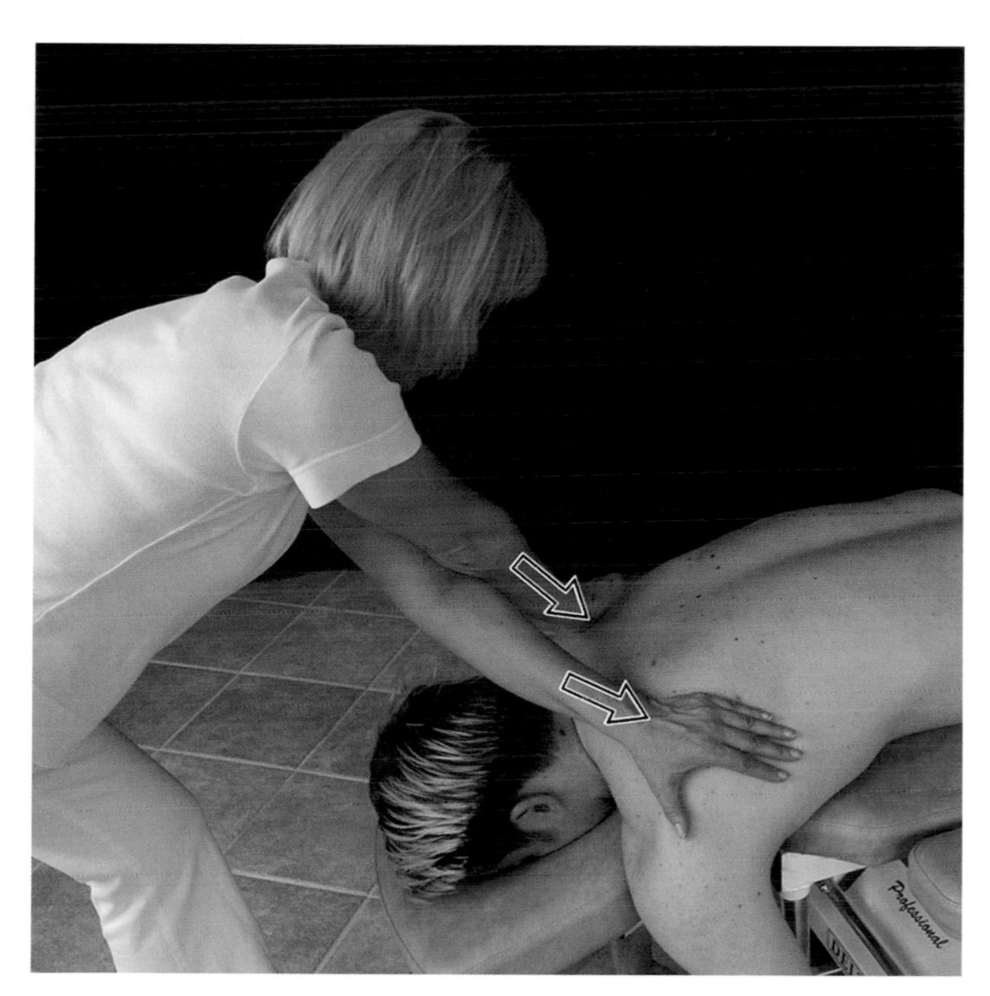

Stretching technique B:

Patient is lying on stomach with the arm to be treated hanging down over the sides of the table. Therapist applies pressure with the thumb of the hand towards the body of muscle away from insertion while using other hand to push on the spine of scapula towards abduction.

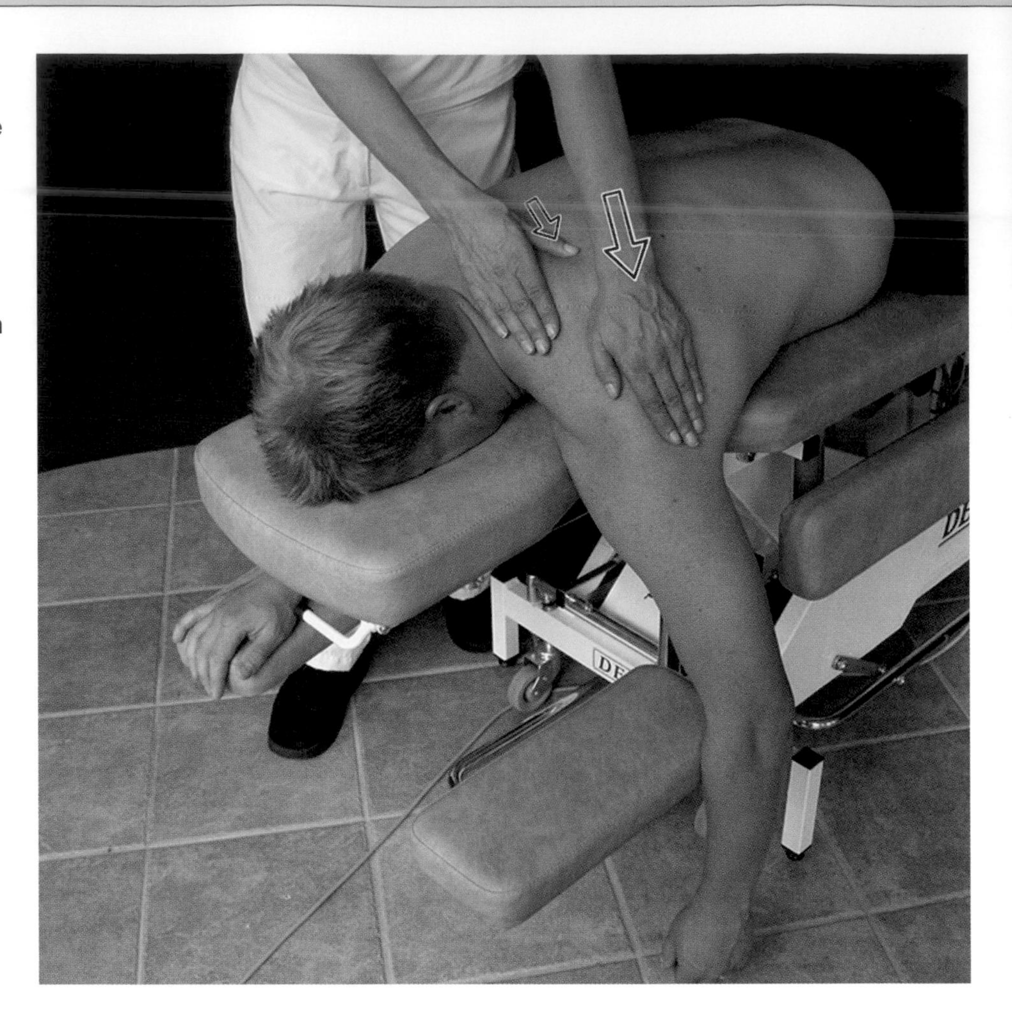

Trapezius

(Inferior ascending part)

Origin: Spinous processes Th6–12.

Insertion: Spine of scapula.

Function: Stabilizes, adducts and draws down scapula.

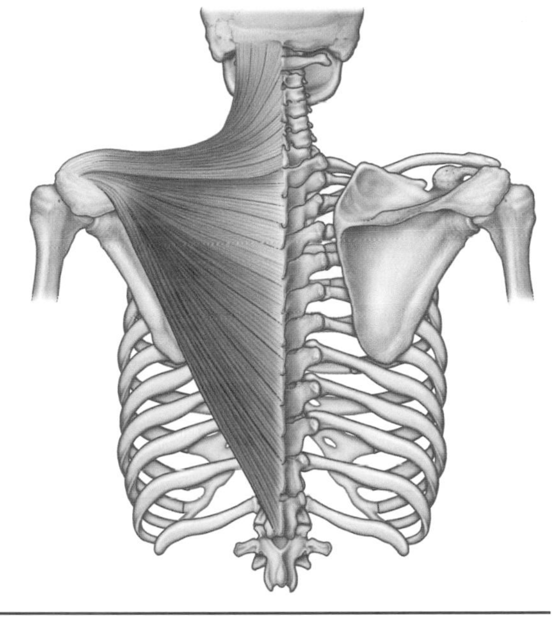

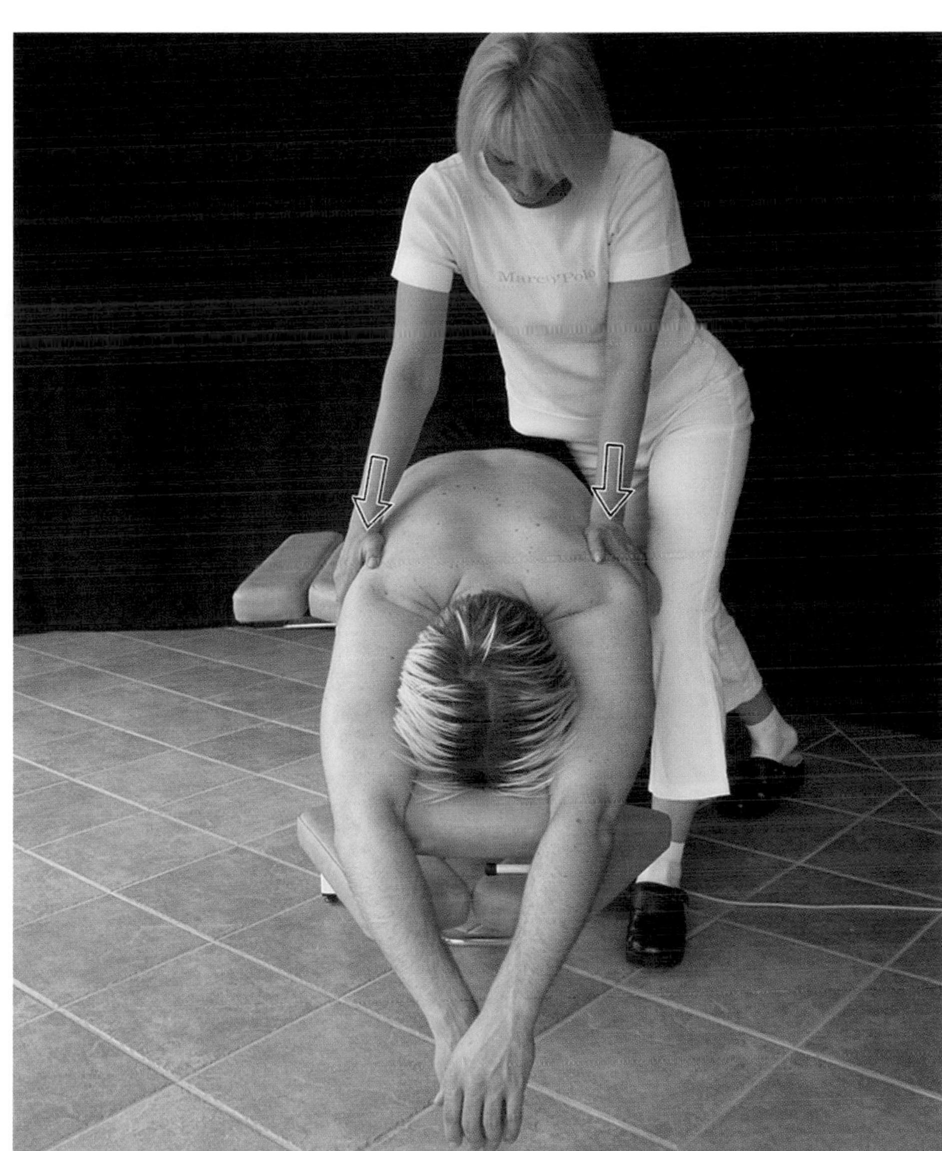

Stretching technique A:

Patient is lying on stomach with the arms above the head. Therapist leans with arms straight to apply pressure on the spine of each scapula, causing them to abduct.

Tension–relaxation technique: Patient tries to adduct both scapulae for 5 sec while therapist resists. Patient is then instructed to gradually relax muscles while therapist applies stretching technique.

Stretching technique B:

Patient is lying on stomach with the arm of side to be treated above head. Therapist pushes the lower end of the scapula upwards, while using the thumb and thenar of the other hand to stretch muscle tissue away from origin at spinous processes.

Tension–relaxation technique: Patient tries to draw the shoulder downwards for 5 sec while therapist resists. Patient is then instructed to gradually relax muscles while therapist applies stretching technique.

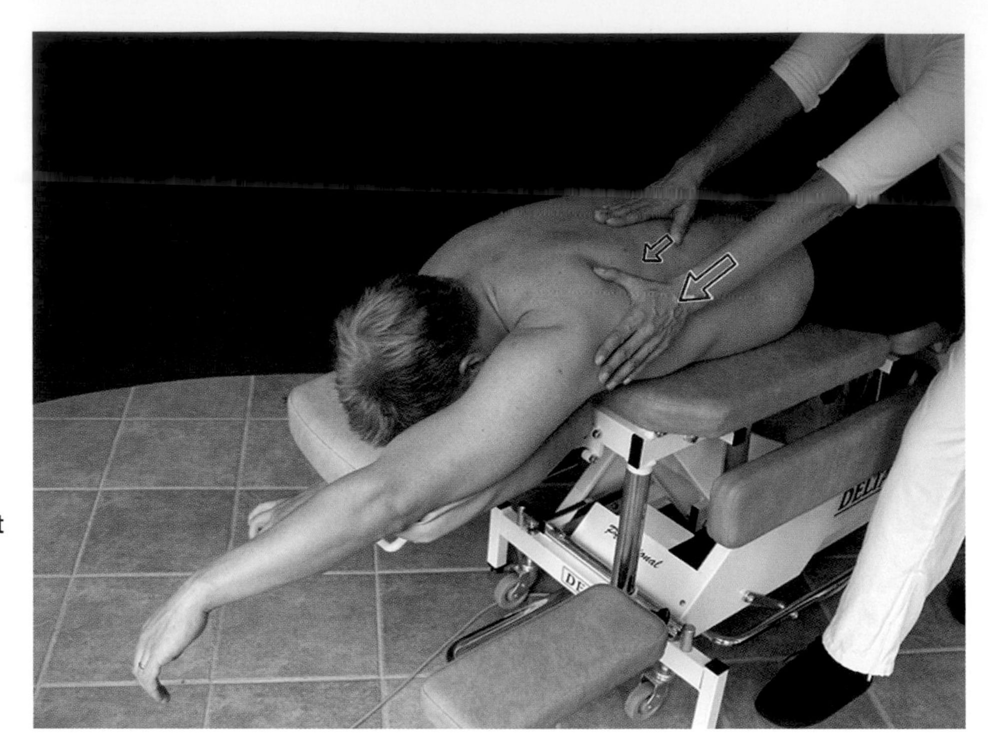

Rhomboid major

Nerve, supply: Dorsal scapular nerve, C4–5.

Origin: Spinous processes Th1–4.

Insertion: Middle medial border of scapula.

Function: Adducts, lifts, rotates down and stabilizes scapula.

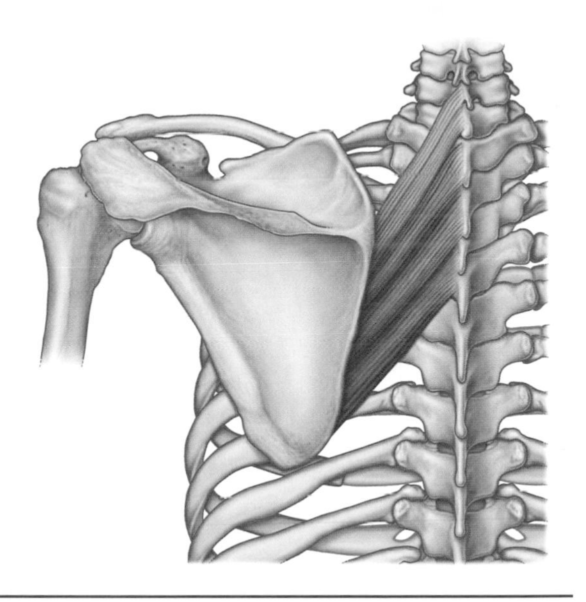

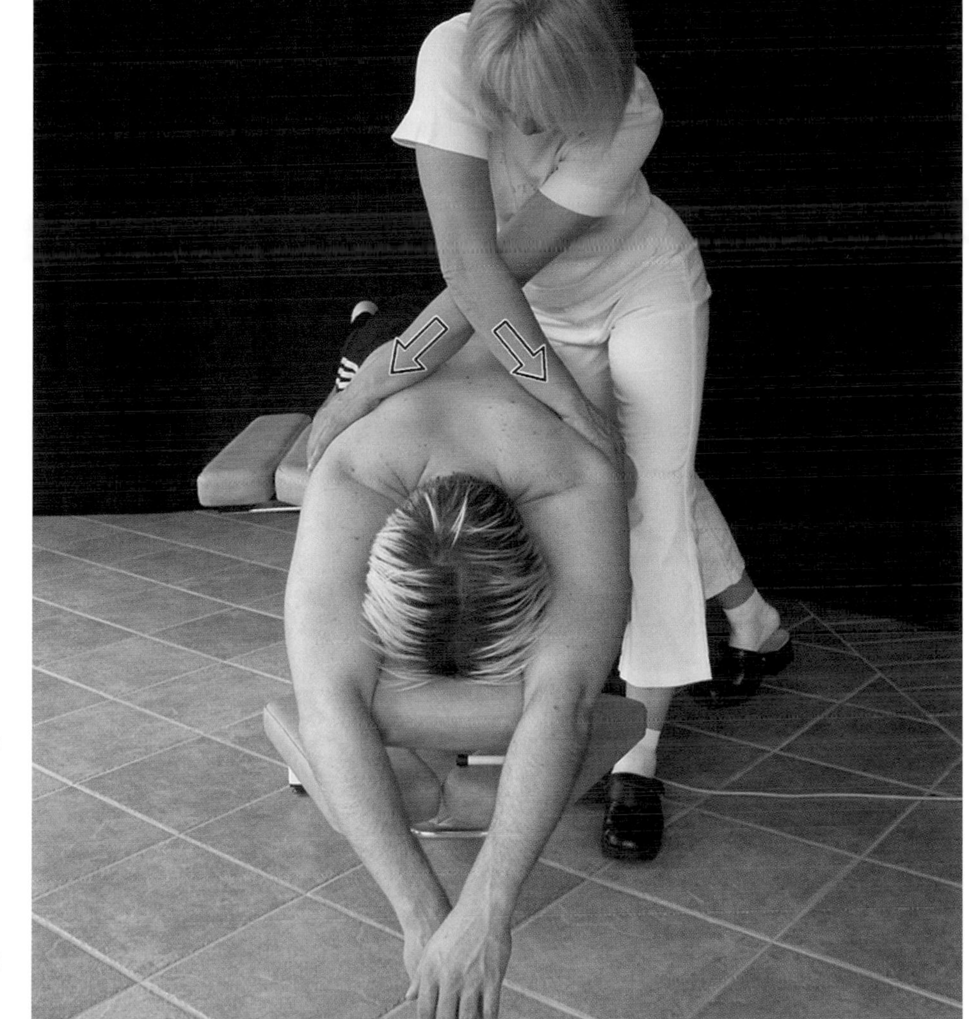

Stretching technique A:

Patient is lying on stomach with arms above the head. Therapist crosses forearms and applies pressure to the medial edge of each scapula by leaning into the stretch so that the scapulae separate.

Tension–relaxation technique: Patient tries to adduct scapulae for 5 sec while therapist resists. Patient is then instructed to gradually relax while therapist pushes scapulae to the sides.

Rhomboid minor

Nerve, supply: Dorsal scapular nerve, C4–5.

Origin: Spinous processes C6–7.

Insertion: Upper medial border of scapula.

Function: Adducts, lifts and stabilizes scapula.

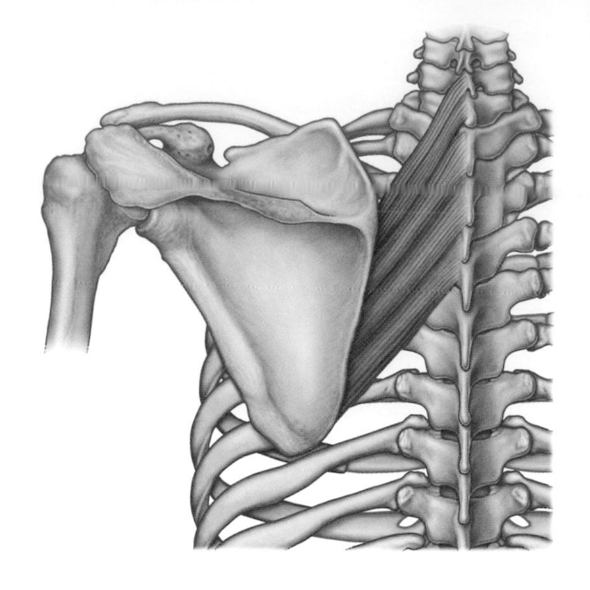

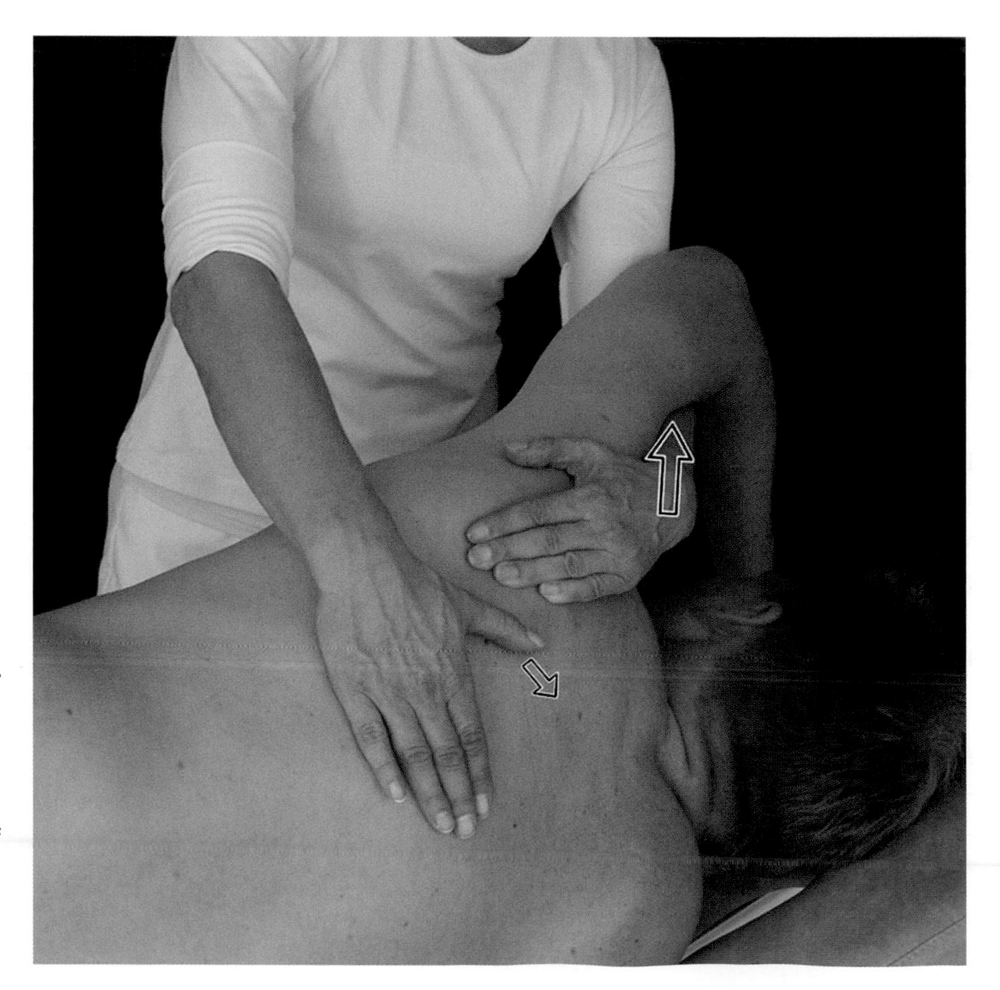

Stretching technique B:

Patient is lying on side with the arm above the head. With forearm under patient's upper arm, therapist grasps the medial edge of the scapula and draws it up diagonally while using the thumb and thenar of the other hand to stretch muscle tissue towards the body of the muscle away from insertion.

Spinalis thoracis

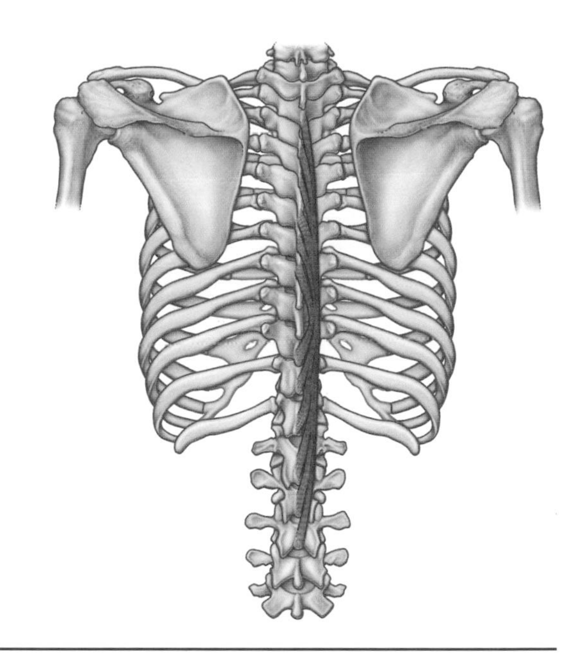

Nerve, supply: Dorsal rami of spinal nerves, Th2–L2.

Origin: Spinous processes Th10–L3.

Insertion: Spinous processes Th2–8 (Shortest muscle fibres run from Th10 to Th8).

Function: Extends thoracic and upper lumbar spine.

Stretching technique:

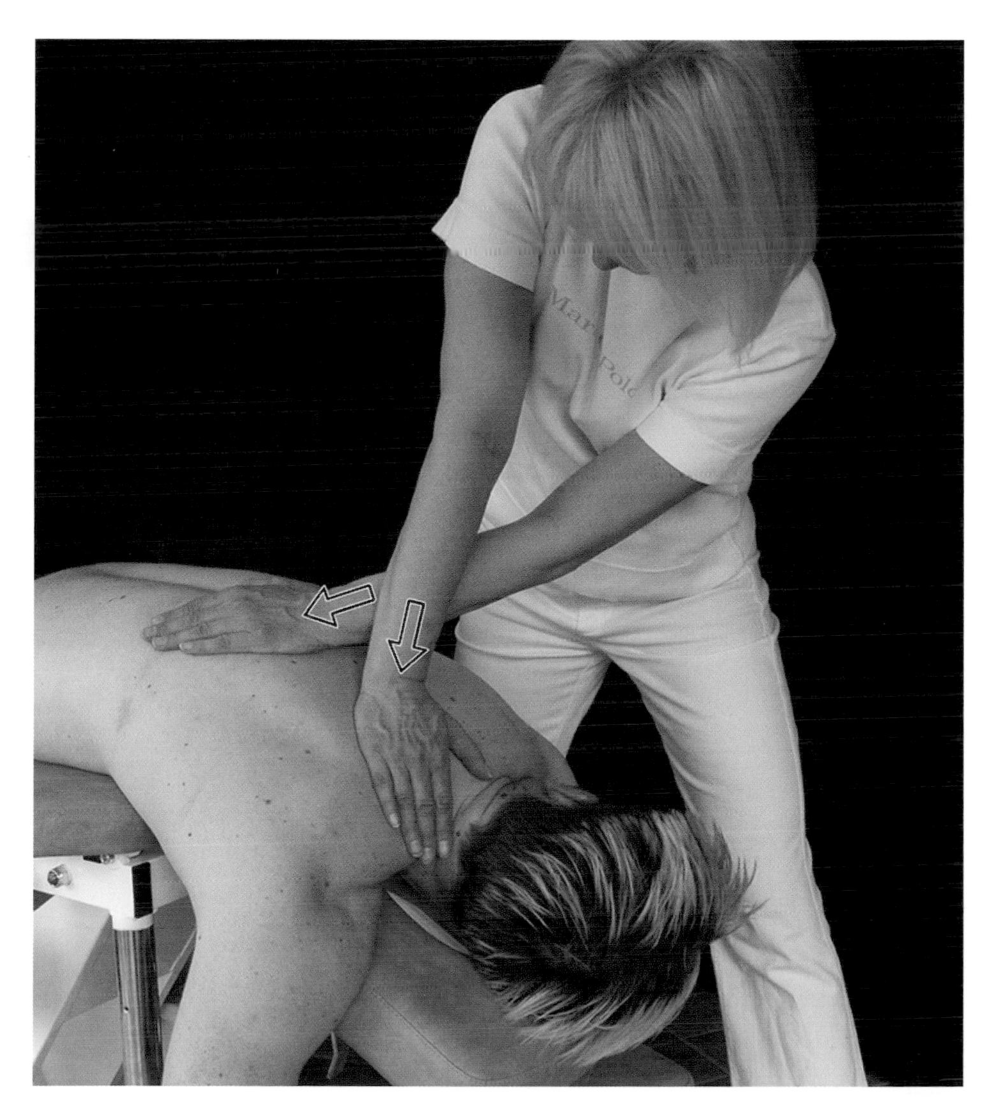

Patient is lying on stomach with the head well lowered down or a pillow under chest to induce flexion of the thoracic spine. Therapist applies pressure with the hypothenar of both hands while arms are crossed. The pressure is aimed on the facet joints at the level Th2–8 diagonally towards the head with one hand while the other hand applies pressure simultaneously at level Th10–L3 diagonally towards the legs.

Tension–relaxation technique: Patient tries to extend thoracic spine for 5 sec while therapist resists. Patient is then instructed to gradually relax muscles while therapist increases pressure to improve stretch.

Iliocostalis thoracis

Nerve, supply: Dorsal rami of spinal nerves, Th1–12.

Origin: Ribs 7–12.

Insertion: Ribs 1–6.

Function: Extends and lateral flexes thoracic spine.

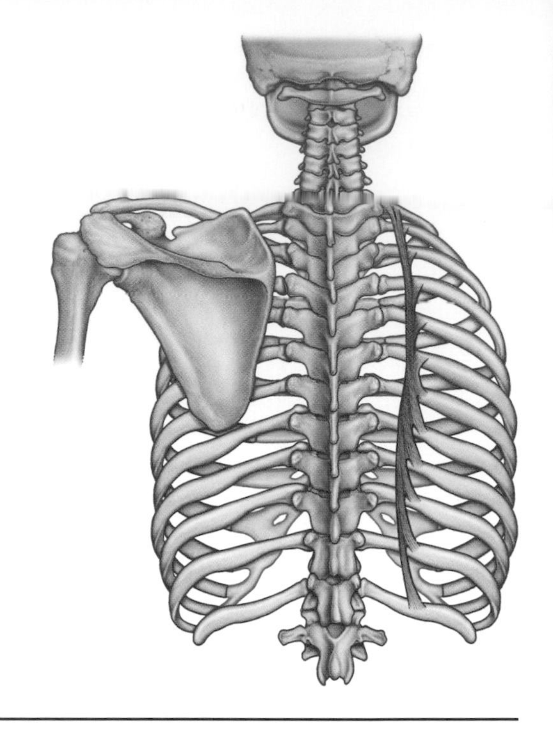

Stretching technique:

Patient is lying on stomach with pillow under chest or table bent up in centre. One arm is raised above head with thoracic spine bent to side opposite to the muscle to provide pre-stretch position. The inferior part can be pre-stretched by moving the legs to same side causing curvature in the lower thoracic spine. Therapist places both hands in the convex side and then presses with hypo-thenar of the hand ribs 1–6 diagonally up towards the head while with the hypo-thenar of the other hand presses on ribs 7–12 diagonally down towards the legs. The arms of the therapist are crossed, and substantial pressure can be achieved by leaning into the stretch.

Tension–relaxation technique: Patient tries to extend thoracic spine for 5 sec while therapist resists. Patient is then instructed to gradually relax muscles while therapist increases stretch.

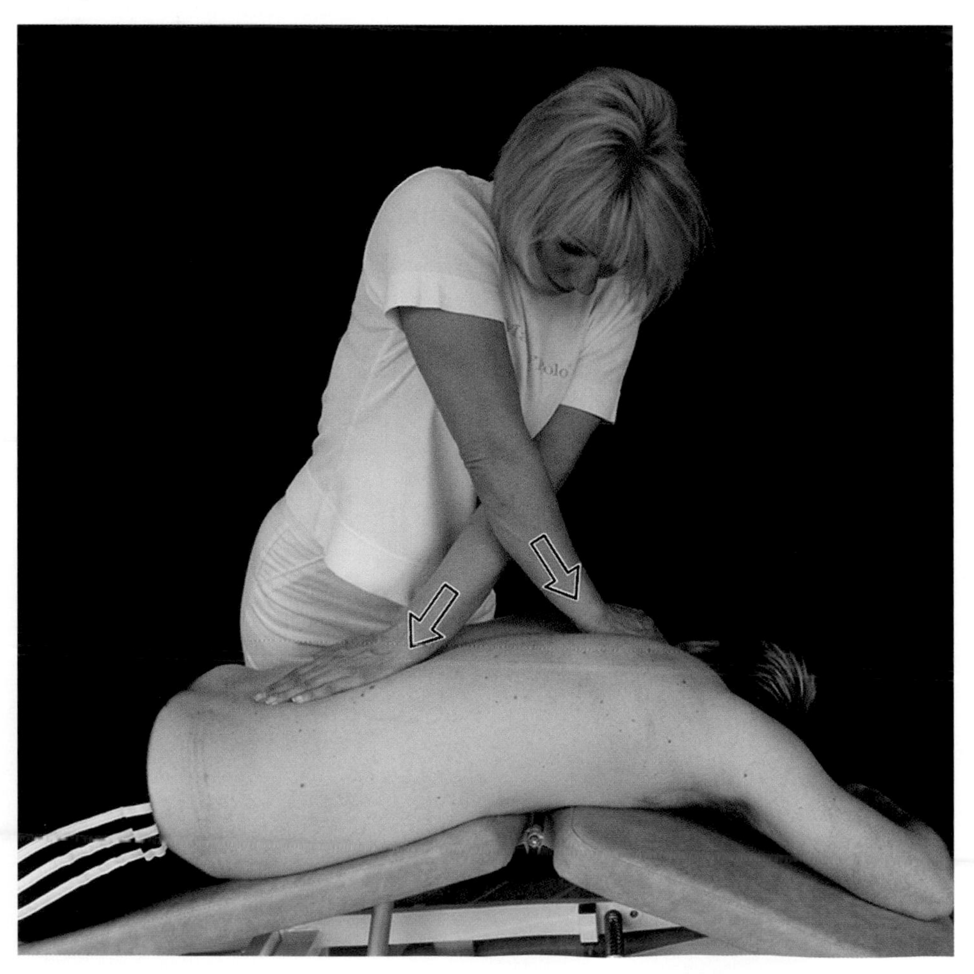

Iliocostalis lumborum

Nerve, supply: Dorsal rami of spinal nerves, Th6–L3.

Origin: Sacrum, iliac crest and thoracolumbar fascia.

Insertion: Transverse processes of L1–3 and ribs 5–12.

Function: Extension and lateral flexion of thoracic and lumbar spine.

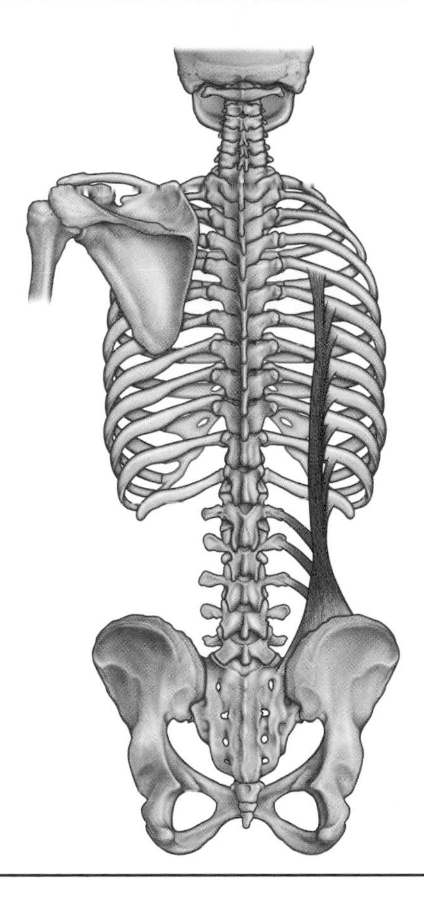

Stretching technique:

Patient is lying on stomach with a pillow under abdomen or table bent up. Arm is raised above head and thoracic spine bent to side away from the muscle to provide pre-stretch position. Legs can be adjusted to same side to stretch out lumbar part. Therapist presses with the hypothenar of the hand in the convex side on ribs 6–12 diagonally up towards the head while the hypothenar of the other hand applies pressure to the iliac crest diagonally down towards the legs. Therapist's arms are crossed and the stretch is achieved by leaning forward.

Tension–relaxation technique: Patient tries to extend lower back for 5 sec while therapist resists. Patient is then instructed to gradually relax while therapist increases stretch.

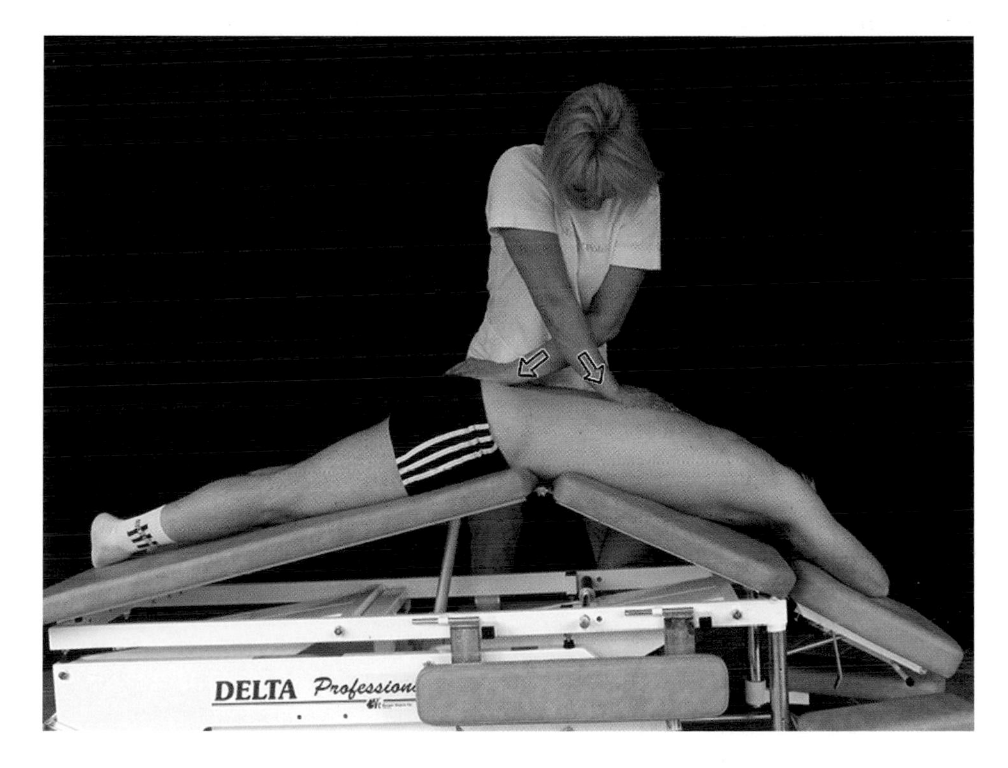

Longissimus thoracis

Nerve, supply: Dorsal rami of spinal nerves, Th1–L5.

Origin: Spinous processes of L1–S4, mamillary processes of L1–2 and transverse processes of Th7–12.

Insertion: Costal and accessory processes of lumbar vertebrae, transverse processes of thoracic vertebrae and ribs.

Function: Extension and lateral flexion of lumbar and thoracic spine.

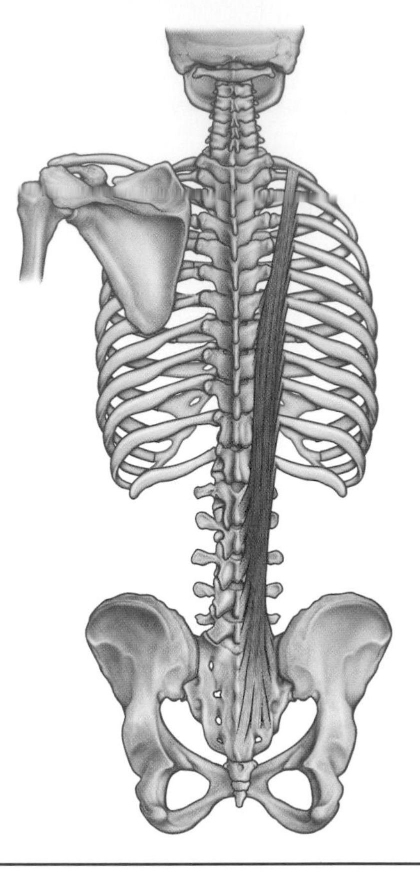

Stretching technique:

Patient is lying on stomach with pillow under abdomen or table bent to flex spine. Arm is raised above the head and thoracic spine bent to side away from the muscle to provide pre-stretch position. Legs are moved to the same side to stretch out lumbar part. Therapist places the thenar of the hand next to transverse processes of thoracic vertebrae in the convex side and applies pressure diagonally towards the head while the hypothenar of the other hand on the sacrum applies pressure diagonally towards the legs. The arms of the therapist are crossed, and substantial pressure can be achieved by leaning into the stretch.

Tension–relaxation technique: Patient tries to extend thoracic spine for 5 sec against resistance by the therapist. Patient then gradually releases tension while therapist allows the stretch to increase under the pressure applied.

Warning ❗ Intense pressure should be avoided, especially in cases of osteoporosis due to risk of rib fracture.

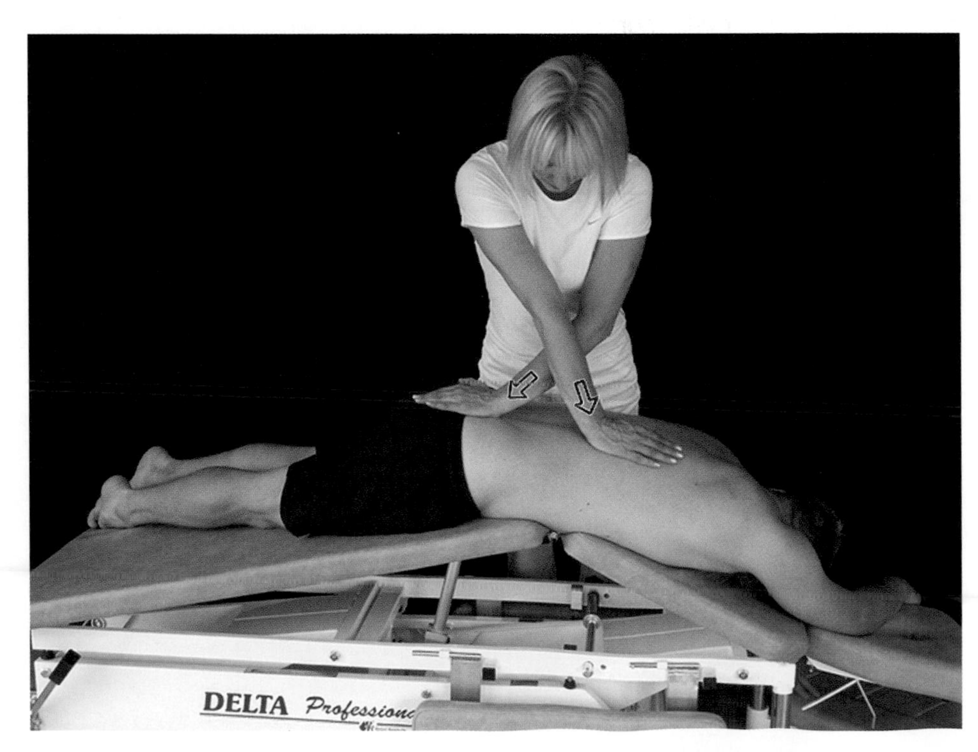

Serratus Posterior inferior

Nerve, supply: Intercostal nerves, Th9–12.

Origin: Thoracolumbar fascia in the region of spinous processes of Th11–L3 and

Insertion: Ribs 9–12.

Function: Draws ribs down. Assists in deep exhalation.

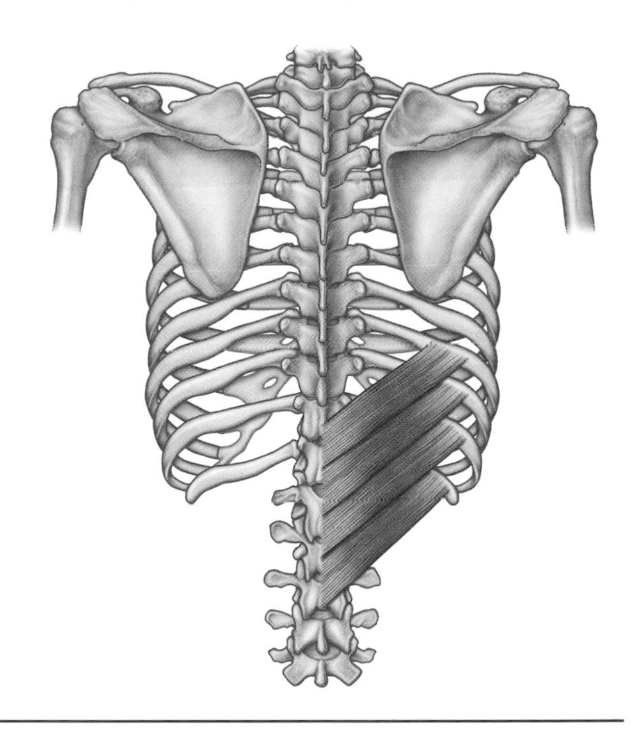

Stretching technique:

Patient is lying on stomach with pillow under abdomen or table bent to flex spine. Arm is raised above the head and thoracic spine bent to side away from the muscle to provide pre-stretch position. Legs are moved to the same side to stretch out lumbar part. Therapist presses with the hand on ribs 9–12 diagonally towards the shoulder while the hypothenar of the other hand, on the facet joints next to the spinous processes of Th11–L3, on the same side applies stretch diagonally down towards the legs. The arms of the therapist are crossed, and substantial pressure can be achieved by leaning into the stretch.

Tension–relaxation technique: Patient takes a deep breath and then proceeds to forcefully exhale by blowing out to empty the lungs. Therapist then instructs patient to inhale normally and relax muscles while performing stretching technique.

Notice: Stretch is not done during deep exhalation because the posterior inferior serratus assists in deep exhalation. The stretch is used during normal respiration or towards the end of inhalation.

Warning ! This stretch is contraindicated in cases of osteoporosis or if other conditions of bone deterioration are suspected.

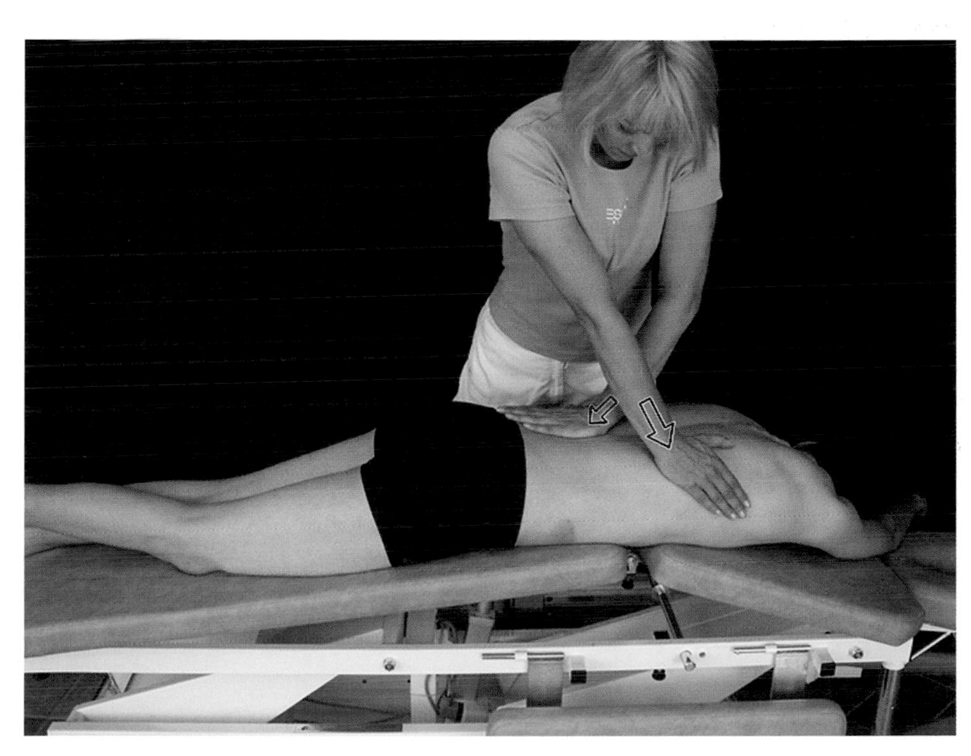

Quadratus lumborum

Nerve, supply: Dorsal rami of spinal nerves, Th12–L3.

Origin: Inner lip of iliac crest, iliolumbar ligament and costal process of transverse processes of L1–4.

Insertion: Transverse processes of L1–4 and twelth rib.

Function: Lateral flexion and stabilization of body and draws twelth rib down. Assists in deep exhalation.

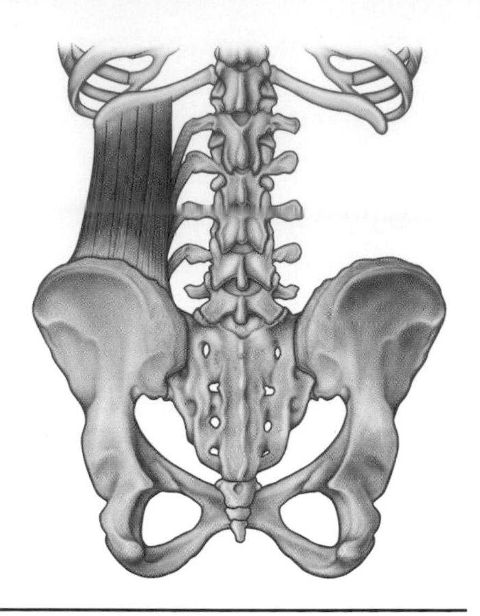

Stretching technique:

Patient is lying on side with the top foot hooked around the calf of the other leg and arm above head. Lumbar spine stretched out by raising centre of table or by placing pillow under the waist. By leaning downwards, therapist presses hip down and forwards with the forearm, while the other forearm presses upper body down and backwards. Hands are used simultaneously to stretch muscle by pulling the origin and insertion away from each other.

Tension–relaxation technique: Patient tries to raise upper body to the side for 5 sec while therapist resists. Patient is then advised to gradually relax muscles while therapist applies pressure to separate pelvis from rib cage.

Notice: Stretching is not performed during exhalation but during normal respiration or towards the end of inhalation as the muscle in question assists in deep exhalation.

Warning ! This stretch is contraindicated in cases of osteoporosis or if there is suspicion of bone deterioration.

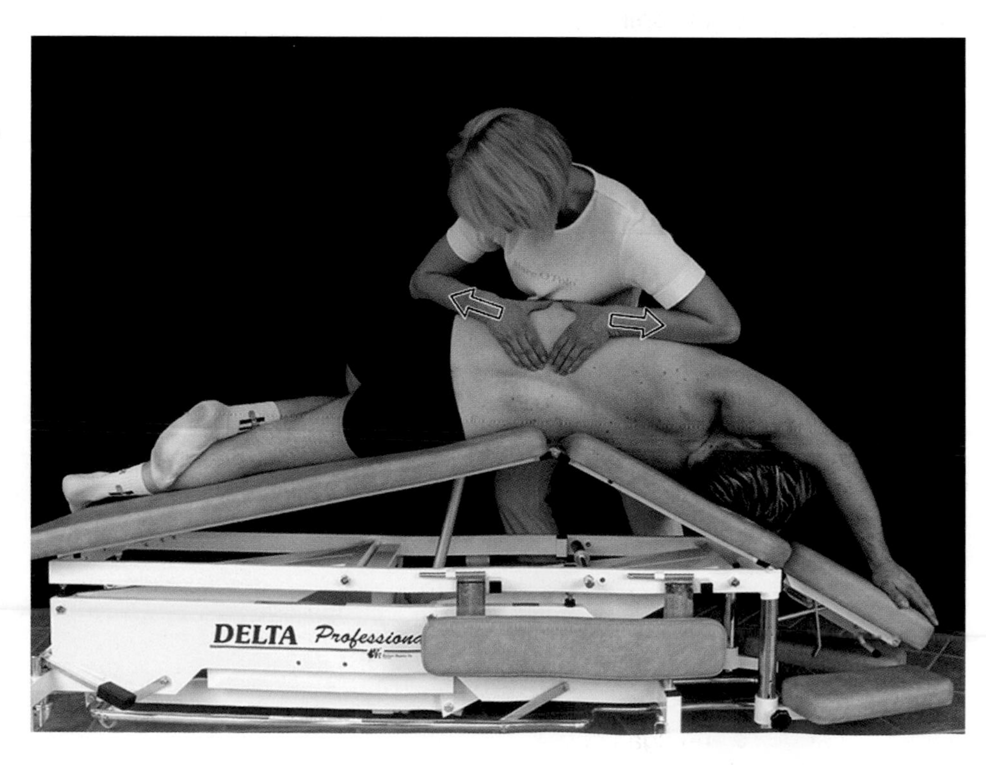

Interspinales thoracis

(Two pairs of muscles)

Nerve, supply: Dorsal rami of spinal nerves, Th11–12.

Origin: Spinous processes of Th11–Th12.

Insertion: Spinous processes of next vertebrae below.

Function: Stabilization and extension of thoracic spine.

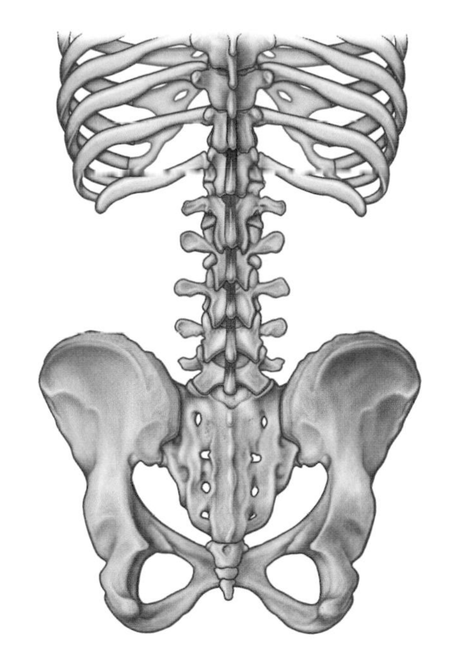

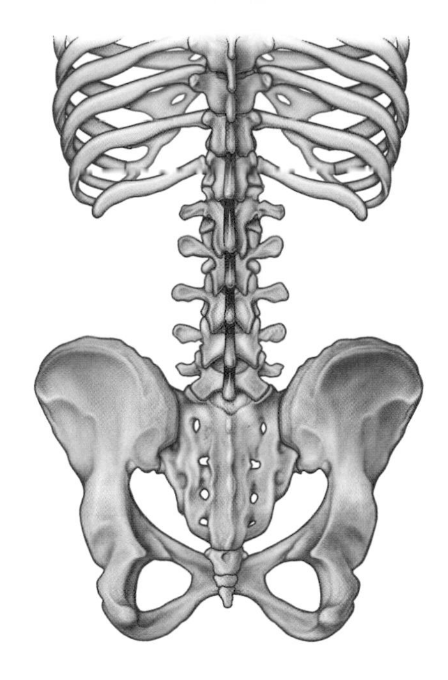

Interspinales lumborum

(Five pairs of muscles)

Nerve, supply: Dorsal rami of spinal nerves, L1–5.

Origin: Spinous processes L1–5.

Insertion: Spinous processes of next vertebrae below.

Function: Stabilization and extension of lumbar spine.

Stretching technique:

Patient is lying on stomach with pelvic hanging over edge of table and feet on the floor. Therapist places the hypothenar of the upper hand on one side of the spinous processes and the thenar on the other side and applies stretch on both sides towards the head, and the other hand presses the sacrum downwards. The arms of the therapist are crossed, and substantial pressure can be achieved by leaning into the stretch.

Tension–relaxation technique: Patient tries to extend lumbar spine for 5 sec while therapist resists. Patient is then instructed to gradually relax muscles while therapist increases stretch.

Warning ❗ Stretch effect is intense in the lumbar discs and ligaments if done while sitting or standing. Disc degeneration is commonly located between L4–5 and L5–S1 and is susceptible to damage in these positions. Pressure is especially focused on the lower joint, and discs while bending forward in a sitting position. It is therefore contraindicated in cases of disc hernia or if there is suspicion of disc rupture.

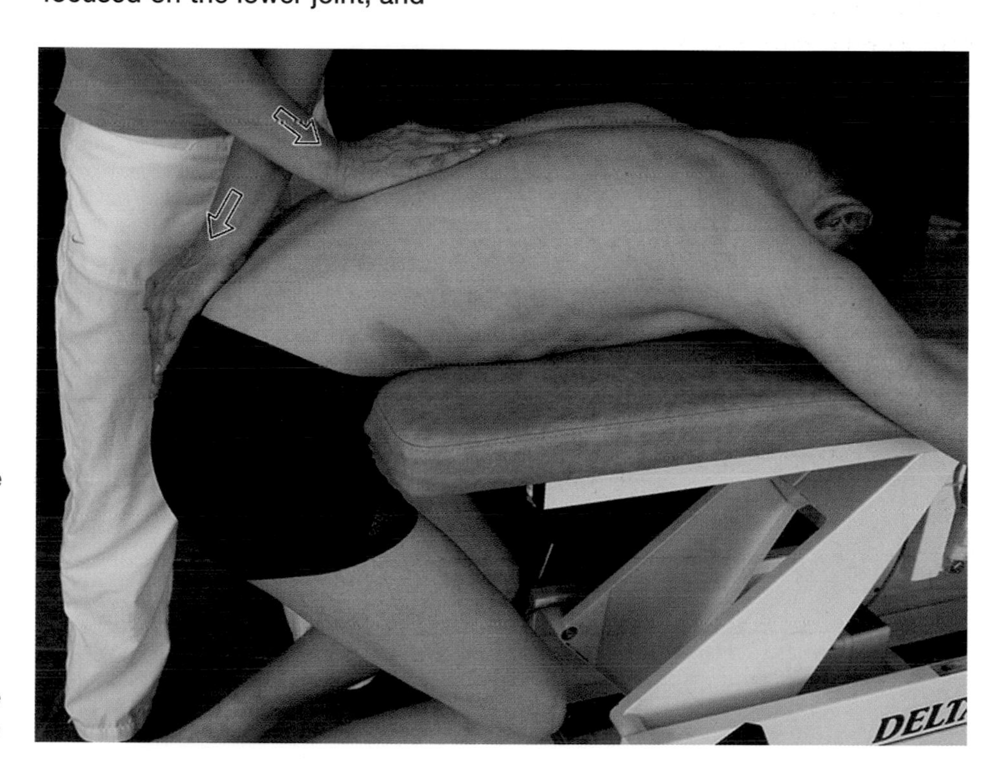

Rotatores thoracis

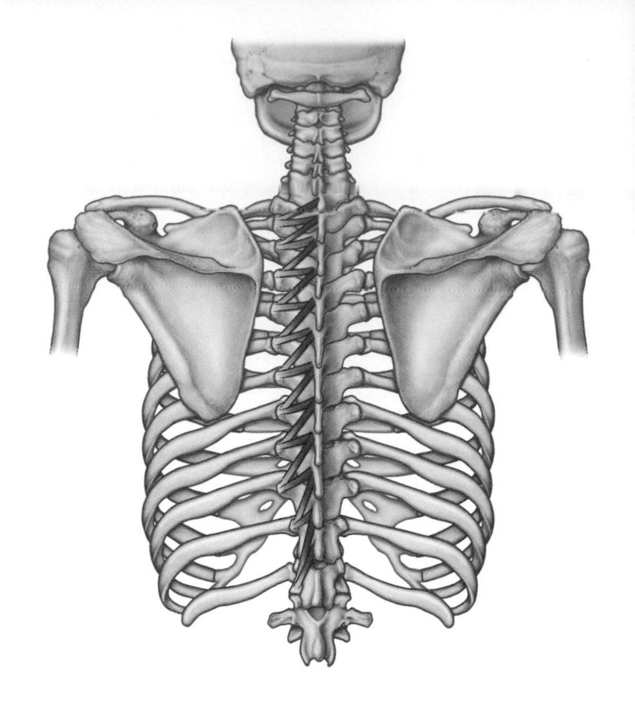

Nerve, supply: Dorsal rami of spinal nerves, Th1–11

Origin: Transverse processes of vertebrae Th1–12

Insertion of short rotators: Lamina, base of spinous process of next higher vertebrae.

Insertion of long rotators: Lamina, base of spinous process of second higher vertebrae.

Function: Stabilize, rotate and lateral flex vertebrae.

Multifidus thoracis

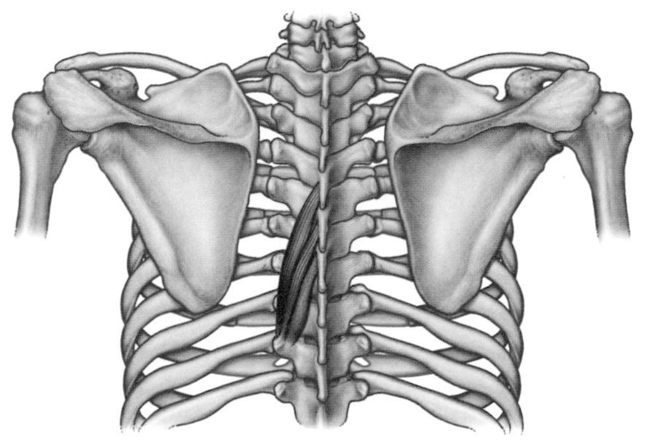

Nerve, supply: Dorsal rami of spinal nerves, C4–Th11.

Origin: Transverse processes of vertebrae Th 1–12 and superficial aponeurosis of longissimus muscle.

Insertion: Each muscle crosses 2–4 vertebrae to insert on the spinous processes of superior vertebrae.

Function: Stabilize, extend, rotate and lateral flex vertebrae.

Stretching technique A:

Patient is lying on side with the hips and knees flexed. Thoracic spine stretched out by raising centre of table or by placing pillow under the lower rib cage. Bottom shoulder and arm are brought forward to rotate rib cage backwards and the patient's hand placed under the head. Top upper arm is next to body with the elbow flexed 90°. Therapist's hand presses shoulder diagonally backwards and towards head to rotate rib cage backwards while using other hand to stretch muscles by pulling away from insertion with fingertips.

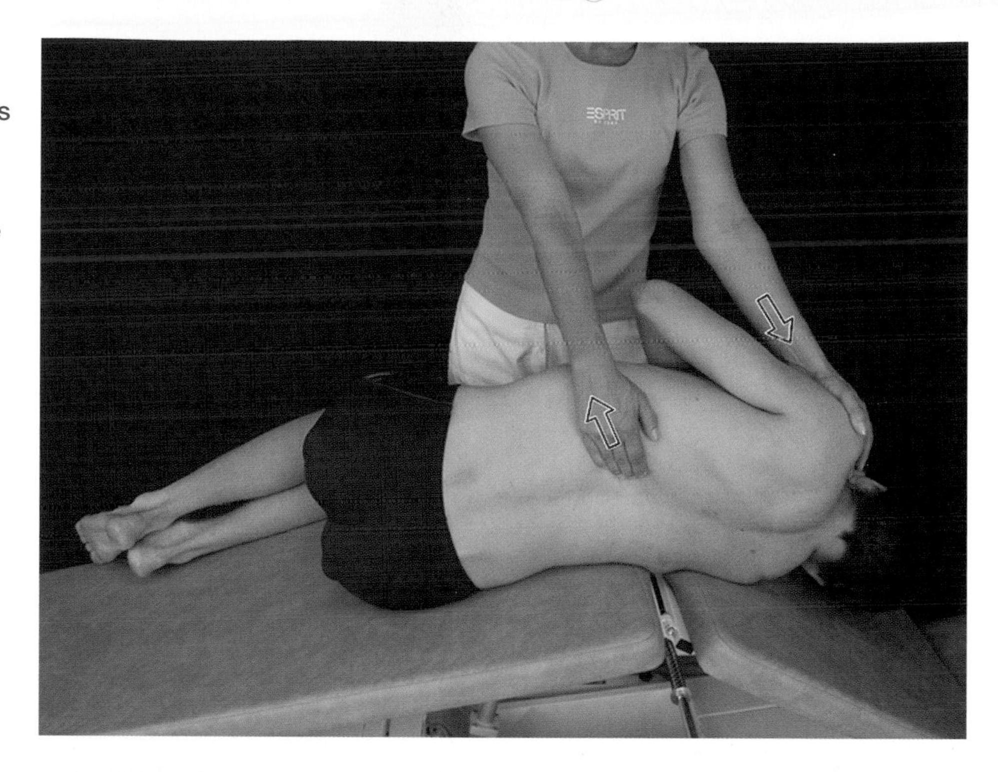

Tension–relaxation technique: Patient tries to push the upper shoulder forwards for 5 sec while therapist resists. Patient is then instructed to relax completely while therapist allows stretch to increase.

Warning ❗ Excessive use of pressure can cause rib fracture, especially in cases of osteoporosis.

Stretching technique B:

Patient is lying on side with the hips and knees flexed. Thoracic spine stretched out by raising centre of table or by placing pillow under the lower rib cage. Bottom shoulder and arm are brought forward to rotate rib cage backwards and patient's hand placed under the head. Top upper arm is next to the body with the elbow flexed 90°. Therapist presses shoulder diagonally backwards and towards head to rotate rib cage with the forearm while using the other forearm to rotate lower thoracic spine and pelvis forwards.

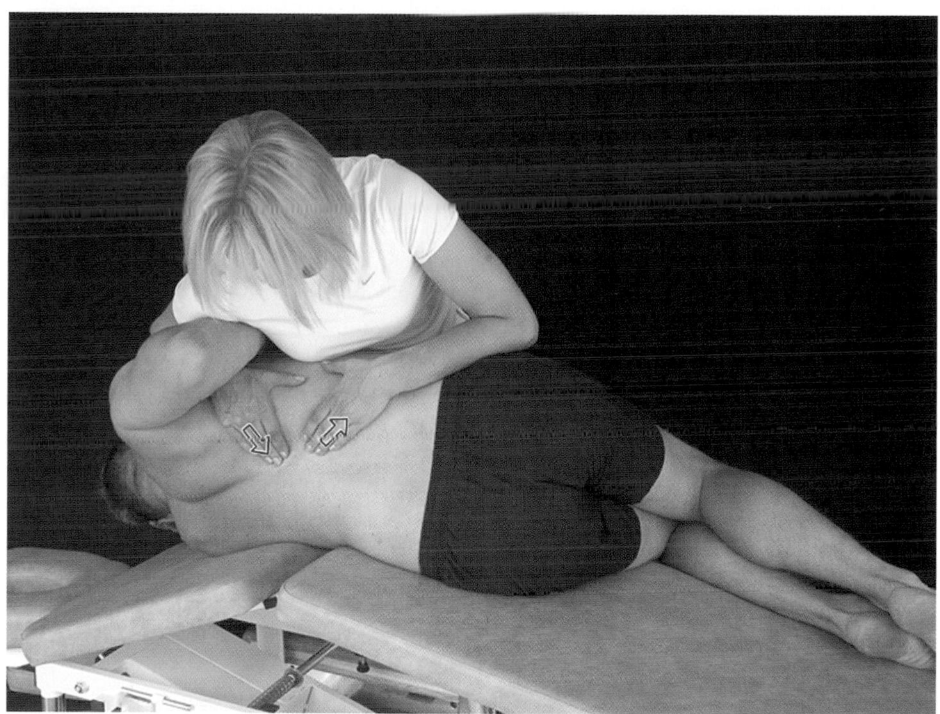

Hands are used simultaneously to stretch muscles by pulling the origin and insertion away from each other with fingertips.

Intertransversarii thoracis

Nerve, supply: Dorsal rami of spinal nerves.

Origin: Transverse processes.

Insertion: Transverse processes of next vertebrae below.

Function: Stabilize spine. Lateral flex vertebrae.

Notice: Usually absent.

Intertransversarii mediales lumborum

Nerve, supply: Dorsal rami of spinal nerves, L1–5.

Origin: Mamillary processes of transverse processes L1–5.

Insertion: Mamillary processes of transverse processes of next vertebra below and sacrum.

Function: Stabilize spine. Lateral flex vertebrae.

Intertransversarii lateral's lumborum

Nerve, supply: Dorsal rami of spinal nerves, L1–5.

Origin: Costal processes of transverse processes of L1–5.

Insertion: Costal processes of next vertebra below and sacrum.

Function: Stabilize spine. Lateral flex vertebrae.

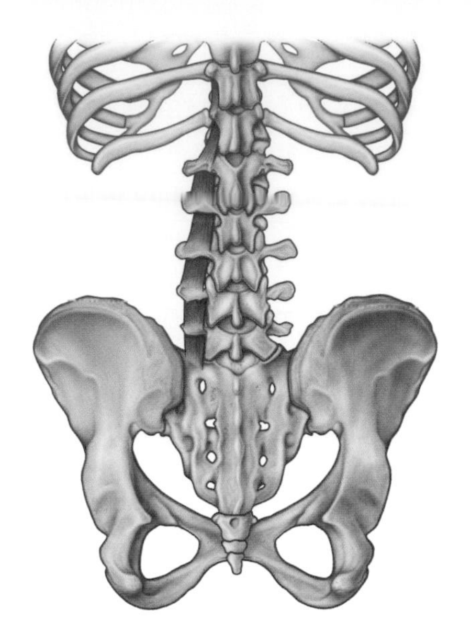

Multifidus lumborum

Nerve, supply: Dorsal rami of spinal nerves, Th12–L5.

Origin: Sacrum and mamillary processes of transverse processes L1–5.

Insertion: Each muscle crosses over 2–4 vertebrae to insert on the spinous processes of superior vertebrae.

Function: Stabilize spine. Extend, lateral flex and rotate vertebrae.

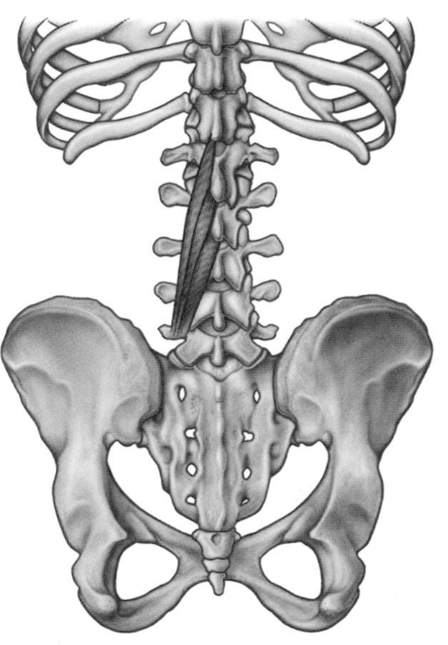

Rotatores breves and longi lumborum

Nerve, supply: Dorsal rami of spinal nerves, Th12–L5.

Origin: Mamillary processes of transverse processes of L1–S1.

Insertion of short muscles: Base of spinous process of next higher vertebrae.

Insertion of long muscles: Base of spinous process of second higher vertebrae.

Function: Stabilization, rotation and lateral flexion of vertebral joints.

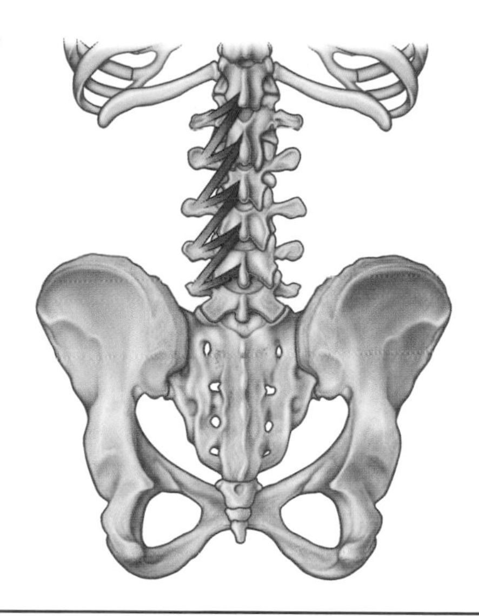

Stretching technique:

Patient is lying on side with the top foot hooked around the calf of the other leg. Lumbar spine stretched out by raising centre of table or by placing pillow under the waist. Lower shoulder and arm in front of body to rotate rib cage backwards and top arm next to body with elbow flexed 90°. Therapist uses forearm to increase rotation of rib cage backwards, while using other forearm to push pelvis forward. By leaning downward, therapist presses hip down and further forward and upper body down and further back. Fingers of both hands next to the spinous processes pull in opposite directions and intensify stretch.

Tension–relaxation technique: Patient tries to rotate the upper body forwards for 5 sec while therapist resists. Patient is then instructed to gradually relax while therapist presses rib cage back and pelvis forward to improve stretch effect.

Warning ! In patients with compression of the nerve root intense rotation may cause further pressure on the nerve root and result in pain and numbness in the leg and in these cases stretch is contraindicated.

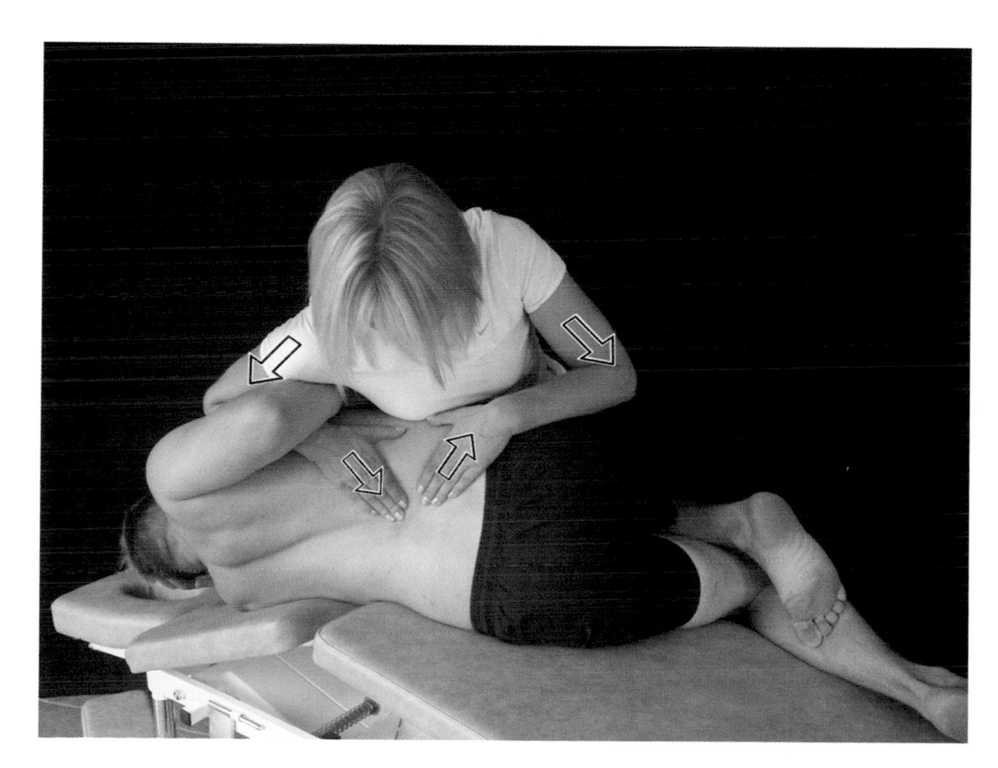

Levatores costarum breves

Nerve, supply: Dorsal rami of spinal nerves, C8–Th11.

Origin of breves: Transverse processes of C7–Th11.

Insertion: Costal angle of next lower rib.

Function: Assist in deep inhalation.

Levatores costarum longi

Nerve, supply: Dorsal rami of spinal nerves, C8–Th11.

Origin of longi: Transverse processes of C7–Th10.

Insertion: Costal angle of second lower rib.

Function: Assist in deep inhalation.

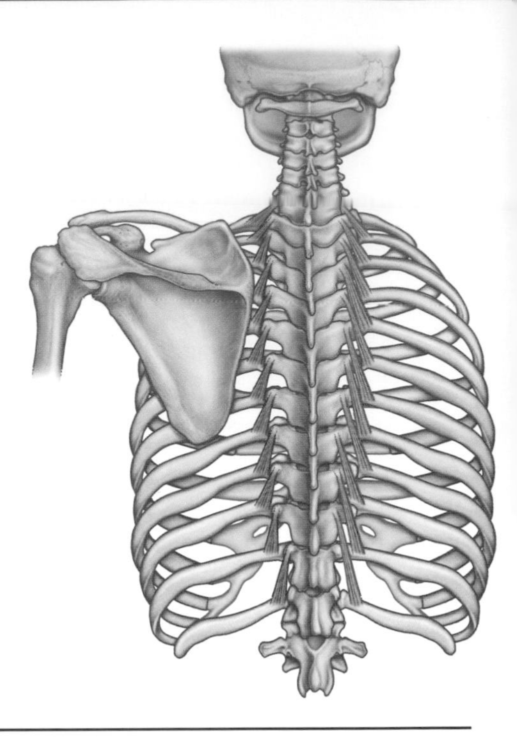

Stretching technique:

Patient is lying on stomach and thoracic spine flexed by raising centre of table or by placing pillow under the chest. Arm above the head, and bend away from the side of the muscle.Legs brought to same side to provide pre-stretch position in sidebending. Therapist applies pressure with the hypothenar of the hand next to the spinous processes on facet joints to stabilize vertebrae, while using hypothenar of the other hand to push on rib of the next or second vertebrae below diagonally in lateral direction towards the hip to stretch muscles on the other side. Arms of therapist cross over each other and stretching is achieved by leaning forward.

Warning ! Ribs are under considerable pressure during this technique and care should be taken to avoid excessive force. The risk of rib fracture increases if the contact is not just beside the vertebrae, but is too far side on the rib. This stretch is contraindicated in cases of osteoporosis or if bone deterioration is suspected due to other reasons.

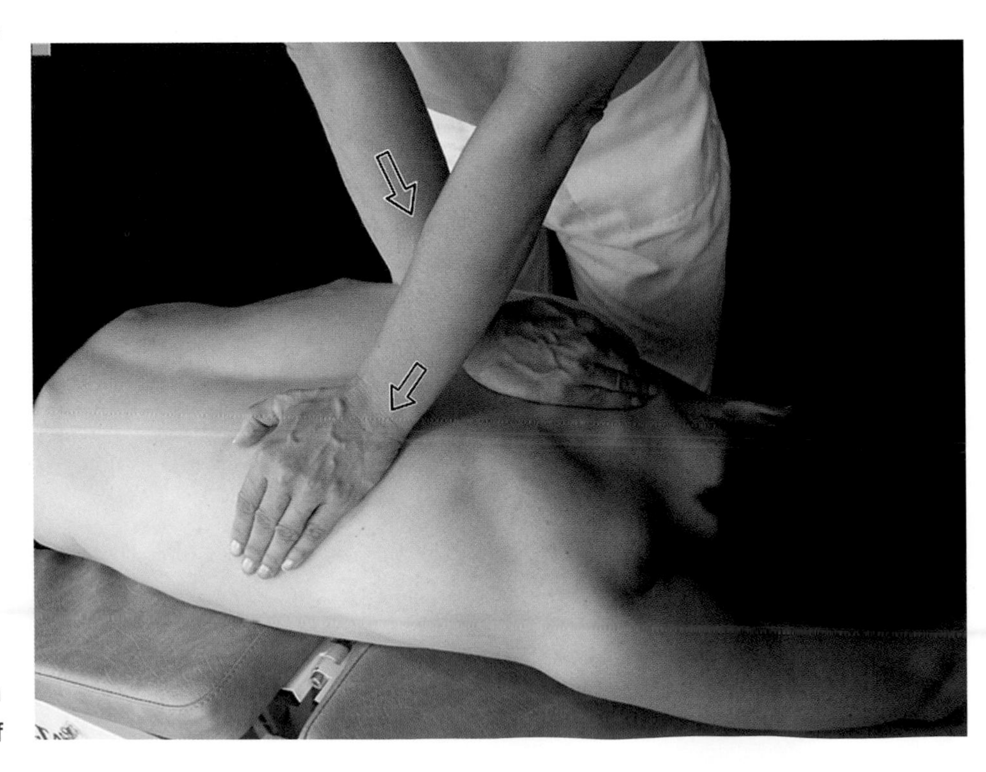

External intercostals

Nerve, supply: Intercostal nerves, Th1–11.

Origin: Inferior surface of ribs.

Insertion: Superior surface of adjacent rib below. Fibre direction is diagonally down and forward.

Function: Elevate ribs and expand rib cage. Assist in deep inhalation.

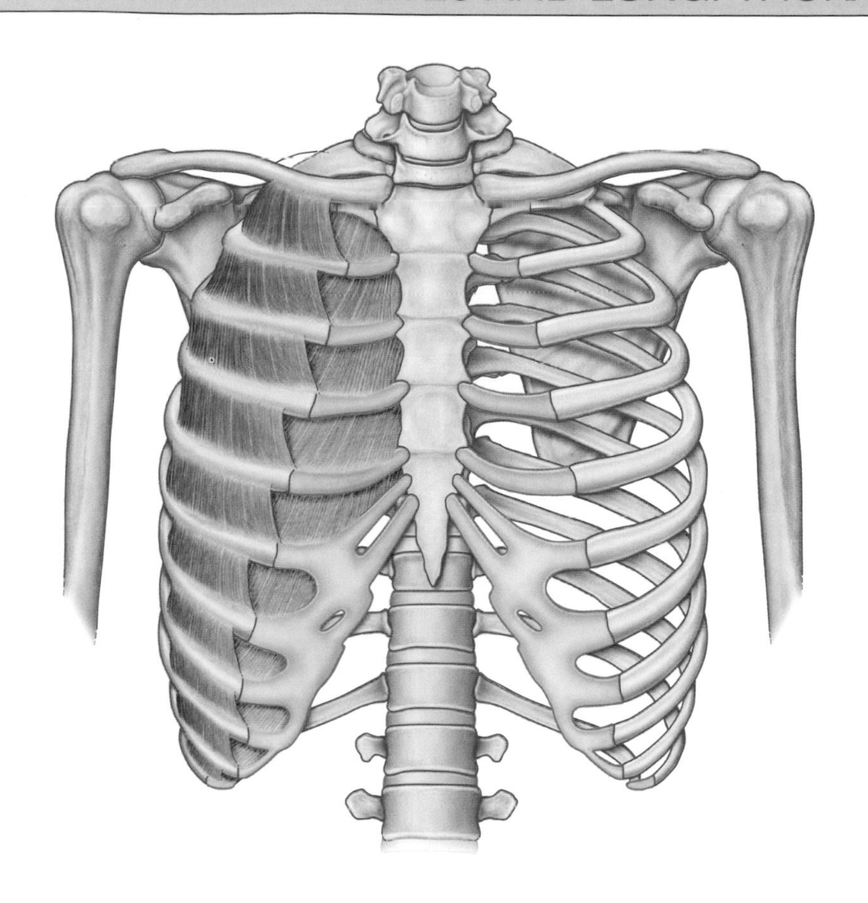

Internal intercostals

Nerve, supply: Intercostal nerves, Th1–11.

Origin: Inferior surface of ribs.

Insertion: Superior surface of adjacent rib. Fibre direction is diagonally down and back.

Function: Lower ribs and contract rib cage. Assist in deep exhalation.

Intercostales intimi

A deep layer of internal intercostals.

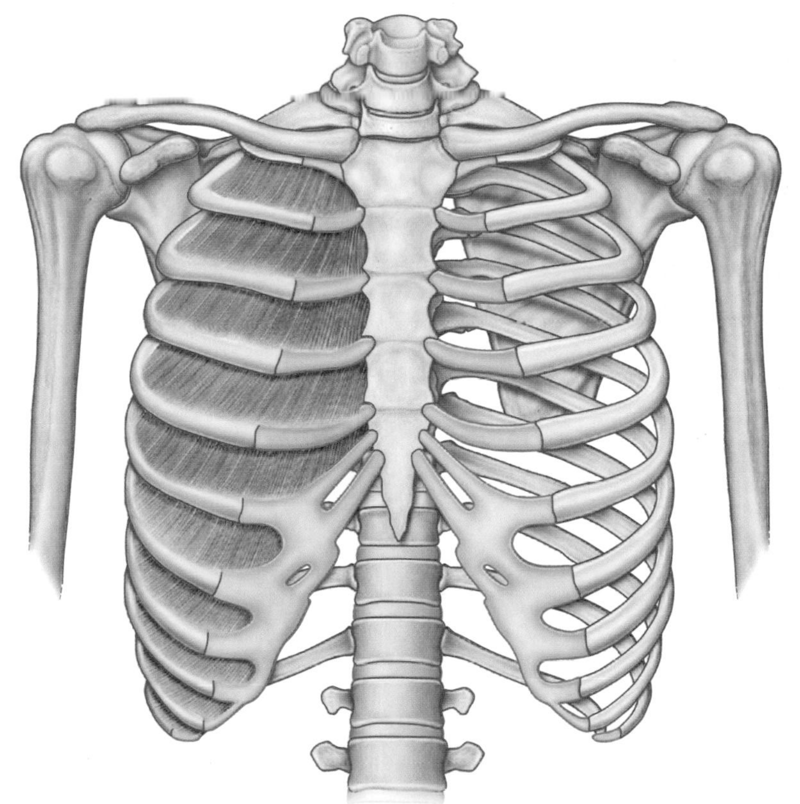

Stretching technique A:

Superior ribs move forward and up during inhalation and this is known as the pump handle movement. Thus, intercostal spaces between 1–5 costae are stretched from the front.

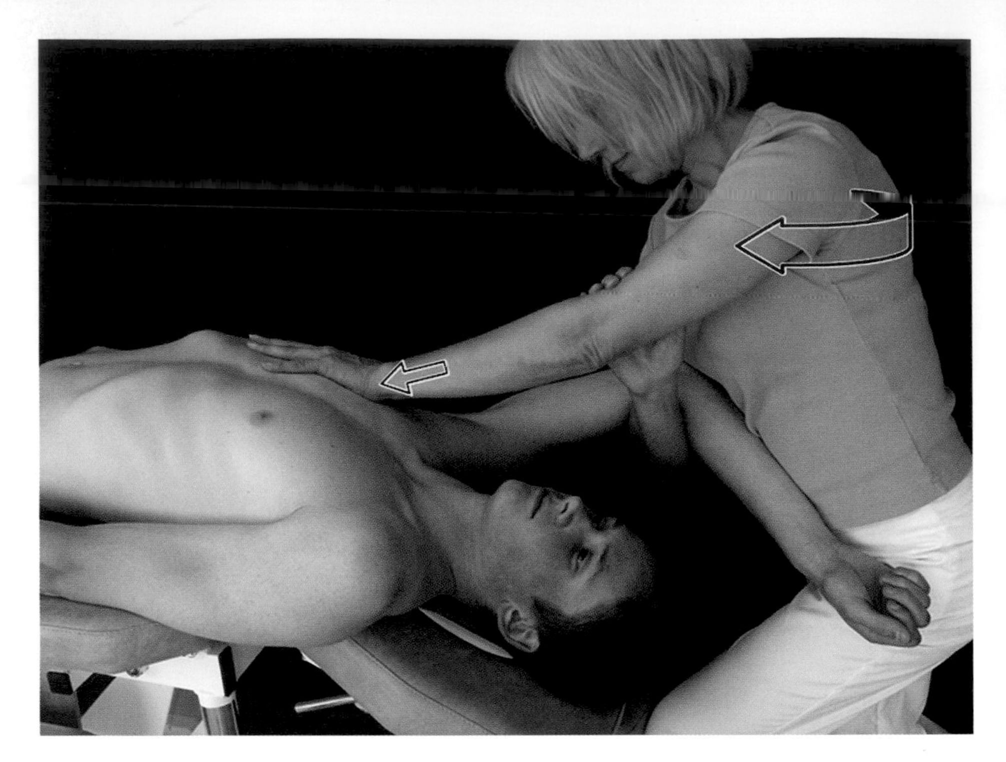

Patient is lying on back with arm above the head and elbow flexed 90°. Therapist supports patient's forearm against own body with the aid of own forearm. The hold is reinforced by grasping the other arm. Which is important to notice! The thenar and hypothenar of this hand are placed between the ribs. Stretching is not applied by pressing down, but the therapist rotates own body while maintaining hold of patient's arm and pushes the rib away from the one above. Stretching is performed during normal shallow exhalation or when patient stops breathing for a short moment.

Warning ❗ This technique to stretch intercostal muscles is contraindicated in cases of osteoporosis or if bone deterioration is suspected.

Stretching technique B:

Inferior ribs move to the side during inhalation and this is known as the bucket handle movement. Thus, intercostal spaces between 6–10 costae are stretched from the side.

Patient is lying on side with lower hand under the head. Therapist supports patient's forearm against own body with aid of own forearm and reinforces the hold by grasping the other arm. The thumb, metacarpal bone and thenar of this hand are placed between the ribs. Stretching is not applied by pressing down, but the therapist rotates own body while maintaining hold of patient's arm and pushes the rib away from the one above. Stretching is performed during normal shallow breathing or when patient stops breathing for a short moment.

Notice: Deep exhalation will activate internal intercostals and in deep inhalation external intercostals are activated, making the stretch futile; this is a common mistake. Thus, breathing should be normal during stretching or stop breathing during the spend for stretching.

Notice: Stretching is directed only in the one intercostal space at a time in both techniques for intercostal muscles.

Warning ❗ This technique to stretch intercostal muscles is contraindicated in cases of osteoporosis or if bone deterioration is suspected.

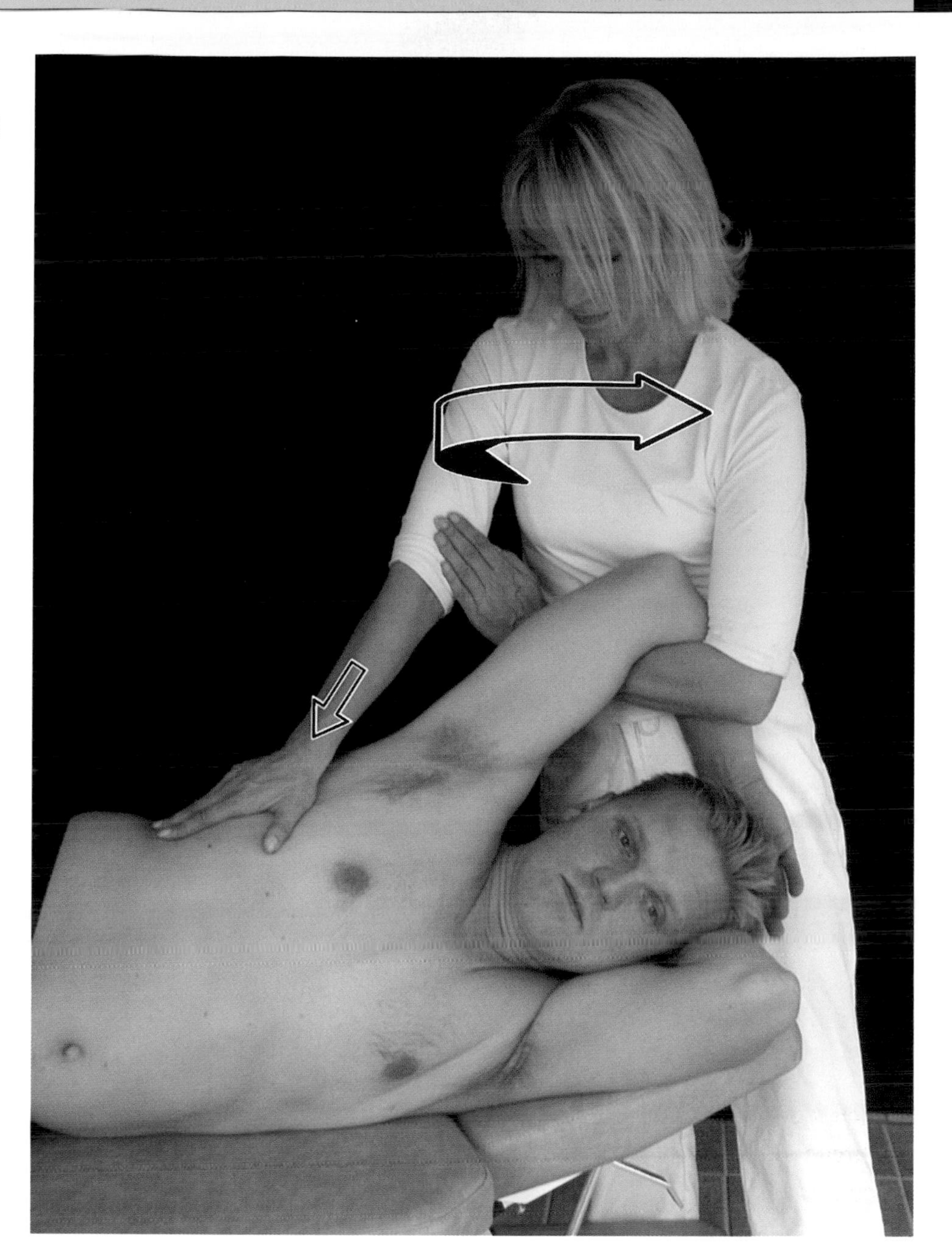

Diaphragm

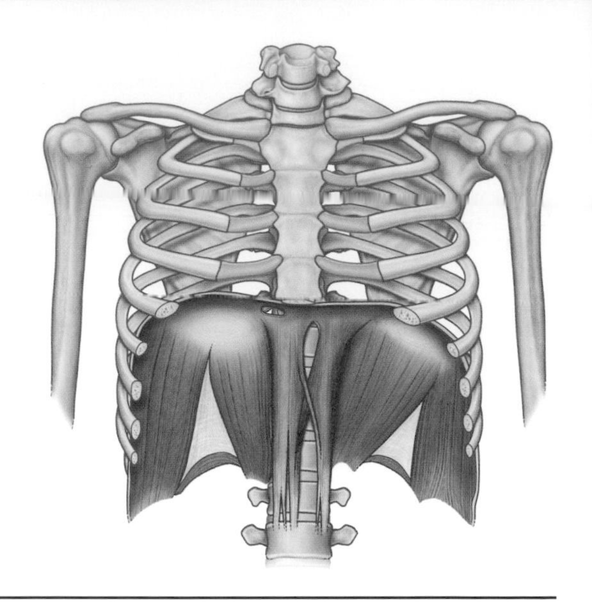

Nerve, supply: Phrenic nerve, C3–5.

Origin: Inner surface of xiphoid process, ribs 7–12, inner surfaces of lumbar vertebrae L1–4 on the right side and L1–3 on the left side, psoas arcade, medial and lateral arcuate ligament.

Insertion: Central tendon.

Function: Inhalation.

Stretching technique:

Patient is lying on back with arms at sides and hips and knees flexed. Therapist grasps the costal arches of cartilages at the level of ribs 6–8. Patient breathes in deeply so that the diaphragm drops down and costal arches lift up and ribcage expands. Therapist 'locks' position of rib cage while patient exhales normally, causing diaphragm to pull down on the ribs. By preventing the return to the resting position the diaphragm undergoes an intense stretch.

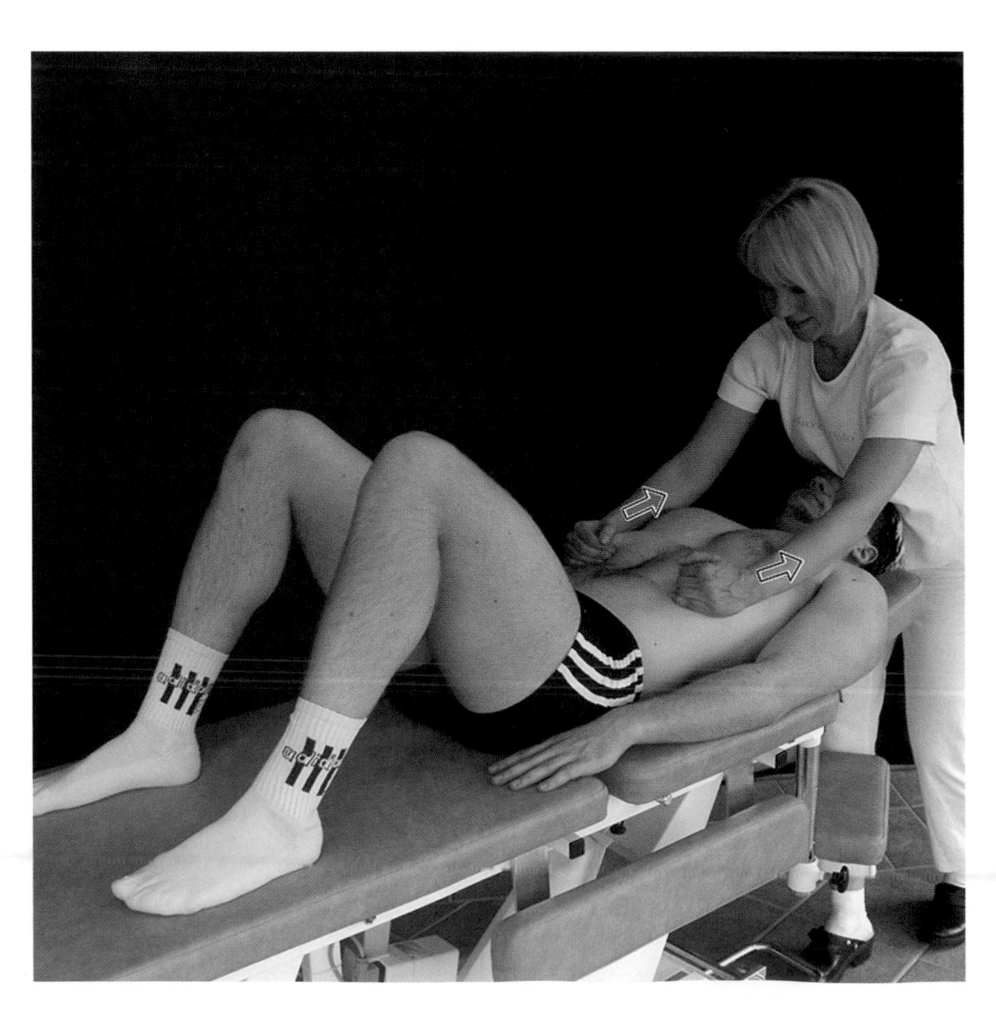

Warning ❗ Grasping of the costal arches too far at the sides should be avoided as this could damage intercostal cartilage or the intercostal nerve.

Warning ❗ The possibility of fracture with this technique is of considerable risk in cases of osteoporosis or if bone deterioration is suspected.

Rectus abdominis

Nerve, supply: Intercostal nerves, Th5–12.

Origin: Outer surface of cartilages of ribs 5–7, xiphoid process and the intervening ligaments.

Insertion: Pubic crest.

Function: Forward bending and trunk support; assists deep exhalation.

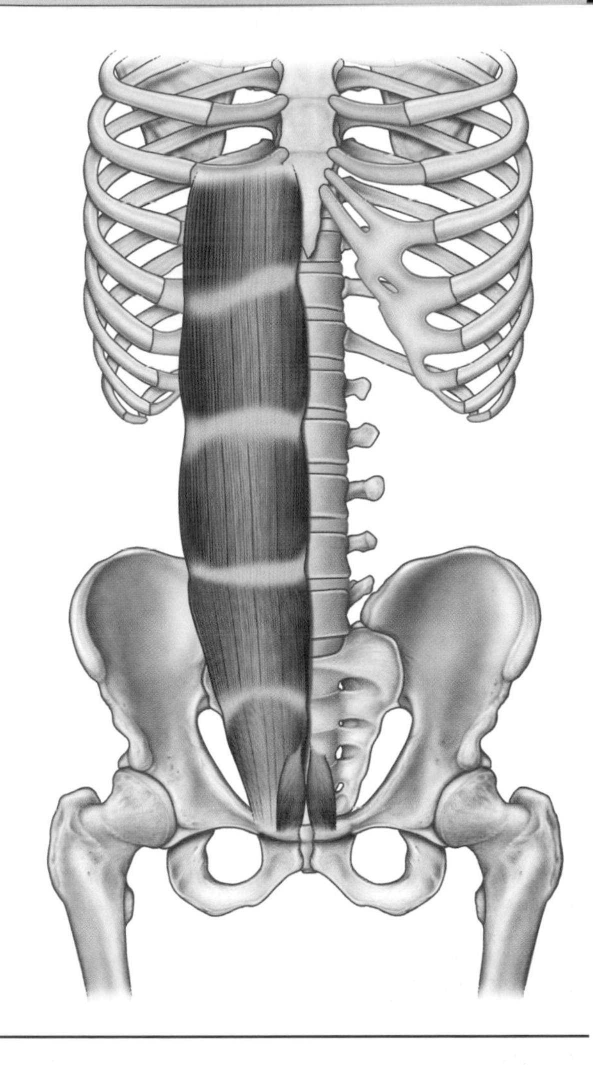

Stretching technique:

Patient is lying on back with arms above head. Rectus abdominis is pre-stretched by raising centre of table or using large therapy ball. Patient breathes in deeply, extending back, expanding rib cage outwards with the aid of the diaphragm and relaxing abdominal muscles. By leaning forwards therapist applies downward pressure at the pubic bone with the forearm, while simultaneously the other hand on xiphoid process presses obliquely towards the head to stretch muscle by pushing the origin and insertion away from each other.

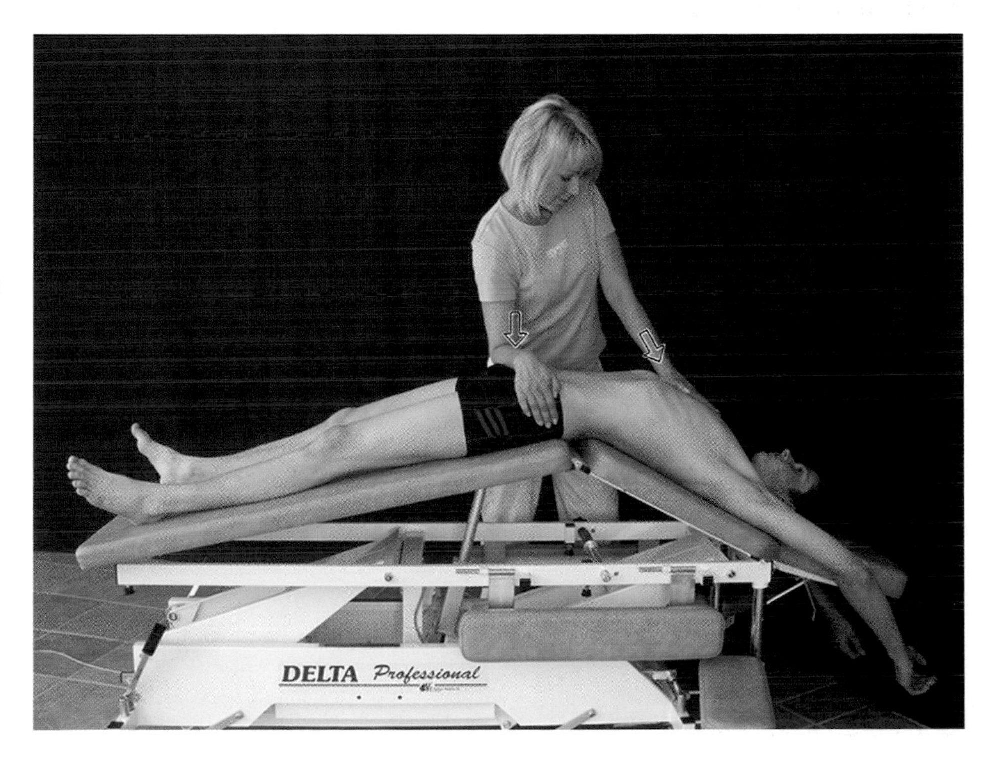

External oblique abdominis

Nerve, supply: Intercostal nerves, Th5–12.

Origin: Outer surface of ribs 5–12.

Insertion: Via aponeuroses to rectus sheath, inguinal ligament, iliac crest.

The direction of fibres is towards inferomedially.

Function: Forward and lateral flexion of the trunk. Assists in deep exhalation.

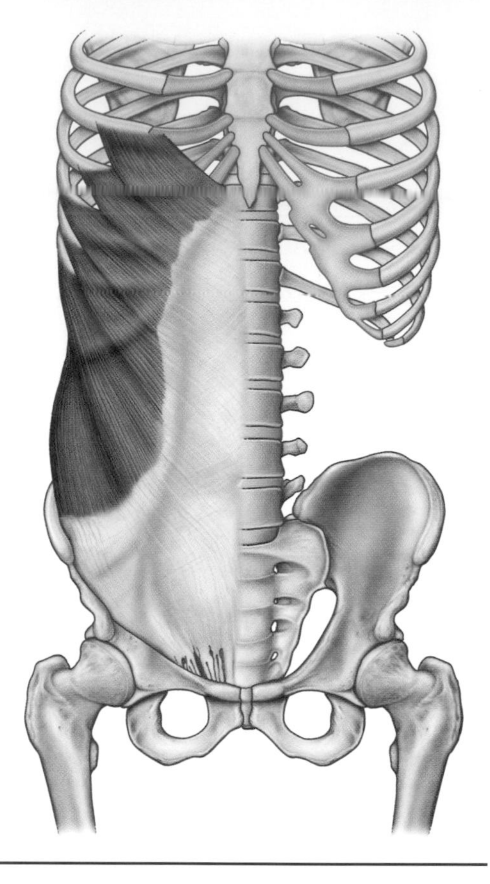

Stretching technique:

Patient is lying on side with upper arm above head, lower hand under the head, bottom leg flexed to give support and top leg hangs out over the back edge of table. Oblique abdominal muscles are pre-stretched by raising centre of table or by placing pillow under the waist. By leaning downwards, therapist presses hip down and forwards with the hand while the other hand presses the rib cage down and back. Hands are used simultaneously to stretch muscle by pushing the origin and insertion away from each other.

Tension–relaxation technique: Patient tries to rotate chest forwards 5 sec while therapist resists. Then gradually relaxes while therapist allows the stretch to increase under the pressure supplied by the hands.

Warning ❗ This technique has a noticeable fracture risk in cases of osteoporosis or if bone deterioration due to other reasons is suspected.

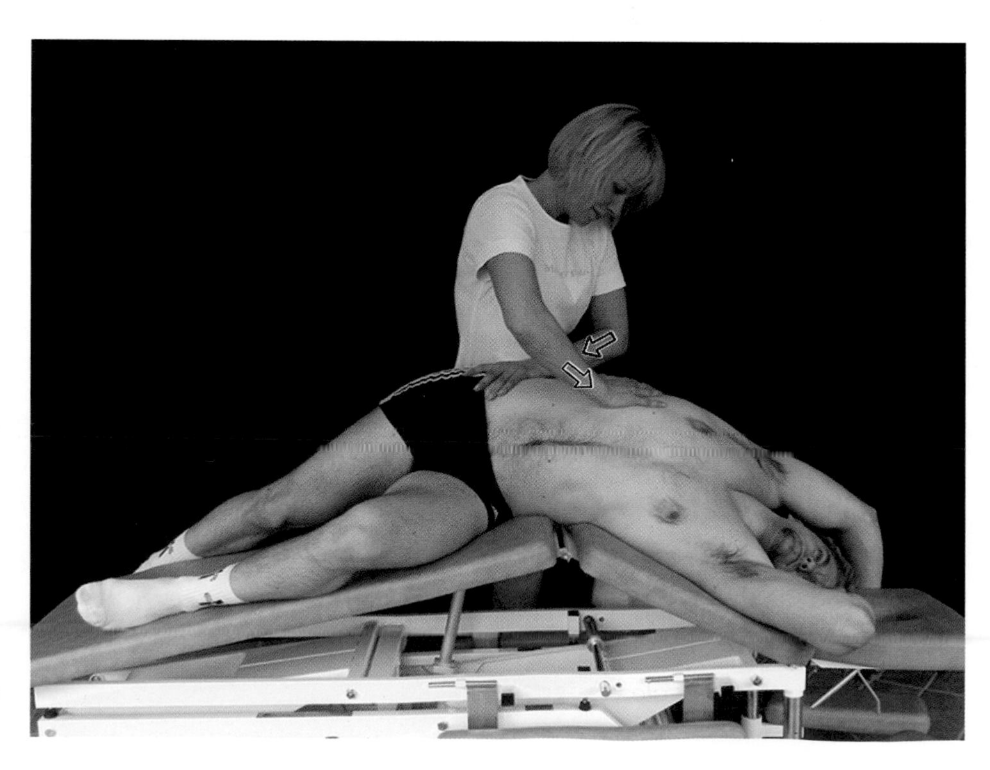

Internal oblique abdominis

Nerve, supply: Intercostal nerves, Th10–L1.

Origin: Thoracolumbar fascia, iliac crest, anterior superior iliac spine and inguinal ligament.

Insertion: Ribs 8–12 and via aponeuroses to rectus sheet.

Function: Forward and lateral flexion of the trunk. Assists in deep exhalation.

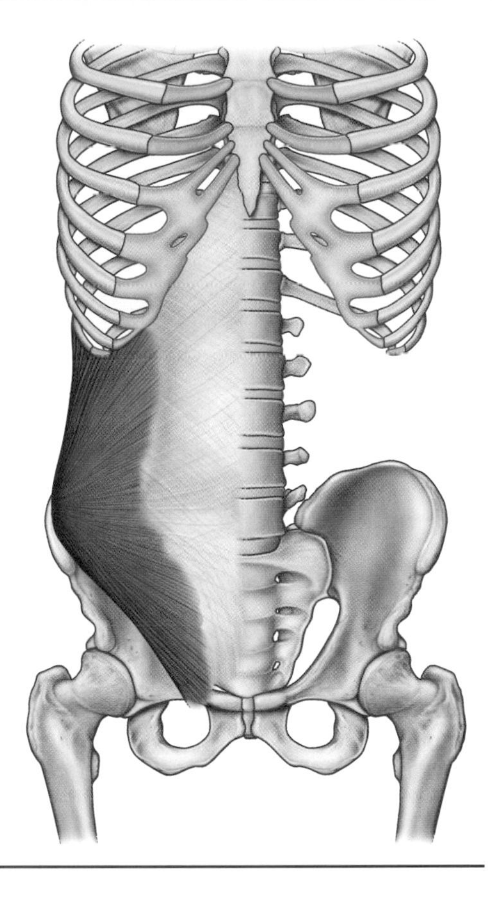

Stretching technique A:

(Upper part)

Patient is lying on side with upper arm above the head and lower arm under the head. Bottom leg flexed to give support while other leg hangs over the back edge of the table. Therapist pulls the hip backwards with hand leans forwards and presses with forearm to increase hand down foreward rotation of the chest while using hands to stretch the muscle fibres.

Tension–relaxation technique: Patient tries to rotate upper body backwards 5 sec while therapist resists. Patient then relaxes gradually while therapist allows the stretch to increase under the pressure supplied by the arms.

Notice: Abdominal muscles are not stretched during deep exhalation when muscles contract, but during inhalation or normal shallow breathing.

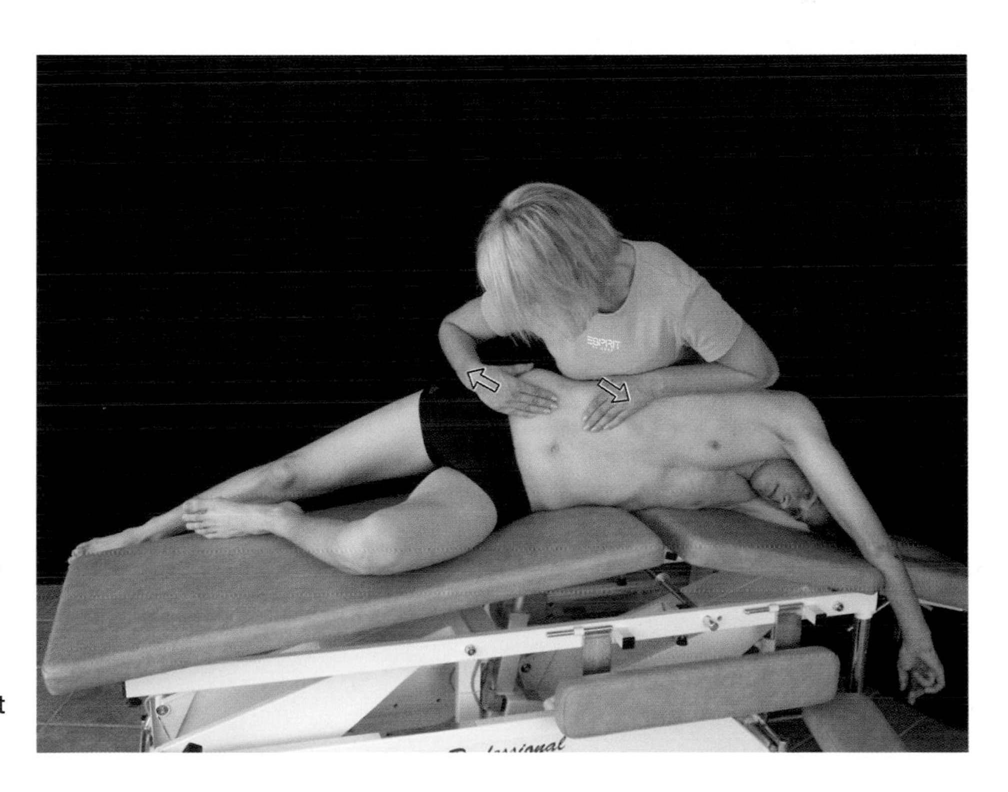

Stretching technique B:

(Lower part)

Patient is lying on the other side with one arm straight out in front of body and the other hand supporting the head. Bottom leg flexed to provide overall support and top leg hanging over the back edge of table. Chest is rotated forwards while pelvis is rotated backwards. Therapist presses pelvis down and backwards with one hand while using the other hand and forearm to pull rib cage down and forwards.

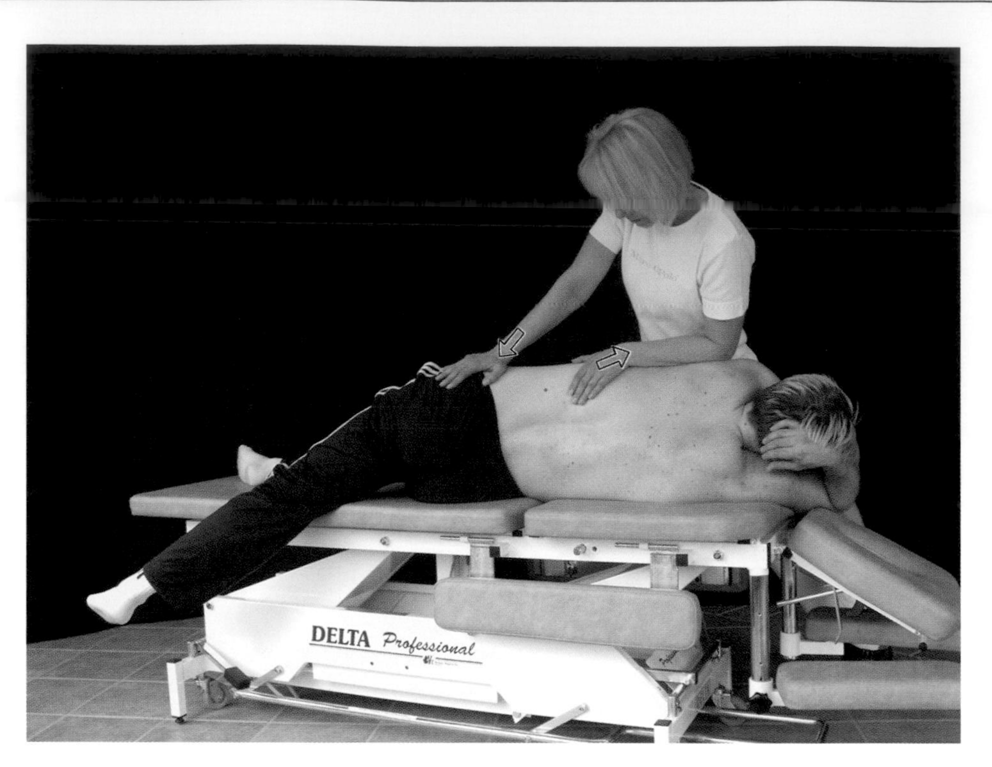

Tension–relaxation technique: Patient tries to rotate upper body backwards for 5 sec while therapist resists. Patient is then instructed to gradually relax muscles while therapist allows stretch to increase under the sustained pressure.

Pyramidalis

Nerve, supply: Intercostal nerves, Th12–L1.

Origin: Pubic crest.

Insertion: Linea alba in the middle of rectus abdominis.

Function: Tense linea alba.

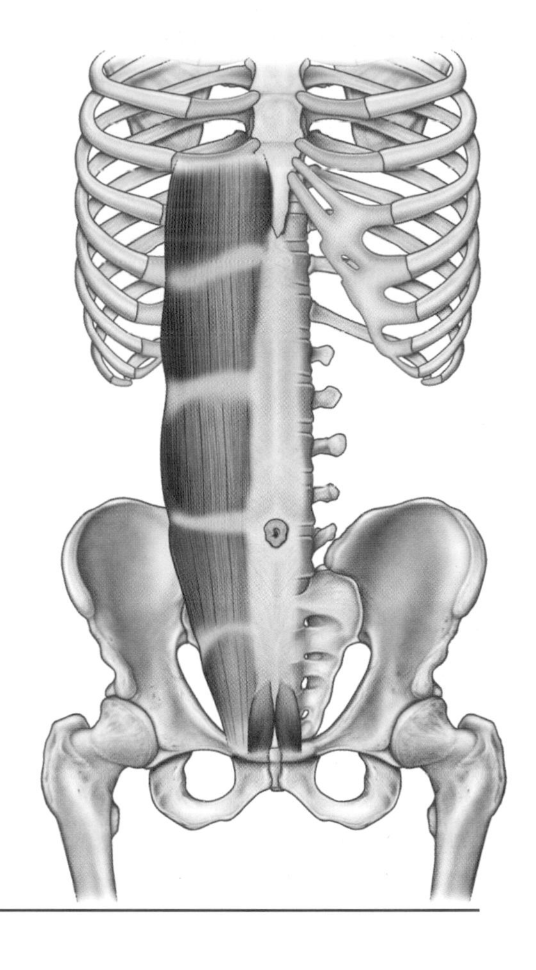

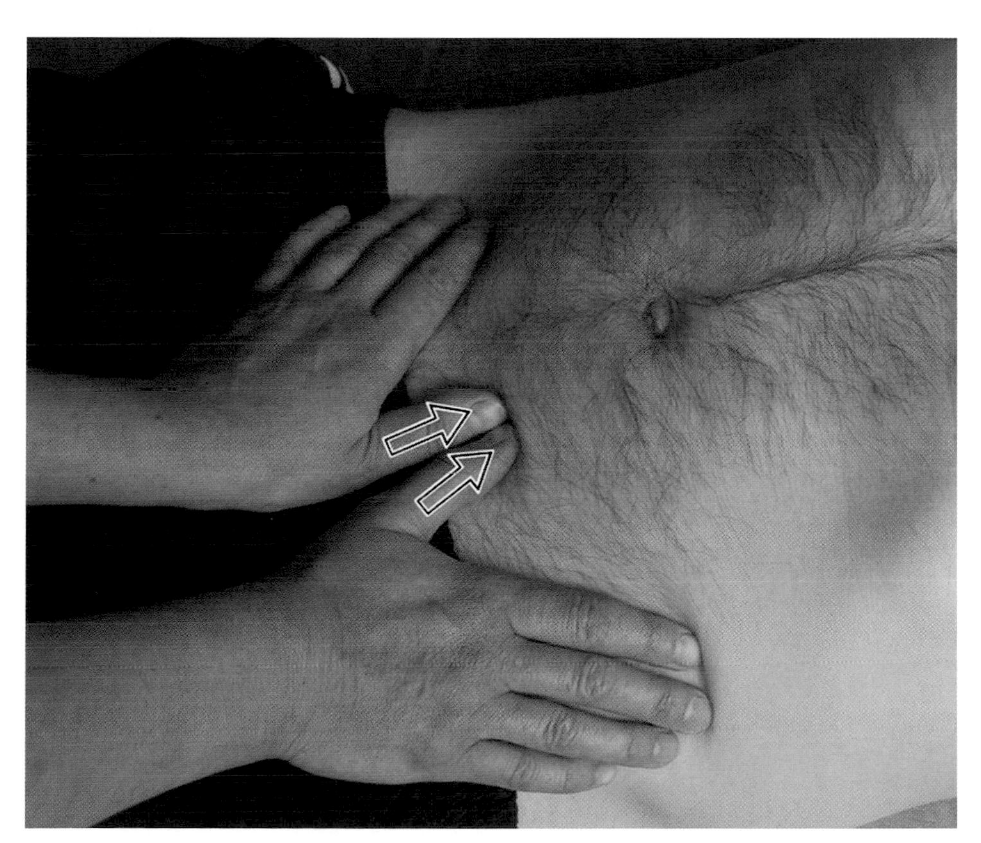

Stretching technique:

Patient is lying on back with arms at side. The stretch is applied with both thumbs towards the body of muscle away from origin. Rectus abdominis may be tensed to achieve a better stretch on pyramidalis.

Transversus abdominis

Nerve, supply: Intercostal nerves, Th7–L1.

Origin: Ribs 7–12, thoracolumbar fascia, iliac crest, anterior superior iliac spine and inguinal ligament.

Insertion: Via aponeuroses to rectus sheet.

Function: Stabilizes trunk and abdomen.

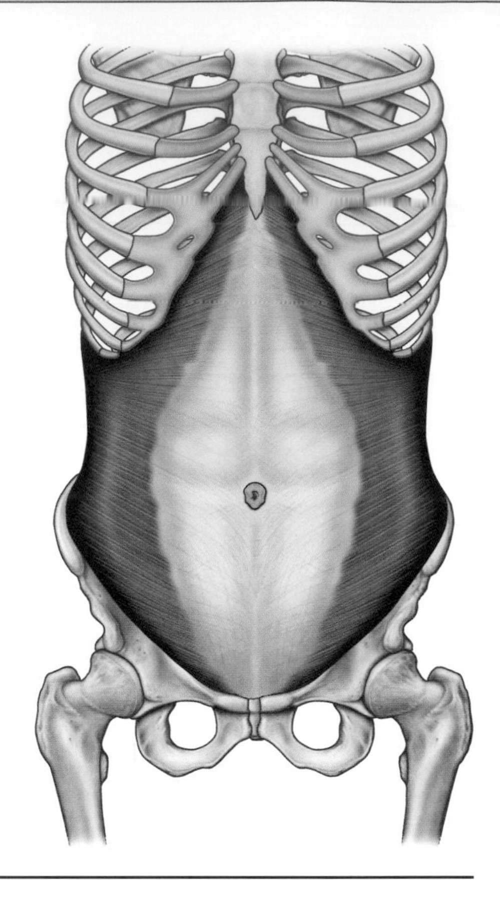

Stretching technique:

This muscle is commonly stretched by eating too much. Thus, it is the main muscle to prevent the abdomen from hanging out. Tightness of abdominal muscles is commonly considered to be beneficial and not a problem.

Traditional stretching of the abdominal muscles can be performed only on those who are extensively trained and have shortened muscles. Most patients have, on the contrary, lengthened muscles and suffer only local muscle tension or trigger points without any general increase in muscle tension.

A decrease in back mobility may also limit stretching of the abdominal muscles and thus stretching massage is the only effective way to release muscle tension.

Traditional abdominal massage does not usually directly affect the muscles in this area, as the patient is lying on their back with the abdomen in a relaxed state. Manual treatment of abdominal muscles requires special stroking and deep friction techniques, which have been described previously by Ylinen and Cash (1988). Stretching massage concentrates on small problem areas of muscle tissue that are causing pain.

Pain due to muscles occurs usually both in the upper and lower abdominal areas and may lead to extensive radiologic examinations and scopies of gastrointestinal tract and urogenital organs, if the muscles are not considered as the source of pain and not treated. Thus, an enormous amount of money is wasted due to inadequate and clinical examinations missing treatment.

Gluteus maximus

Nerve, supply: Inferior gluteal nerve, L5–S2.

Origin: Iliac crest, posterior superior iliac spine, ala of ilium, thoracolumbar fascia, sacrum, coccyx, sacrotuberal ligament and gluteal aponeurosis.

Insertion: Iliotibial tract and gluteal tuberosity.

Function: Extends, externally rotates, abducts and adducts hip. Extends and stabilizes pelvis. Starts to contract only with greater loads. Assists in contraction of pelvic floor muscles.

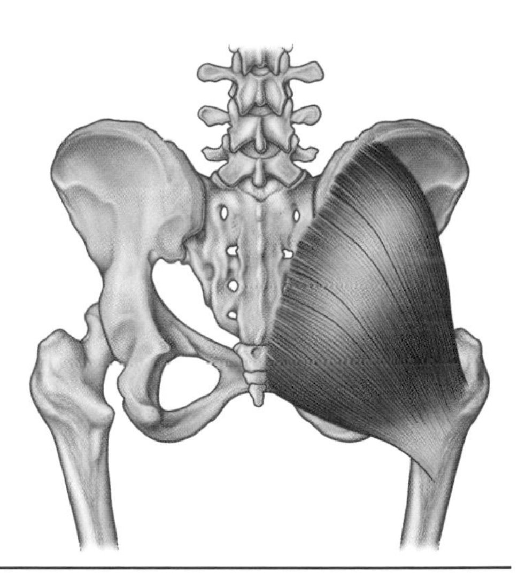

Stretching technique A (flexion + adduction + external rotation):

Patient is lying on back with hip and knee joints flexed and thigh externally rotated about 20–30°. Therapist grasps the knee and leans with the forearm on the leg to bring adduction in slight while using the thenar of the other hand to stretch muscle fibres away from the gluteal tuberosity towards the body of muscle.

Tension–relaxation technique: Patient tries to extend hip joint for 5 sec while therapist resists. Patient is then instructed to gradually relax while therapist allows stretch to increase under the applied pressure.

Notice: The hip joint should not be rotated or adducted too much in the beginning of the stretch, because it restricts movement in flexion. Intense adduction may also cause uncomfortable squeezing of soft tissues of the anterior hip joint area. If there is pain in the groin area, therapist should use less adduction. The angle depends on the position of the acetabulum and thus varies individually.

Notice: Posterior parts of the gluteus medius and minimus, which lie under the gluteus maximus, will be also treated with this technique.

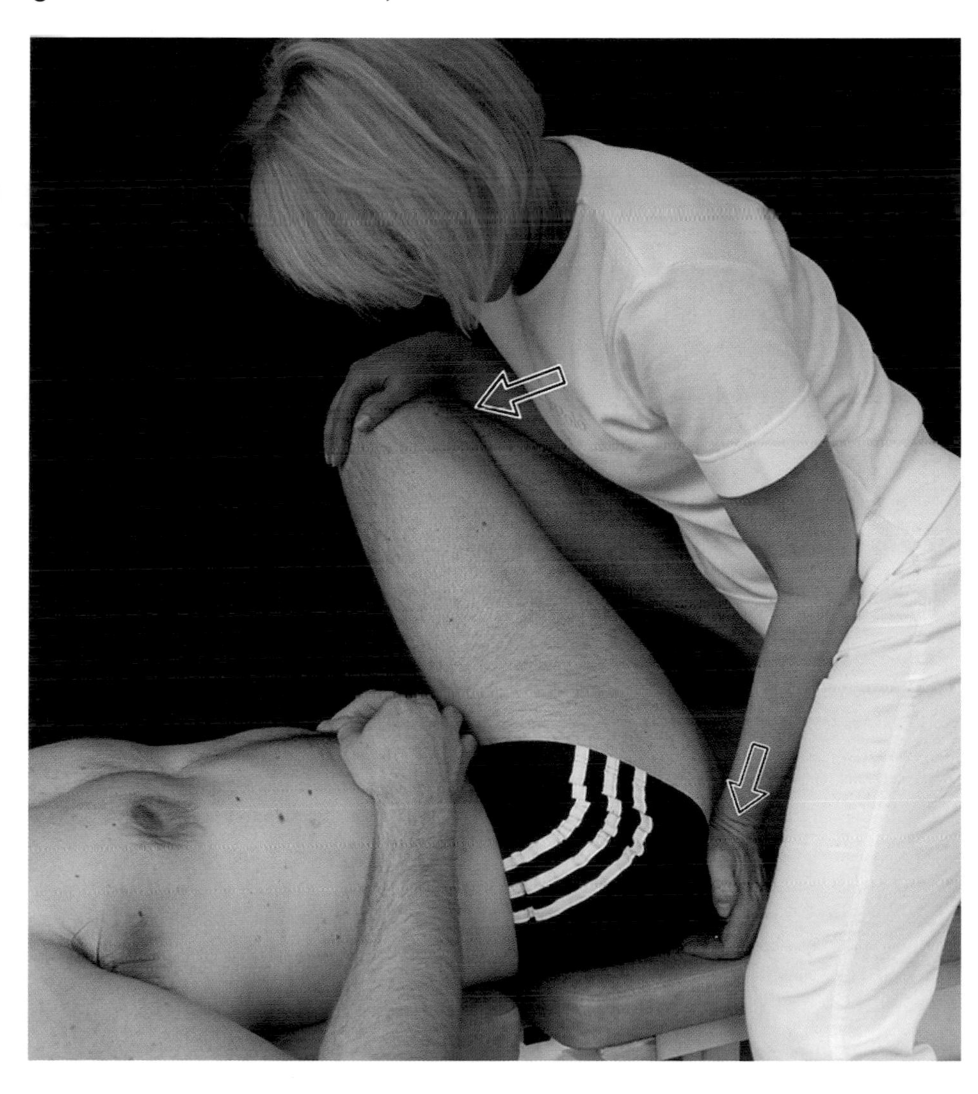

Gluteus medius

Nerve, supply: Superior gluteal nerve, L4–5.

Origin: Lateral surface of ilium, iliac crest and gluteal aponeurosis.

Insertion: Greater trochanter.

Function: Abduction, extension, flexion, internal and external rotation of hip.

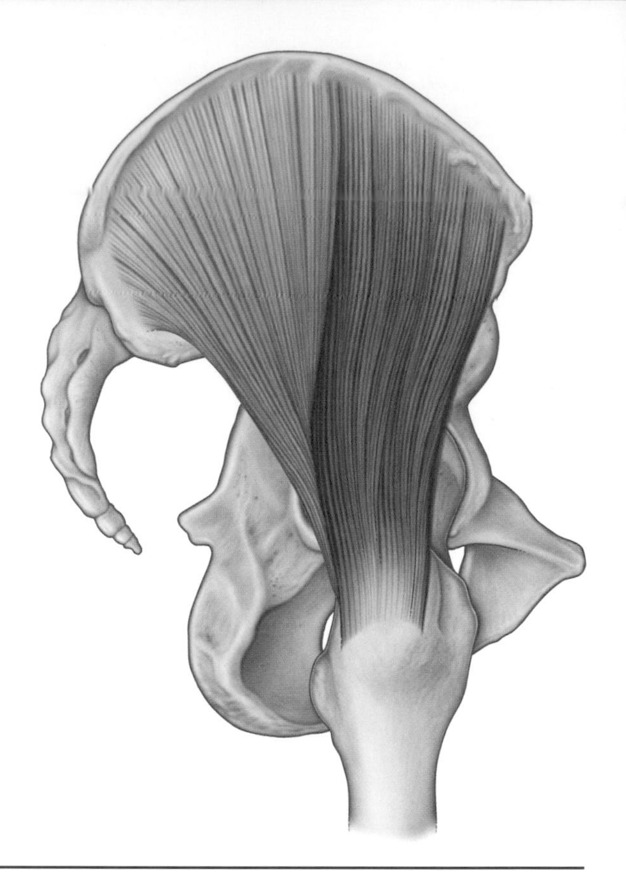

Stretching technique B:

Patient is lying on stomach with foot of side to be treated on floor. Table is lowered so that the hip is almost in full flexion. Therapist stabilizes the pelvis with pressure of the hand to the opposite iliac crest while applying pressure with the thenar of the other hand on the side to be treated below and away from the iliac crest and sacrum towards the body of muscle.

Tension–relaxation technique: Patient tries to extend hip joint for 5 sec while therapist resists by leaning down on pelvis. Patient is then instructed to gradually relax while therapist allows stretch to increase under the applied pressure. Therapist may also lower the treatment table further to increase stretch.

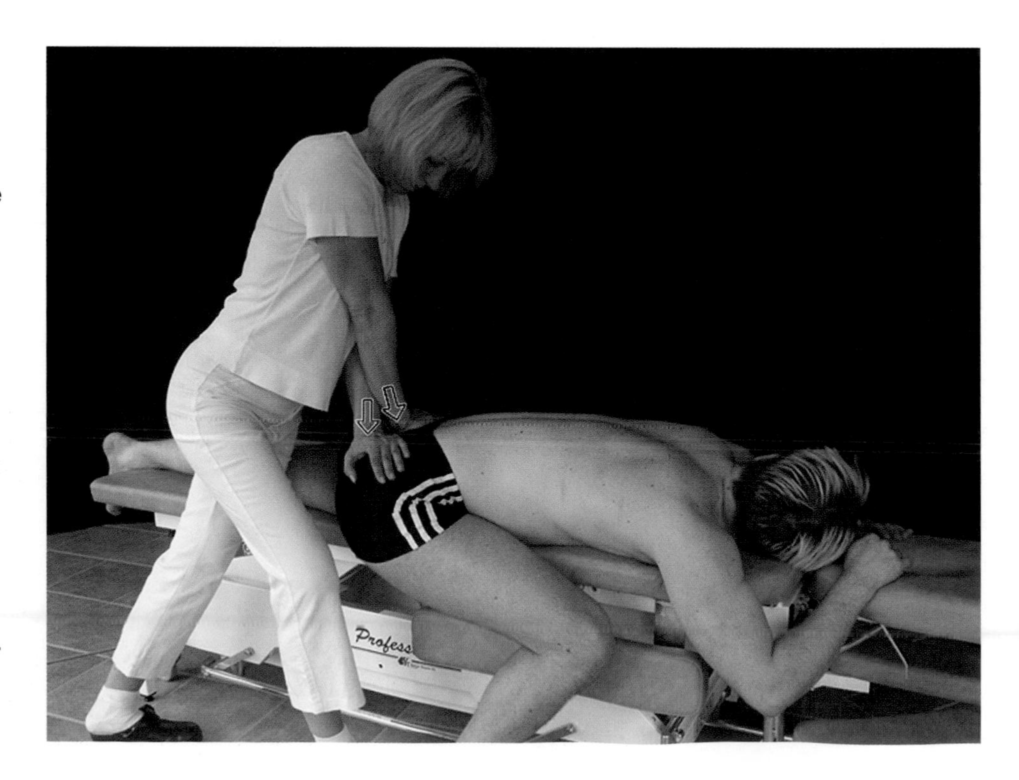

Gluteus minimus

Nerve, supply: Superior gluteal nerve, L4–S1.

Origin: Lateral surface of ilium.

Insertion: Greater trochanter.

Function: Abduction, extension, flexion, internal and external rotation of hip.

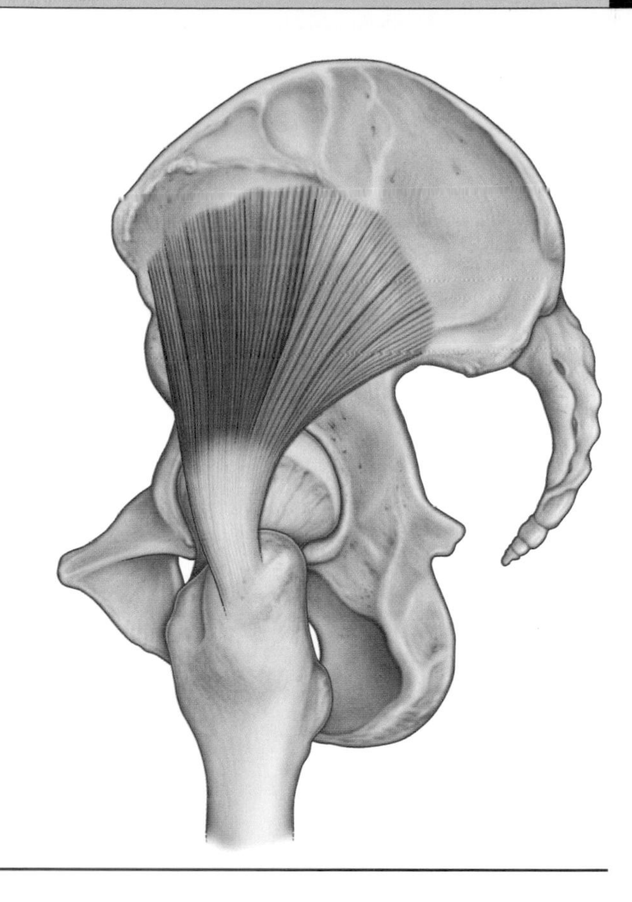

Stretching technique (extension + adduction + internal rotation):

Patient is lying on side with the hip and knee of bottom leg well flexed to stabilize the pelvis. Hip of top leg straight, knee flexed 70°–90°. Therapist grasps the knee, applies pressure at the knee and supports the foot with the thigh. Therapist presses the knee down to internally rotate the hip and draws it by moving her body backwards to extend the hip while the thenar of the other hand is used to stretch muscle fibres away from the insertion towards the body of muscle.

Tension–relaxation technique: Patient tries to abduct thigh for 5 sec while therapist resists. Patient is then instructed to gradually relax muscles while therapist increases adduction, extension and internal rotation.

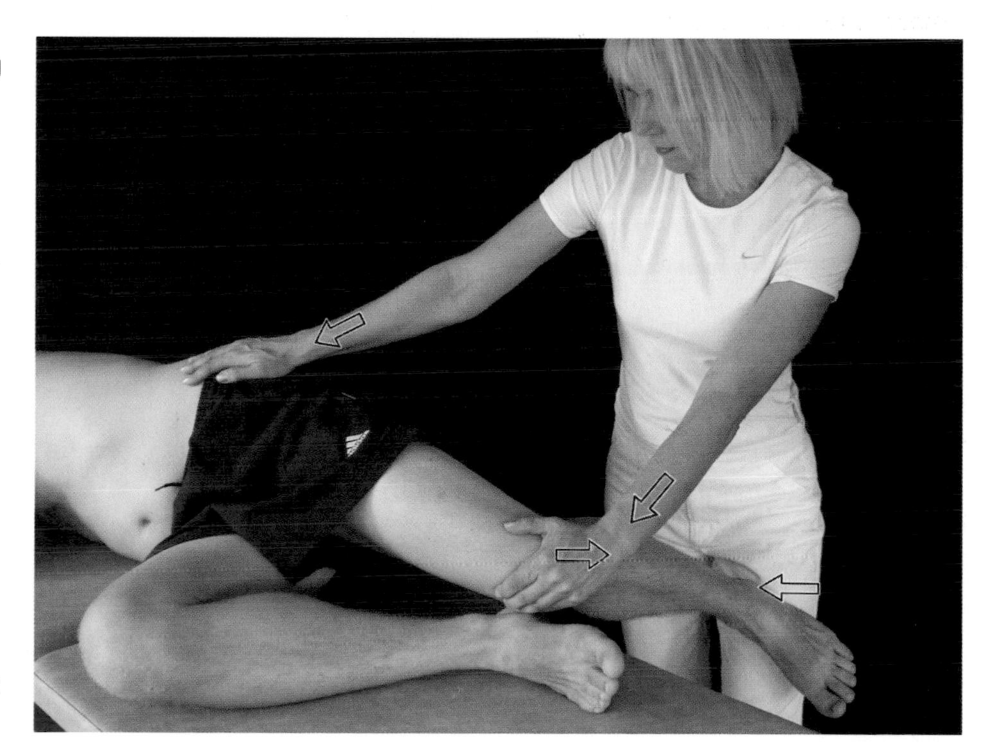

Piriformis

Nerve, supply: Sacral plexus L5–S2.

Origin: Greater sciatic notch of the margin of ilium and ischium and anterior surface of sacrum, lateral to sacral foramina.

Insertion: Anterio-medial surface of greater trochanter.

Function: Abduction, extension and external rotation of hip.

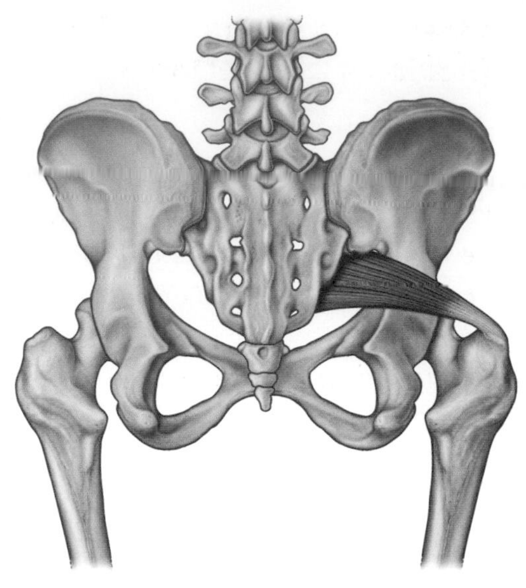

Stretching technique A (flexion + adduction + external rotation):

Patient is lying on back with hip and knee of leg to be treated both in flexion. Therapist grasps the knee, flexes the hip as far as it goes freely, externally rotates the hip to 45–60° and adducts it with the forearm on the lower leg. Pressure should also be downwards to prevent hip from rising off table. The other hand is used to stretch muscle fibres towards the body of muscle away from the insertion.

Tension–relaxation technique: Patient tries to internally rotate thigh for 5 sec while therapist resists. Patient is then instructed to gradually relax muscles while therapist flexes, adducts and externally rotates hip further.

Notice: Although piriformis in the upright posture functions as an external rotator, the hip joint is not rotated internally during this stretch, because this pear-shaped muscle changes to an internal rotator while the hip is in flexion over 90° (Kapandji 1982).

Notice: Intense adduction of thigh may squeeze the soft tissues anteromedial to the hip joint, and in this case less adduction should be used and more flexion and rotation.

Notice: The muscle may be absent and thus the stretch cannot be felt.

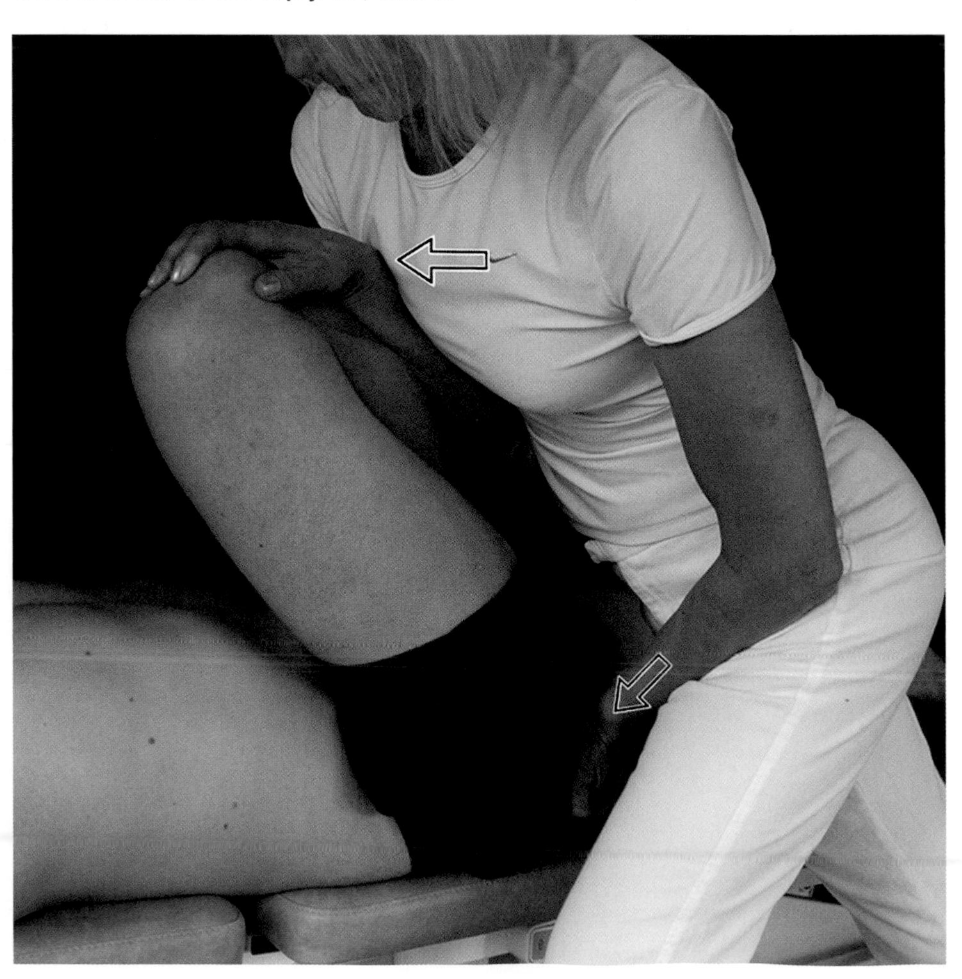

Stretching technique B (flexion + adduction + internal rotation):

Patient is lying on back with the knee flexed to 90° and hip of leg to be treated in flexion to about 45°. Therapist grasps the knee and adducts and internally rotates the leg. The other hand is used to stretch muscle fibres towards the body of muscle away from insertion.

Notice: This technique stretches more the posterior capsule of the hip joint and stretching of the piriformis is often minimal or non-existent. However, in some cases, especially hypermobility of the hip joint, the piriformis muscle may be treated also with this technique.

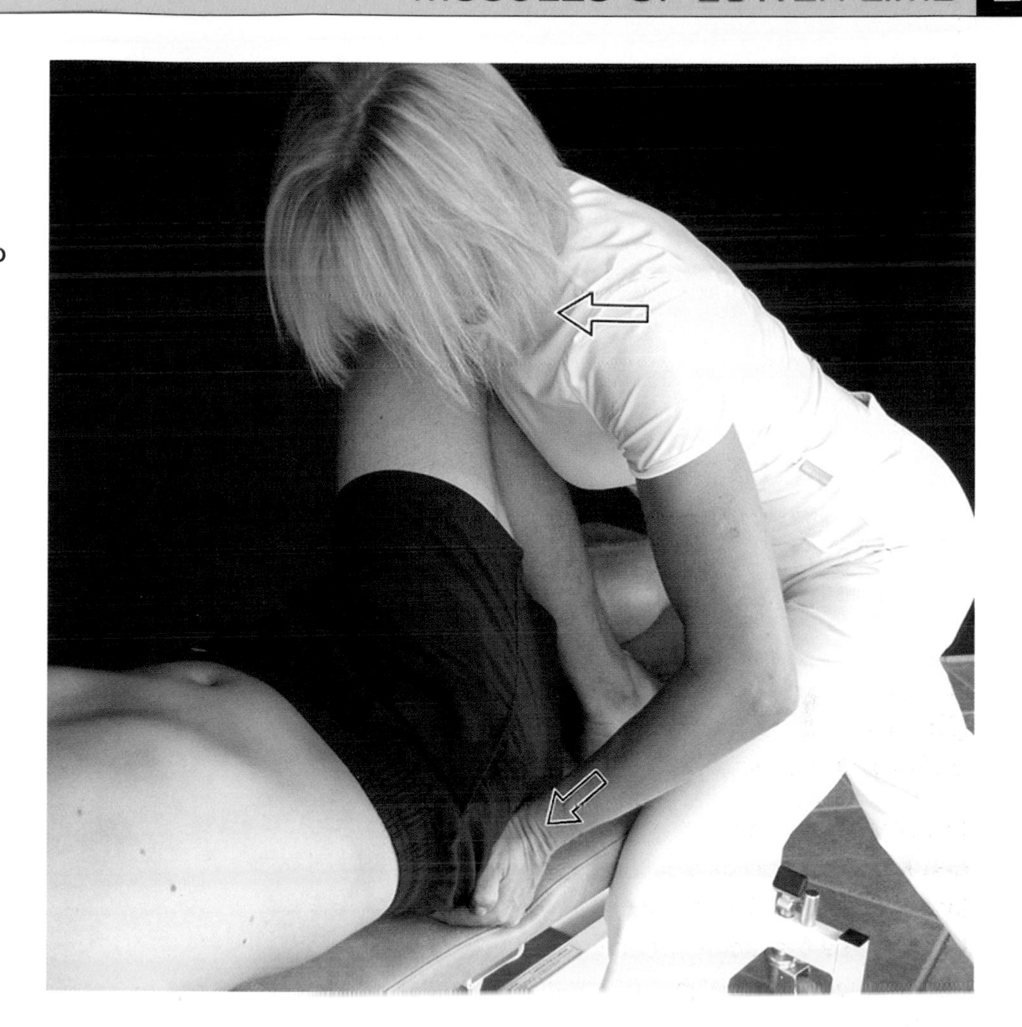

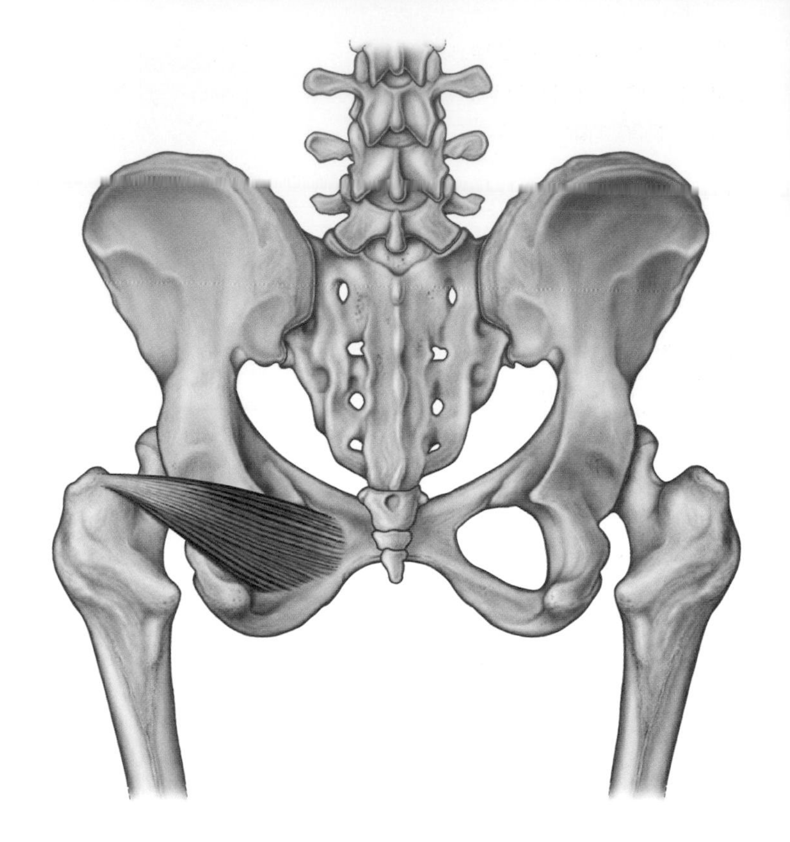

Obturator internus

Nerve, supply: Inferior gluteal nerve, sacral plexus, L5–S2.

Origin: Obturator membrane and around it from inner surface of ischium and pubic bones of hip.

Insertion: Trochanteric fossa.

Function: External rotation of hip and abduction of flexed hip.

Gemellus superior

Nerve, supply: Inferior gluteal nerve, sacral plexus, L5–S2.

Origin: Ishial spine.

Insertion: Trochanteric fossa.

Function: External rotation of hip and abduction of flexed hip.

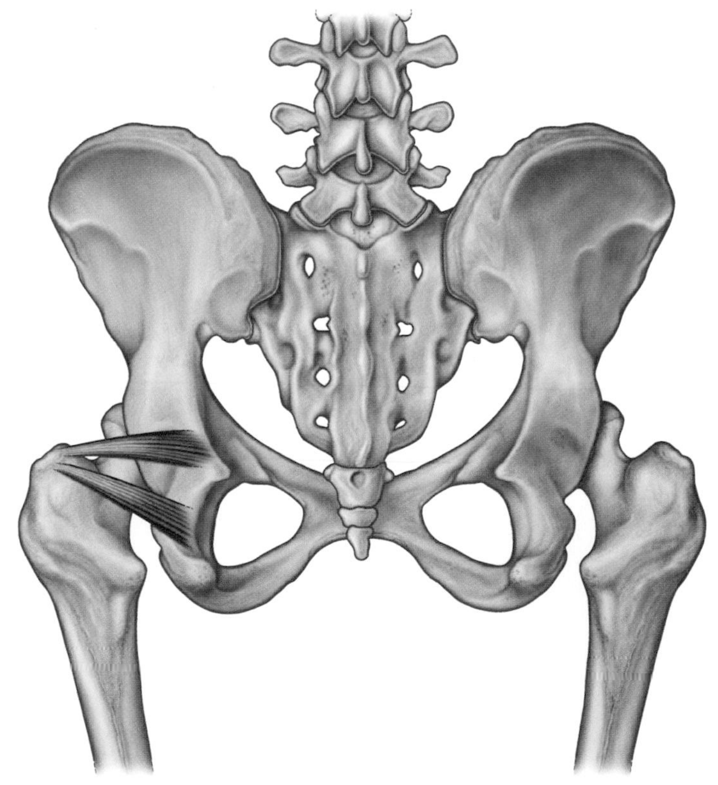

Gemellus inferior

Nerve, supply: Inferior gluteal nerve, sacal plexus, L5–S2.

Origin: Ishial tuberosity.

Insertion: Trochanteric fossa.

Function: External rotation of hip and abduction of flexed hip.

Notice: One or both muscles may be absent.

Stretching technique (flexion + adduction + internal rotation):

Patient is lying on side with bottom leg flexed to stabilize the body. Hip of top leg is flexed to 45° and knee to 90°. Therapist grasps above the ankle and internally rotates the hip by lifting ankle up, and adducts by pressing on knee with own thigh. The thenar of the other hand is used to stretch along muscle away from insertion.

Tension–relaxation technique: Patient tries to externally rotate thigh for 5 sec while therapist resists. Patient is then instructed to gradually relax muscles while therapist applies further stretching.

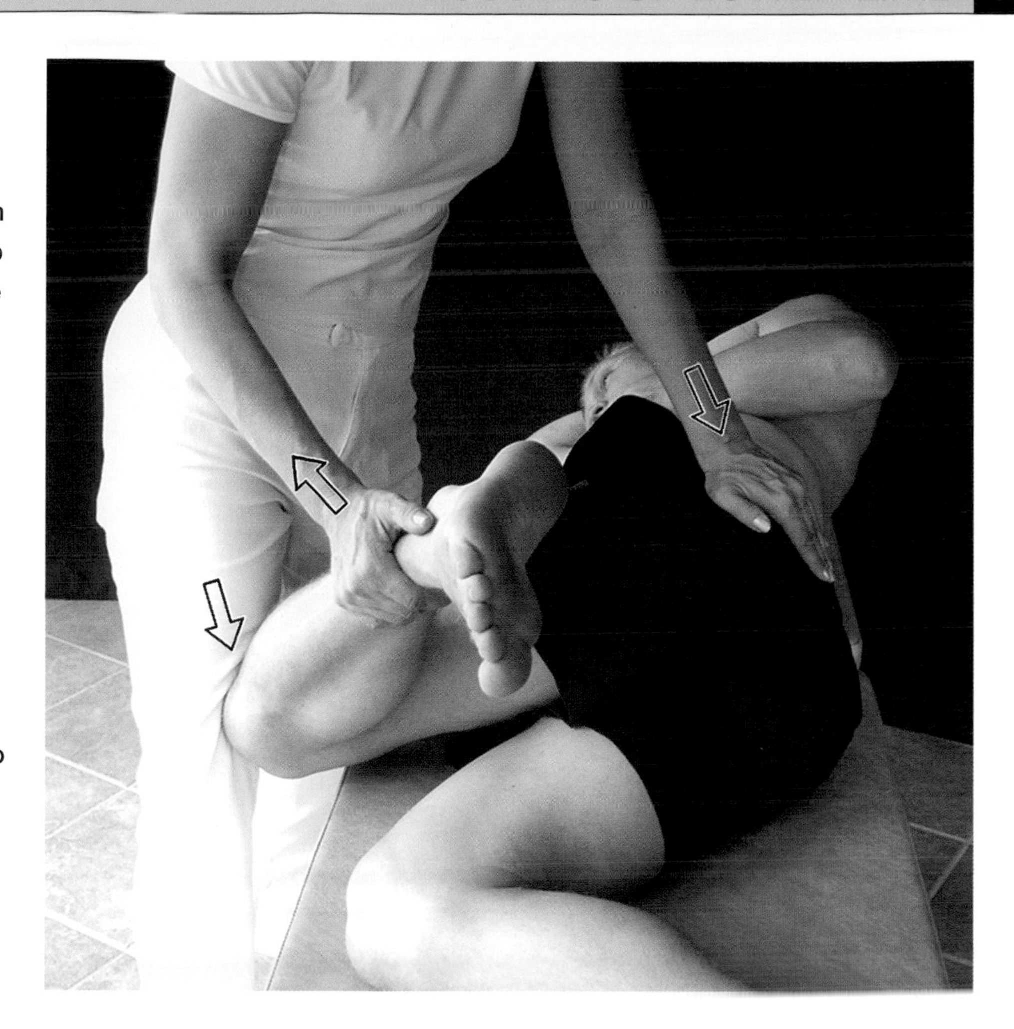

Obturator externus

Nerve, supply: Obturator nerve, L1–4.

Origin: Obturator membrane and around it from external surface of ischium and pubic bones of hip.

Insertion: Trochanter fossa and in some cases joint capsule of hip.

Function: External rotation of hip and weak adductor.

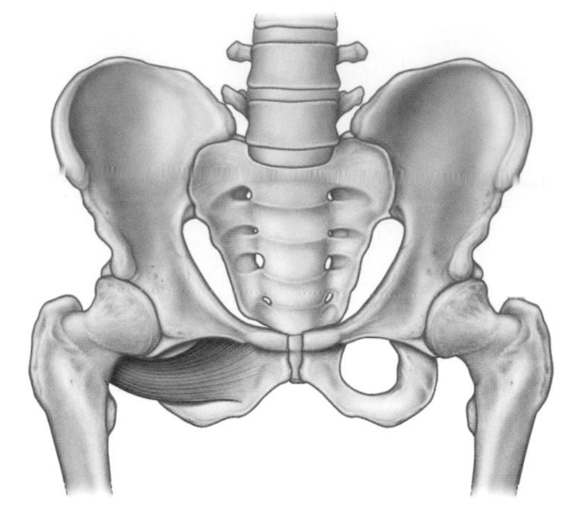

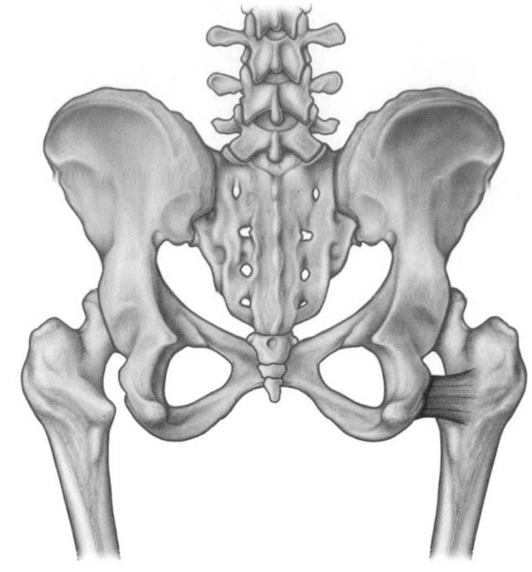

Quadratus femoris

Nerve, supply: Inferior gluteal nerve, sacral plexus L5–S2.

Origin: Lateral side of ischial tuberosity.

Insertion: Intertrochanteric crest.

Function: External rotation of hip and weak adductor.

Stretching technique (abduction + internal rotation):

Patient is lying on stomach with the knee flexed 90°. Therapist grasps at knee and supports lower leg against own body. Therapist moves thigh into abduction while internally rotating the hip. The thenar of the other hand is used to stretch muscle tissue away from insertion by turning the body towards it, while the elbow is supported against therapist's hip to be able to push with sufficient force.

Tension–relaxation technique: Patient tries to externally rotate thigh for 5 sec while therapist resists. Patient is then instructed to gradually relax while therapist allows abduction and internal rotation to increase.

Notice: Outer part of the obturator externus is covered by the quadratus femoris muscle and thus treated at the same time.

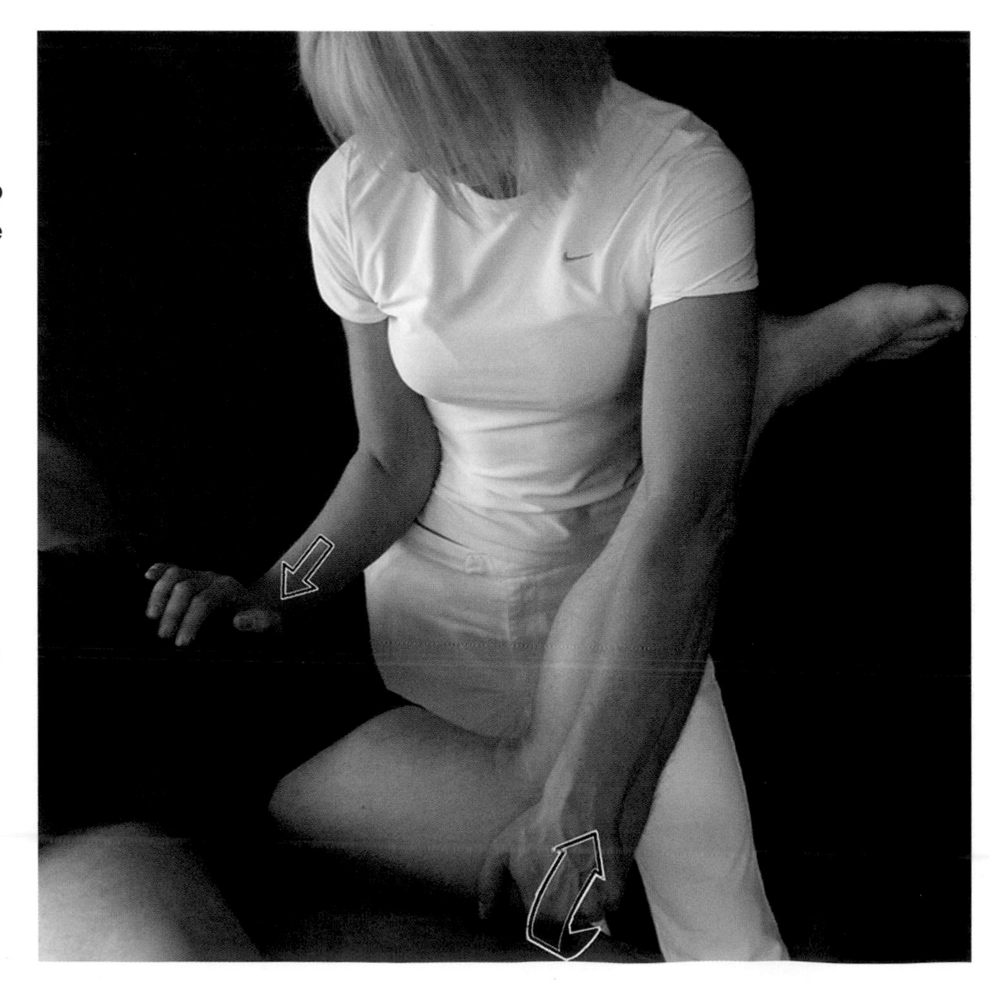

Tensor of fascia lata

Nerve, supply: Superior gluteal nerve, L4–5.

Origin: Anterior superior iliac spine.

Insertion: Inferior to greater trochanter into the fascia latae (iliotibial tract), which is inserted on lateral tibial condyle.

Function: Abduction, flexion and internal rotation of hip. Flexion, extension and final external rotation of knee.

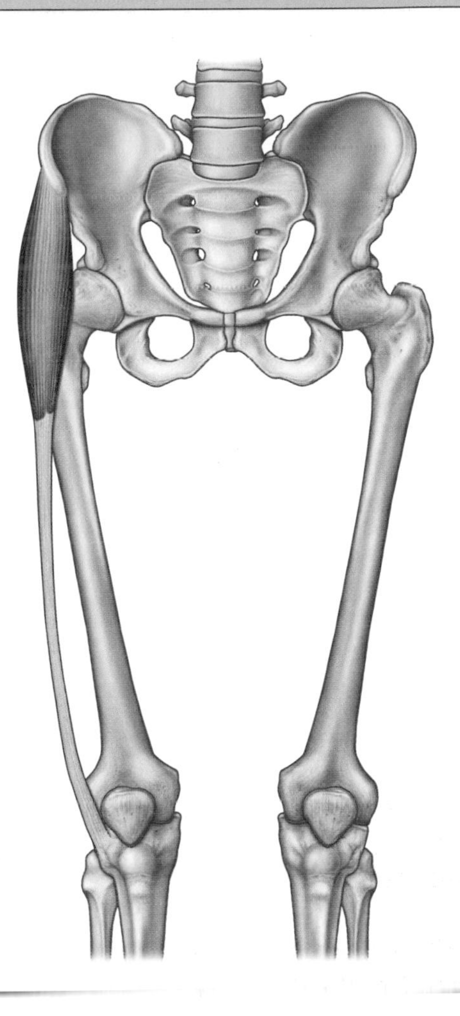

Stretching technique A: (extension + adduction + external rotation):

Patient is lying on stomach with legs over the edge of table and feet on the floor. Therapist grasps above the knee, flexes it to 90° and supports the lower leg with the forearm and shoulder. Therapist extends, adducts and rotates hip externally. The hypothenar of the other hand is used to stretch muscle tissue away from the tendon–muscle junction towards the body of the muscle.

Tension–relaxation technique: Patient tries to abduct the thigh for 5 sec while therapist resists. Patient is then instructed to relax muscles gradually while therapist allows adduction and external rotation to increase further.

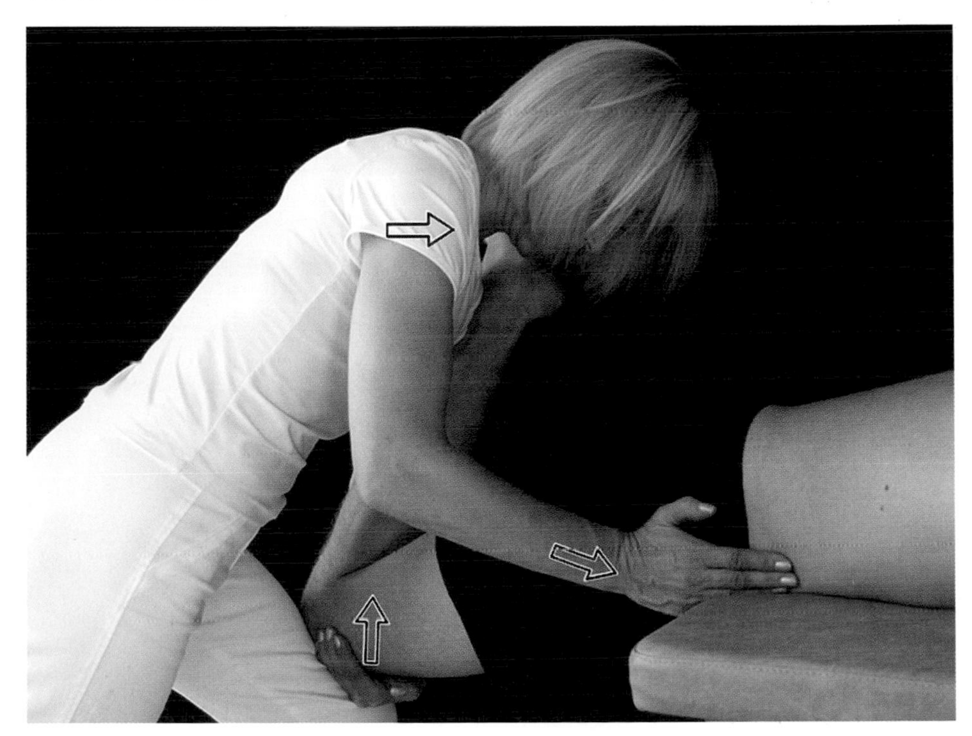

Stretching technique B (extension + adduction + external rotation):

Patient is lying on back, hands wrapped around knee to support knee and hip in flexion while the other leg hangs freely over edge of table. Therapist adducts the hip and presses down on knee with the hand, and using own thigh therapist presses against lower leg to externally rotate hip. The thenar of the other hand is used to stretch along muscle away from tendon–muscle junction towards the body of muscle.

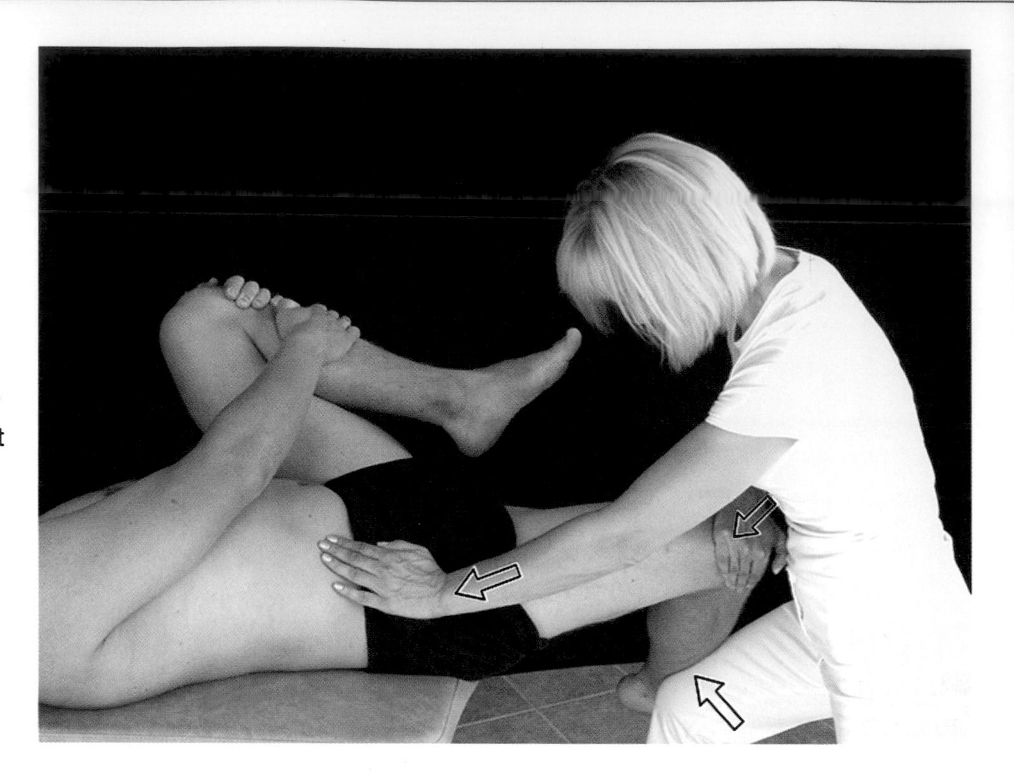

Tension–relaxation technique: Patient tries to abduct the thigh for 5 sec while therapist resists. Patient is then instructed to relax muscles gradually while therapist allows adduction and external rotation to increase further.

Iliopsoas

(Divided into three sections: iliacus, psoas major and minor)

1. Iliacus

Nerve, supply: Femoral nerve, lumbar plexus L1–3.

Origin: Iliac fossa and anterior inferior iliac spine.

Insertion: Lesser trochanter.

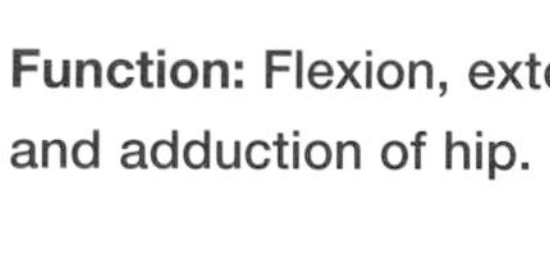

Function: Flexion, external rotation and adduction of hip.

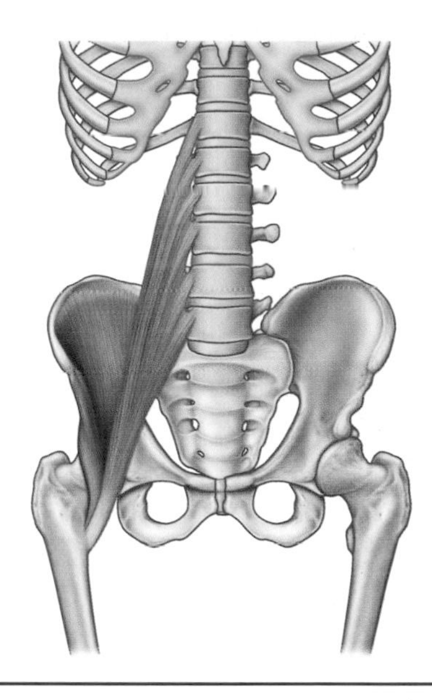

Stretching technique (extension + abduction + internal rotation):

Patient is lying on back with hands wrapped around knee to support knee and hip in flexion and the other leg hangs freely over edge of table. Therapist presses knee down and to the side with hand to increase extension and abduction, while using own lower leg to push patient's lower leg laterally and to press thigh to internal rotation. The other hand is used to stretch towards the body of muscle away from insertion.

Tension–relaxation technique: Patient tries to flex hip for 5 sec while therapist resists. Patient is then advised to gradually relax muscles while therapist increases extension.

Notice: Patient's knee on side treated should not be flexed by the therapist, because this would direct the stretch effect to the rectus fomaris muscle instead of the iliopsoas. Therapist needs to watch that patient does not release the knee and allow pelvis to rise up from table, as this would significantly lessen the effectiveness of the stretch and affect back.

Warning ! Extension of the lumbar spine due to lack of support to keep pelvis in position may cause symptoms of pain in this area.

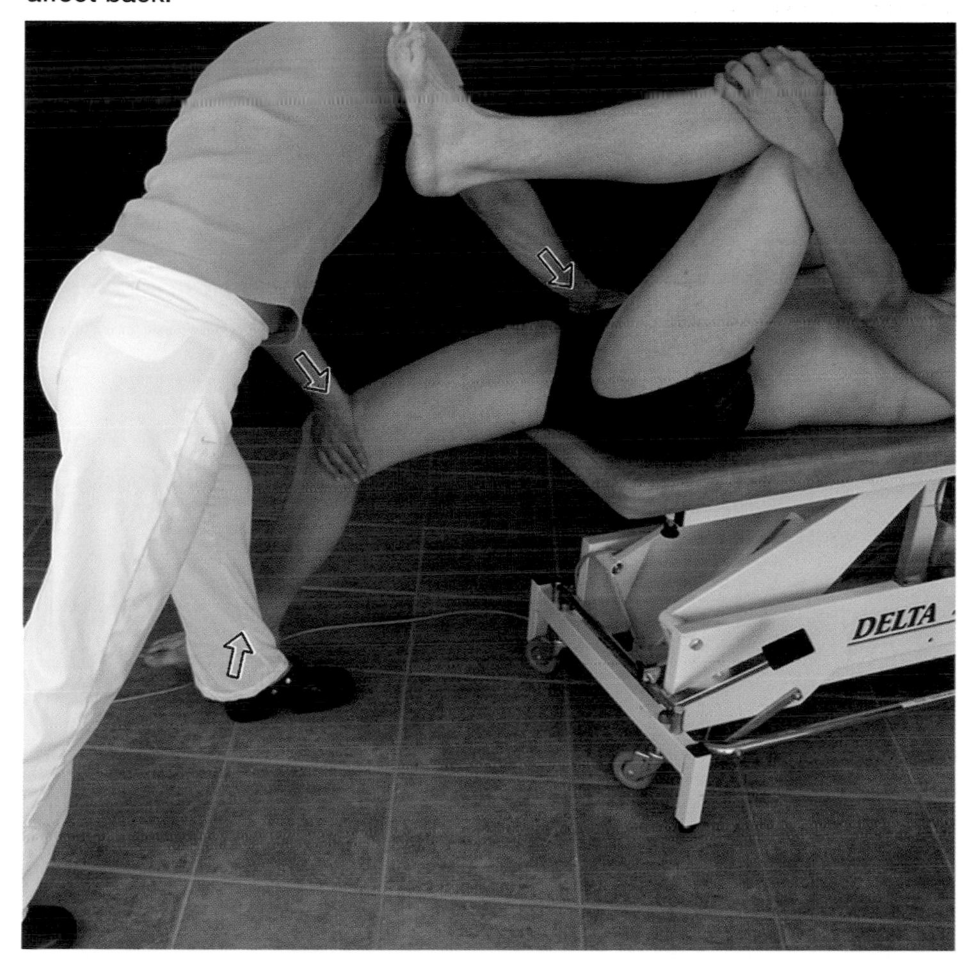

2. Psoas major

Nerve, supply: Lumbar plexus, L1–3.

Origin: Superficial layer from lateral surfaces of vertebral bodies of Th12–L4 and deeper layer from costal processes of L1–5.

Insertion: Lesser trochanter.

Function: Stabilization of the lumbar spine. Flexion and lateral flexion of lumbar spine. Flexion, adduction and external rotation of thigh. In the recumbent position lift the upper body or legs.

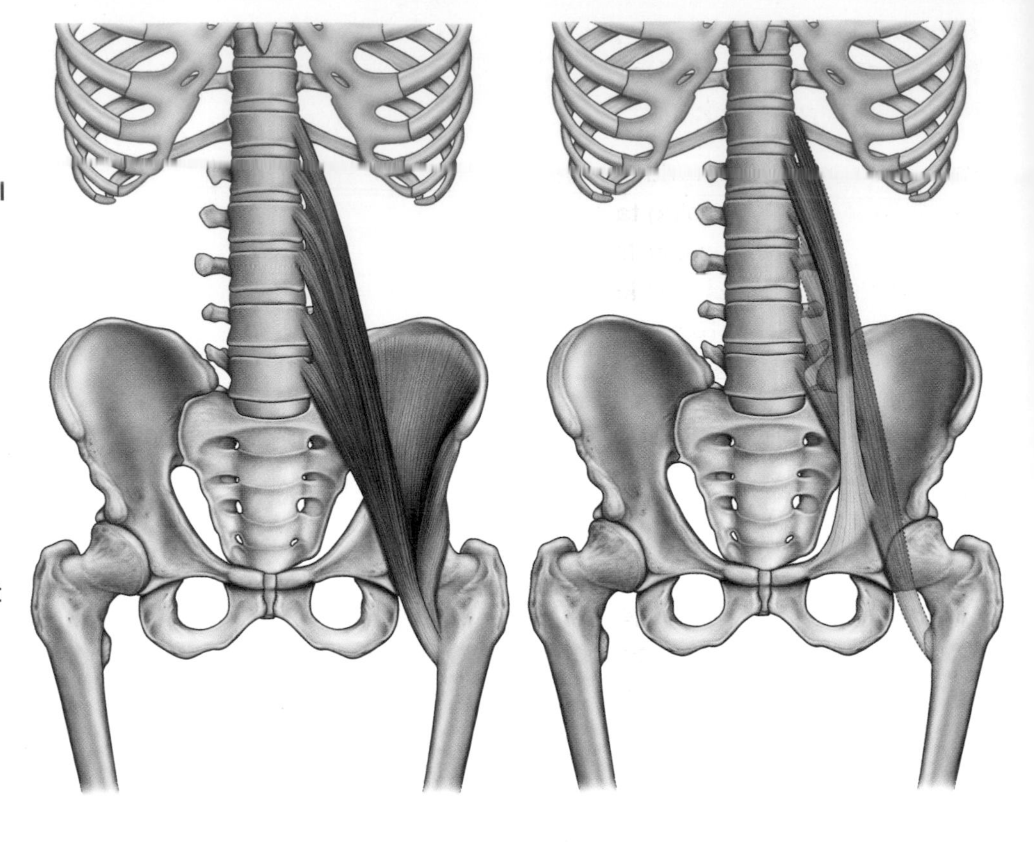

3. Psoas minor

Nerve, supply: Lumbar plexus, L1–3.

Origin: Vertebrae Th12–L1.

Insertion: Iliac fascia, iliopubic eminence, and iliopectineal arch.

Function: Stabilization of the lumbar spine.

Notice: Present in less than 50% of population.

Stretching technique A (extension + abduction + internal rotation):

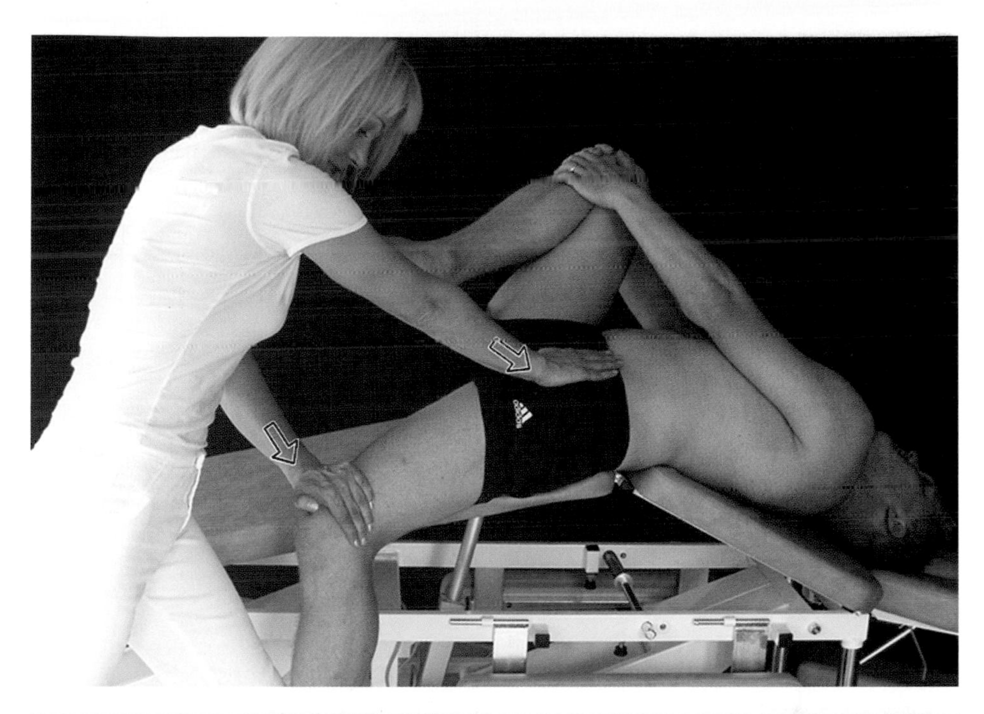

Patient is lying on back with lumbar spine extended by bending table or use of pillows placed under the back. Patient supports own knee in flexion. The other leg hangs freely over the side of the table. Therapist presses knee down and to the side to increase extension and abduction. Pressing with therapist's own lower leg against the medial side of patient's ankle the therapist can internally rotate the hip joint. The other hand is used to stretch towards the body of muscle away from insertion.

Tension–relaxation technique: Patient tries to flex hip for 5 sec while therapist resists. Patient is then instructed to gradually relax muscles while therapist allows extension to increase under the pressure.

Stretching technique B:

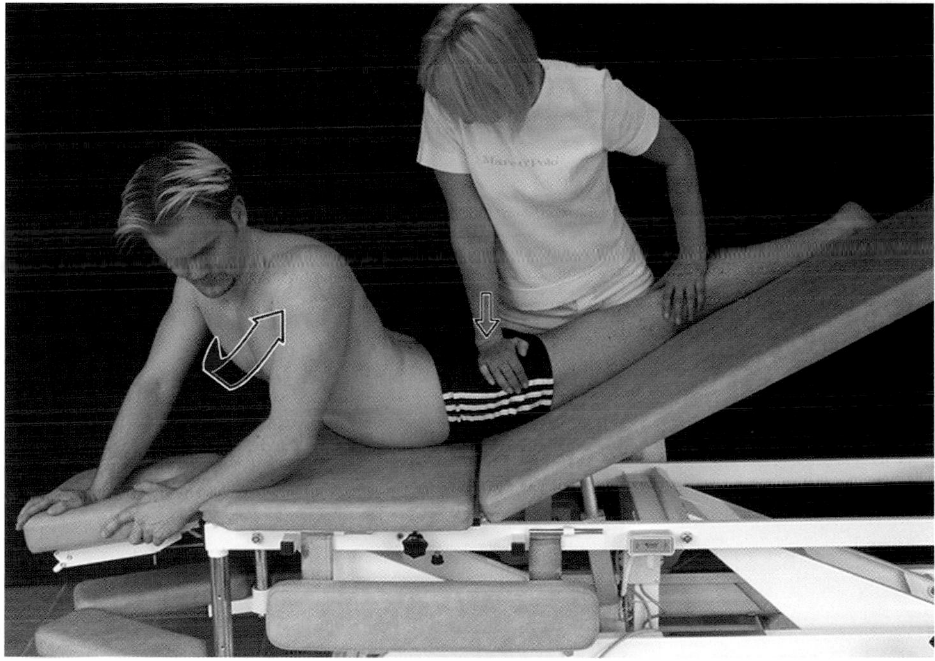

Patient is lying on stomach with the leg hanging freely over the side of the table and the foot on the floor. The lower part of the table is elevated with the other leg so that the hip is almost in full extension. Therapist stabilizes the pelvis with pressure of the hand on the ischial tuberosity and thus increases the hip extension. Patient presses his upper body up and rotates it to the side of the treated muscle.

Warning ! This technique should be used with caution especially in cases of disc disease and hypermobility, because extension of the lumbar spine may sometimes increase back pain. Thus, if there is increased local pain in the lower back, the stretch should be stopped and lower back must be straightened and stabilized before stretching.

Warning ! Therapist should not press on the lower back, which may cause hyperextension.

Notice: liopsoas is the only stabilizing muscle in the front side of the back, when the superficial abdominal muscles are not tensed. Thus, there is often extra tension and shortening, and painful conditions are also common, which may appear as chronic back pain or hip pain syndrome. Moreover, shortened muscle is difficult to stretch effectively by oneself. Thus, it is essential that the therapist knows the proper stretching technique.

Quadriceps femoris

(Divided into four sections: vastus medialis, intermedius and lateralis and rectus femoris).

Nerve, supply: Femoral nerve, L2–4.

1. Vastus medialis

Origin: Posterior and medial surface of femur from medial lip of linea aspera.

Insertion: Via quadriceps tendon to tibial tuberosity.

Function: Extension of knee.

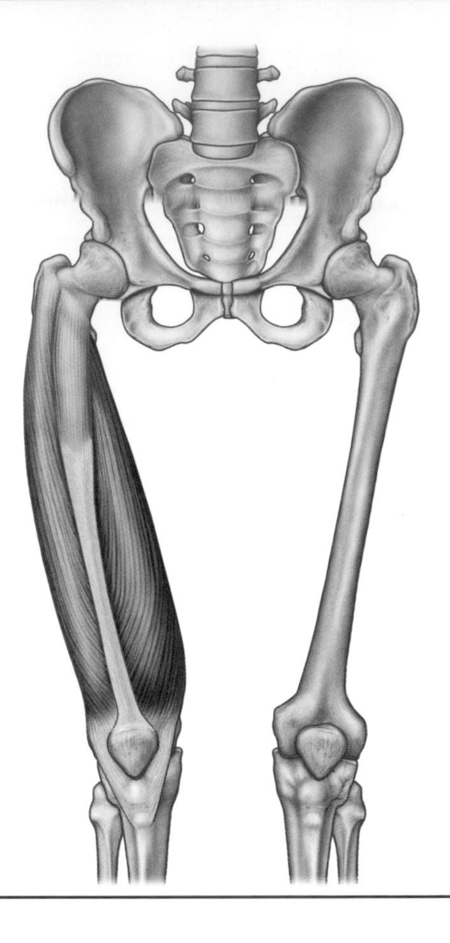

Stretching technique:

Patient is lying on back with one leg straight and the other over side of table. The therapist grasps the lower leg and flexes the knee 90° and the hip is flexed 20–30°. Therapist presses with thigh against patient's lower leg to increase knee flexion. The hypothenar of the other hand is used to stretch along muscle away from the tendon–muscle junction.

Tension–relaxation technique: Patient tries to extend knee for 5 sec while therapist resists. Patient is then instructed to gradually relax while therapist allows knee to flex further.

Notice: Hip joint should remain flexed, because extension of hip would direct the stretch to the iliopsoas and rectus femoris muscles instead of the quadriceps.

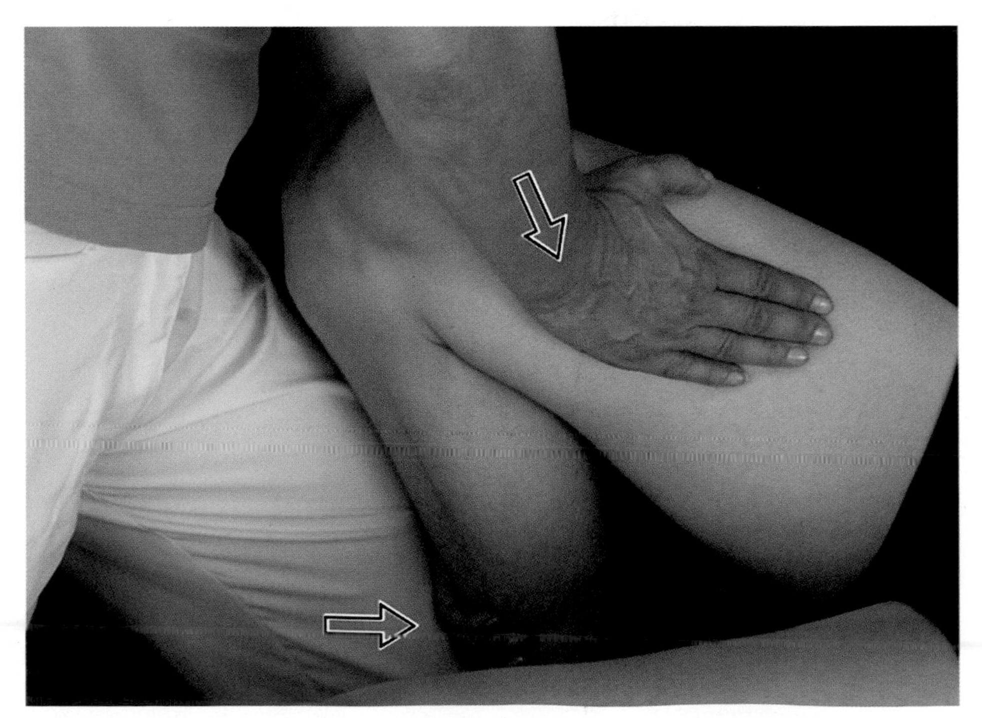

2. Vastus intermedius

Origin: Anterior and lateral surface of femur.

Insertion: Via the quadriceps tendon to the tibial tuberosity.

Function: Extension of knee.

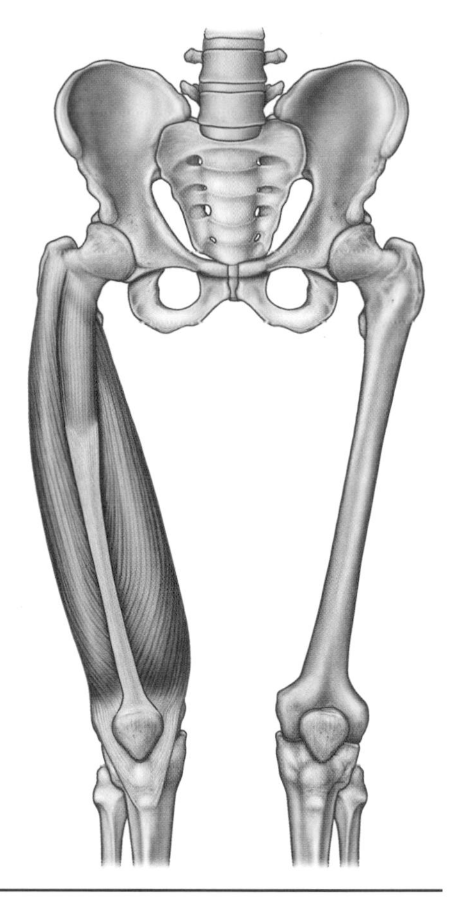

Stretching technique:

Patient is lying on back with one leg straight and the other over side of table. The therapist supports forearm on her thigh and grasps the lower leg and flexes the knee 90° and the hip is flexed 20° to relax the overlying rectus femoris muscle. Therapist presses with the leg against patient's lower leg to increase knee flexion. The thenar of the other hand is used to stretch along muscle away from the tendon–muscle junction.

Tension–relaxation technique: Patient tries to extend knee for 5 sec while therapist resists. Patient is then instructed to gradually relax while therapist increases knee flexion.

Notice: Hip joint should remain flexed, because extension of hip would direct the stretch to the iliopsoas and rectus femoris muscles instead of the quadriceps.

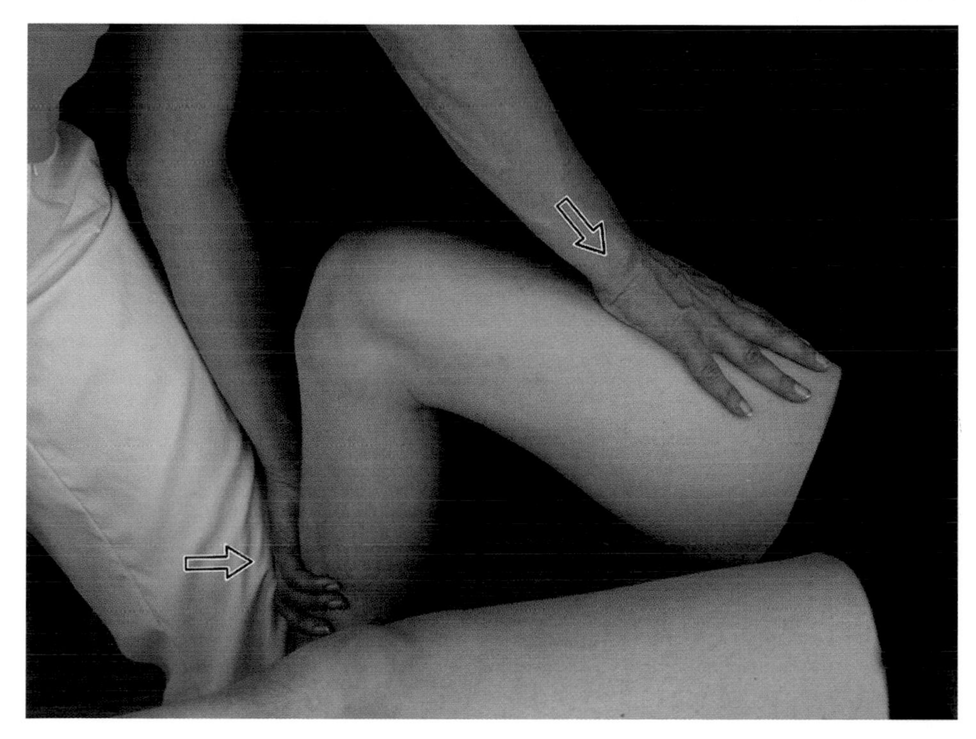

3. Vastus lateralis

Origin: Lateral surface of greater trochanter, intertrochanter line, gluteal tuberosity and posterior and lateral side of femur from the lateral lip of linea aspera.

Insertion: Via the quadriceps tendon to the tibial tuberosity.

Function: Extension of knee.

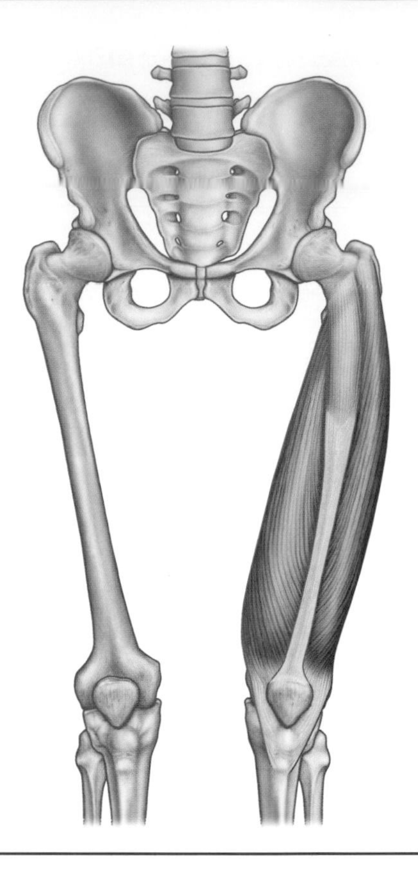

Stretching technique:

Patient is lying on back with one leg straight and the other over side of table. The therapist grasps the lower leg and flexes the knee 90° and the hip is flexed 20–30°. Therapist presses with thigh against patient's lower leg to increase knee flexion. The hypothenar of the other hand is used to stretch along muscle away from the tendon–muscle junction.

Tension–relaxation technique: Patient tries to extend knee for 5 sec while therapist resists. Patient is then instructed to gradually relax while therapist allows knee flexion to increase under the pressure.

Notice: Hip joint should remain flexed, because extension of hip would direct the stretch to the iliopsoas and rectus femoris muscles instead of the quadriceps.

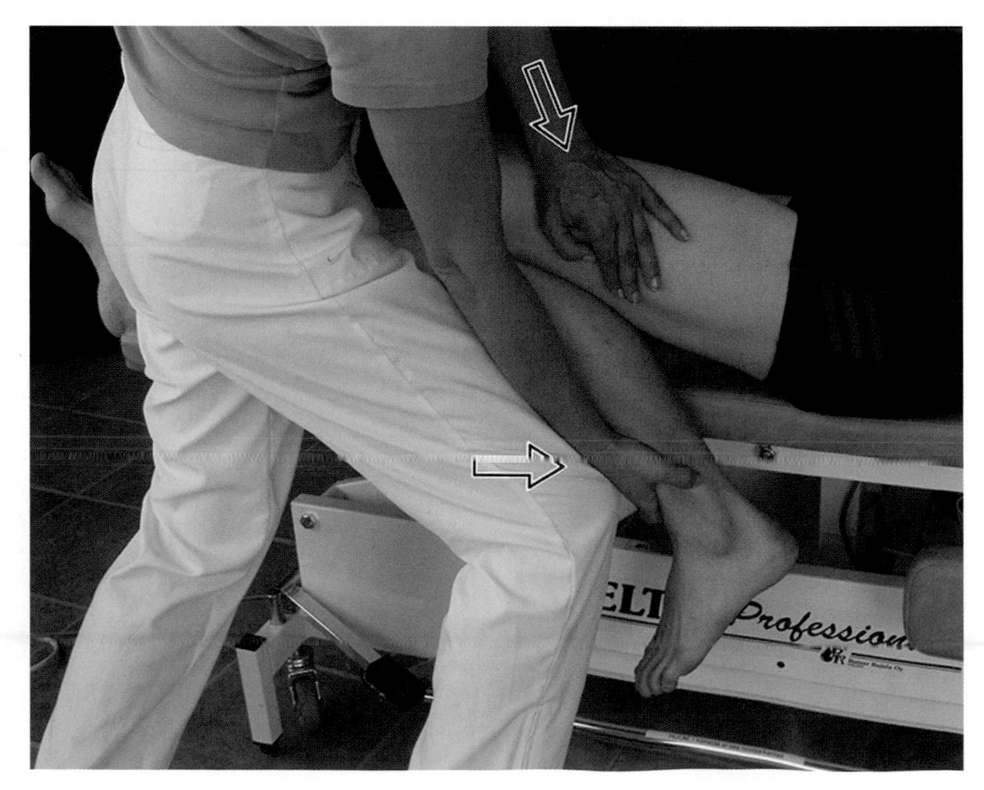

4. Rectus femoris

Origin: Anterior inferior iliac spine and supra-acetabular groove.

Insertion: Via the quadriceps tendon to the tibial tuberosity.

Function: Flexion of hip and extension of knee.

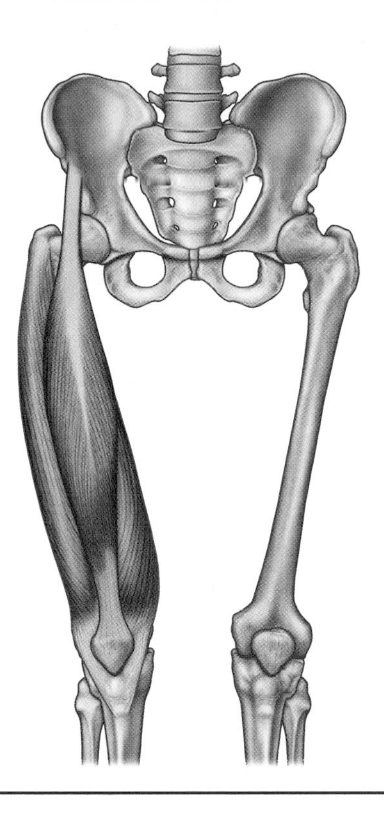

Stretching technique A:

Patient is lying on back with the untreated leg flexed on the table to stabilize the pelvis. The other leg is over the edge of the table with the hip in extension and the knee in flexion. The therapist grasps the lower leg and flexes the knee 90°. Therapist presses with thigh against patient's lower leg to increase knee flexion. The thenar of the other hand is used to stretch along muscle away from the tendon–muscle junction and to press the hip in extension.

Tension–relaxation technique: Patient tries to extend knee for 5 sec while therapist resists. Patient is then instructed to gradually relax muscles while therapist increases knee flexion and hip extension.

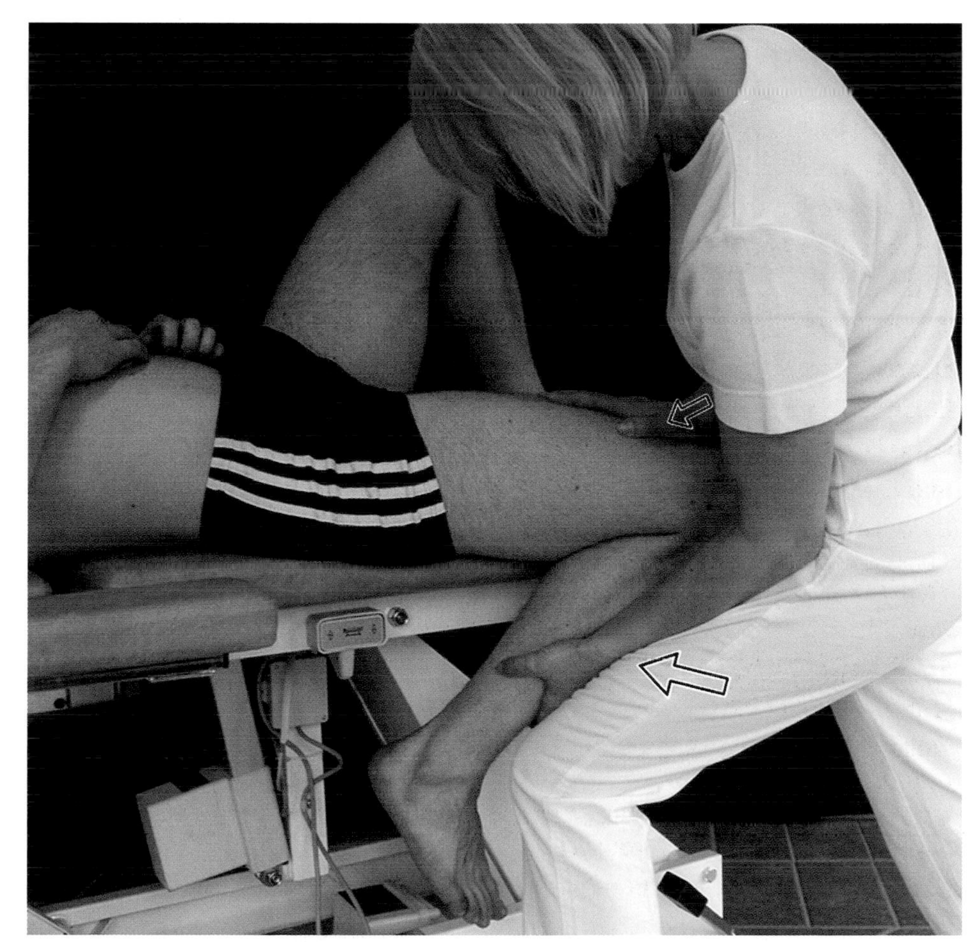

Stretching technique B:

Patient is lying on back with the untreated leg flexed on the table to stabilize the pelvis and the other leg hanging over the edge of the table with the hip in extension. Therapist grasps the lower leg and flexes the knee. Therapist uses the hypothenar of the other hand to apply pressure along the body of muscle away from the origin and to extend hip while simultaneously increasing knee flexion.

Tension–relaxation technique: Patient tries to extend knee for 5 sec while therapist resists. Patient is then instructed to gradually relax while therapist allows stretch to increase.

Notice: Also several other muscles may be stretched manually in both directions (techniques A and B).

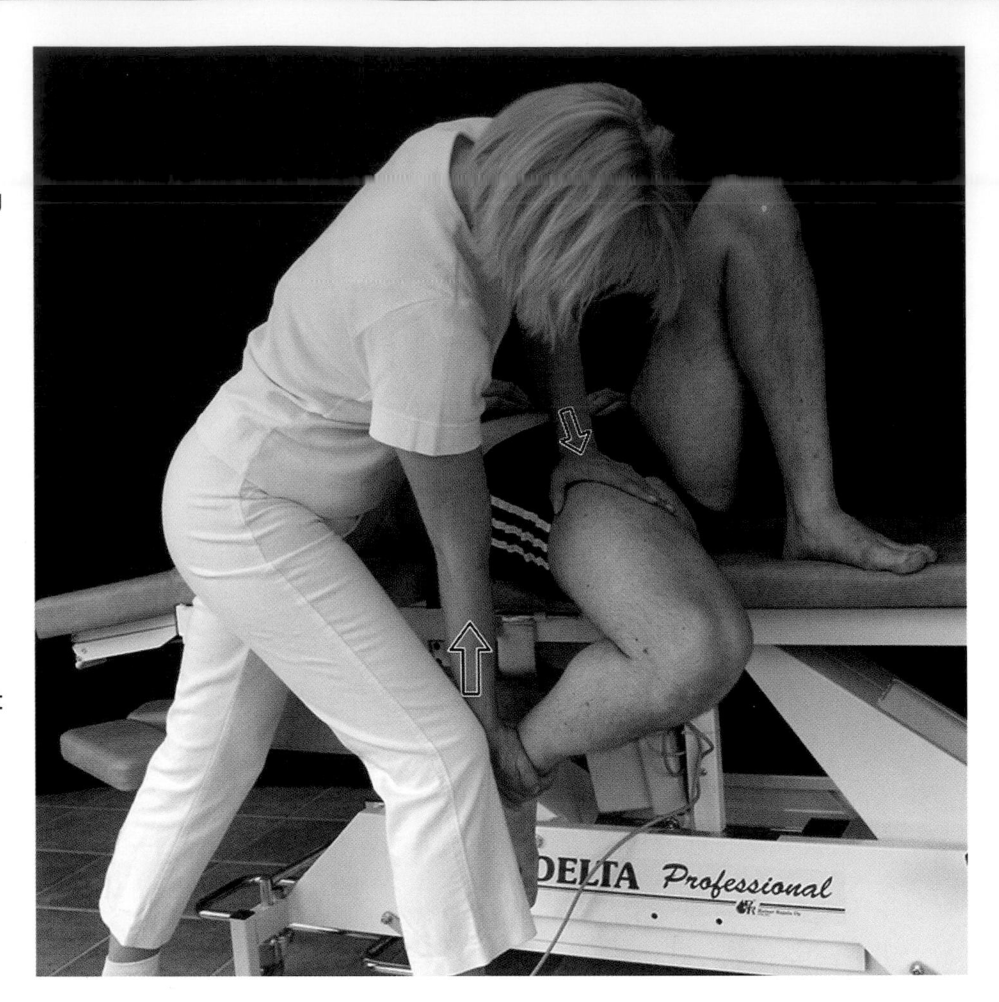

Sartorius

Nerve, supply: Femoral nerve, L2–3.

Origin: Anterior superior iliac spine.

Insertion: Medial to tibial tuberosity.

Function: Flexion, abduction and external rotation of hip. Flexion and internal rotation of knee.

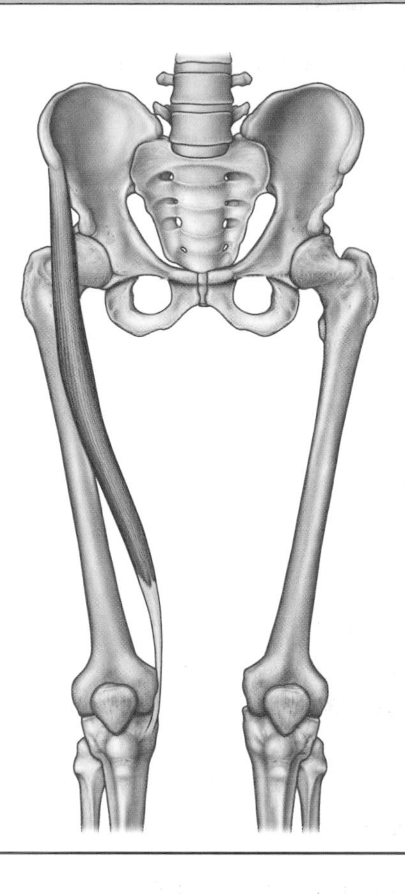

Stretching technique (extension + internal rotation + adduction):

Patient is lying on back with hands wrapped around the knee to support the hip and knee in flexion and the other leg extends over the end of the table with both hip and knee extended. Therapist grasps around the ankle and internally rotates the leg with forearm. Therapist also adducts leg by pulling it medially while using the thenar of other hand to apply pressure away from the tendon–muscle junction towards the body of the muscle and pressing the hip to further extension.

Warning ! It is important that patient holds the knee in flexion properly, as otherwise the lower back may bend to hyperextension and become painful.

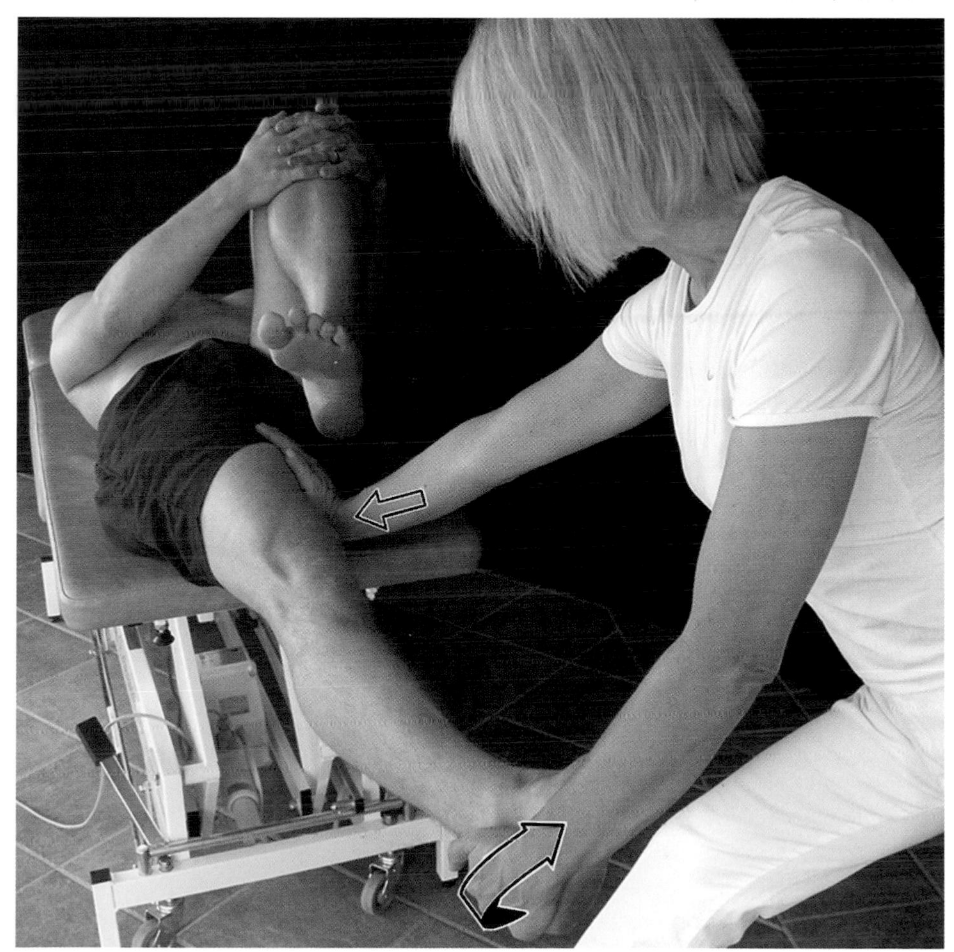

Articularis genus

Nerve, supply: Femoral nerve, L3–4.

Origin: Anterior, inferior surface of femur.

Insertion: Superior edge of joint capsule.

Function: Tightens joint capsule.

Notice: The muscle may be absent.

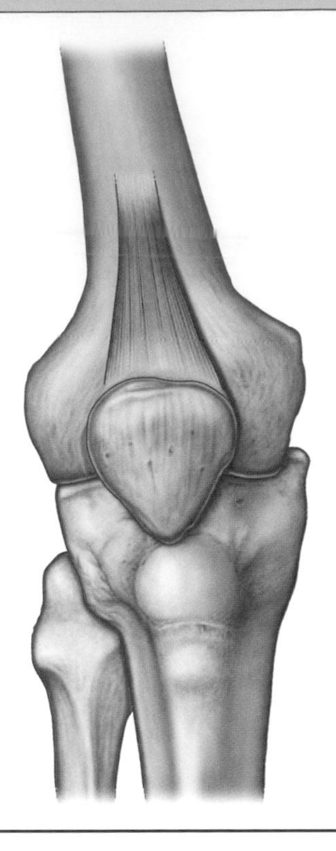

Stretching technique:

Patient is on back with one leg straight and the other at the edge of table with knee in flexion. The therapist grasps the upper leg and the hip is flexed 20°. Therapist presses with the thigh against patient's lower leg to increase knee flexion. The thumbs of both hands are used to stretch along muscle away from insertion towards the body of muscle.

Tension–relaxation technique: Patient tries to extend knee for 5 sec while therapist resists. Patient is then instructed to gradually relax while therapist allows knee flexion to increase under the pressure.

Notice: Hip is flexed and should not be straightened, because it will tense the rectus femoris muscle overlying the articularis genus muscle and stretching would not be specifically directed on the articularis genus muscle.

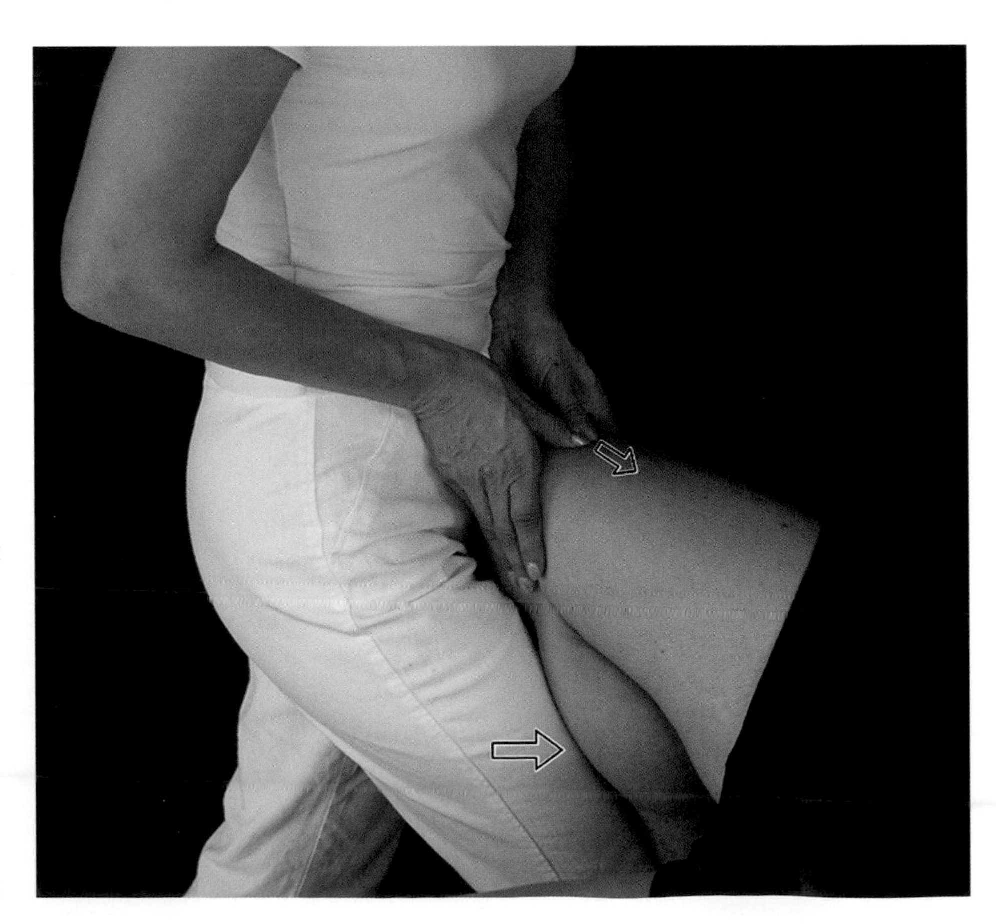

Gracilis

Nerve, supply: Obturator nerve, L2–3.

Origin: Inferior ramus of the pubis near the symphysis.

Insertion: Medial surface of tibia.

Function: Adduction of hip and extension when hip is in flexion and flexion when hip is in extension. Flexion and internal rotation of knee.

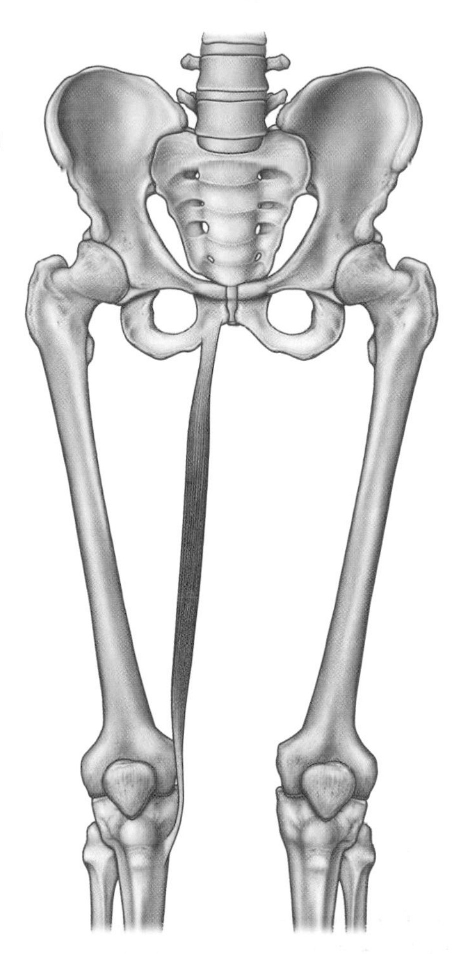

Stretching technique (abduction + extension):

Patient is on back with hands wrapped around knee to stabilize pelvis and the leg to be treated hanging freely over edge of table. Therapist grasps the lower leg above the ankle extends knee joints and steps aside to induce hip abduction with his/her body. The thenar of other hand is used to stretch away from the tendon–muscle junction towards the body of the muscle while preventing knee flexion and allowing for hip extension and abduction with the pressure.

Tension–relaxation technique: Patient tries to adduct thigh for 5 sec while therapist resists. Patient is then instructed to gradually relax while therapist allows abduction to increase under the pressure.

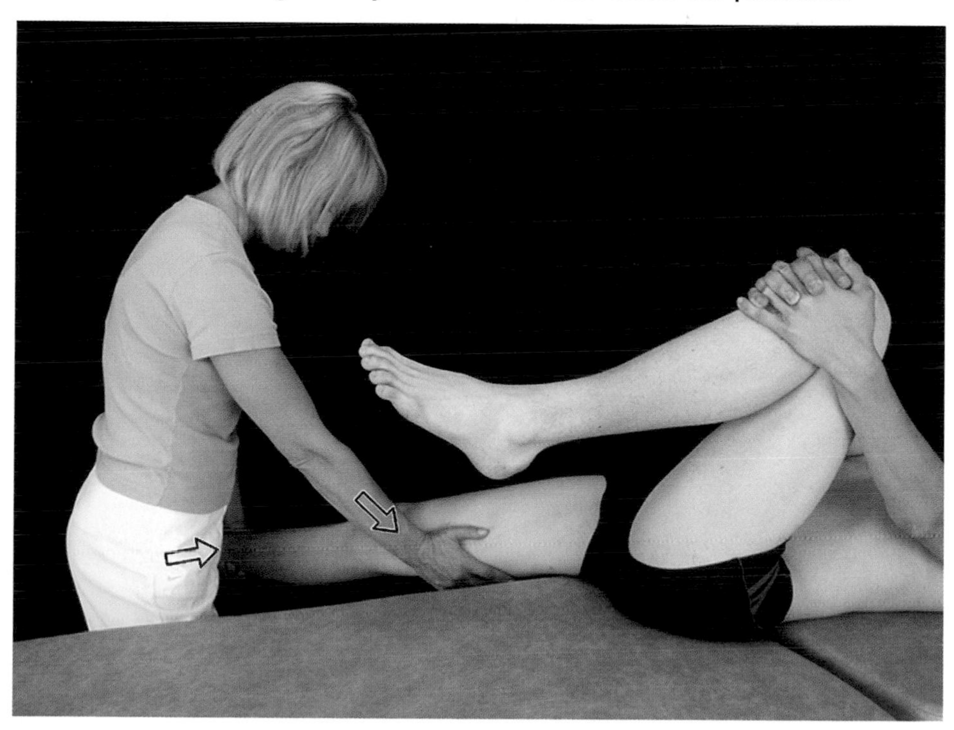

Adductor magnus

Nerve, supply: Obturator nerve, L2–4 and tibial nerve, L3–5.

Origin: Anterior surface of inferior ramus of pubis and inferior ramus of ischium as far as ischial tuberosity.

Insertion: Linea aspera on the posterior surface of femur and by tendon to the adductor tubercle of the medial epicondyle.

Function: Adduction and external rotation of hip. Hip extension when hip is in flexion and hip flexion when hip is in extension. Part inserting at medial epicondyle is an internal rotator when hip is in flexion and externally rotated.

Function: Adduction and external rotation of hip. Hip extension when hip is in flexion and hip flexion when hip is in extension.

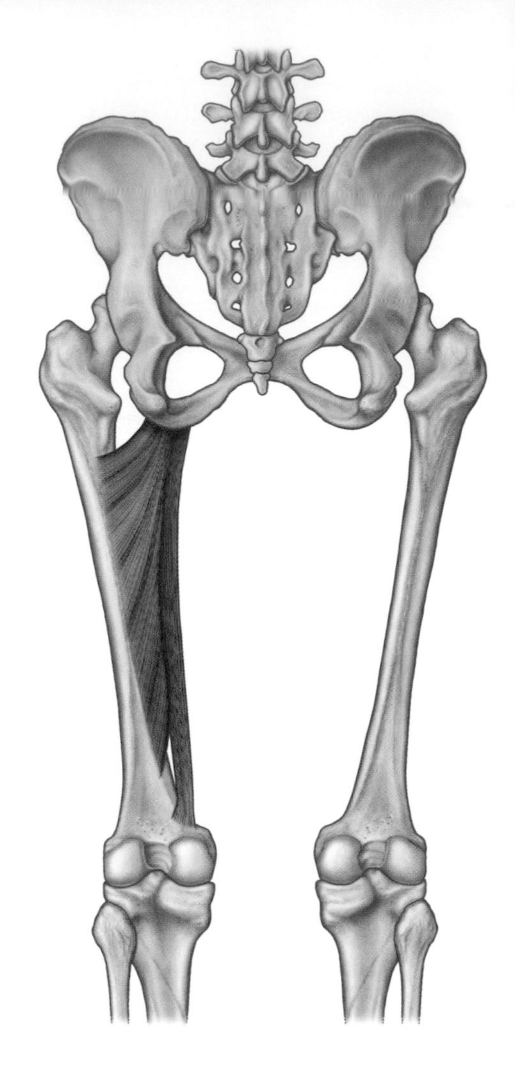

Adductor longus

Nerve, supply: Obturator nerve, L2–4.

Origin: Anterior surface of superior ramus of pubis.

Insertion: Medially to middle third of linea aspera on posterior surface of femur.

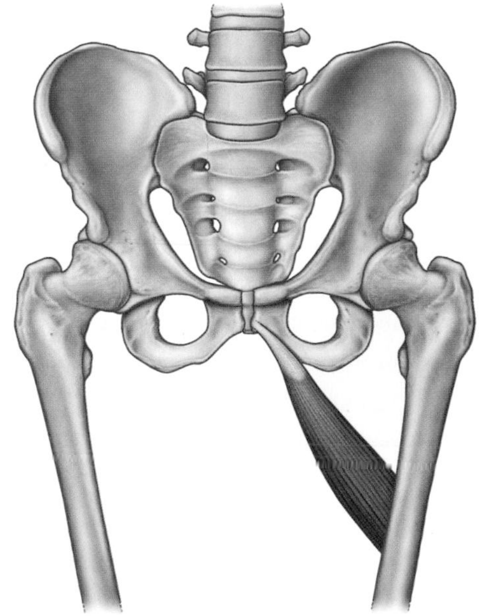

Adductor brevis

Nerve, supply: Obturator nerve, L2–4.

Origin: Anterior surface of inferior ramus of pubis near symphysis.

Insertion: Superior third of linea aspera on posterior surface of femur.

Function: Adduction and external rotation of hip. Hip extension when hip is in flexion and hip flexion when hip is in extension.

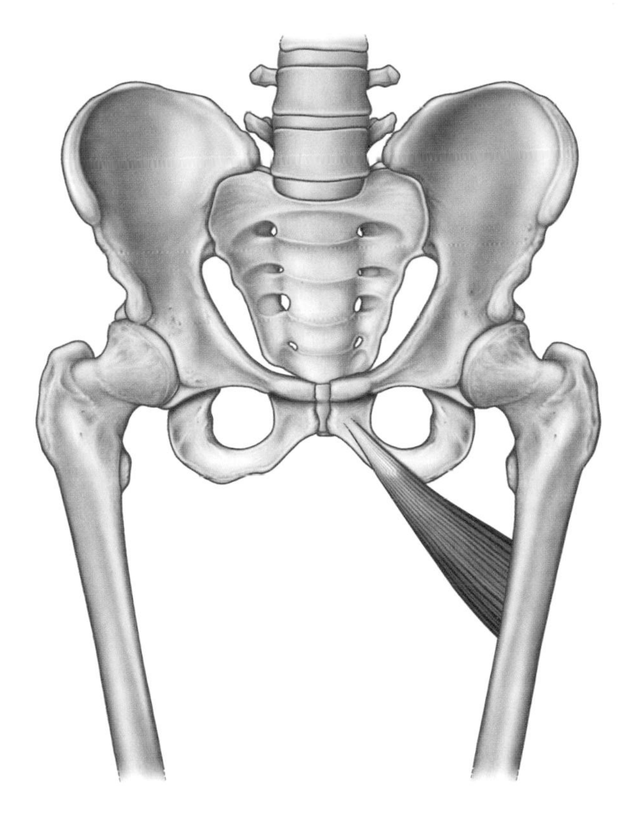

Pectineus

Nerve, supply: Femoral nerve, L2–3 and obturator nerve, L2–4.

Origin: Iliopubic eminence along pecten pubis of superior ramus of pubis.

Insertion: Pectineal line below the lesser trochanter and superior part of linea aspera on posterior surface of femur.

Function: Adduction and external rotation of hip. Hip extension when hip is in flexion and hip flexion when hip is in extension.

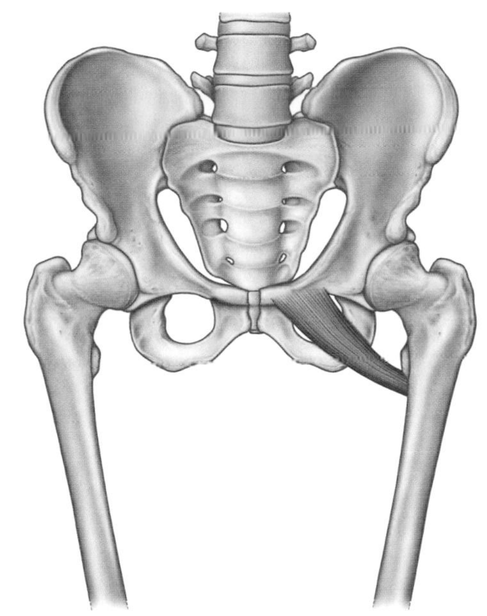

Adductor minimus

Nerve, supply: Obturator nerve, L3–5.

Origin: Inferior ramus of pubis.

Insertion: Linea aspera on posterior surface of femur.

Function: Adduction and external rotation of hip. Hip extension when hip is in flexion and hip flexion when hip is in extension.

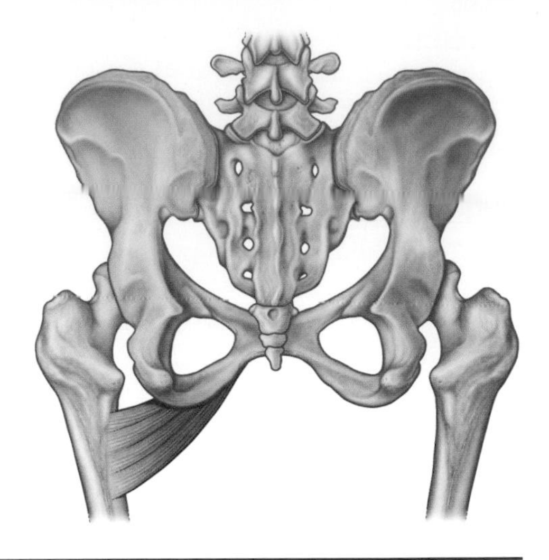

Stretching technique (abduction + internal rotation + extension):

Patient is on back with hands wrapped around knee in flexion to stabilize pelvis and leg to be treated hangs freely over edge of table. Therapist's hand presses down and to the side on the knee to increase hip extension and abduction. Therapist applies pressure with own lower leg against medial side of lower leg of patient to internally rotate hip joint. The thenar of other hand is used to stretch along body of muscle away from insertion and to increase abduction.

Tension–relaxation technique: Patient tries to adduct leg for 5 sec while therapist resists. Patient is then instructed to gradually relax while therapist allows extension and abduction to increase under the pressure.

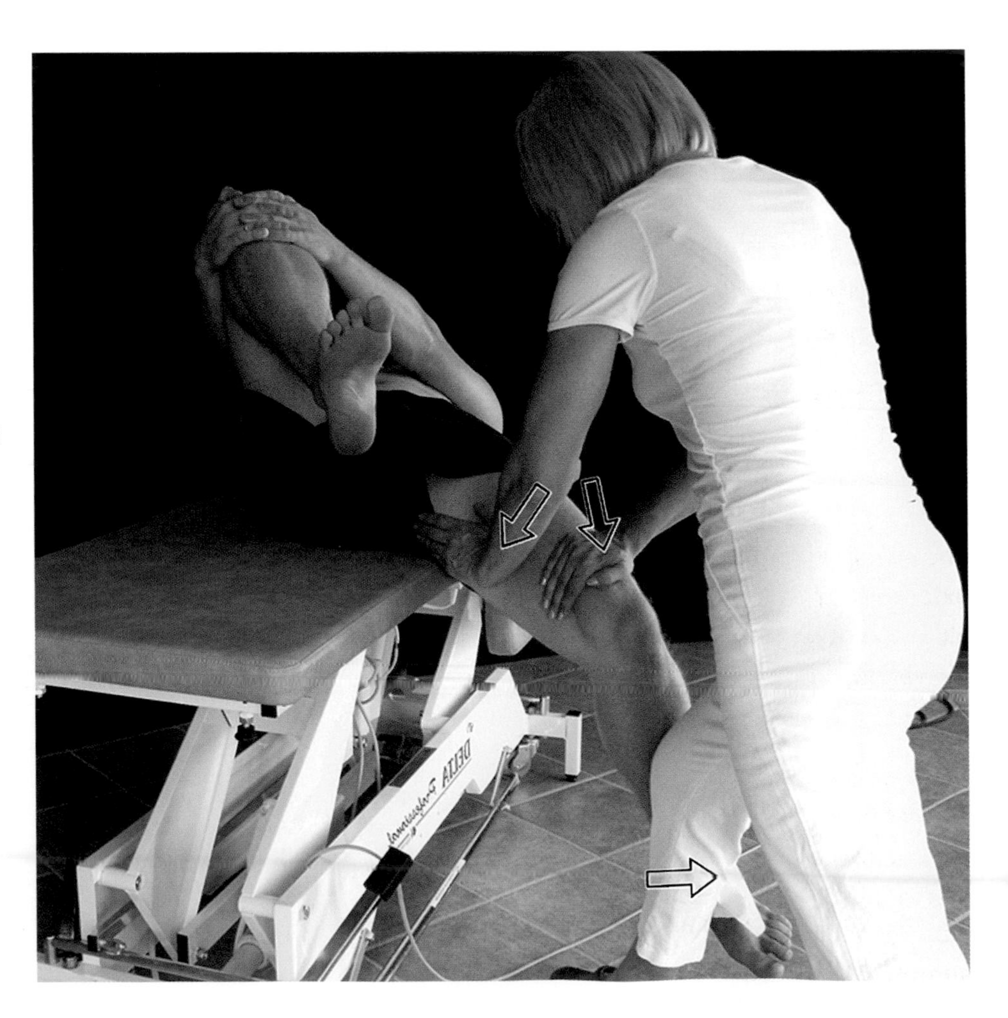

Biceps femoris/ Caput longum

Nerve, supply: Tibial nerve, L5–S2.

Origin: Ishial tuberosity.

Insertion: Head of fibula.

Function: Extension, adduction and external rotation of hip. Knee flexion. External rotation of knee, when knee is flexed.

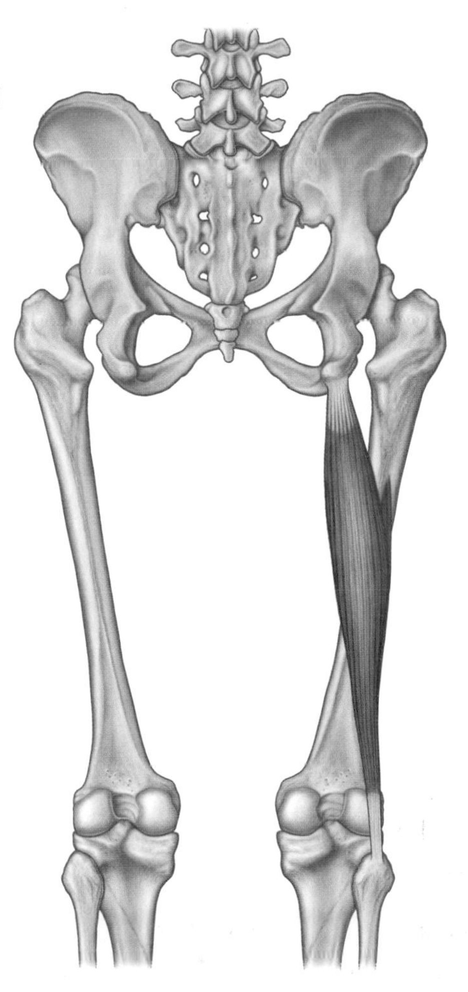

Stretching technique A (flexion + abduction):

Patient is lying on back with one leg straight on the table. Therapist lifts the other leg up and holds the lower leg in the armpit to flex and abduct hip joint while knee remains extended. The other hand stretches along body of muscle away from the tendon–muscle junction towards the body of the muscle.

Tension–relaxation technique: Patient tries to extend hip for 5 sec while therapist resists. Patient is then instructed to gradually relax muscles while therapist allows stretch to increase.

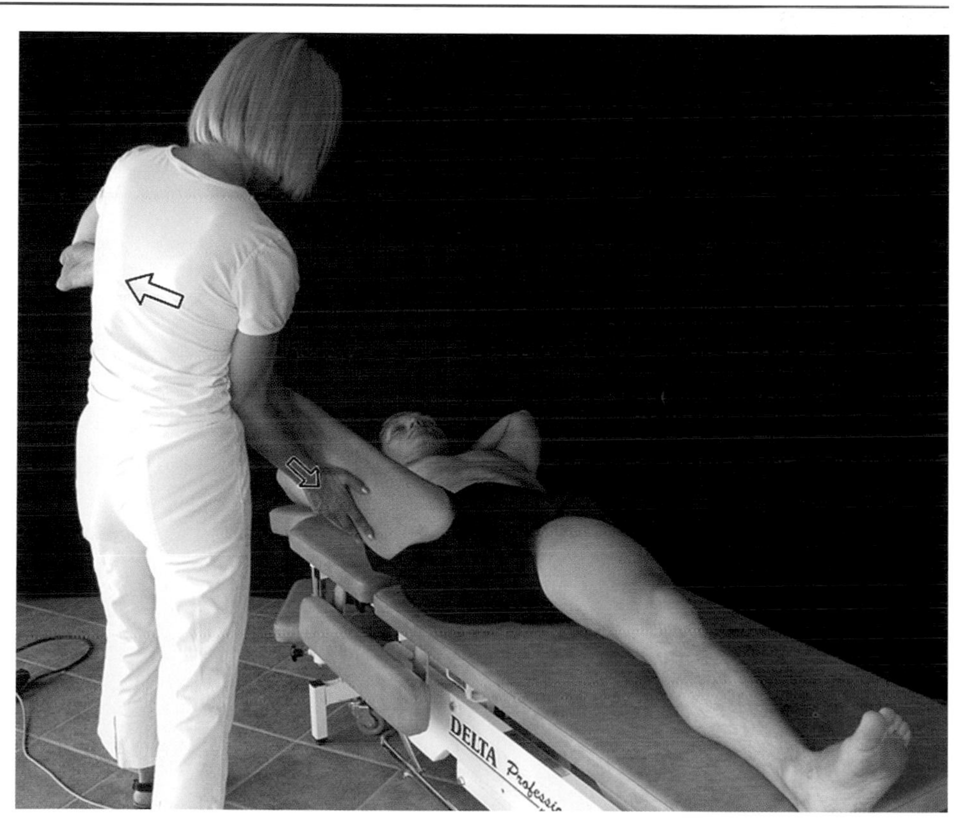

Stretching technique B (flexion + abduction):

Patient is lying on stomach with one leg straight on the table and the other leg straight on the floor in slight abduction. Therapist pushes with the foot patient's leg forward as far as possible. Therapist stretches with thenar of the hand along the body of muscle away from origin.

Tension–relaxation technique: Patient tries to flex knee for 5 sec while therapist resists. Patient is then instructed to gradually relax while therapist increases stretch.

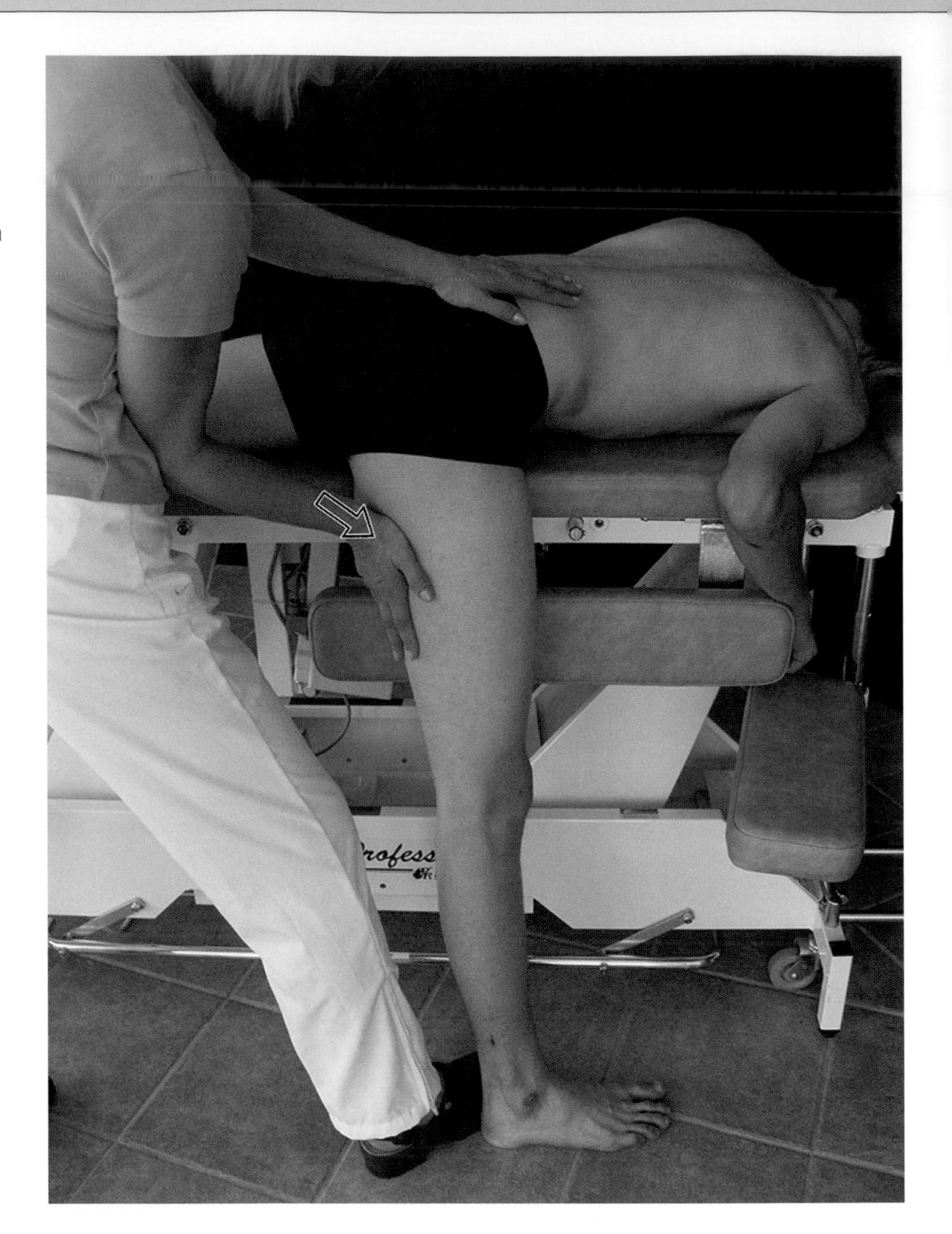

Stretching technique C (flexion + abduction):

Patient is lying on side, bottom leg with hip and knee in flexion for support. Therapist grasps upper leg and lifts it into abduction and supports against the body so that knee is extended while pressing the hip into flexion. The thenar of the other hand stretches along the body of muscle away from insertion.

Tension–relaxation technique: Patient tries to extend hip for 5 sec while therapist resists. Patient is then instructed to gradually relax while therapist allows stretch to increase.

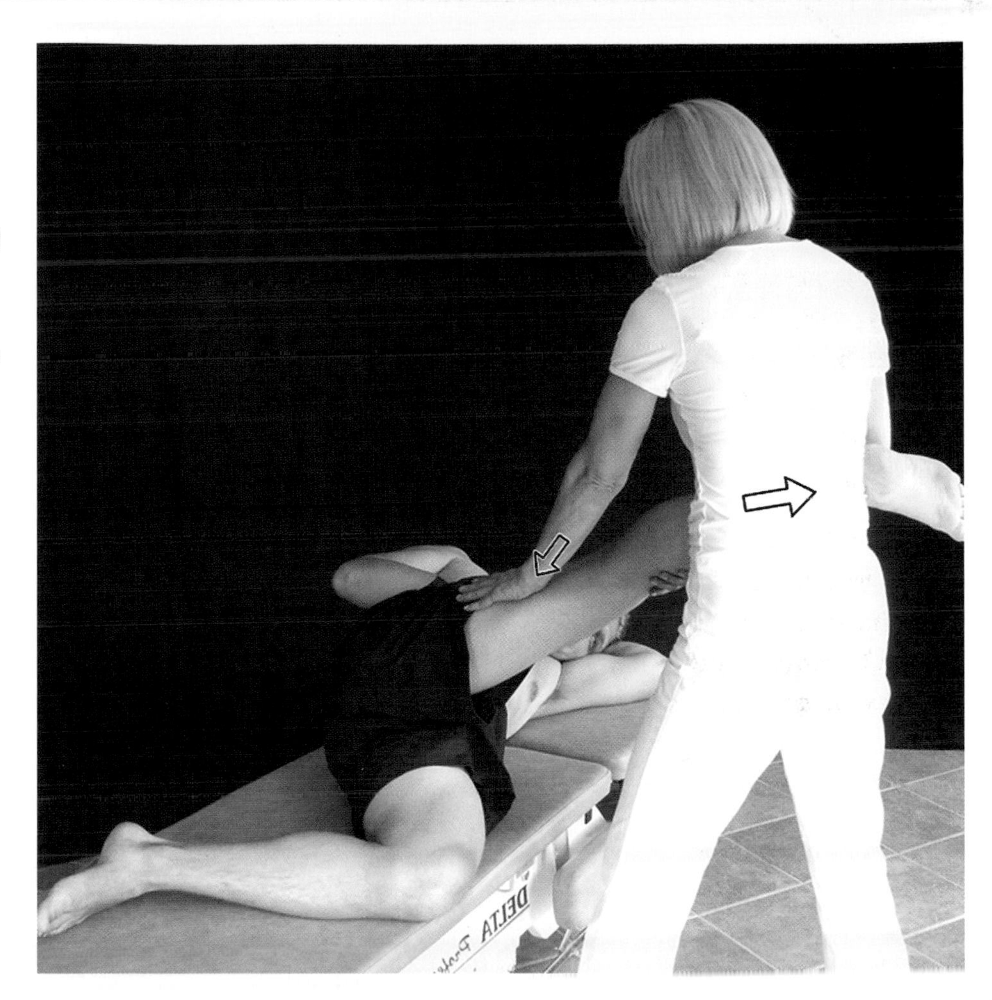

Biceps femoris/ Caput breve

Nerve, supply: Common fibular nerve, S1–2.

Origin: Middle third of lateral lip of linea aspera and the intermuscular septum.

Insertion: Head of fibula.

Function: Flexion of knee. External rotation of knee, when knee is flexed.

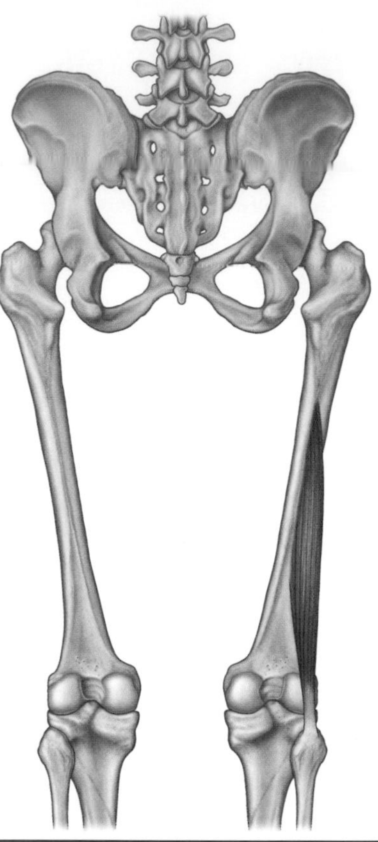

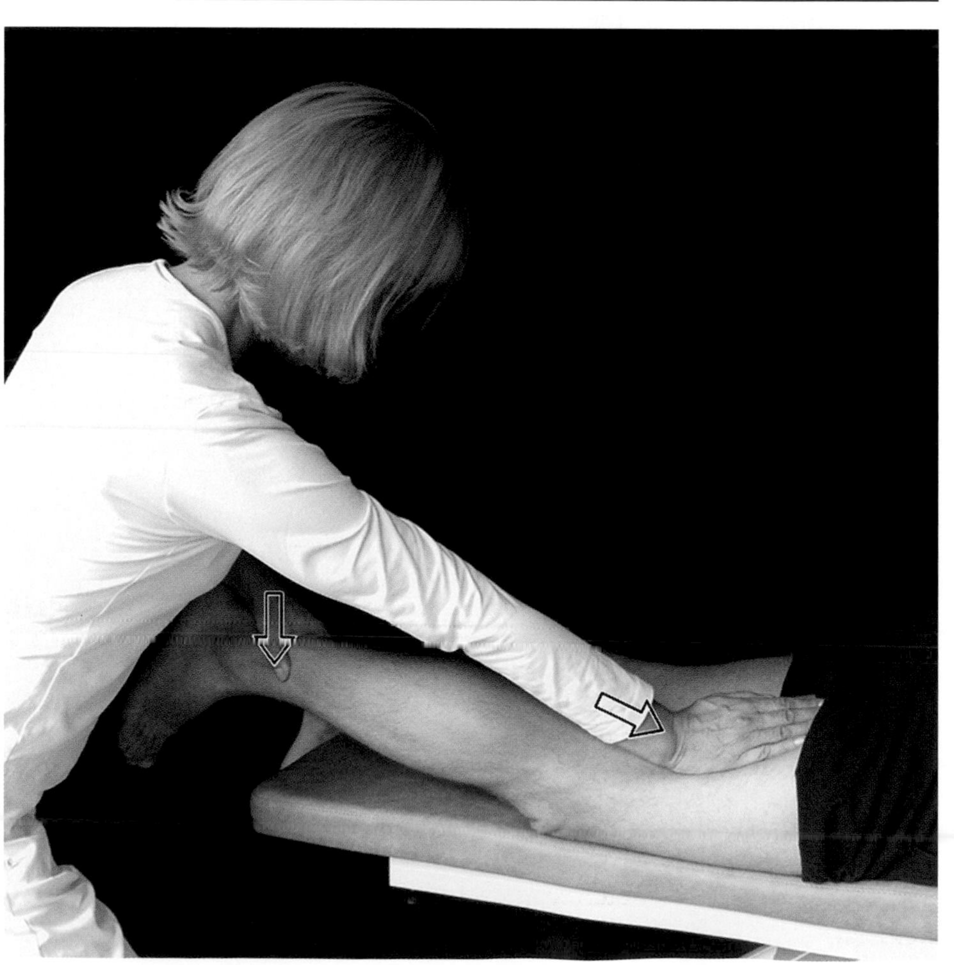

Stretching technique:

Patient is lying on stomach with one leg straight and the other one with knee flexed to 45°. Therapist grasps above the ankle to extend the knee while simultaneously applying pressure with the hypothenar of other hand along the belly of the muscle away from insertion.

Tension–relaxation technique: Patient tries to flex knee for 5 sec while therapist resists. Patient is then instructed to gradually relax while therapist allows stretch to increase.

Semitendinosus

Nerve, supply: Tibial nerve, L5–S2.

Origin: Ishial tuberosity.

Insertion: Medial condyle of tibia.

Function: Extension, adduction and internal rotation of hip. Flexion and internal rotation of knee.

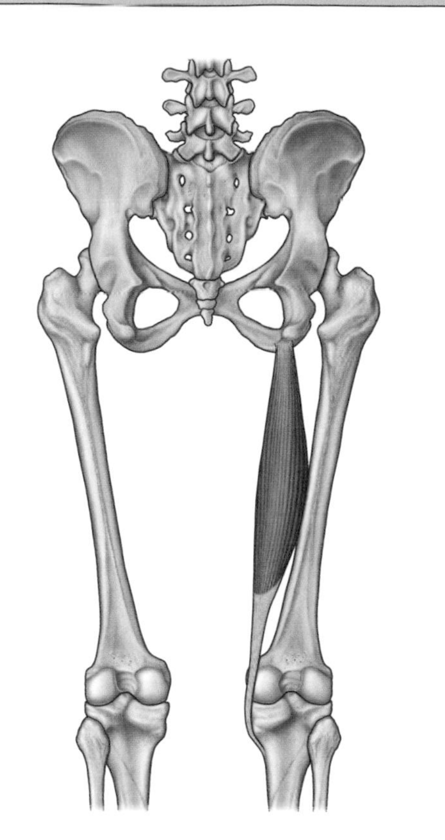

Semimembranosus

Nerve, supply: Tibial nerve, L5–S2.

Origin: Ishial tuberosity.

Insertion: Medial condyle of tibia, oblique popliteal ligament, posterior, medial knee joint capsule and medial meniscus.

Function: Extension, adduction and internal rotation of hip. Flexion and internal rotation of knee. Tenses knee joint capsule.

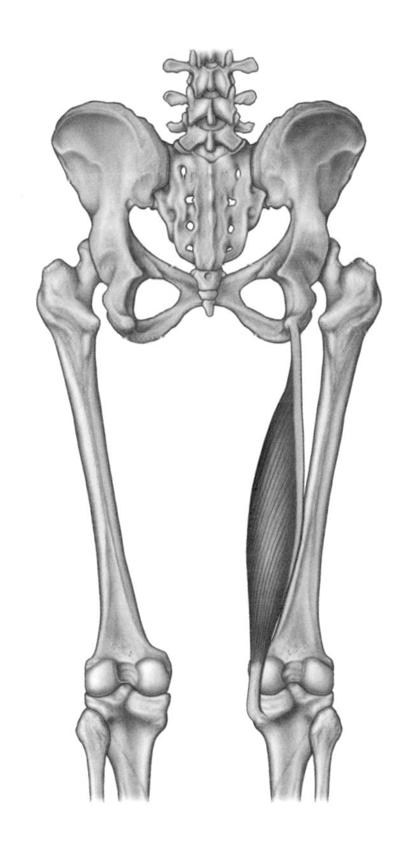

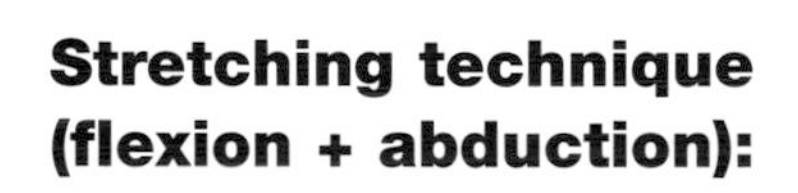

Stretching technique (flexion + abduction):

Patient is lying on back with legs out straight. Therapist lifts one leg on her shoulder and grasps around the knee to lock it in extension position. The leg is moved into abduction about 30–45°. Therapist uses the thenar of the other hand to stretch towards the body of muscle from the tendon–muscle junction.

Tension–relaxation technique: Patient tries to extend hip for 5 sec while therapist resists. Patient is then instructed to gradually relax while therapist allows stretch to increase.

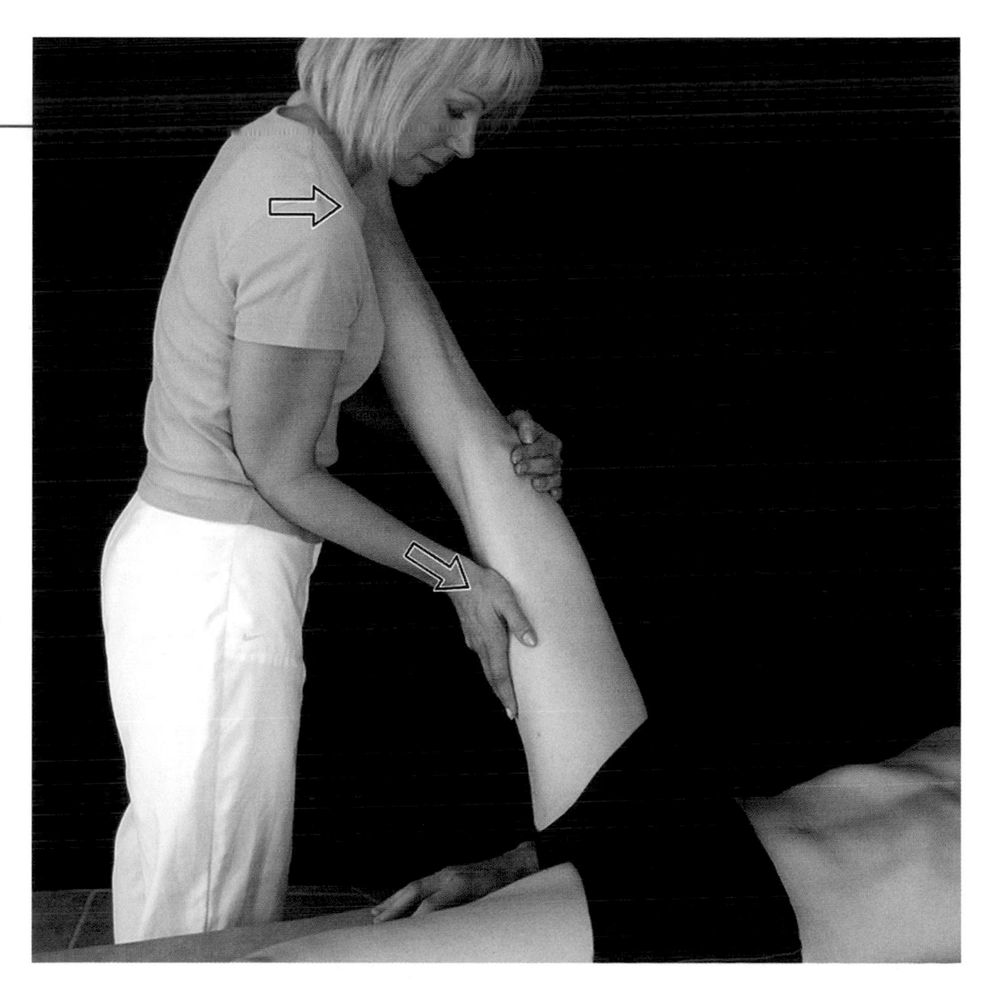

Popliteus

Nerve, supply: Tibial nerve, L4–S1.

Origin: Lateral femoral epicondyle

Insertion: Posterior, superior surface of tibia, posterior, lateral knee joint capsule and lateral meniscus.

Function: Flexion and internal rotation of knee.

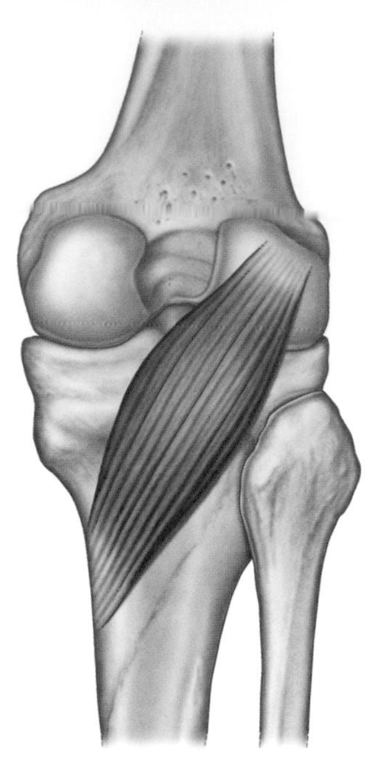

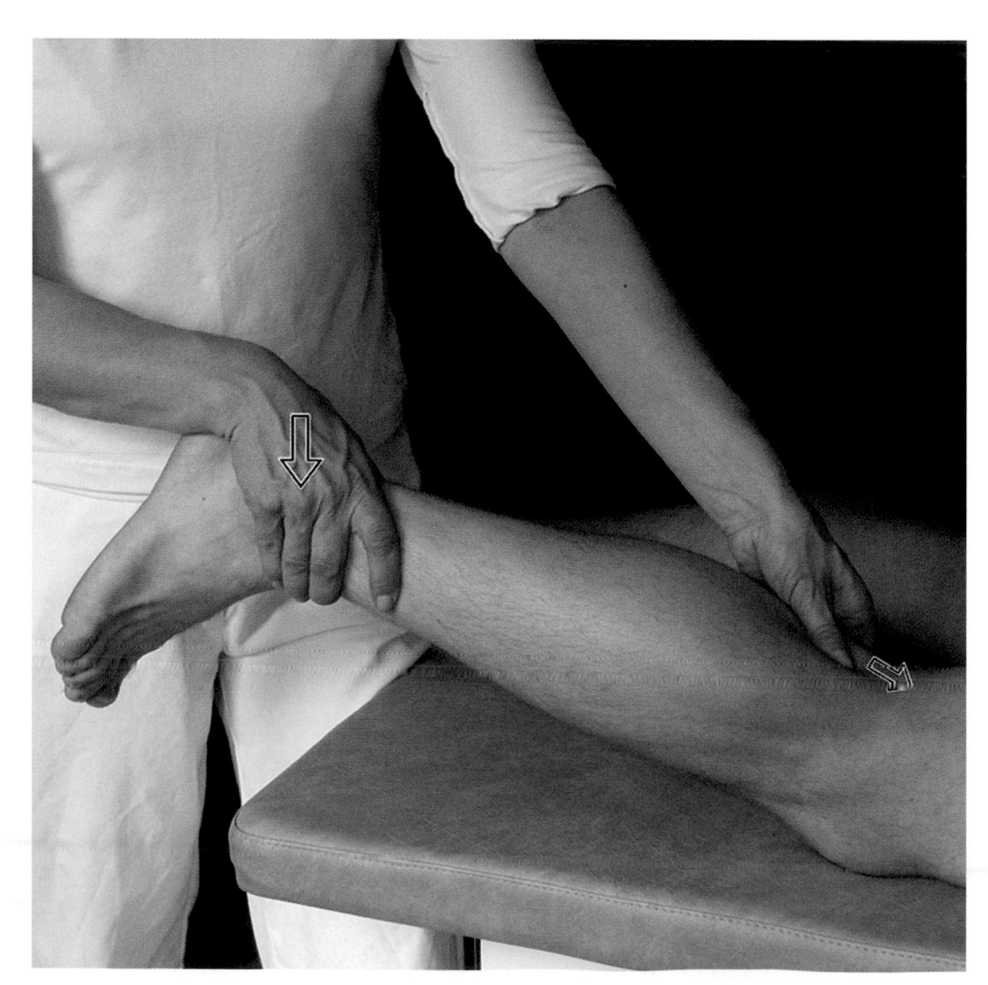

Stretching technique:

Patient is lying on back with legs out straight. Therapist grasps lower leg above the ankle and knee is flexed to 45°. Therapist uses the thumb of the other hand to stretch muscle tissue away from insertion towards belly of the muscles while simultaneously extending the knee.

Tension–relaxation technique: Patient tries to flex knee for 5 sec while therapist resists. Patient is then advised to gradually relax muscles while therapist allows stretch to increase under pressure.

Tibialis anterior

Nerve, supply: Fibular nerve, L4–5.

Origin: Lateral surface of tibia, interosseous membrane and crural fascia.

Insertion: Medial plantar surface of medial cuneiform and medial surface of first metatarsal.

Function: Dorsiflexion and supination of ankle.

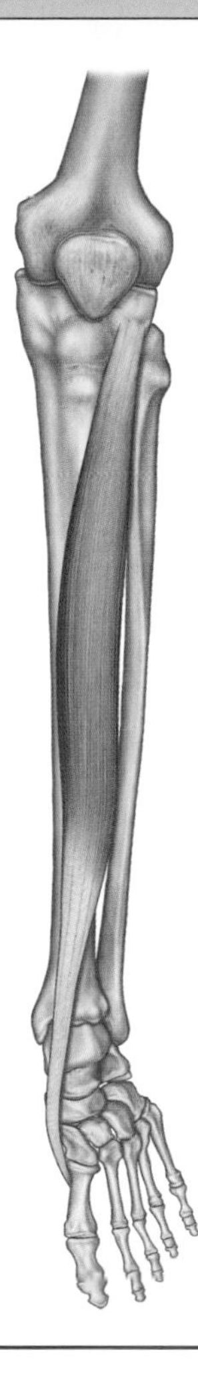

Stretching technique (plantar flexion + pronation):

Patient is lying on back. Therapist grasps the foot at the cuneiform and first metatarsal bones and applies pressure obliquely down to achieve plantar flexion and pronation. Therapist uses the thenar of the other hand to stretch along body of muscle away from insertion.

Tension–relaxation technique: Patient tries to dorsiflex the foot for 5 sec against resistance by the therapist. Patient is then instructed to gradually relax while therapist allows stretch to increase.

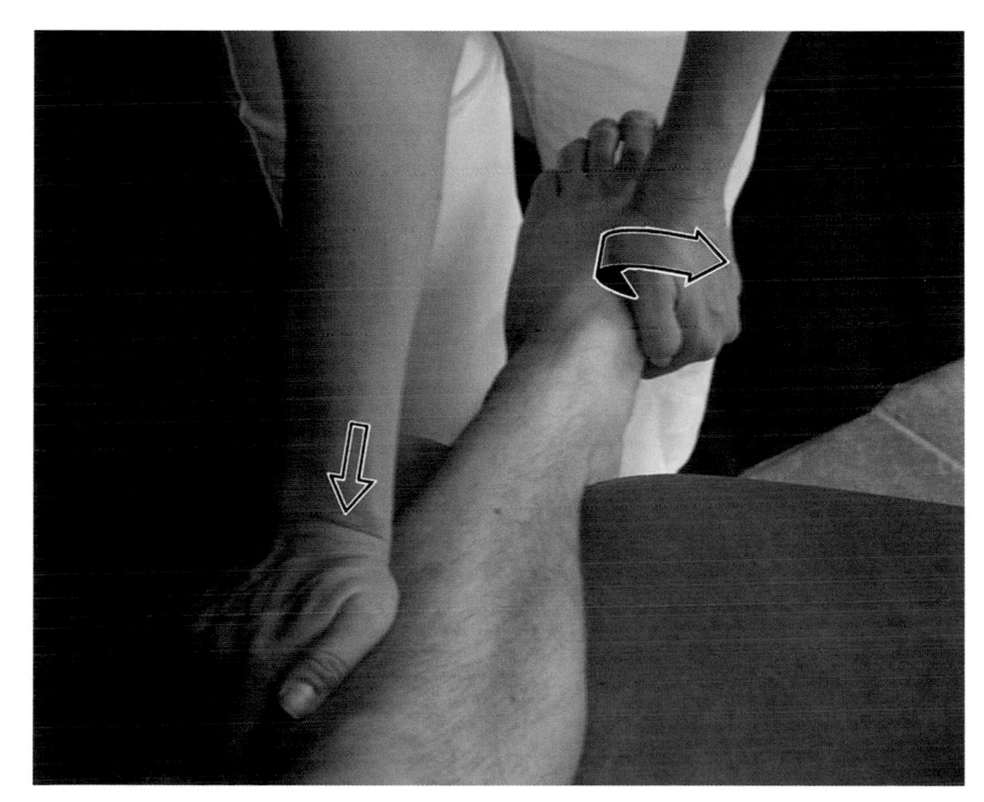

Extensor digitorum longus

Nerve, supply: Fibular nerve, L5–S1.

Origin: Lateral condyle of tibia, anterior crest of fibula, deep crural fascia and interosseous membrane.

Insertion: Via dorsal aponeurosis to the bases of middle and distal phalanges of toes 2–5.

Function: Dorsiflexion of toes. Dorsiflexion and pronation of ankle.

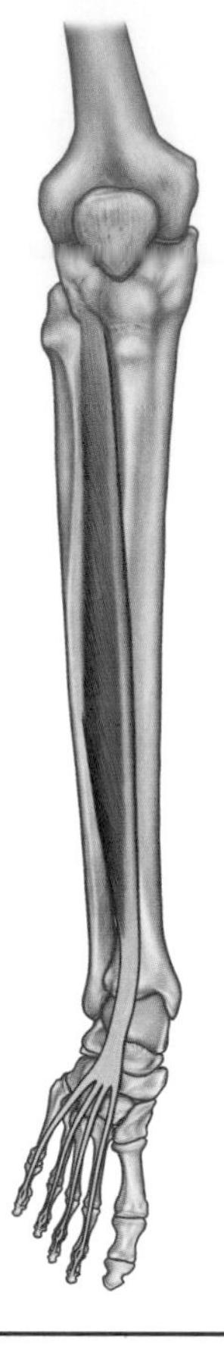

Stretching technique (plantar flexion + supination):

Patient is lying on back. Therapist grasps at flexed toes 2–5 and presses the foot in plantar flexion and supination. The thenar of the other hand is used to stretch along body of muscle away from insertion.

Tension–relaxation technique: Patient tries to dorsiflex toes for 5 sec while therapist resists. Patient is then instructed to gradually relax while therapist applies further stretch.

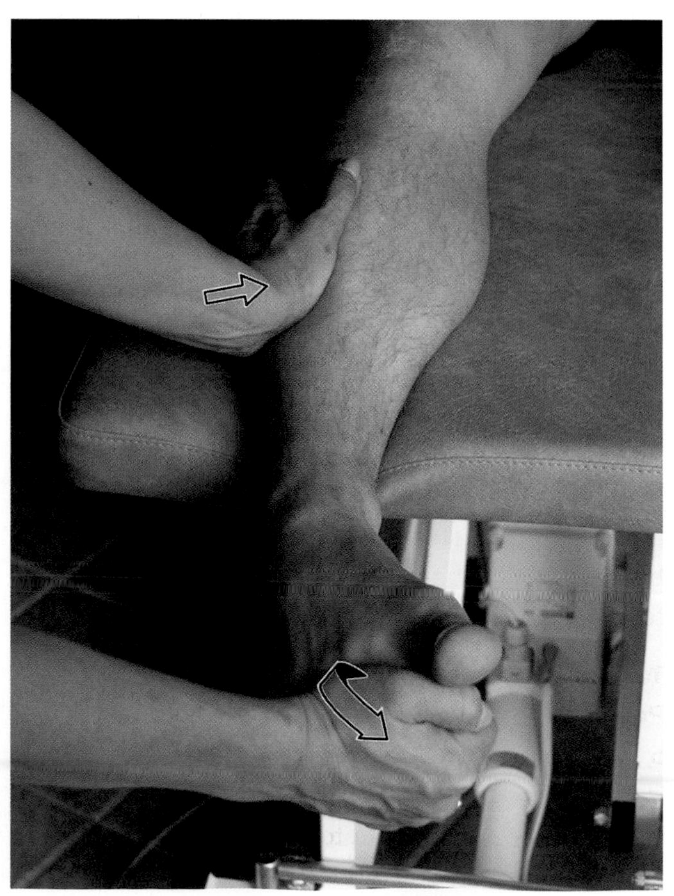

Extensor hallucis longus

Nerve, supply: Deep fibular nerve, L4–S1.

Origin: Medial surface of fibula and interosseous membrane.

Insertion: Base of distal phalax of first toe.

Function: Dorsiflexion of big toe. Dorsifloxion of ankle and supination.

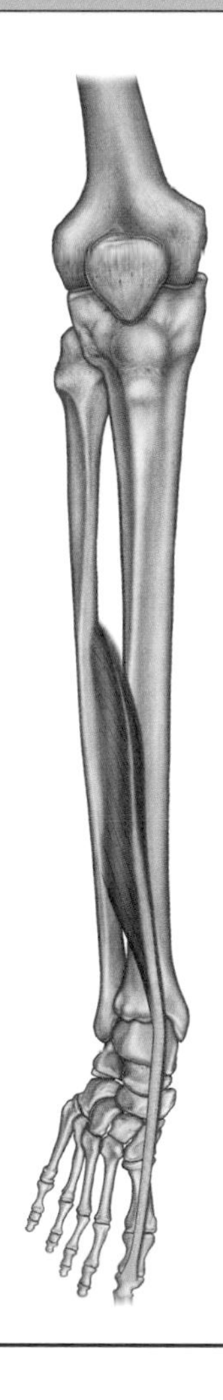

Stretching technique (plantar flexion and pronation):

Patient is lying on back. Therapist grasps the flexed big toe and presses the foot into plantar flexion and pronation. The thenar of other hand stretches muscle tissue along the body of muscle away from the tendon–muscle junction.

Tension–relaxation technique: Patient tries to dorsiflex big toe for 5 sec while therapist resists. Patient is then instructed to gradually relax while therapist allows stretch to increase.

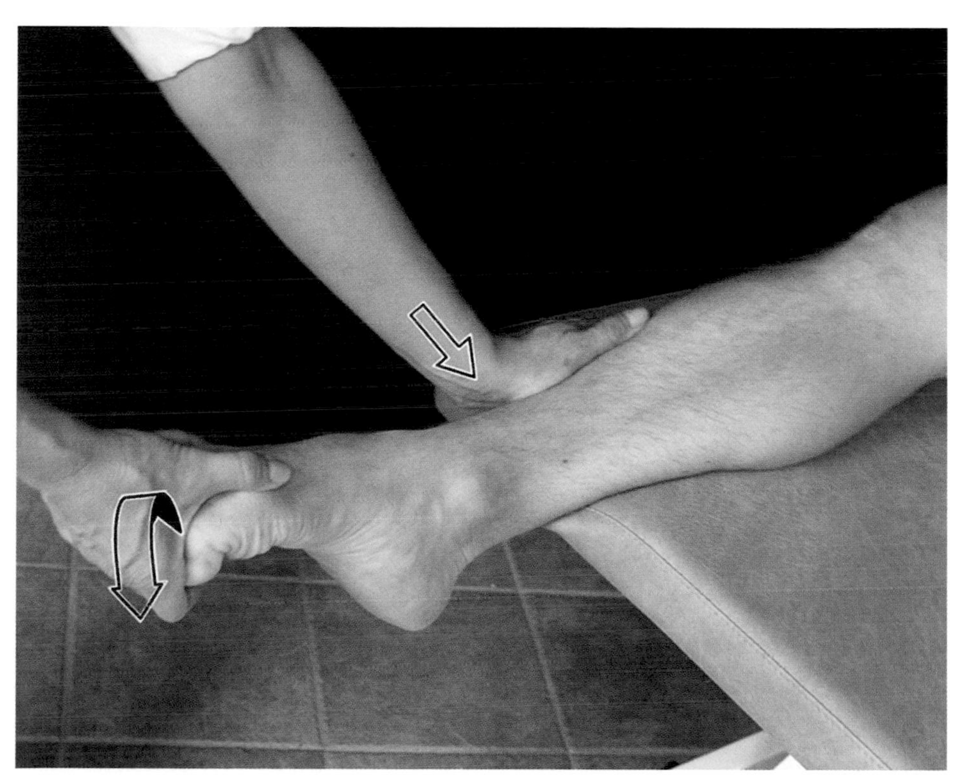

Fibularis longus

Nerve, supply: Superficial fibular nerve, L5–S1.

Origin: Superior surface of fibula and capsule of tibiofibular joint.

Insertion: Plantar surface of medial cuneiform and base of first metatarsal.

Function: Plantar flexion and pronation of foot.

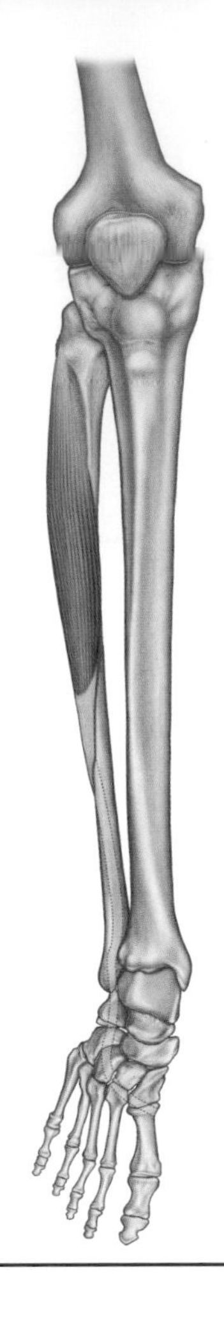

Stretching technique (dorsiflexion + supination):

Patient is lying on stomach. Therapist grasps medial surface of foot around the medial cuneiform and the first metatarsal and lifts the lower leg to 45° angle. Therapist presses the foot in dorsiflexion and supination. The thenar of other hand stretches along body of muscle away from the tendon–muscle junction.

Tension–relaxation technique: Patient tries to plantar flex foot for 5 sec while therapist resists. Patient is then instructed to gradually relax while therapist allows stretch to increase.

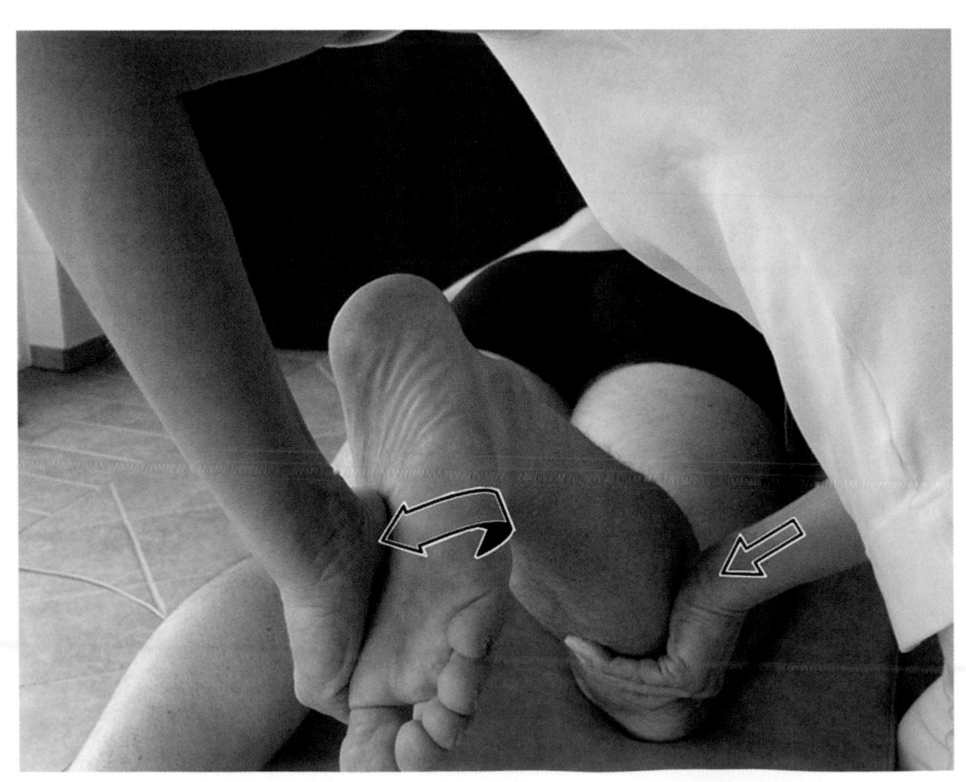

Fibularis brevis

Nerve, supply: Superficial fibular nerve, L5–S1.

Origin: Middle and lower third of lateral surface of fibula.

Insertion: Laterally base of fifth metatarsal.

Function: Plantar flexion and pronation of foot.

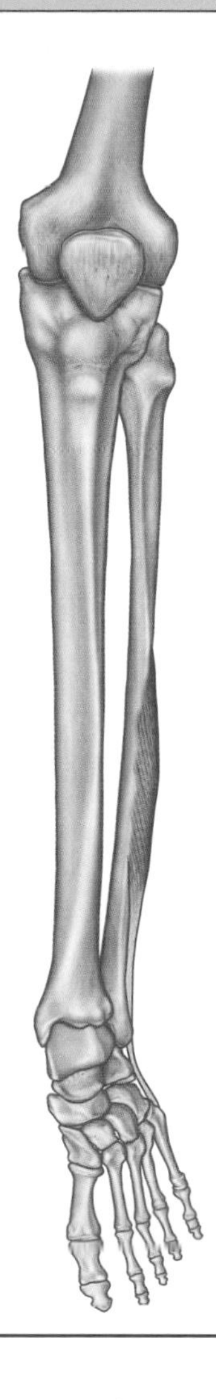

Stretching technique (dorsiflexion + supination):

Patient is lying on side with straight leg and the top foot over the edge of the table. Therapist grasps the foot and twists it in supination while pressing with thigh on to the patient's sole to cause dorsiflexion. Therapist uses other hypothenar of the hand to stretch along body of muscle away from the tendon–muscle junction.

Tension–relaxation technique: Patient tries to plantar flex the foot for 5 sec while therapist resists. Patient is then instructed to gradually relax while therapist allows stretch to increase.

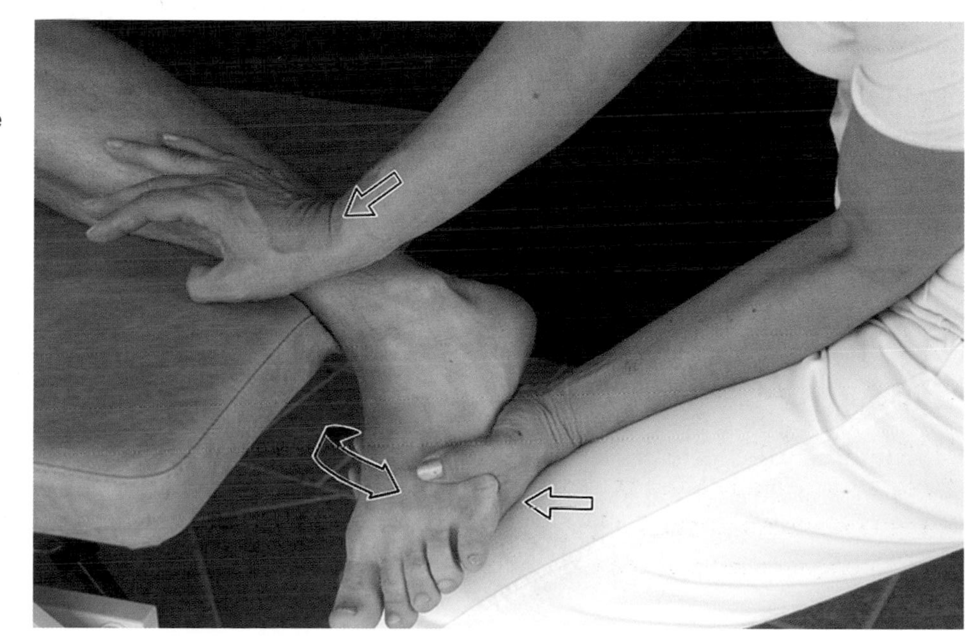

Fibularis tertius

Nerve, supply: Deep fibular nerve, L5–S1.

Origin: Inferior third of lateral surface of fibula.

Insertion: Dorsal surface at base of fifth metatarsals and sometimes also fourth metatarsal.

Function: Dorsiflexion and pronation of foot.

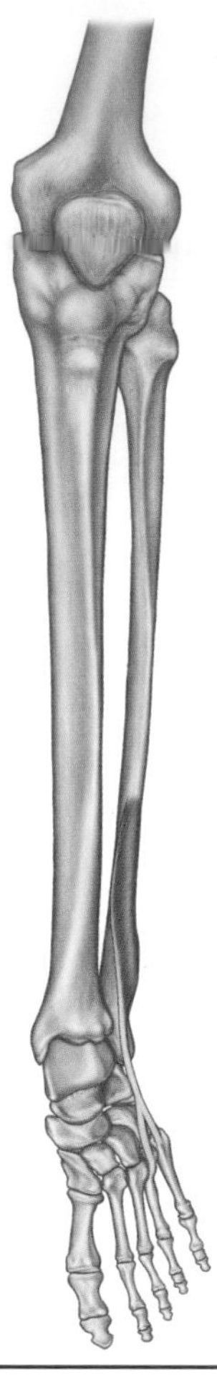

Stretching technique (plantar flexion + supination):

Patient is lying on side with foot over the edge of the table. Therapist grasps foot on dorsal side with thenar of the hand over the base of metatarsals 4–5. Pressure is applied to plantar flex ankle and the foot is twisted externally. The hypothenar of other hand stretches along the body of muscle away from the tendon–muscle junction.

Tension–relaxation technique: Patient tries to dorsiflex the ankle for 5 sec while therapist resists. Patient is then instructed to gradually relax while therapist allows stretch to increase.

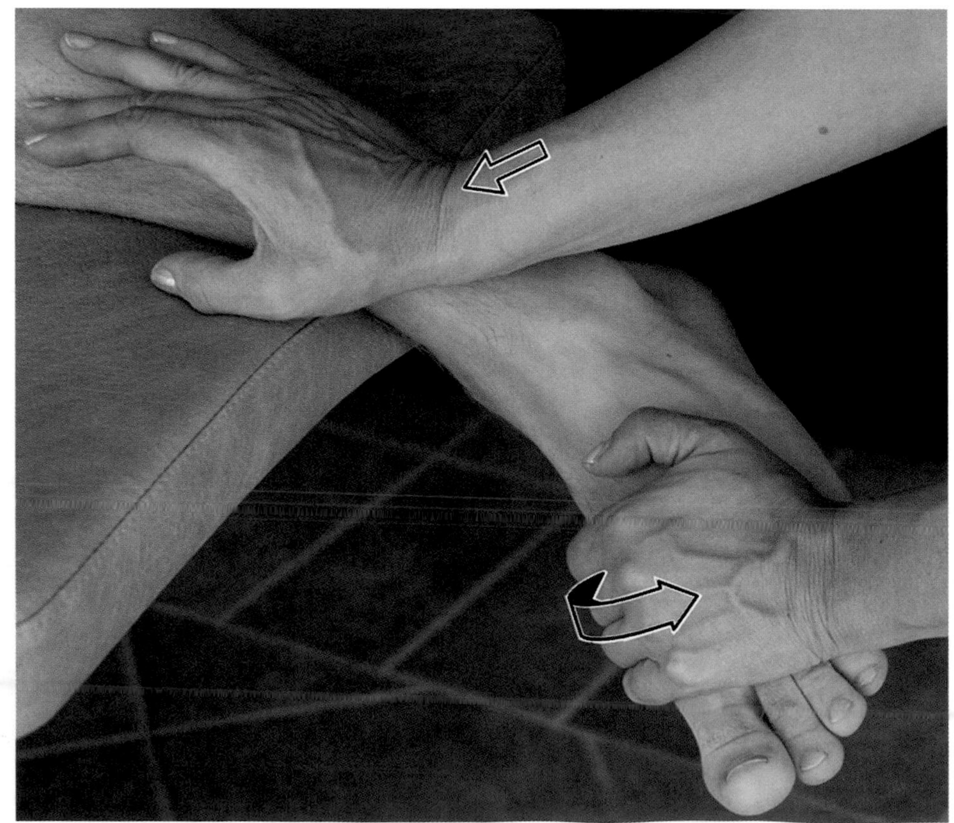

Plantaris

Nerve, supply: Tibial nerve, S1–2.

Origin: Lateral femoral condyle and joint capsule.

Insertion: Via Achilles tendon to the superior medial border of tuber of calcaneus.

Function: Assists in flexion of knee and plantar flexion of ankle.

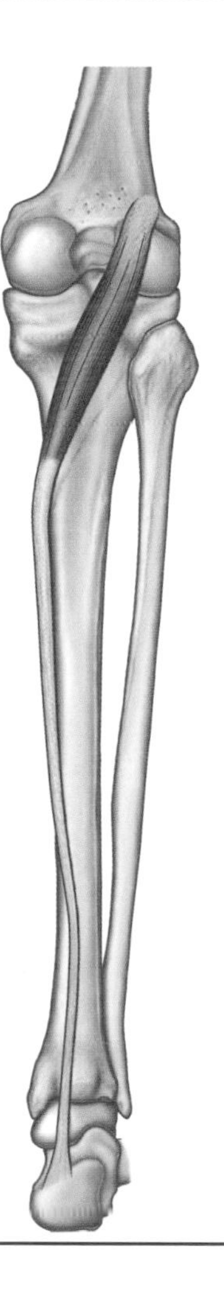

Stretching technique (dorsiflexion):

Patient is lying on stomach with feet over the edge of the table. Therapist grasps the sole of foot and flexes the knee about 30°. Therapist presses with thigh on the sole of the foot to cause dorsiflexion. Then she lowers the foot while the hypothenar of other hand is used to stretch along the body of muscle away from the tendon–muscle junction.

Tension–relaxation technique: Patient tries to plantar flex ankle for 5 sec while therapist resists. Patient is then instructed to gradually relax muscles while therapist allows stretch to increase under pressure.

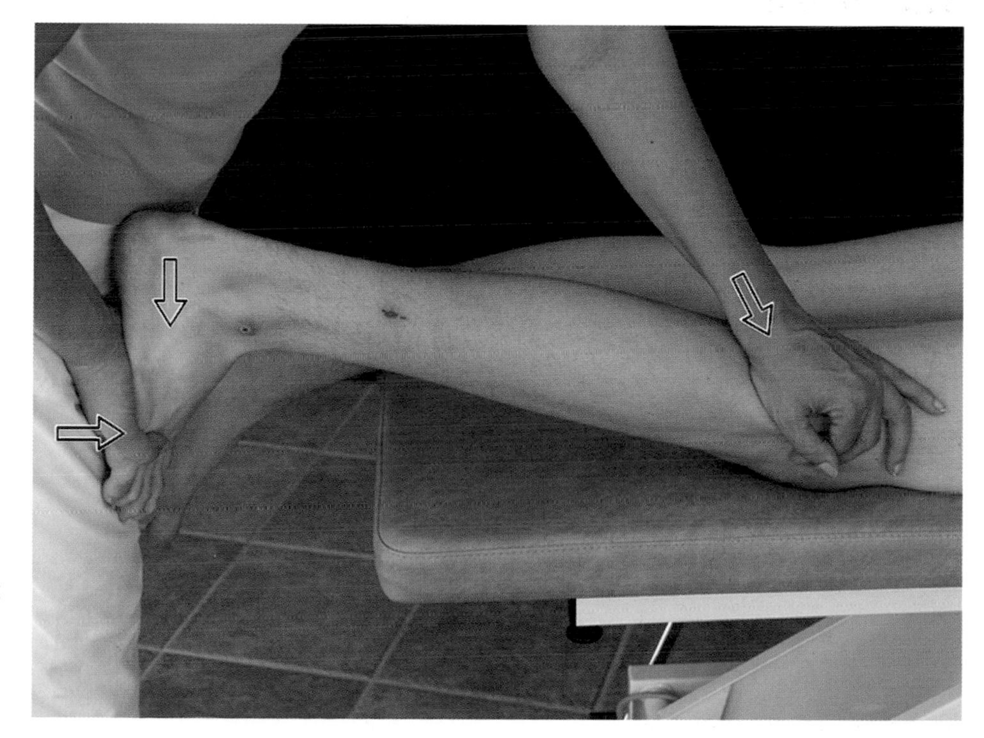

Triceps surae

(Composed of two muscles: gastrocnemius and soleus)

Gastrocnemius

Nerve, supply: Tibial nerve, S1–2.

Origin: Two heads arising from the lateral and medial femoral condyles and posterior capsule of knee joint.

Insertion: Via the Achilles tendon to the tuber of calcaneus.

Function: Flexion of knee and plantar flexion and supination of ankle.

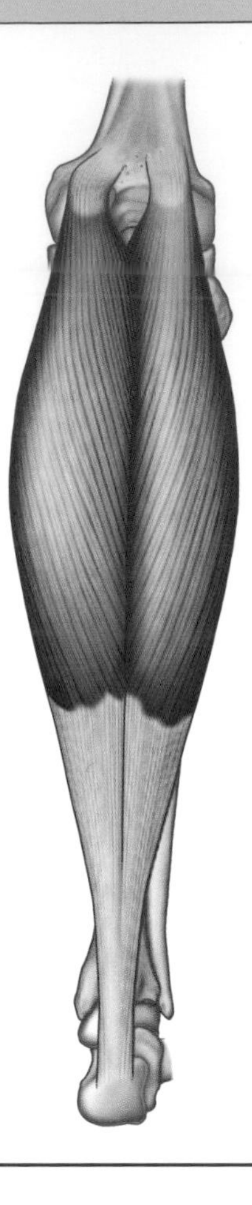

Stretching technique (dorsiflexion):

Patient is lying on stomach with the leg straight and well over the edge of the table. Therapist applies pressure to sole of foot with the thigh while using thenars of both hands to stretch along body of muscle away from tendon–muscle junction.

Tension–relaxation technique: Patient tries to plantar flex foot for 5 sec while therapist resists. Patient is then instructed to gradually relax while therapist allows stretch to increase.

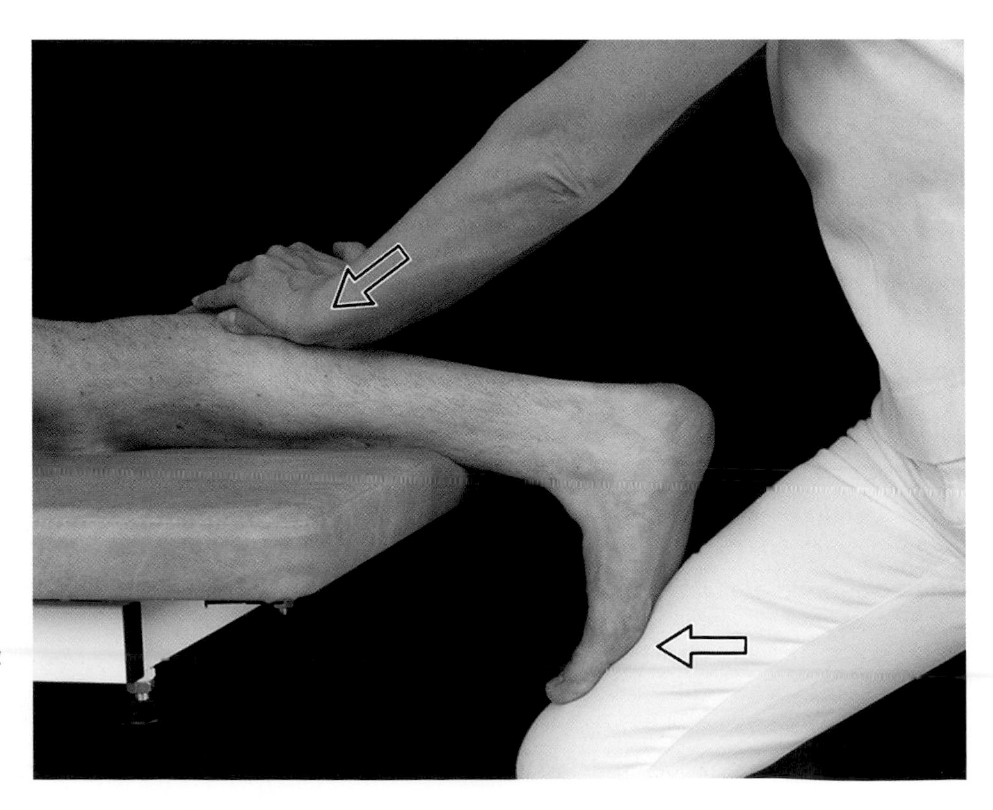

Soleus

Nerve, supply: Tibial nerve, S1–2.

Origin: Upper third of posterior surfaces on tibia and fibula.

Insertion: Via the Achilles tendon to the tuber of the calcaneus.

Function: Plantar flexion and supination of ankle.

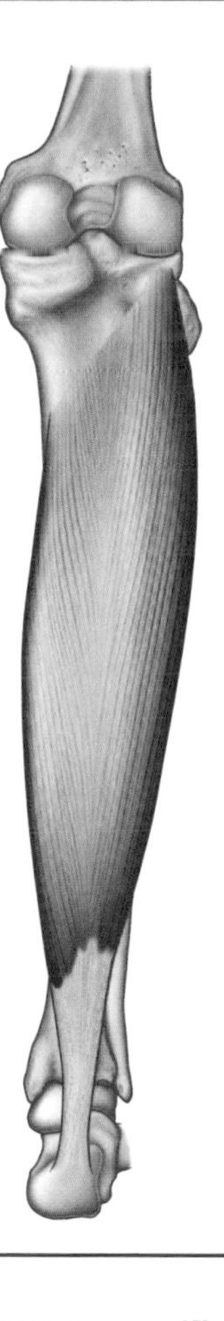

Stretching technique (dorsiflexion + pronation):

Patient is lying on stomach with feet over the edge of the table. Therapist grasps the sole of foot and flexes the knee about 20°. Therapist presses with thigh on the sole of the foot to cause dorsiflexion and stretches with the thenars of both hands along the body of muscle away from the tendon–muscle junction.

Tension–relaxation technique: Patient tries to plantar flex foot for 5 sec while therapist resists. Patient is then instructed to gradually relax while therapist allows stretch to increase under pressure.

Notice: Knee is flexed and should not be straightened, because it will tense the gastrocnemius overlying the soleus and then stretching would not be specifically directed on the soleus muscle.

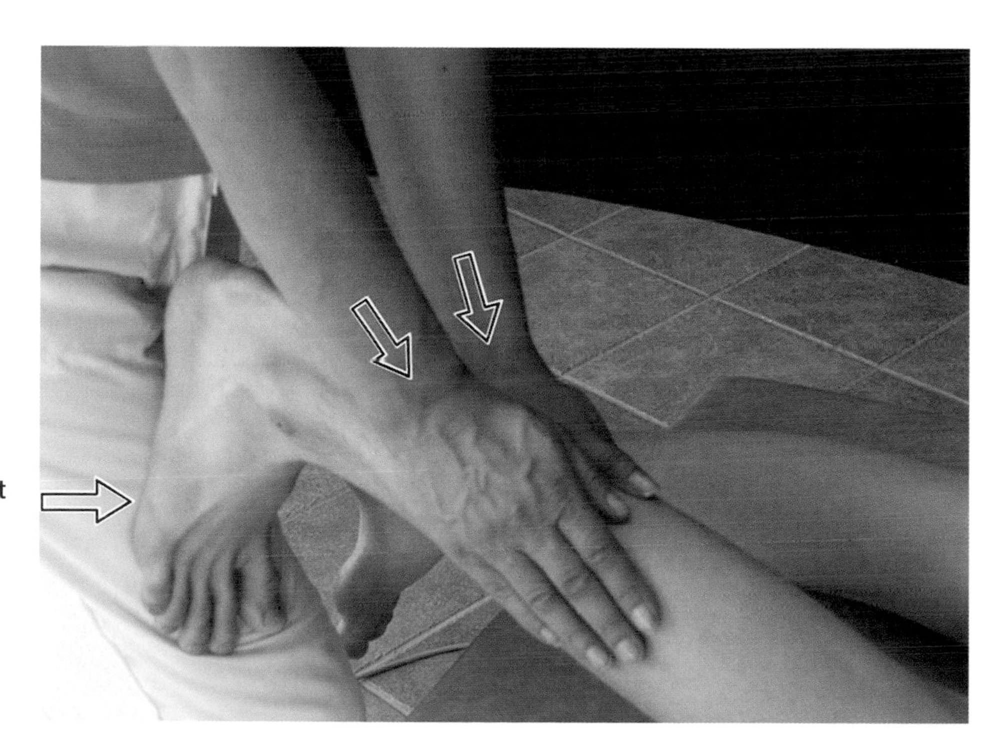

Tibialis posterior

Nerve, supply: Tibial nerve, L4–5.

Origin: Upper and middle third of tibia, fibula and interosseous membrane.

Insertion: Navicular, three cuneiforms cuboid and base of metatarsals 2–4.

Function: Plantar flexion and supination.

Notice: The muscle may be absent.

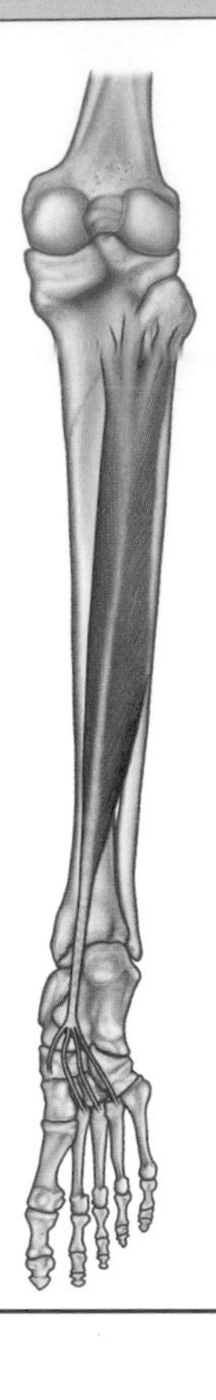

Stretching technique (dorsiflexion + pronation):

Patient is lying on stomach with knee flexed about 20° and ankle supported with bolster. Therapist grasps the sole of the foot at the lateral tarsals and metatarsals to dorsiflex the ankle and to twist the foot into pronation. Therapist applies stretch with the hypothenar of the other hand along the body of the muscle away from the tendon–muscle junction.

Tension–relaxation technique: Patient tries to plantar flex ankle for 5 sec while therapist resists. Patient is then instructed to gradually relax while therapist allows stretch to increase.

Notice: Knee is held in flexion to relax overlying gastrocnemius muscle and thus to be able to direct the manual stretch into deeper muscle layers.

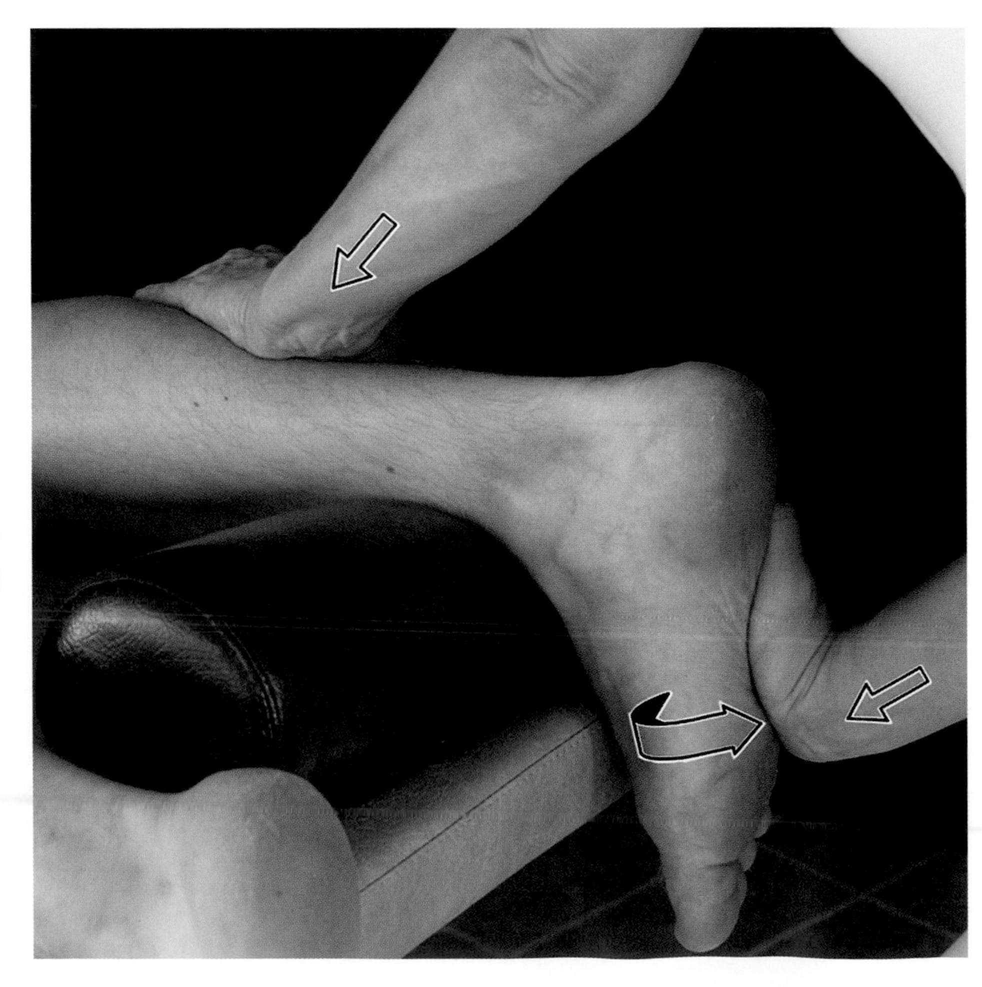

Flexor hallucis longus

Nerve, supply: Tibial nerve, S1–3.

Origin: Distal two thirds of posterior surface of fibula, interosseous membrane and intermuscular septum.

Insertion: Base of distal phalanx of the first digit.

Function: Plantar flexion of big toe. Plantar flexion and pronation of foot.

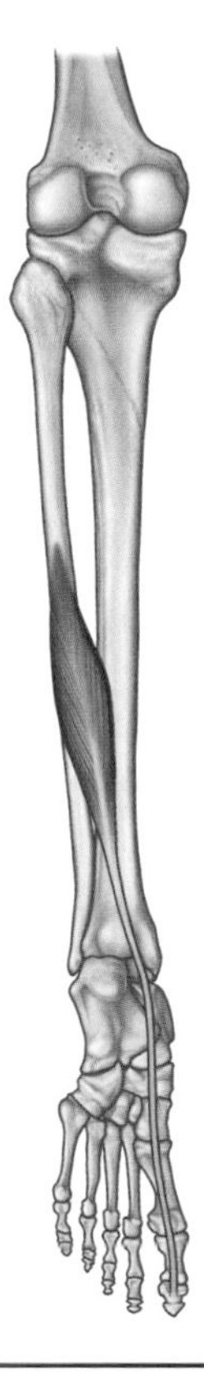

Stretching technique (dorsiflexion + supination):

Patient is lying on stomach with the knee supported in flexed position by therapist's forearm. Therapist grasps big toe to extend it and to dorsiflex the ankle. The hypothenar of the other hand is used to stretch along the body of muscle away from the tendon–muscle junction.

Tension–relaxation technique: Patient tries to plantar flex big toe for 5 sec while therapist resists. Patient is then instructed to gradually relax muscles while therapist allows stretch to increase.

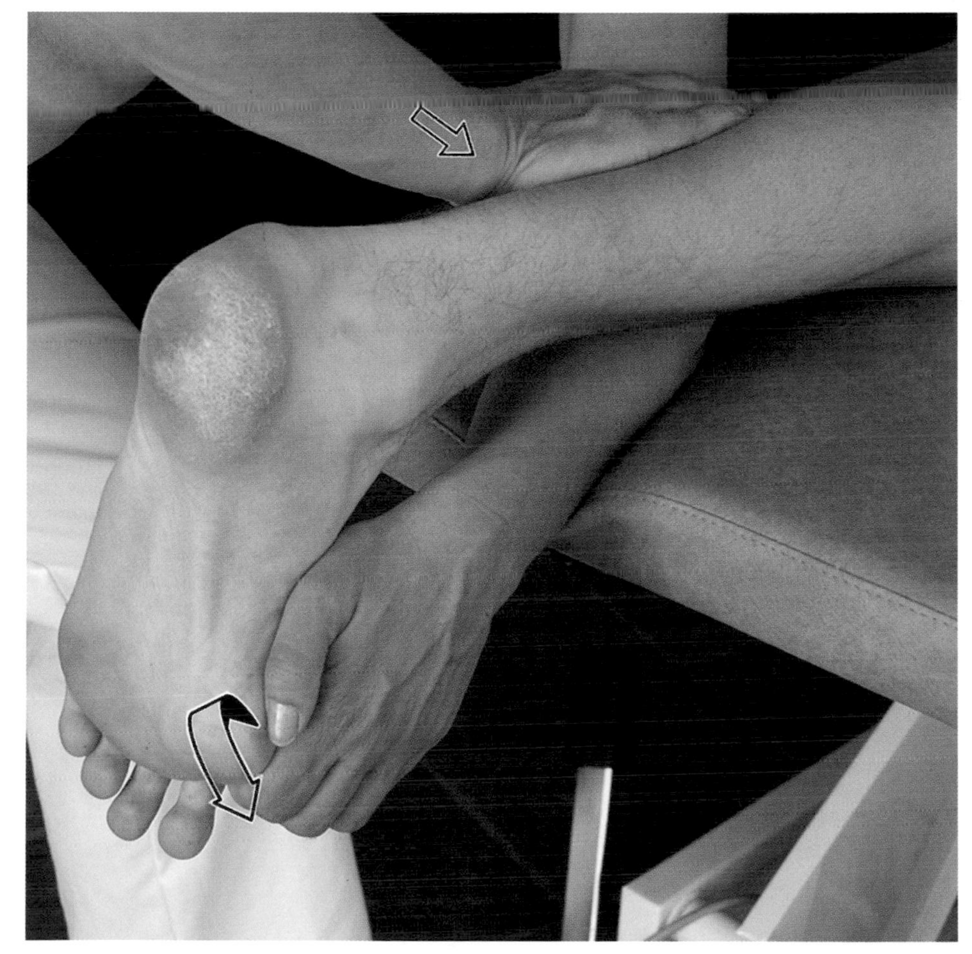

Flexor digitorum longus

Nerve, supply: Tibial nerve, S1–3.

Origin: Posterior surface of tibia.

Insertion: Distal phalanges of toes 2–5.

Function: Plantar flexion of toes 2–5, plantar flexion and supination of ankle and supports plantar arch.

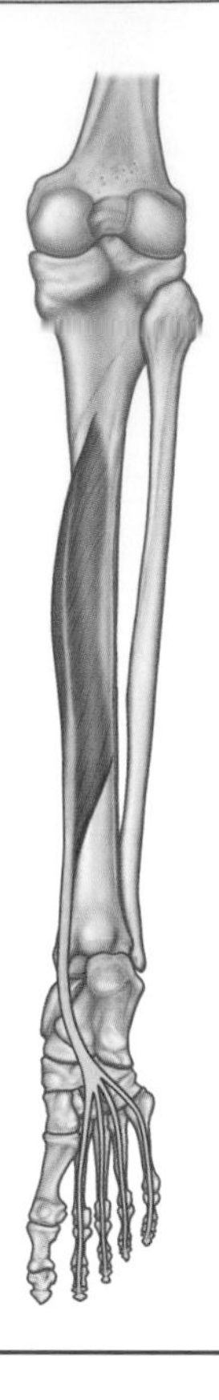

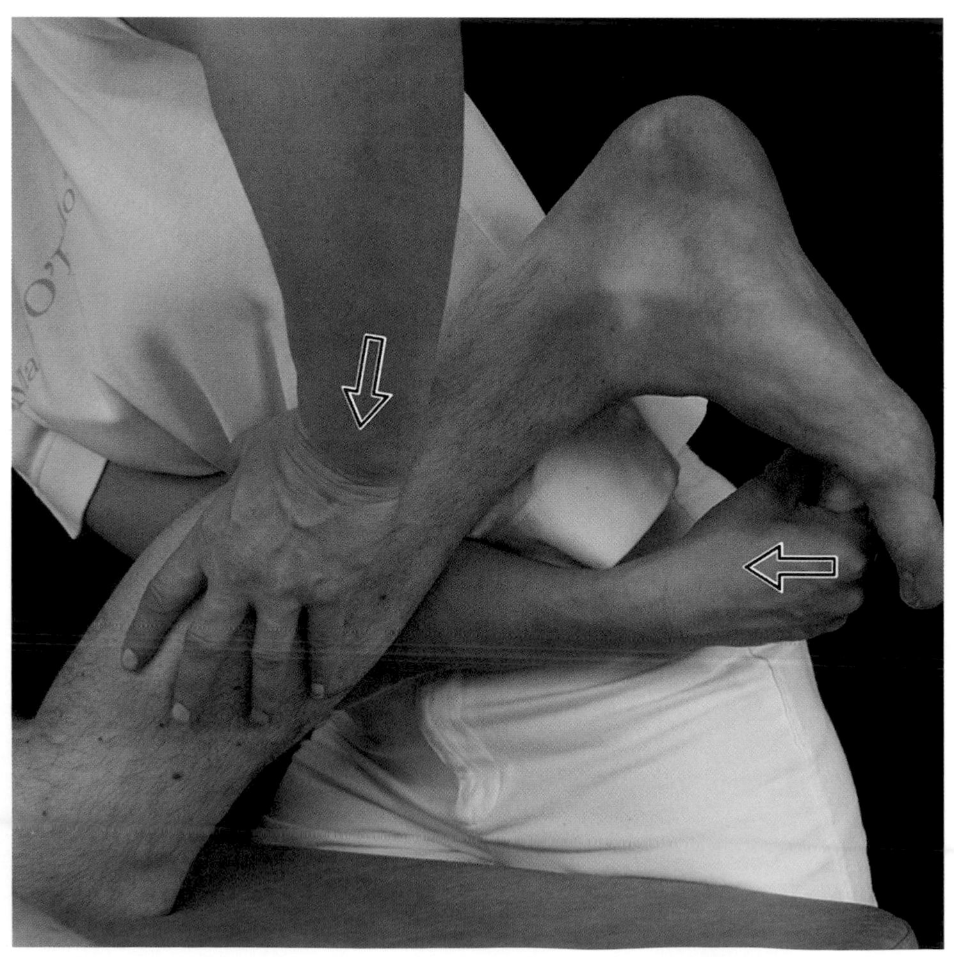

Stretching technique (dorsiflexion + pronation):

Patient is lying on stomach with the knee flexed. Therapist grasps toes 2–5 and applies pressure to dorsiflex them and the ankle. The thenar of the other hand is used to stretch along the body of muscle away from the tendon–muscle junction.

Tension–relaxation technique: Patient tries to plantar flex toes for 5 sec while therapist resists. Patient is then instructed to gradually relax muscles while therapist increases dorsiflexion and internal rotation.

Extensor hallucis brevis

Nerve, supply: Deep fibular nerve, S1–2.

Origin: Superior surface of calcaneus and extensor retinaculum.

Insertion: Base of the proximal phalanx of first toe.

Function: Dorsiflexion of big toe.

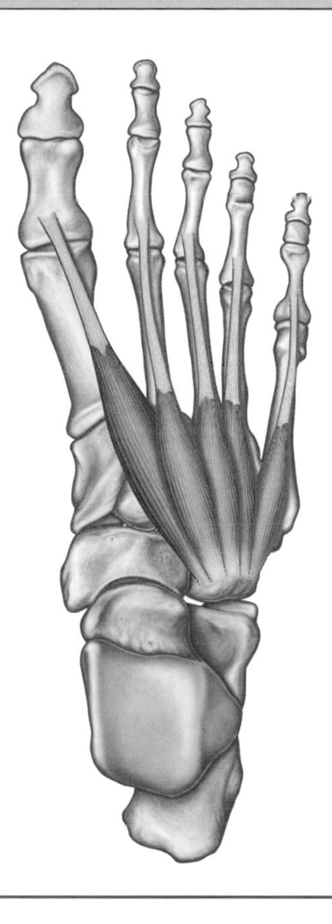

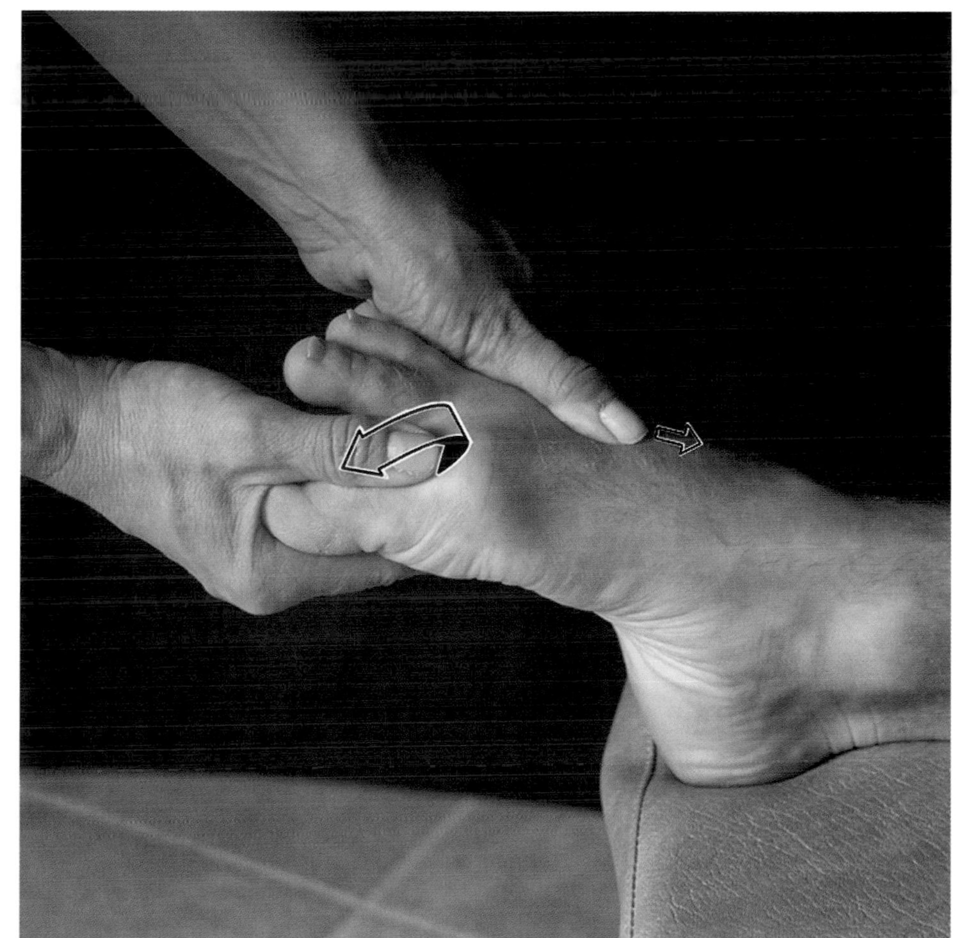

Stretching technique:

Therapist grasps the proximal phalanx of the big toe and pulls it in order to avoid compression of metatarsophalangeal joint. Therapist plantar flexes the big toe while using the thumb of the other hand to stretch along the body of muscle away from the tendon–muscle junction.

Extensor digitorum brevis

Nerve, supply: Deep fibular nerve, S1–2.

Origin: Superior surface of calcaneus and extensor retinaculum.

Insertion: Via the extensor aponeurosis to bases of middle and distal phalanges of toes 2–5.

Muscle to fifth toe is only occasionally present.

Function: Dorsiflexion of toes.

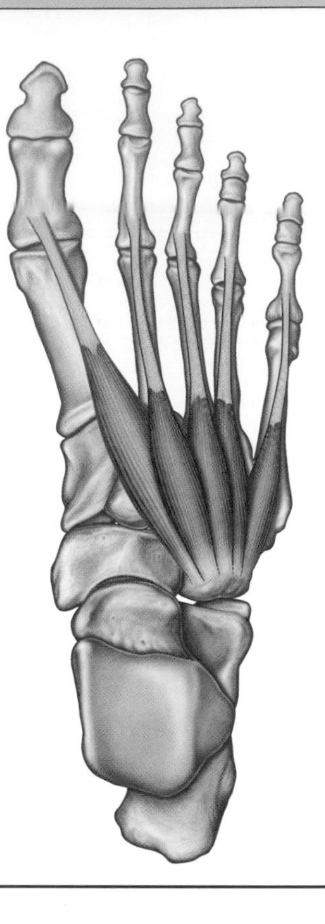

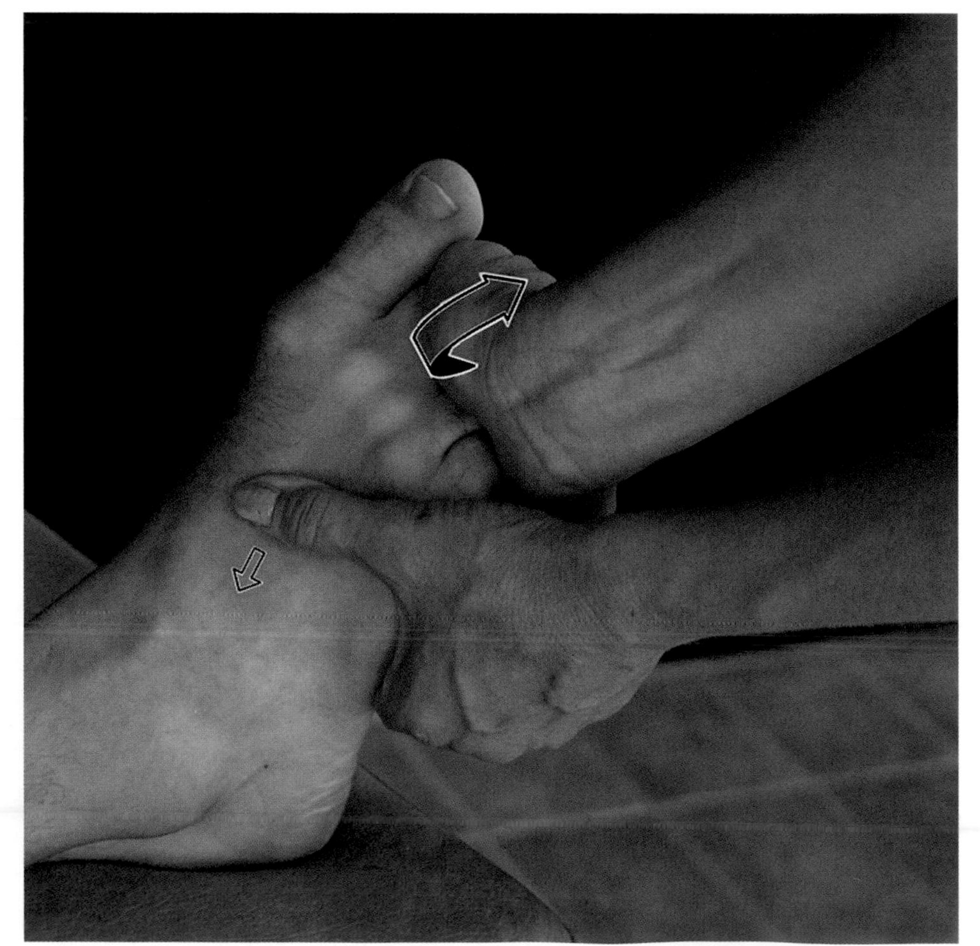

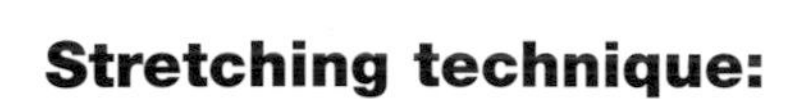

Stretching technique:

Therapist grasps toes and pulls them in order to avoid compression of metatarsophalangeal joints. Therapist plantar flexes toes while using the thumb of the other hand to stretch along body of muscle away from tendon–muscle junction.

Interossei dorsales

(Four muscles between metatarsals)

Nerve, supply: Lateral plantar nerve, S1–2.

Origin: Each arising from two metatarsal bones and from long plantar ligament.

Insertion: Base of the proximal phalanges of the second toe on the medial side and from the second to fourth toes on the lateral side.

Function: Abduction of toes and plantar flexion of metatarsophalangeal joints.

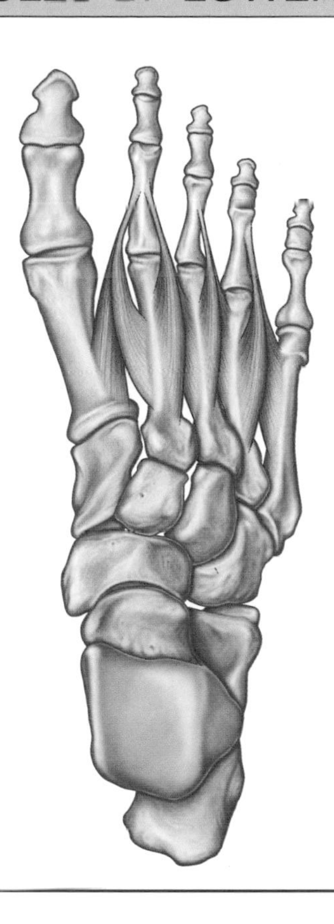

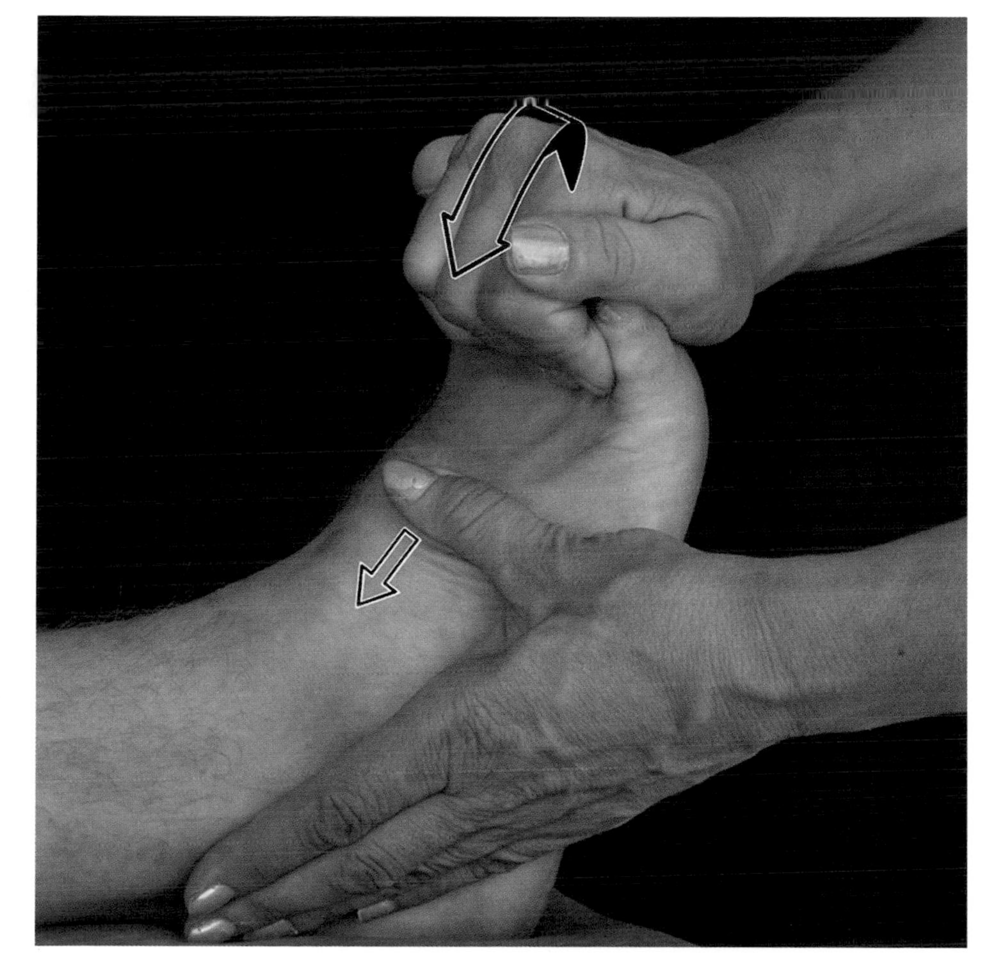

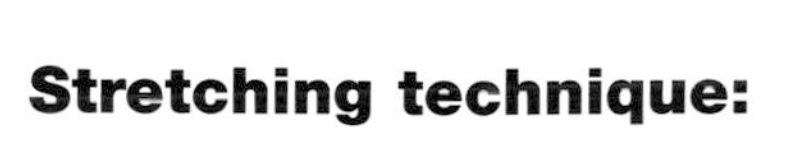

Stretching technique:

Therapist grasps toes and pulls them in order to avoid compression of metatarsophalangeal joints. Therapist bends toes into dorsiflexion while using the thumb of the other hand to stretch between the metatarsals along the bodies of the muscles.

Quadratus plantae (flexor accessories)

Nerve, supply: Lateral plantar nerve, S1–2.

Origin: Calcaneus.

Insertion: Lateral surface of the tendon of flexor digitorum longus inserting at the bases of distal phalanges of toes 2–5.

Function: Plantar flexion of toes. Support longitudinal arch of foot.

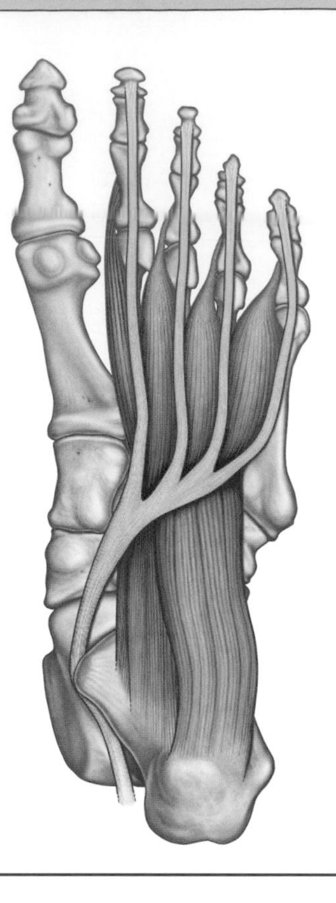

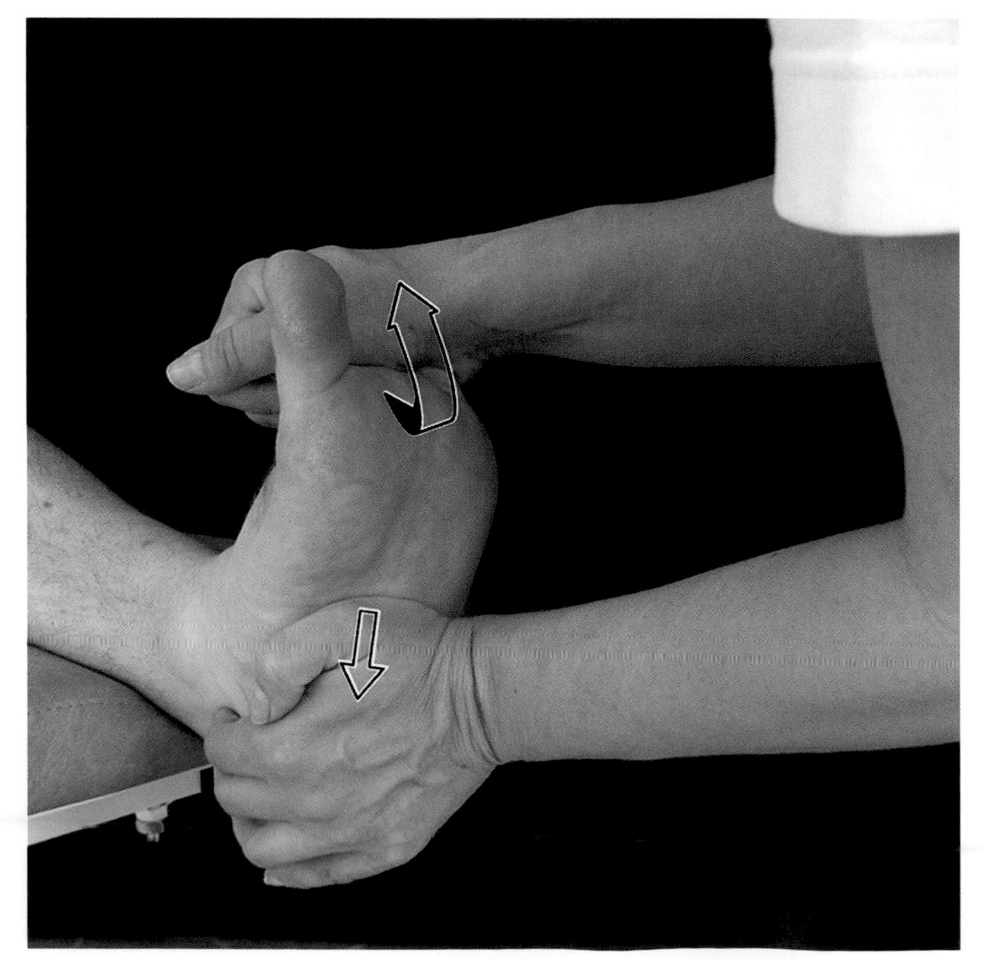

Stretching technique:

Therapist grasps toes 2–5 and pulls them in order to avoid compression of metatarsophalangeal joints. Therapist bends toes into dorsiflexion while using the thenar of the other hand to stretch down along body of muscle away from insertion.

Lumbricales

(Four muscles)

Nerve, supply: Medial plantar nerve, and lateral plantar nerve, L5–S2.

Origin: Arise from the medial surfaces of the individual tendons of the flexor digitorum longus.

Insertion: Medial margin of bases of proximal phalanges of toes 2–5 and extension aponeurosis.

Function: Plantar flexion of metacarpophalangeal joints and adduction towards big toe. Support longitudinal arch of foot.

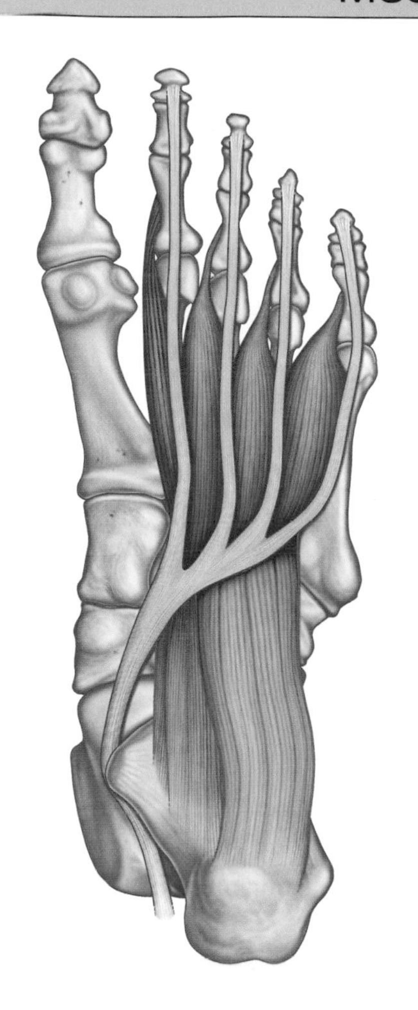

Interossei plantares

(Three muscles between metatarsal bones)

Nerve, supply: Lateral plantar nerve, S1–2.

Origin: Medial surface of metatarsals 3–5 and partially from the long plantar ligament.

Insertion: Medial surface of corresponding proximal phalanges.

Function: Plantar toe flexion and adduct toes together.

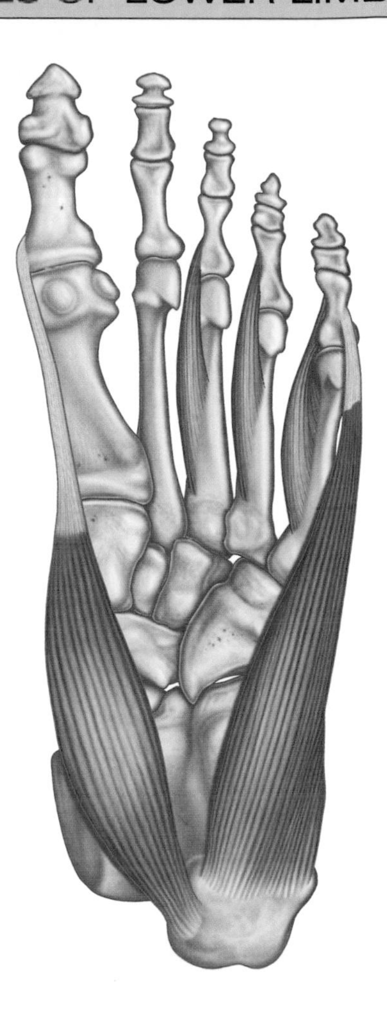

Stretching technique:

Therapist abducts toes from each other by placing fingers in between and bending them into dorsiflexion. The thumb of the other hand is used to stretch between metatarsals along the bodies of the muscles.

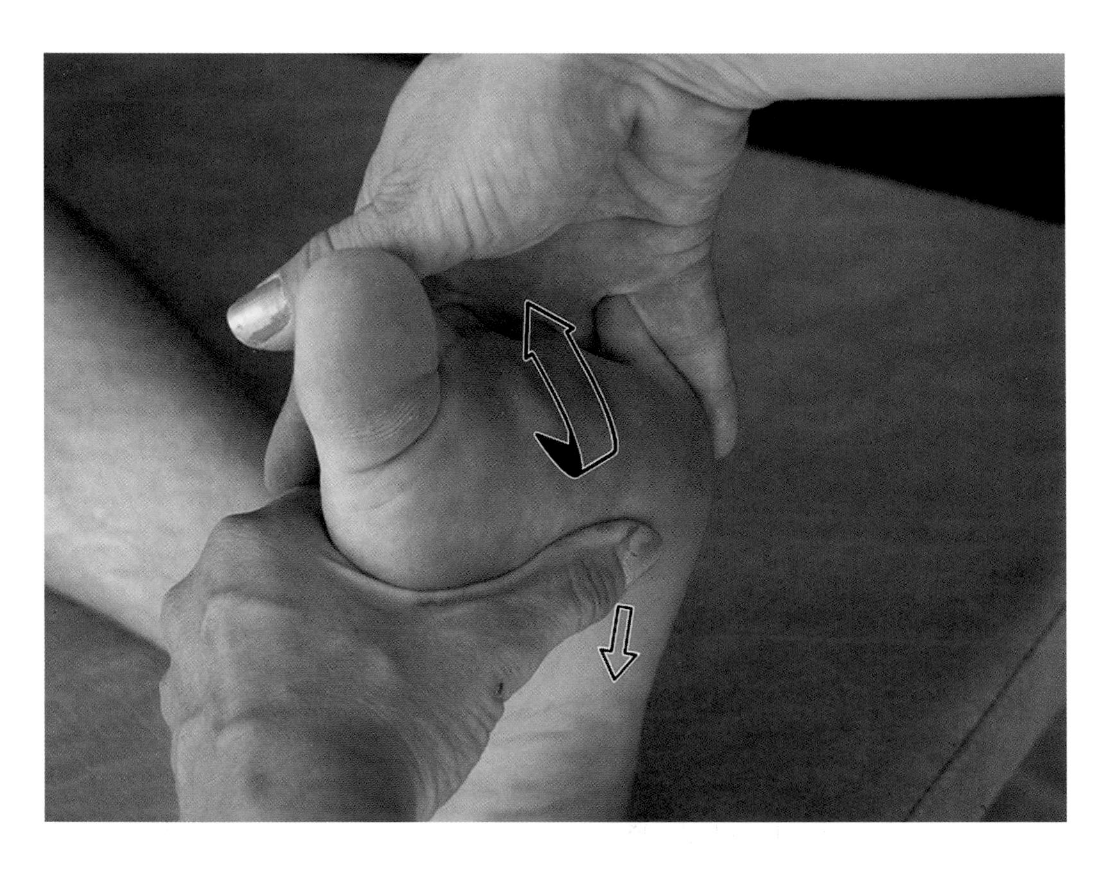

Flexor digitorum brevis

Nerve, supply: Medial plantar nerve, L5–S1.

Origin: Anterior edge of tuber calcanei and proximal part of plantar aponeurosis.

Insertion: Middle phalanges of toes 2–5 via divided tendons.

The muscle to 5th digit may be abcont.

Function: Plantar toe flexion. Supports longitudinal arch of foot.

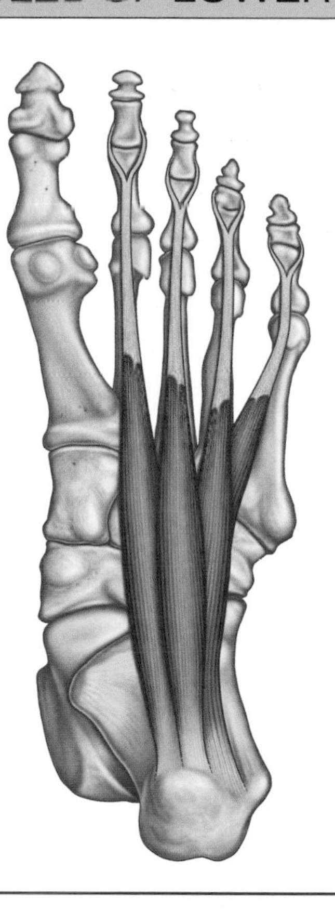

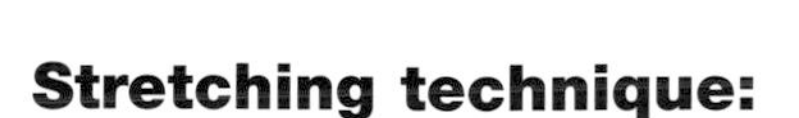

Stretching technique:

Therapist grasps toes and pulls them in order to avoid compression of metatarsophalangeal joints. Therapist stretches toes into dorsiflexion while using the thenar of the other hand to stretch along the muscle down from the tendon–muscle junction.

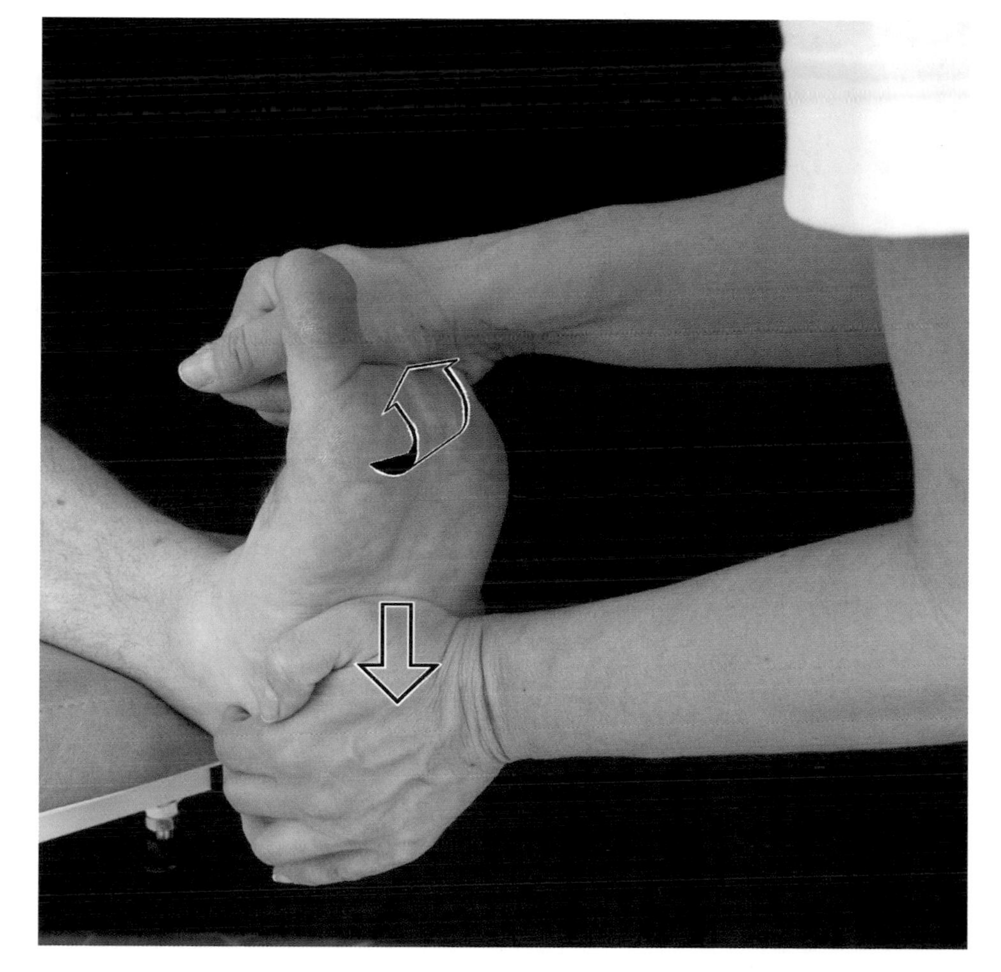

Flexor hallucis brevis

Nerve, supply: Medial plantar nerve, L5–S1.

Origin: Medial cuneiform bone, long plantar ligament, tendon of the tibialis posterior and plantar aponeuroses.

Insertion: Via two heads at base of proximal phalanx and to the medial and lateral sesamoid bones located on the proximal phalanx of big toe.

Function: Plantar flexion of big toe. Supports longitudinal arch of foot.

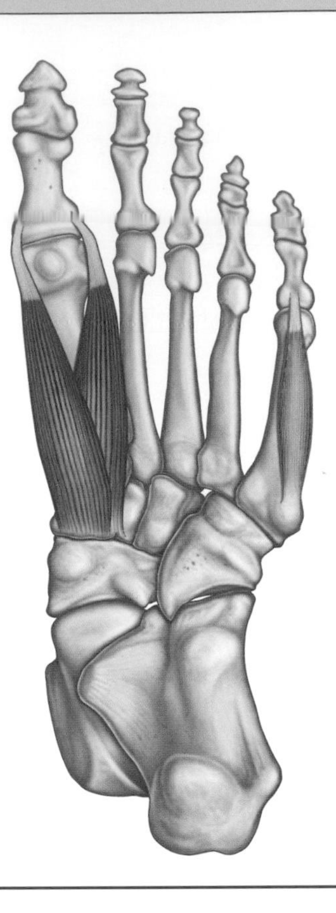

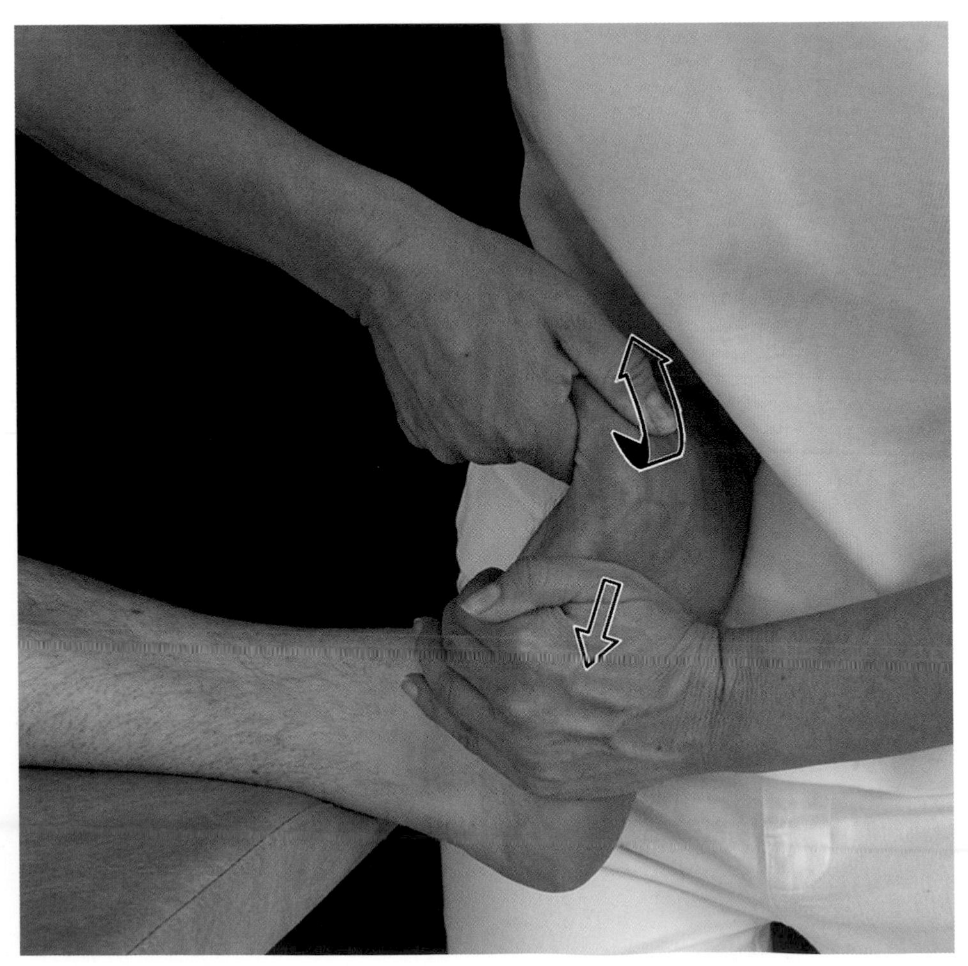

Stretching technique:

Therapist grasps the big toe and pulls it in order to avoid compression of metatarsophalangeal joint. Therapist dorsi flexes big toe while the thenar of the other hand is used to stretch along the muscle body away from the insertion.

Warning ! Pressure on the metatarsophalangeal joint of the big toe should be avoided, as this can lead to joint pain.

Abductor hallucis

Nerve, supply: Medial plantar nerve, L5–S1.

Origin: Medial process of tuber calcanei, flexor retinaculum, and plantar aponeurosis.

Insertion: Medial base of proximal phalanx and medial sesamoid bone of big toe.

Function: Abduction and plantar flexion of big toe. Supports longitudinal arch of foot.

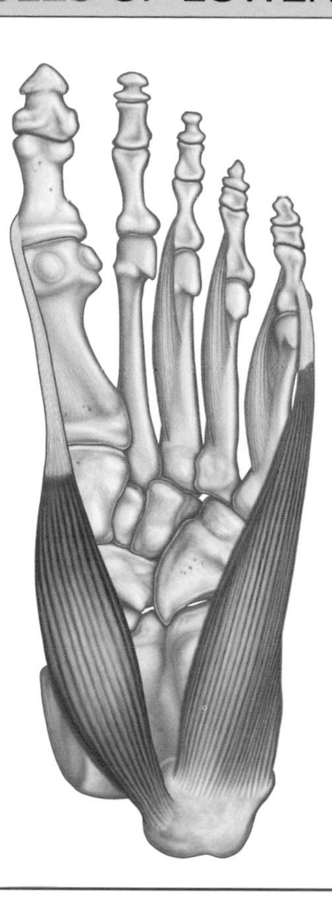

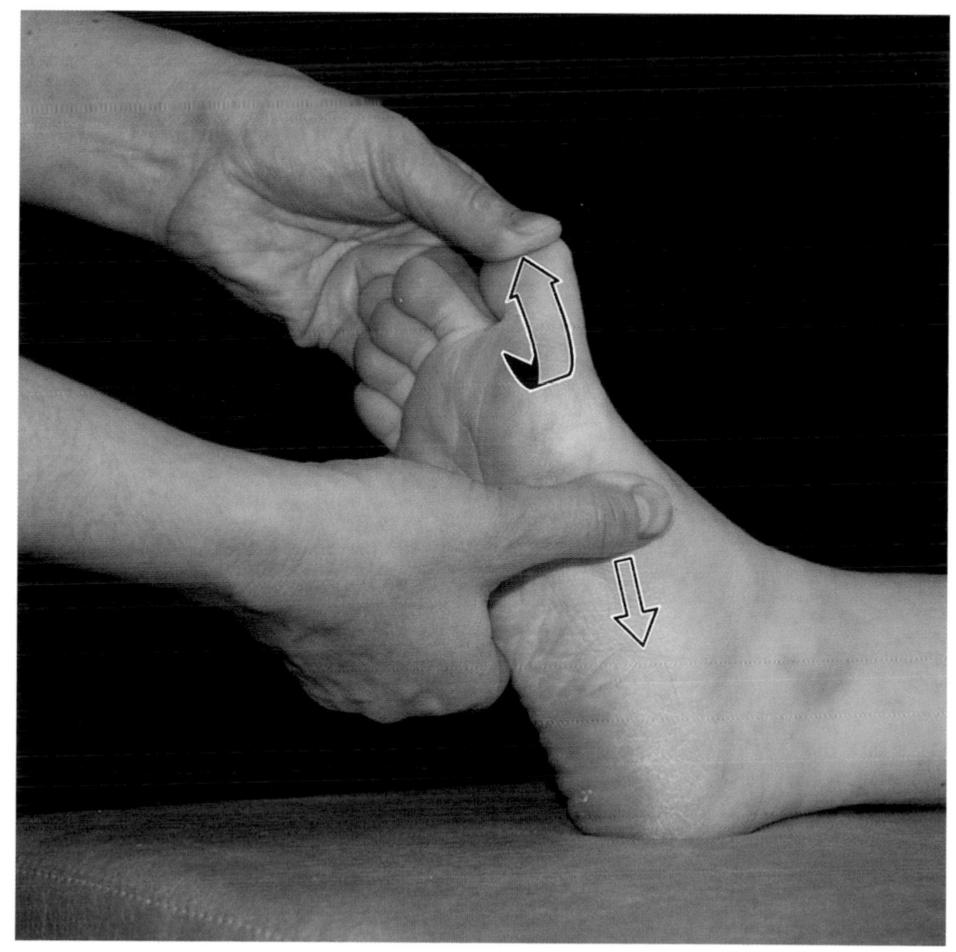

Stretching technique:

Therapist lifts adducts and dorsiflexes the big toe while using the thumb of the other hand to stretch along body of muscle.

Warning ❗ Pressure on the metacarpophalangeal joint of the big toe should be avoided, as this can lead to joint pain.

Adductor hallucis

Nerve, supply: Lateral plantar nerve, S1–2.

Origin: Oblique head from cuboid and lateral cuneiform and bases of metatarsals 2–4, plantar calcaneocuboidal ligament, long plantar ligament and tendon of peroneus longus. Transverse head from capsular ligaments of metatarsophalangeal joint of toes 3–5 and the deep transverse metatarsal ligament.

Insertion: Lateral base of proximal phalanx and lateral sesamoid bone of big toe.

Function: Adduction and plantar flexion of big toe. Supports longitudinal arch of foot.

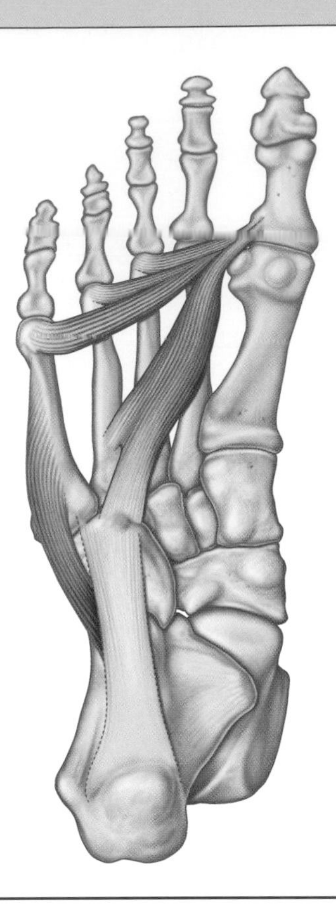

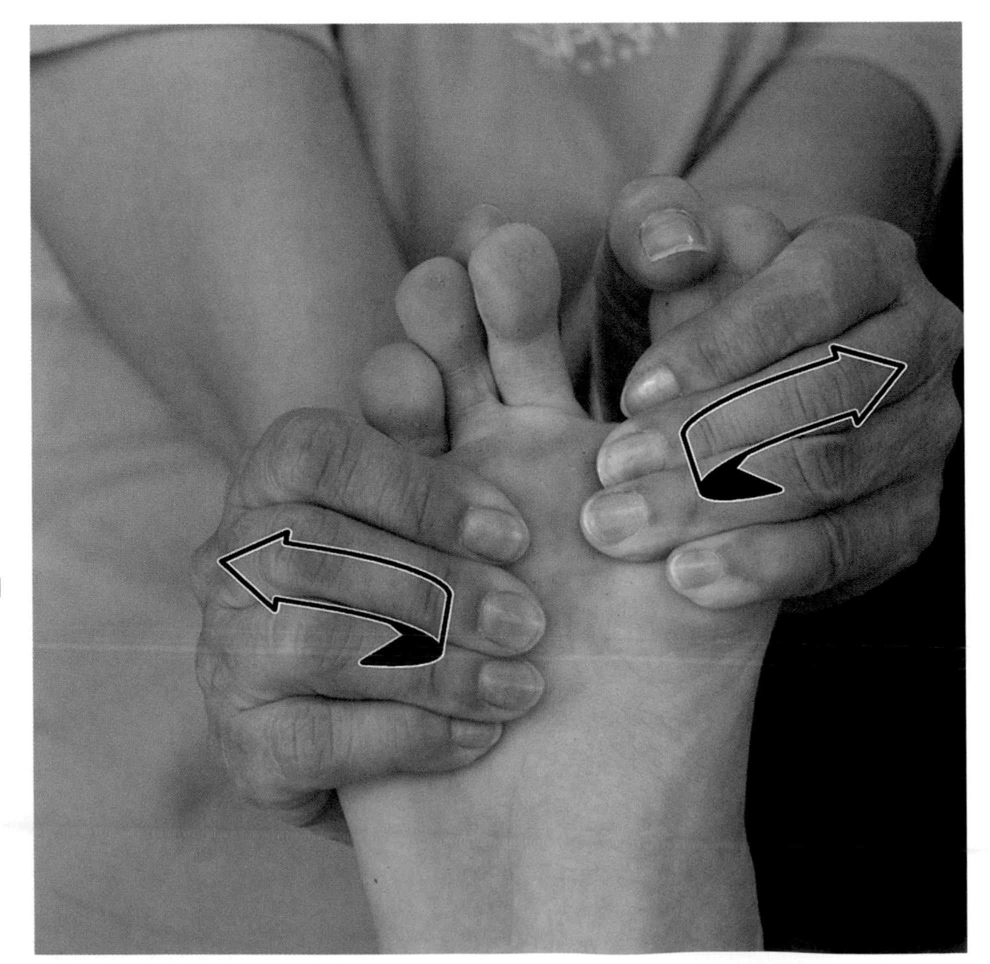

Stretching technique:

Therapist grasps the first metatarsal and big toe she pulls it in order to avoid compression of metatarsophalangeal joint. Therapist abducts and dorsiflexes the big toe. The other hand grasps metatarsals 3–5 and by twisting hands away from each other, the therapist stretches the adductor muscles between the fingers.

Flexor digiti minimi

Nerve, supply: Lateral plantar nerve, S1–2.

Origin: Laterally on base of fifth metatarsal, long plantar ligament and tendon of peroneus longus.

Insertion: Laterally on base of proximal phalanx of little toe.

Function: Flexion and abduction of little toe.

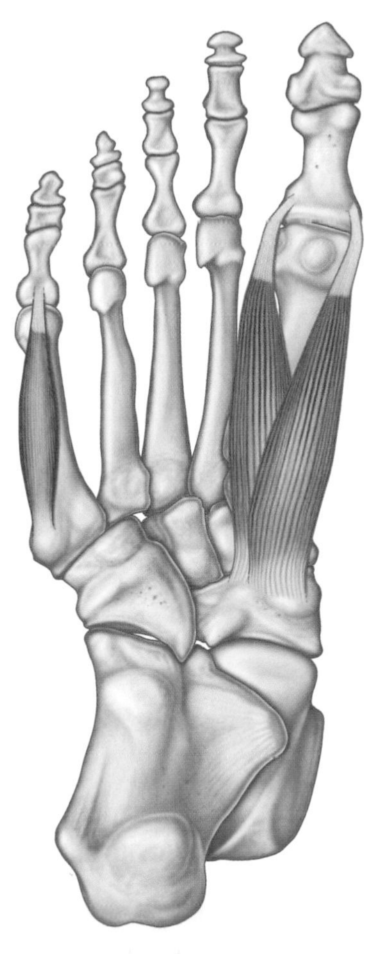

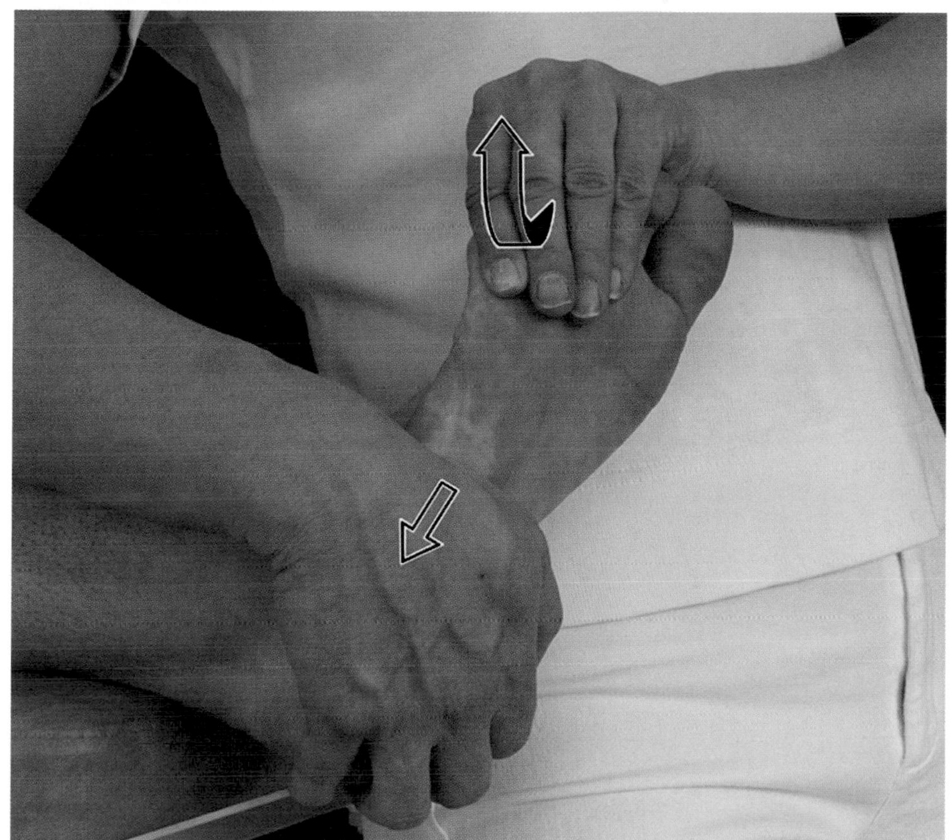

Stretching technique:

Therapist grasps the little toe and the head of fifth metatarsal and dorsiflexes them and adducts the little toe while using the thenar of the other hand to stretch along body of muscle away from insertion.

Abductor digiti minimi pedis

Nerve, supply: Lateral plantar nerve, S1–2.

Origin: Anterior, inferior edge of calcaneous, base of fifth metatarsal and plantar aponeurosis.

Insertion: Laterally on base of proximal phalanx of little toe.

Function: Abduction and flexion of little toe.

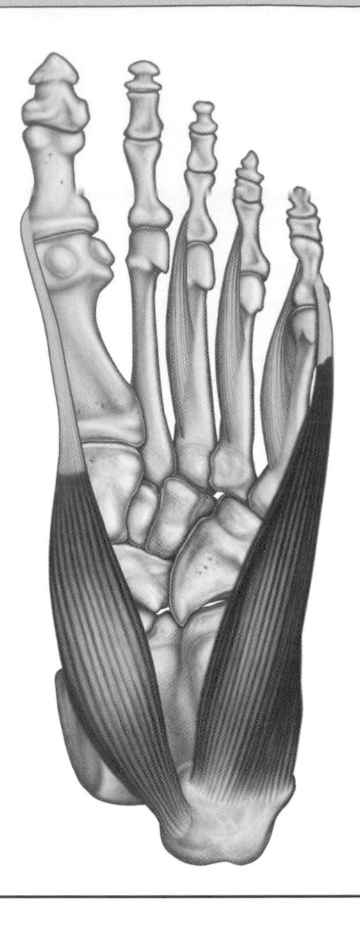

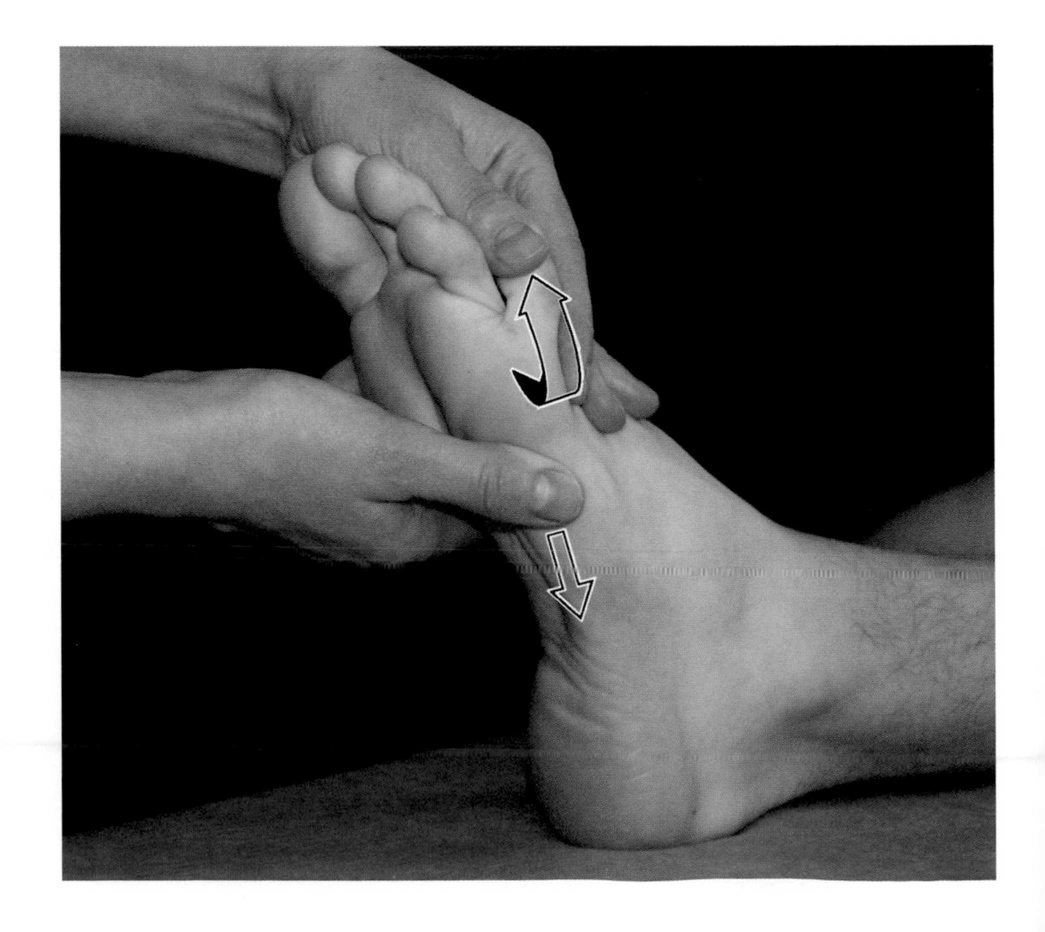

Opponens digiti minimi

Origin: Long plantar ligament and tendon of peroneus longus.

Insertion: Distally on lateral side of fifth metatarsal.

Function: Flex 5th metatarsal and supports lateral arch of foot.

Notice: Opponens digiti minimi is often absent.

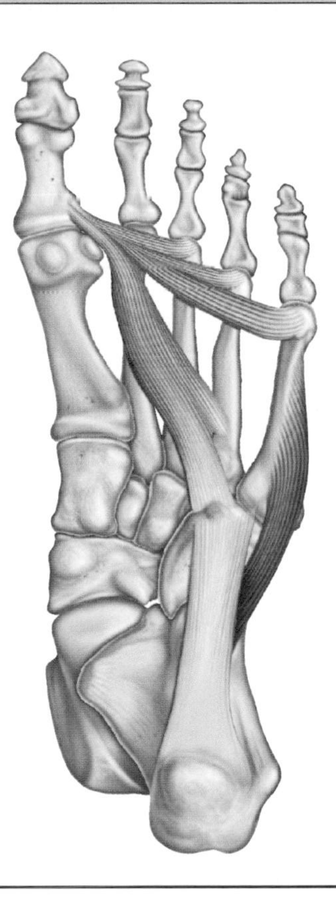

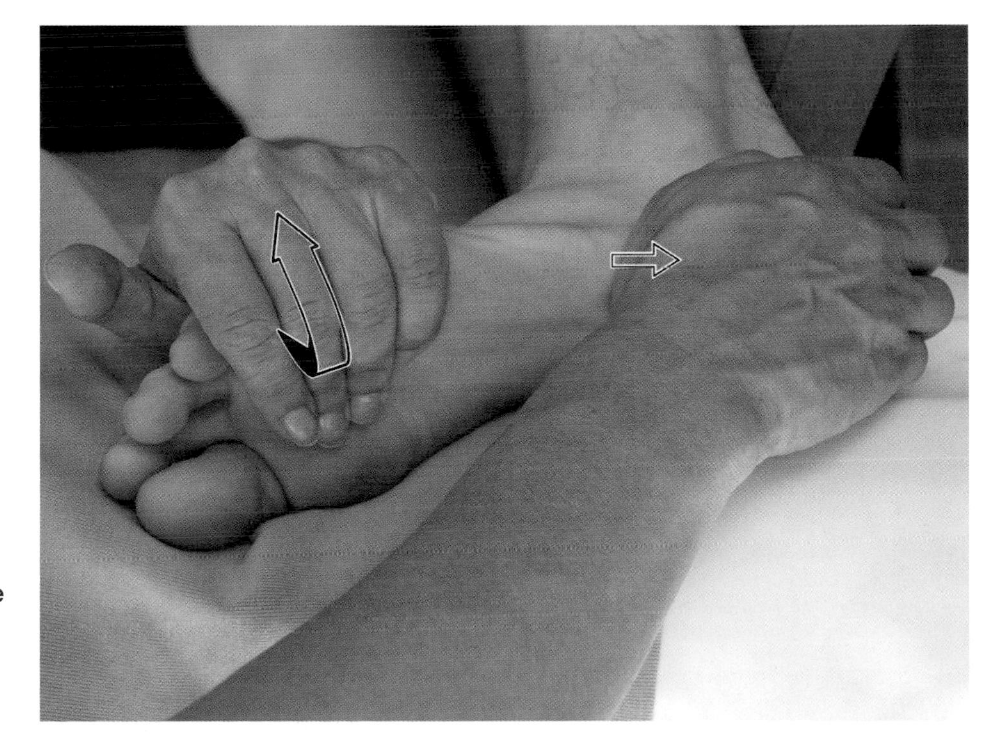

Stretching technique:

Therapist extends and adducts little toe with the thumb while using the thenar of the other hand to stretch along body of muscle.

REFERENCES

Alexander RM, Bennet-Clark HC 1977 Storage of elastic strain energy in muscles and other tissues. Nature 265:114–117

Avela J 1998 Stretch-reflex adaptation in man: interaction between load, fatigue and muscle stiffness. Thesis no 57 University of Jyväskylä, Jyväskylä

Avela J, Kyrüläinen H, Komi PV 1999 Altered reflex sensitivity after repeated and prolonged passive muscle stretching. Journal of Applied Physiology 86:1283–1291

Bandy WD, Irion JIM 1994 The effect of time on static stretch on the flexibility of the hamstring muscles. Physical Therapy 74:845–852

Bandy WD, Irion JIM, Briggler M 1997 The effect of time and frequency of static stretching on flexibility of the hamstring muscles. Physical Therapy 77:1090–1096

Bandy WD, Irion JM, Briggler M 1998 The effect of static stretch and dynamic ROM training on the flexibility of the hamstring muscles. Journal of Orthopaedic and Sports Physical Therapy 27:295–300

Basur RL, Shephard E, Mouzas GI 1976 A cooling method in the treatment of ankle sprains. Practitioner 216:708–711

Baxter MP, Dulberg C 1988 'Growing pains' in childhood a proposal for treatment. Journal of Pediatric Orthopedics 8:402–406

Behm DG, Button DC, Butt JC 2001 Factors affecting force loss with prolonged stretching. Canadian Journal of Applied Physiology 26:262–272

Beighton P, Grahame R, Bird H 1983 Hypermobility of joints. Springer-Verlag, Berlin

Bixler B, Jones RL 1992 High-school football injuries: effects of a post-halftime warm-up and stretching routine. Family Practice Research Journal 12:131–139

Björklund M, Hamberg J, Crenshaw AG 2001 Sensory adaptation after 2-week stretching regimen of the rectus femoris muscle. Archives of Physical Medicine and Rehabilitation 82:1245–1250

Bohannon RW 1984 Effect of repeated eight-min muscle loading on the angle of straight-leg raising. Physical Therapy 64:491–497

Bonebrake AR 1994 A treatment for carpal tunnel syndrome: results of follow-up study. Journal of Manipulative and Physiological Therapeutics 8:565–567

Borms J, Van Roy PV, Santens JP, Haentjens A 1987 Optimal duration of static stretching exercises for improvement of coxo-femoral flexibility. Journal of Sports Science 5:39–47

Bressel E, McNair 2002 The effect of prolonged static and cyclic stretching on ankle joint stiffness, torque relaxation, and gait in people with stroke. Physical Therapy 82:880–887

Brodowicz GR, Welsch R, Wallis J 1996 Comparison of stretching with ice, stretching with heat, or stretching alone on hamstring flexibility. Journal of Athletic Training 31:324–327

Buroker KC, Schwane JA 1989 Does postexercise static stretching alleviate delayed muscle soreness? Physician and Sportsmedicine 17:65–83

Carter AM, Kinzey SJ, Chitwood LF, Cole J 2000 Proprioceptive neuromuscular facilitation decreases muscle activity during the stretch reflex in selected posterior thigh muscles. Sport Rehabil 9:269–278

Chan J, Hong Y, Robinson PD 2001 Flexibility and passive resistance of the hamstrings of young adults using two different static stretching protocols. Scandinavian Journal of Medicine and Science in Sports 11:81–86

Chleboun GS, Howell JN, Conatser RR, Giesey JJ 1997 The relationship between elbow flexor volume and angular stiffness at the elbow. Clinical Biomechanics (Bristol, Avon) 12:383–392

Cipriani D, Abel B, Pirrwitz D 2003 A comparison of two stretching protocols on hip ROM: implications for total daily stretch duration. Journal of strength and conditioning research/National Strength & Conditioning Association 17:274–278

Clark S, Christiansen A, Hellman DF, Hugunin JW, Hurst KM 1999 Effect of ipsilateral anterior thigh soft tissue stretching on passive unilateral straight-leg raise. Journal of Orthopaedic and Sports Physical Therapy 29:4–12

Clarke DH, Stelmach GE 1966 Muscular fatigue and recovery curve parameters at various temperatures. Research Quarterly 37:468–479

Condon SM, Hutton RS 1987 Soleus muscle electromyographic activity and ankle dorsiflexion ROM during four stretching procedures. Physical Therapy 67:24–30

Cook AC, Szabo RM, Birkholz SW, King EF 1995 Early mobilization following carpal tunnel release. A prospective randomized study. Journal of Hand Surgery 2(B):228–230

Cornelius WL, Hinson MM 1984 The relationship between isometric contractions of hip extensors and subsequent flexibility in males. Journal of Sports Medicine and Fitness 20:75–80

Cornelius WL, Ebrahim K, Watson J, Hill DW 1992 The effects of cold application and modified PNF stretching techniques on hip joint flexibility in college males. Research Quarterly for Exercise and Sport 63:311–314

Cornwell A, Nelson AG, Heise GD, Sidaway B 2001 Acute effects of passive muscle stretching on vertical jump performance. Journal of Human Movement Studies 40:307–324

Cornwell A, Nelson AG, Sidaway B 2000 Acute effects of stretching on the neuromechanical properties of the triceps surae muscle complex. European Journal of Applied Physiology 86:428–434

Crosman LJ, Chateauvert SR, Weisberg J 1984 The effects of massage to the hamstring muscle group on the ROM. Journal of Orthopaedic and Sports Physical Therapy 6:168–172

Dalenbring S, Schuldt K, Ekholm J, Stenroth 1999 Location and intensity of focal and referred pain provoked by maintained extreme rotation position of the cervical spine in healthy females. Eur J Phys Med Rehabil 8:170–177

De Vries H 1962 Evaluation of static stretching procedures for improvement of flexibility. Research Quarterly 3:222–229

De Weijer VC, Gorniak GC, Shamus E 2003 The effect of static stretch and warm-up exercise on hamstring length over the course of 24 hs. Journal of Orthopaedic and Sports Physical Therapy 33:727–733

Draper DO, Castro JL, Feland B, Schulthies S, Eggett D 2004 Shortwave diathermy and prolonged stretching increase hamstring flexibility more than prolonged stretching alone. Journal of Orthopaedic and Sports Physical Therapy 34:13–20

Draper DO, Ricard MD 1995 Rate of temperature decay in human muscle following 3 MHz ultrasound: the stretching window revealed. Journal of Athletic Training 30:304–307

Duong B, Low M, Moseley AM, Lee RY, Herbert RD 2001 Time course of stress relaxation and recovery in human ankles. Clinical Biomechanics 16:601–607

Dyck P 1984 Lumbar nerve root: the enigmatic eponyms. Spine 9:3–6

Ekstrand J, Giliquist J, Liljedahl SO 1983 Prevention of soccer injuries: supervision by doctor and physiotherapist. American Journal of Sports Medicine 11:116–120

Ekstrand J, Wiktorsson M, Öberg B, Gillquist J 1982 Lower extremity goniometric measurements: a study to determine their reliability. Archives of Physical Medicine and Rehabilitation 63:171–175

Elnaggar IM, Nordin M, Sheikhzadeh A, Parniapour M, Kahanovitz N 1991 Effects of spinal flexion and extension exercises on low-back pain and spinal mobility in chronic mechanical low-back pain patients. Spine 16:967–972

Enoka RM 1994 Neuromechanical basis of kinesiology. Human Kinetics, Champaign, IL

Etnyre BR, Abraham LD 1986 Gains in range of ankle dorsiflexion using three popular stretching techniques. American Journal of Physical Medicine 65:189–196

Etnyre BR, Abraham LD 1986 H-reflex changes during static stretching and two variations of proprioceptive neuromuscular facilitation techniques. Electroencephalography and Clinical Neurophysiology 63:174–179

Etnyre BR, Lee EJ 1988 Chronic and acute flexibility of men and women using three different stretching techniques. Research Quarterly in Exercise and Sport 59:222–228

Feland JB, Marin HN 2004 Effect of submaximal contraction intensity in Contract-relax proprioceptive neuromuscular facilitation stretching. British Journal of Sports Medicine 38:e18

Feland JB, Myrer JW, Merrill RM 2001a Acute changes in hamstring flexibility: PNF versus static stretch in senior athletes. Physical Therapy Sport 2:186–193

Feland JB, Myrer JW, Schulthies SS, Fellingham GW, Meason GW 2001b The effect of duration of stretching of the hamstring muscle group for increasing range of motion in people aged 65 years or older. Physical Therapy 81:1110–1117

Feretti G, Ishii M, Moia C, Ceretelli P 1992 Effects of temperature on the maximal instantaneous muscle power of humans. Journal of Applied Physiology 63:112–116

Fowles JR, Sale DG, MacDougall JD 2000 Reduced strength after passive stretch of the human plantar flexors. Journal of Applied Physiology 89:1179–1188

Frankeny IR, Holly RG, Ashmore R 1983 Effects of graded duration of stretch on normal and dystrophic skeletal muscle. Muscle Nerve 6:269–277

Frisen M, Magi M, Viidik A 1969 Rhelogical analysis of collagenous tissue: part I. Journal of Biomechanics 2:13–20

Funk D, Swank AM, Adams KJ, Treolo D 2001 Efficacy of moist heat pack application over static stretching on hamstring flexibility. Journal of

Strength and Conditioning Research/National Strength & Conditioning Association 15:123–126
Gajdosik RL 1991 Effects of static stretching on the maximal length and resistance to passive stretch of short hamstring muscles. Journal of Orthopedic and Sports Physical Therapy 14:250–255
Garfinkel MS, Singhal A, Katz WA, Allan DA, Reshetar R, Schumacher HR Jr 1998 Yoga-based intervention for carpal tunnel syndrome: a randomized trial. JAMA: Journal of the American Medical Association 11(280): 1601–1603
Garrett WE, Nikolaou PK, Ribbeck BM, Glisson RR, Seaber AV 1988 The effect of muscle architecture on the biomechanical failure properties of skeletal muscle under passive extension. American Journal of Sports Medicine 16:7–12
Gerritsen AA, de Vet HC, Scholten RJ, Bertelsmann FW, de Krom MC, Bouter LM 2002 Splinting vs surgery in the treatment of carpal tunnel syndrome: a randomized controlled trial. JAMA: Journal of the American Medical Association 11:288:1245–1251
Girouard CK, Hurley BF 1995 Does strength training inhibit gains in ROM from flexibility training in older adults? Medicine and Science in Sports and Exercise 27:1444–1449
Gleim GW, Stachenfeld NS, Nicholas JA 1990 The influence of flexibility on the economy of walking and jogging. Journal of Orthopaedic Research 8:814–823
Godges JJ, MacRae H, Longdon C 1989 The effects of two stretching procedures on hip range of motion and gait economy. Journal of Orthopedic Sports Physical Therapy 10:350–357
Godges JJ, MacRae PG, Engelke K 1993 Effects of exercise on hip ROM, trunk muscle performance, and gait economy. Physical Therapy 73:468–477
Goldspink G, Scutt A, Loughna PT, Wells DJ, Jaenicke T, Gerlach GF 1992 Gene expression in skeletal muscle in response to stretch and force generation. American Journal of Physiology 262:356–363
Goldspink G, Tabary C, Tabary JC 1974 Effect of denervation on the adaptation of sarcomere number and muscle extensibility to the functional length of the muscle. Journal of Physiology 236:733–742
Grady JF, Saxena A 1991 Effects of stretching the gastrocnemius muscle. Journal of Foot Surgery 30:465–469
Guissard N, Duchateau J, Hainaut K 1988 Muscle stretching and neuron excitability. European Journal of Applied Physiology 58:47–52
Guissard N, Duchateau J, Hainaut K 2001 Mechanisms of decreased motoneurone excitation during passive muscle stretching. Experimental Brain Research 137:163–169
Gunn CC 1996 The Gunn approach to the treatment of chronic pain. Churchill Livingstone, Edinburgh
Göeken LN, Hof AL 1991 Instrumental straight-leg raising: a new approach to Lasegue's test. Archives of Physical Medicine and Rehabilitation 72:959–967
Haggmark E, Jansson E, Eriksson E 1981 Fibre type and metabolic potential of the thigh muscle in man after knee surgery and immobilization. International Journal of Sports Medicine 2:12–17
Halar EM, Stolov WC, Venkatesh B, Brozovich RV, Harley JD 1978 Gastrocnemius muscle belly and tendon length in stroke patients and able-bodied persons. Archives of Physical Medicine and Rehabilitation 59:476–484
Halbertsma JPK, Göeken LN 1994 Stretching exercises: effect on passive extensibility and stiffness in short hamstrings of healthy subjects. Archives of Physical Medicine and Rehabilitation 75:976–981
Halbertsma JPK, Göeken LNH, Hof AL, Groothoff JW, Eisma WH 2001 Extensibility and stiffness of the hamstrings in patients with nonspecific low back pain. Archives of Physical Medicine and Rehabilitation 82:232–238
Halbertsma JPK, Mulder I, Göeken LNH, Eisma WH 1999 Repeated passive stretching: acute effect on the passive muscle moment and extensibility of short hamstrings. Archives of Physical Medicine and Rehabilitation 80:407–414
Halbertsma JPK, van Bolhuis AI, Göeken LN 1996 Sport stretching: effect on passive muscle stiffness of short hamstrings. Archives of Physical Medicine and Rehabilitation 77:688–692
Hardy L 1985 Improving active range of hip flexion. Research Quarterly for Exercise and Sport 56:111–114
Harms-Ringdahl K, Ekholm J 1986 Intensity and character of pain and muscular activity levels elicitated by maintained extreme flexion position of the lower cervical and upper thoracic spine. Scandinavian Journal of Rehabilitation Medicine 18:117–126
Hartig DE, Henderson JM 1999 Increasing hamstring flexibility decreases lower extremity overuse injuries in military basic trainees. American Journal of Sports Medicine 27:173–176
Hartley-O'Brien SJ 1980 Six mobilization exercises for active range of hip flexion. Research Quarterly for Exercise and Sport 51:625–635
Harvey LA, Batty J, Crosbie J, Poulter S, Herbert RD 2000 A randomized trial assessing the effects of 4 weeks of daily stretching on ankle mobility in patients with spinal cord injuries. Archives of Physical Medicine and Rehabilitation 81:1340–7
Harvey LA, Byak AJ, Ostrovskaya M, Glinsky J, Katte L, Herbert R 2003 Randomised trial of the effects of four weeks of daily stretch on extensibility of hamstring muscles in people with spinal cord injuries. Australian Journal of Physiotherapy 49:176–181
Henricson A, Larsson A, Olsson E, Westlin N 1983 The effect of stretching on the ROM of the ankle joint in badminton players. Journal of Orthopedic Sports Physical Therapy 5:74–77
High DM, Howley ET, Franks BD 1989 The effects of static stretching on prevention of DOMS. Research Quarterly Exercise and Sports 60:357–361
Hocutt J, Jaffe R, Rylander CR, Bebbe JK 1982 Cryotherapy in ankle sprains. American Journal of Sports Medicine 10:316–319
Holt LE, Smith RK 1983 The effects of selected stretching programs on active and passive flexibility. In: Terauds J (ed) Biomechanics in sport: 54–67
Holt LE, Travis TM, Okita T 1970 Comparative study of three stretching techniques. Perceptual and Motor Skills 31:611–616
Hoover HV 1958 Functional technic. Acad Appl Osteop Yearbook 47–51
Hornsby T, Nicholson G, Gossman M, Culpepper M 1987 Effect of inherent muscle length on isometric plantar torque in healthy women. Physical Therapy 67:1991–1997
Hortobagyi T, Faludi J, Tihanyi J, Merkely B 1985 Effects of intense stretching — flexibility training on the mechanical profile of the knee extensors and on the ROM of the hip joint. International Journal of Sports Medicine 6:317–321
Howell DW 1984 Musculoskeletal profile and incidence of musculoskeletal injuries in lightweight women rowers. American Journal of Sports Medicine 12:278–282
Hugh MP, Magnusson SP, Gleim GW, Nicholas JA 1992 Viscoelastic stress relaxation in human skeletal muscle. Medicine and Science in Sports and Exercise 24:1375–1382
Issurin VB, Lieberman VG, Tenenbaum G 1994 Effect of vibratory stimulation training on maximal force and flexibility. Journal of Sports Science 12:561–566
Jayaraman et al 2004 MRI evaluation of topical heat and static stretching as therapeutic modalities for the treatment of eccentric exercise-induced muscle damage. In press
Johansson PH, Lindström L, Sundelin G, Lindström B 1999 The effect of pre-exercise stretching on muscular soreness, tenderness and force loss following heavy eccentric training. Scandinavian Journal of Medicine and Science in Sports 9:219–225
Johns RJ, Wright V 1962 Relative importance of various tissues in joint stiffness. Journal of Applied Physiology 17:824–828
Jones AM 2002 Running economy is negatively related to sit-and-reach test performance in international-standard distance runners. International Journal of Sports Medicine 23:40–43
Jones LH 1981 Strain and counterstrain. American Academy of Osteopathy, Colorado Springs
Khalil TM, Asfour SS, Martinez LM, Waly SM, Rosomoff RS, Rosomoff HL 1992 Stretching in rehabilitation of low-back pain patients. Spine 17:311–317
Kjær M, Langberg H, Skovgaard D, Olesen J. Bulow J, Krogsgaard M, Boushel R 2000 In vivo studies of peritendinous tissue exercise. Scand J Med Sci :326–331
Klinge K, Magnusson SP, Simonsen EB, Aagaard P, Klausen K, Kjær M 1997 The effect of strength and flexibility training on skeletal muscle EMG, stiffness and viscoelastic response. American Journal of Sports Medicine 25:710–716
Knight CA, Rutledge CR, Cox ME, Acosta M, Hall SJ 2001 Effect of superficial heat, deep heat, and active exercise warm-up on the extensibility of the plantar flexors. Physical Therapy 81:1206–1214
Knott M, Voss DE 1968 Proprioceptive neuromuscular facilitation, 2nd edn. Harper and Row, New York
Kokkonen J, Nelson AG, Cornwell A 1998 Acute muscle stretching inhibits maximal strength performance. Research Quarterly in Exercise and Sports 69:411–415
Krivickas LS, Feinberg JH 1996 Lower extremity injuries in college athletes: relation between ligamentous laxity and lower extremity muscle tightness. Archives of Physical Medicine and Rehabilitation 77:1139–1143

Kroll PG, Goodwin ME, Nelson TL, Ranelli DM, Roos K 2001 The effect of increased hamstring flexibility on peak torque, work, and power production in subjects with seventy degrees or greater of straight leg raise. Physical Therapy 81:A2

Kubo K, Kanehisa H, Kawakami Y, Fukunaga T 2000a Elasticity of tendon structures of the lower limbs in sprinters. Acta Physiologica Scandinavica 168:327–335

Kubo K, Kanehisa H, Takeshita D, Kawakami Y, Fukashiro, Fukunaga T 2000b In vivo dynamics of human medial gastrocnemius muscle-tendon complex during stretch-shortening cycle exercise. Acta Physiologica Scandinavica 170:127–135

Kubo K, Kawakami Y, Fukunaga T 1999 The influence of elastic properties of tendon structures on jump performance in humans. Journal of Applied Physiology 87:2090–2096

Kubo K, Kanehisa H, Fukunaga T 2002 Effects of transient muscle contractions and stretching on the tendon structures in vivo. Acta Physiologica Scandinavica 175:157–164

Kyröläinen H, Belli A, Komi PV 2001 Biomechanical factors affecting running economy. Medicine and Science in Sports and Exercise 33:1330–1337

Læssøe U, Voigt M 2004 Modification of stretch tolerance in a stooping position. Scandinavian Journal of Medicine and Science in Sports 14:239–244

Lehmann JF, Masock AJ, Warren CG, Koblanski JN 1970 Effect of therapeutic temperatures on tendon extensibility. Archives of Physical Medicine and Rehabilitation 51:481–487

Leivseth G, Torstensson J, Reikerrås O 1989 Effect of passive muscle stretching in osteoarthritis of the hip joint. Clinical Science 76:113–117

Lentell G, Hetherington T, Eagan J, Morgan M 1992 The use of thermal agents to influence the effectiveness of a low-load prolonged stretch. Journal of Orthopaedic and Sports Physical Therapy 16:200–207

Li Y, Mc Cure PW, Pratt N 1996 The effect of hamstring muscle stretching on standing posture and on lumbar and hip motions during forward bending. Physical Therapy 26:836–849

Lin YH 2003 Effects of thermal therapy in improving the passive range of knee motion: comparison of cold and superficial heat applications. Clinical Rehabilitation 17:618–623

Lucas R, Koslow R 1984 Comparative study of static, dynamic and proprioceptive neuromuscular facilitation stretching techniques on flexibility. Perceptual and Motor Skills 58:615–618

Lund H, Vestergaard-Poulsen P, Kanstrup I-L, Sejrsen E 1998 The effects of passive stretching on delayed onset muscle soreness, and other detrimental effects following eccentric exercise. Scandinavian Journal of Medicine and Science in Sports 8:216–221

Madding S, Wong JG, Hallum A, Medeiros JM 1987 Effect of duration of passive stretch on hip abduction range of motion. Journal of Orthopaedic and Sports Physical Therapy 8:409–416

Magnusson PA 1998 Biomechanical evaluation of human skeletal muscle during stretch. Thesis, Kobenhavns Universitet, Lageforeningens forlag

Magnusson SP, Aagaard, P, Simonsen EB, Bojsen-Møller F 2000 Passive tensile stress and energy of the human hamstring muscles in vivo. Scandinavian Journal of Medicine and Science in Sports 10:351–359

Magnusson SP, Simonsen EB, Aagaard P 1996 A mechanism for altered flexibility in human skeletal muscle. Journal of Physiology 497:291–298

Magnusson SP, Simonsen EB, Aagaard P, Dyhre-Poulsen P, McHugh MP, Kjaer M 1996 Mechanical and physiological responses to stretching with and without preisometric contraction in human skeletal muscle. Archives of Physical Medicine and Rehabilitation 77:373

Magnusson SP, Simonsen EB, Aagaard P, Gleim GW, McHugh MP, Kjær M 1995 Viscoelastic response to repeated static stretching in the human hamstring muscle. Scandinavian Journal of Medicine and Science in Sports 5:342–347

McCarthy PW, Olsen JP, Smeby IH 1997 Effects of contract-relax stretching procedures on active range of motion of the cervical spine in the transverse plane. Clinical Biom 12:136–138

McGlynn GH, Laughlin NT, Rowe V 1979 Effect of electromyographic feedback and static stretching on artificially induced muscle soreness. American Journal of Physical Medicine 58:139–148

McHugh MP, Kremenic IJ, Fox MB, Gleim GNL 1998 The role of mechanical and neural restraints to joint range of motion during passive stretch. Medicine and Science in Sports and Exercise 30:928–932

McNair PJ, Dombroski EW, Hewson DJ, Stanley SN 2000 Stretching at the ankle joint: viscoelastic responses to holds and continuous passive motion. Medicine and Science in Sports and Exercise 33:354–358.

McNair PJ, Stanley SN 1996 Effect of passive stretching and jogging on the series elastic muscle stiffness and range of motion of the ankle joint. British Journal of Sports Medcine 30:313–318 Lisää??

Medeiros JM, Smidt GL, Burmeister LF, Soderberg G 1977 The influence of isometric exercise and passive stretch on hip joint motion. Physical Therapy; 57:518–523

Melzack R, Wall PD 1965 Pain mechanisms: a new theory. Science 150:971–979

Merrick MA, Bernard KD, Devor ST, Williams JM 2003 Identical 3-MHz ultrasound treatments with different devices produce different intramuscular temperatures. Journal of Orthopaedic and Sports Physical Therapy 33:379–385

Mitchell F Jnr, Moran PS, Pruzzo N 1979 An evaluation and treatment manual of osteopathic muscle energy procedures. Valley Park, IL

Moore M, Hutton R 1980 Electromyographic investigation of muscle stretching techniques. Medicine and Science in Sports and Exercise 12:322–329

Möller M, Ekstrand J, Öberg B, Gillquist J 1985 Duration of stretching effect on range of motion in lower extremities. Archives of Physical Medicine and Rehabilitation 66:171–173

Möller MH, Öberg B, Gillquist J 1985 Stretching exercise and soccer: effect of stretching on range of motion in the lower extremity in connection with soccer training. International Journal of Sports Medicine 6:50–52

Nelson AG, Kokkonen J, Eldredge C, Cornwell A, Glickman-Weiss E 2001 Chronic stretching and running economy. Scandinavian Journal of Medicine and Science in Sports 11:260–265

Newham DJ, McPhail G, Mills KR, Edwards RHT 1983 Ultrastructural changes after concentric and eccentric contractions of human muscle. Journal of the Neurological Sciences 61:109–122

Noonan TJ, Best TM, Seaber AV, Garrett WE 1993 Identification of a threshold for skeletal muscle injury. American Journal of Sports Medicine 22:257–261

Osternig L, Robertson R, Troxel R, Hansen P 1987 Muscle activation during proprioceptive neuromuscular facilitation (PNF) stretching techniques. American Journal of Physical Medicine 66:298–307

Osterning LR, Robertson RN, Troxel RK, Hansen P 1990 Differential responses to proprioceptive neuromuscular facilitation (PNF) stretch techniques. Medicine and Science in Sports and Exercise 22:106–111

Payne J, Morin S, Seibeneicher S, Langois M 2003 Comparison of three stretching techniques of the hamstring muscles on quadriceps and hamstring muscle strength. Journal of Orthopaedic and Sports Physical Therapy 33:A–39

Pope RP, Herbert RD, Kirwan JD, Graham BJ 1998 Effects of ankle dorsiflexion range and pre-exercise calf muscle on injury risk in army recruits. Aus J Phys 44:165–172

Pope RP, Herbert RD, Kirwan JD, Graham BJ 2000 A randomized trial of preexercise stretching for prevention of lower-limb injury. Medicine and Science in Sports and Exercise 32:271–277

Prentice WE 1983 A comparison of static and PNF stretching for improvement of hipjoint flexibility. Athletic Training 18:56–59

Reid J 1960 Effects of extension movements of the head and spine upon the spinal cord and nerve roots. J Neurol Neurosurg Psychiatry 23:214–221

Rosenbaum D, Hennig E 1995 The influence of stretching and warm-up exercises on Achilles tendon reflex activity. Journal of Sports Science 13:481–490

Rozmaryn LM, Dovelle S, Rothman ER, Gorman K, Olvey KM, Bartko JJ 1998 Nerve and tendon gliding exercises and the conservative management of carpal tunnel syndrome. Journal of Hand Therapy 11:171–179

Sady J, Wortman M, Blanke D 1982 Flexibility training: ballistic, static, or PNF? Archives of Physical Medicine and Rehabilitation 63:261–263

Sawyer PC, Uhl TL, Mattacola CG, Johnson DL, Yates JW 2003 Effects of moist heat on hamstring flexibility and muscle temperature. Journal of Strength and Conditioning Research 17: 285–290

Seradge H, Jia YC, Owens W 1993 In vivo measurement of carpal tunnel pressure in the functioning hand. Journal of Hand Surgery 20A:855–859

Simons DG, Travell JG, Simons LS 1999 Travell & Simons' myofascial pain and dysfunction: the trigger point manual, 2nd edn. Williams & Wilkins, Baltimore

Smith LL, Brunetz MH, Chenier T 1993 The effects of static and ballistic stretching on DOMS and creatine kinase. Research Quarterly for Exercise and Sport 64:103–107

Solveborn SA 1997 Radial epigondyalgia ('tennis elbow'): treatment with stretching on forearm band. A prospective study with long-term follow-up including range of motion measurements. Scandinavian Journal of Medicine and Science in Sports 7:229–237

Starring DT, Gossman MR, Nicholson GG, Lemons J 1988 Comparison of cyclic and sustained passive stretching using a mechanical device to increase resting length of hamstring muscles. Physical Therapy 68:314–320

Steffen TM, Mollinger LA 1995 Low-load, prolonged stretch in the treatment of knee flexion contractures in nursing home residents. Physical Therapy 75:886–895

Sucher BM, Hinrichs R 1998 Manipulative treatment of carpal tunnel syndrome: biomechanical and osteopathic intervention to increase the length of the transverse carpal ligament. Journal of the American Osteopathic Association 12:679–686

Sullivan MK, Dejulia JJ, Worrell TW 1992 Effect of pelvic position and stretching method on hamstring muscle flexibility. Medicine and Science in Sports and Exercise 24:1383–1389

Swank AM, Funk MP, Durham MP, Roberts S 2003 Adding weights to stretching exercise increases passive ROM for healthy elderly. Journal of Strength and Conditioning Research 17:374–378

Tabary JC, Tabary C, Tardieu C, Tardieu G, Goldspink G 1972 Physiological and structural changes in the cat's soleus muscle due to immobilization at different lengths by plaster casts. Journal of Physiology 224:231–244

Tanigawa MC 1972 Comparison of the hold–relax-procedure and passive mobilization on increasing muscle length. Physical Therapy 52:725–735

Taylor DC, Dalton JD, Seaber AV, Garret WE 1990 Viscoelastic properties of the muscle tendon unit: the biomechanical effects of stretching. American Journal of Sports Medicine 18:300–309

Thigpen LK, Moritani T, Thiebaud R, Hargis JL 1985 The acute effects of static stretching on alpha motoneuron excitability. In: Winter et al Biomechanics IX-A. Human Kinetics, Champaign, IL

Toft E, Espersen GT, Kålund S, Sinkjaer T, Hornemann BC 1989 Passive tension of the ankle before and after stretching. American Journal of Sports Medicine 17:489–494

Todnem K, Lundemo G 2000 Median nerve recovery in carpal tunnel syndrome. Muscle Nerve 23:1555–1560

Valente R, Gibson H 1994 Chiropractic manipulation in carpal tunnel syndrome. Journal of Manipulative and Physiological Therapeutics 4:246–249

Vallbö AB 1974 Afferent discharge from human muscle spindles in non-contracting muscles. Steady state impulse frequency as a function of the joint angle. Acta Physiologica Scandinavica 90:303–318

Vandenburgh HH 1987 Motion into mass: how does tension stimulate muscle growth? Med Sci Sports Exercise 19:19 (Suppl):S142–149

Van den Dolder PA, Roberts DL 2003 A trial into the effectiveness of soft tissue massage in the treatment of shoulder pain. Aus J Phys 49:183–188

Van Mechelen W, Hlobil H, Kemper HCG, Voorn WJ, de Jongh R 1993 Prevention of running injuries by warmup, cool-down, and stretching exercises. American Journal of Sports Medicine 21:711–9

Viidik A 1972 Simultaneous mechanical and light microscopic studies of collagen fibers. Zeitschrift fur Anatomie und Entwicklungsgeschichte 136:204–12

Wallin D, Ekblom B, Grahn R, Nordenborg T 1985 Improvement of muscle flexibility: a comparison between two techniques. American Journal of Sports Medicine 13:263–8

Wang XT, Ker R, Alexander RM 1995 Fatigue rupture of wallaby tail tendons. Journal of Experimental Biology 198:847–52

Ward RS, Hayes-Lundy C, Reddy R, Brockway C, Mills P, Saffle JR 1994 Evaluation of topical therapeutic ultrasound to improve response to physical therapy and lessen scar contracture after burn injury. J Burn Care Rehabil 15:74–79

Weldon SM, Hill RH 2003 The efficacy of stretching for prevention of exercise-related injury: a systematic review of the literature. Systematic review. Manual Therapy 8:141–150

Wessel J, Wan A 1994 Effect of stretching on the intensity of DOMS. Clin J Sports Med 4:83–87

Wessling KC, DeVane DA, Hylton CR 1987 Effects of static stretch versus static stretch and ultrasound combined on triceps surae muscle extensibility in healthy women. Physical Therapy 67:674–679

Wiktorsson-Möller M, Oborg B, Ekstrand J, Gillquist J 1983 Effects of warming up, massage, and stretching on ROM and muscle strength in the lower extremity. American Journal of Sports Medicine 11:249–252

Williams PE, Goldspink G 1978 Changes in sacromere length and physiological muscle properties in immobilized muscle. Journal of Anatomy 127:459–468

Williford HN, East JB, Smith FH, Burry LA 1986 Evaluation of warm-up for improvement in flexibility. American Journal of Sports Medicine 14:316–319

Williford HN, Smith JF 1985 A comparison of proprioceptive neuromuscular facilitation and static stretching techniques. Am Con Ther 39:30–33

Willy RW, Kyle BA, Moore SA, Chleboun GS 2001 Effect of cessation and resumption of static hamstring muscle stretching on joint ROM. Journal of Orthopaedic and Sports Physical Therapy 31:138–144

Winkelstein BA, McLendon RE, Barbir A, Myers BS 2001 An anatomical investigation of the human cervical facet capsule, quantifying muscle insertion area. Journal of Anatomy 198:455–461

Witvrouw E, Bellemans J, Lysens R, Danneels L, Cambier D 2001 Intrinsic risk factors for the development of patellar tendinitis in an athletic population: a two years prospective study. American Journal of Sports Medicine 29:190–195

Witvrouw E, Danneels L, Asselman P, D'Have T, Cambier D 2003 Muscle flexibility as a risk factor of developing muscle injuries in professional male soccer players. American Journal of Sports Medicine 31:41–46

Wordsworth P, Ogilvie D, Smith R, Sykes B 1987 Joint mobility with particular reference to racial variation and inherited connective tissue disorders. British Journal of Rheumatology 26:9–12

Wright V, Johns RJ 1961 Quantitative and qualitative analysis of joint stiffness in normal subjects and in patients with connective tissue diseases. Annals of the Rheumatic Diseases 20:36–46

Ylinen J, Cash M 1988 Sports massage. Stanley Paul, London

Ylinen J, Takala E, Nykänen M, Häkkinen A, Mälkiä E, Pohjolainen T, Karppi S, Kautiainen H and Airaksinen O 2003 Active neck muscle training in the treatment of chronic neck pain in women, a randomized controlled trial. JAMA: Journal of the American Medical Association 289:2509–2516

Youdas JW, Krause DA, Egan KS, Therneau TM, Laskowski ER 2003 The effect of static stretching of the calf muscle–tendon unit on active ankle dorsiflexion range of motion. Journal of Orthopaedic and Sports Physical Therapy 33:408–417

FURTHER READING

Adler SS, Beckers D, Buck M 1993 PNF in practice: an illustrated guide. Springer-Verlag, New York

Agre JC, Pierce LE, Raab DM, McAdams M, Smith EL 1998 Light resistance and stretching exercise in elderly women: effect upon stretch. Archives of Physical Medicine and Rehabilitation 69:273–276

Alnaqeeb MA, Al Zaid NS, Goldspink G 1984 Connective tissue changes and physical properties of developing and aging skeletal muscle. Journal of Anatomy 139:677–689

Alter MJ 1996 Science of flexibility. Human Kinetics, Champaign IL

American Academy of Orthopaedic Surgeons 1965 Joint motion: method of measuring and recording. Churchill Livingstone, Edinburgh

Anderson B, Burke ER 1991 Scientific, medical, and practical aspects of stretching. Clinics in Sports Medicine 10:63–86

Arem AJ, Madden JW 1976 Effects of stress on healing wounds: intermittent noncyclical tension. Journal of Surgical Research 20:93–102

Ashmore CR, Summers PJ 1981 Stretch-induced growth of chicken muscles: myofibrillar proliferation. American Journal of Physics 241:C93–97

Askter HA, Granzier HLM, Focant B 1989 Differences in I band structure, sarcomere extensibility, and electrophoresis of titin between two muscle fibre types of the perch. Journal of Ultrastructure and Molecular Structure Research 102:109–121

Aten DW, Knight KT 1987 Therapeutic exercise in athletic training: principles and overview. Athletic Training 13:123–126

Barker D 1974 The morphology of muscle receptors. In: Hunt CC (ed) Handbook of sensory physiology. Muscle receptors, vol. 3. Springer, New York

Barnett CH 1971 The mobility of synovial joints. Rheumatology and Physical Medicine 11:20–27

Barnett JG, Holly RG, Ashmore CR 1980 Stretch-induced growth in chicken wing muscles: biochemical and morphological characterization. American Journal of Physiology, Cell Physiology 8:239–246

Barrack RL, Skinner HB, Brunet ME 1983 Joint laxity and proprioception in the knee. Physician and Sportsmedicine 11:130–135

Basmajian JV, Deluca CJ 1985 Muscles alive. Their functions revealed by electromyography. Williams & Wilkins, Baltimore

Bates RA 1971 Flexibility training: the optimal time period to spend in a position of maximal stretch. Unpublished master's thesis, University of Alberta, Edmonton

Battie MC, Bigos SJ, Fisher LD et al 1990 The role of spinal flexibility in back pain complaints within industry. Spine 15:768–773

Battie MC, Bigos SJ, Sheehy A, Wortley MD 1987 Spinal flexibility and individual factors that influence it. Physican Therapy 67:653–658

Beaulieu JE 1981 Developing a stretching program. Physician and Sportsmedicine 9:59–65

Bell RD, Hoshizaki TB 1981 Relationship of age and sex with ROM of seventeen joint actions in humans. Canadian Journal of Applied Sport Sciences 6:202–206

Belli A, Bosco C 1992 Influence of stretch-shortening cycle on mechanical behaviour of triceps surae during hopping. Acta Physiologica Scandinavica 144:401–408

Bennet MB, Ker RF, Dimery NJ, Alexander RM 1986 Mechanical properties of various mammalian tendons. Journal of Zoology 209:537–548

Bertolasi L, De Grandis D, Bongiovanni LG, Zanette GP, Gasperini M 1993 The influence of muscular lengthening on cramps. Annals of Neurology 33:176–180

Bick EM 1961 Aging in the connective tissues of the human musculoskeletal system. Geriatrics 16:448–453

Bird HA, Brodie DA, Wright V 1979 Quantification of joint laxity. Rheum Rehabil 18:161–166

Bobath B 1955 The treatment of motor disorders of pyramidal and extrapyramidal origin by reflex inhibition and by facilitation of movements. Physiotherapy 41:146–152

Bobbert MP, Hollander AP, Huijing PA 1986 Factors in delayed onset muscular soreness of man. Medicine and Science in Sports and Exercise 18; 75–81

Bohannon RW, Chavis D, Larkin P, Lieber C, Liddick R 1985 Effectiveness of repeated prolonged loading for increasing flexion in knees demonstrating postoperative stiffness. Physical Therapy 65:494–496

Bohannon RW, Gajdosik RL, LeVeau BF 1985 Contribution of pelvic and lower limb motion to increases in the angle of passive straight leg raising. Physical Therapy 1985; 65:474–476

Bohannon RW, Gajdosik RL, LeVeau BF 1985 Relationship of pelvic and thigh motion during unilateral and bilateral hip flexion. Physical Therapy 65:1501–1504

Bohannon RW 1982 Cinematographic analysis of the passive straight-leg raising test for hamstring muscle length. Physical Therapy 1(62):1269–1274

Boone DC, Azen SP, Lin CM 1978 Reliability of goniometric measurements. Physical Therapy 58:1355–1360

Boone DC, Azen SP 1979 Normal ROM of joints in male subjects. Journal of Bone and Joint surgery 61:756–759

Borg TK, Caulfield JB 1980 Morphology of connective tissue in skeletal muscle. Tissue Cell 12:197–207

Bosco C, Montanari G, Tarkka I 1987 The effect of prestretch on mechanical efficiency of human skeletal muscle. Acta physiologica Scandinavica 131:323–329

Botelho SY, Cander L, Guiti N 1954 Passive and active tensionlength diagrams of intact skeletal muscle in normal women of different ages. Journal of Applied Physiology 7:93–95

Botsford DJ, Esses SI, Ogilvie-Harris DJ 1994 In vivo diurnal variation in intervertebral disc volume and morphology. Spine 19:935–940

Brodie DA, Bird HA, Wright V 1982 Joint laxity in selected athletic populations. Medicine and Science in Sports and Exercise 14:190–193

Broer MR, Gales NR 1958 Importance of various body measurements in performance of toe touch test. Research Quarterly 29:253–257

Bromley I 1998 Tetraplegia and paraplegia: a guide for physiotherapists. Churchill Livingstone, New York

Buckwalter JA, Woo SL, Goldberg VM 1993 Soft tissue aging and musculoskeletal function. J Bone Joint Surg Am 75:1533–1548

Burke D, Hagbarth KE, Lofstedt L 1978 Muscle spindle activity in man during shortening and lengthening contraction. Journal of Physiology 277:131–142

Byrnes WC, Clarkson PM 1986 DOMS and training. Clinics in Sports Medicine 5:605–614

Calguneri M, Bird HA, Wright V 1982 Changes in joint laxity occurring during pregnancy. Annals of the Rheumatic Diseases 41:126–128

Cameron DM, Bohannon RW Owen SV 1994 Influence of hip position on measurements of the straight leg raise test. Journal of Orthopaedic and Sports Physical Therapy 9:168–172

Carlsen F, Knappels GG, Buchthal F 1961 Ultrastructure of the resting and contracted striated muscle fibre at different degree of stretch. The Journal of Biophysical and Biochemical Cytology 10:95–118

Chapman EA, de Vries HA, Swezey R 1972 Joint stiffness: effects of exercise on young and old men. Journal of Gerontology 27:A105 218–221

Cheng JCY, Chan PS, Hui PW 1991 Joint laxity in children. Journal of Pediatric Orthopedics 11:752–726

Cherry DB 1980 Review of physical therapy alternatives for reducing muscle contracture. Physical Therapy 60:877–881

Child AH 1986 Joint hypermobility syndrome: Inherited disorder of collagen synthesis. The Journal of Rheumatology 13:239–243

Ciullo JV, Zarins B 1983 Biomechanics of the musculotendinous unit: Relation to athletic performance and injury. Clinics in Sports Medicine 2:71–86

Cleak MJ, Eston RG 1992 DOMS: mechanisms and management. Journal of Sports Science 10:325–341

Clendenlel RA, Gossman MR, Katholl CR 1984 Hamstring muscle length in men and women: Normative data. Physical Therapy 64:716–717

Corbin CB 1984 Flexibility. Clinics in Sports Medicine 3:101–117

Cornelius WL 1983 Stretch evoked activity by isometric contraction and submaximal concentric contraction. Athletic Training 18:106–109

Cornelius WL, Hagemann RW, Jackson AW 1988 A study on placement of stretching within a workout. Journal of Sports Medicine and Physical Fitness 28:234–236

Craib VA, Mitchell KB, Fields TR Cooper R, Hopewell DW 1996 The association between flexibility and running economy in sub–elite male distance runners. Medicine and Science in Sports and Exercise 28:737–743

Cureton TK 1941 Flexibility as an aspect of physical fitness. Research Quarterly 12:381–390

Davidoff RA 1992 Skeletal muscle tone and the misunderstood stretch reflex. Neurology 42:951–963

DeLateur BJ 1994 Flexibility. Physical Medicine and Rehabilitation Clinics of North America 5:295–307

DeLuca C 1985 Control properties of motor units. Journal of Experimental Biology 115:125–136

Denny-Brown D, Doherty MM 1945 Effects of transient stretching of peripheral nerve. Arch Neurol Psych 54:116–122

Diaz MA, Estevez EC, Guijo PS 1993 Joint hyperlaxity and musculoligamentous lesions: study of a population of homogeneous age, sex and physical exertion. British Journal of Rheumatology 32:120–122

Dickenson RV 1968 The specificity of flexibility. Research Quarterly 39:792–794

Docherty D, Bell RD 1985 The relationship between flexibility and linearity measures in boys and girls 6–15 years of age. Journal of Human Movement Studies 11:279–288

Donatelli R, Owens-Burkhart H 1981 Effects of immobilization on the extensibility of periarticular connective tissue. Journal of Orthopaedic Sports Physical Therapy 3:67–72

Draper DO, Miner L, Knight KL, Ricard MD 2002 The carry-over effects of diathermy and stretching in developing hamstring flexibility. Journal of Athletic Training 37:37–42 J Athl Train 1998.

Einkauf DK, Gohdes ML, Jensen GM, Jewell MJ. Changes in spinal mobility with increasing age in women. Physical Therapy 1986; 67:370–375

Ekstrand J. Soccer injuries and their prevention 1982 Thesis no 130, Linköping University

Ekstrand J, Giliquist J 1982 The frequency of muscle tightness and injuries in soccer players. American Journal of Sports Medicine 10:13875–13878

Eldred E, Linsley DE, Buchwald JS 1960 The effect of cooling on mammalian muscle spindles. Experimental Neurology 2:144–157

Etnyre BR, Abraham LD 1988 Antagonist muscle activity during stretching: A paradox re-assessed. Medicine and Science in Sports and Exercise 20:285–289

Etnyre BR, Lee EJ 1987 Comments on proprioceptive neuromuscular facilitation stretching techniques. Research Quarterly for Exercise and Sport 58:184–188

Evjenth O, Hamberg J 1997 Muscle stretching in manual therapy. A clinical manual, 4th edn. Alfta Rehab Förlag

Fairbank JCT, Pynsent PB, van Poortvliet JA, Phillips H 1984 Influence of anthropometric factors and joint laxity in the incidence of adolescent back pain. Spine 9:461–464

Fatney FW, Hirst DG 1978 Cross-bridge detachment and sarcomere 'give' during stretch of active frog's muscle. Journal of Physiology 276:449–465

Faulkner JA, Brooks SV, Opiteck JA 1993 Injury to skeletal muscle fibres during contractions: conditions of occurrence and prevention. Physical Therapy 73:911–921

Feldman H 1968 Relative contribution of the back and hamstring muscles in performance of the toe-touch test after selected extensibility exercises. Research Quarterly 39:518–523

Finni T, Komi PV, Lepola V 2001 In vivo muscle mechanics during locomotion depend on movement amplitude and contraction intensity. European Journal of Applied Physiology 85:170–176

Ford LE, Huxley AF, Simmons RM 1981 The relation between stiffness and filament overlap in stimulated frog muscle fibres. Journal of Physiology 311:219–249

Francis KT 1983 Delayed muscle soreness: a review. Journal of Orthopaedic and Sports Physical Therapy 5:10–13

Fredericson M, Guillet M, DeBenedictis L 2000 Quick solutions for iliotibial band syndrome. Physician and Sportsmedicine 28:5553–5568

Frekany GA, Leslie DK 1975 Effects of an exercise program on selected flexibility measurements of senior citizens. Gerontologist 15:182–183

Friden J, Lieber RL 1992 Structural and mechanical basis of exercise-induced muscle injury. Medicine and Science in Sports and Exercise 24:521–530

Gadjosik RL, Bohannon RW 1987 Clinical measurements of ROM: review of goniometry emphasizing reliability and validity. Physical Therapy 67:1867–1872

Gajdosik R, Lusin G 1983 Hamstring muscle tightness: Reliability of an active-knee-extension test. Physical Therapy 63:1085–1089

Gajdosik R 1985 Rectus femoris muscle tightness: intratester reliability of an active knee flexion test 1985 Journal of Orthopaedic and Sports Physical Therapy 6:289–292

Gajdosik RL, Giuliani CA, Bohannon RW 1990 Passive compliance and length of the hamstring muscles of healthy men and women. Clinical Biomechanics 5:23–29

Gajdosik RL, LeVeau BF, Bohannon RW 1985 Effects of ankle dorsiflexion on active and passive unilateral straight leg raising. Physical therapy 65:1478–1482

Gajdosik RL 1995 Flexibility or muscle length? Physical Therapy 75:238–239

Gajdosik R 1991 Passive compliance and length of clinically short hamstring muscles of healthy men. Clinical Biomechanics 6:239–244

Gareis H, Solomonow M, Baratta R, Best R, D'Ambrosia R 1991 The isometric length-force models of nine different skeletal muscles. Journal of Biomechanics 25:903–916

Garfin SR, Tipton CM, Mubarak SJ, Woo SL-Y, Hargens AR, Akeson WH 1981 Role of fascia in maintenance of muscle tension and pressure. Journal of Applied Physiology 51:317–320

Garrett WE, Safran MR, Seaber AV 1987 Biomechanical comparison of stimulated and nonstimulated skeletal muscle pulled to failure. American Journal of Sports Medicine 15:448–454

Garrett WE 1996 Muscle strain injuries. American Journal of Sports Medicine 24:S2–S8

Germain NW, Blair SN 1983 Variability of shoulder flexion with age, activity and sex. American Corrective Therapy Journal 37:156–160

Gersten JW 1955 Effect of ultrasound on tendon extensibility. American Journal of Physical Medicine 34:368–372

Gifford LS 1987 Circadian variation in human flexibility and grip strength. Aus J Phys 33:3–9

Gleim GW, McHugh MP 1997. Flexibility and its effects on sports injury and performance. Sports Medicine 24:289–299

Glick JM 1980 Muscle strains: prevention and treatment. Physician Sports Medicine 8:73–77

Goldspink G, Williams, PE 1979 The nature of the increased passive resistance in muscle following immobilization of the mouse soleus muscle. Journal of Physiology 289, 55P.

Goodridge JP 1981 Muscle energy technique: definition, explanation, methods of procedure. Journal of the American Osteopathic Association 1:67–72

Gordon AM, Huxley AF, Julian FJ 1966 The variation in isometric tension with sarcomere length in vertebrate muscle fibres. Journal of Physiology 184:170–192.

Gossman MR, Sahrmann SA, Rose SJ 1982 Review of length–associated changes in muscle: experimental evidence and clinical implications. Journal of the American Osteopathic Association 62:1799–1808

Grace TG 1985 Muscle imbalance and extremity injury. Sports Medicine 2:77–82

Grahame R, Jenkins JM 1972 Joint hypermobility-asset or liability? Annals of the Rheumatic Diseases 31:109–111

Grahn R, Nordenborg T, Wallin D, Nyström J, Ekblom B 1981 Improvement of muscle flexibility — comparisons between two techniques. Scandinavian Journal of Sports Science

Guissard N, Duchateau J 2004 Effect of static stretch training on neural and mechanical properties of the human plantar-flexor muscles. Muscle Nerve 29:248–255

Göeken LN, Hof AL 1993 Instrumental straight-leg raising: results in healthy subjects. Archives of Physical Medicine and Rehabilitation 74:194–203

Göeken LN, Hof AL 1994 Instrumental straight-leg raising: results in patients. Archives of Physical Medicine and Rehabilitation 75:470–477.

Göeken LN 1988 Straight-leg raising in 'short hamstrings'. Thesis, University of Groningen, Groningen

Haftek J 1970 Stretch injury of peripheral nerve: Acute effects of stretching on rabbit nerve. Journal of Bone and Joint Surgery 52:354–365

Hagbarth KE, Hägglund JV, Norkin M, Wallin EU 1985 Thixotropic behaviour of human finger flexor muscles with accompanying changes in spindle and reflex responses to stretch. Physiology 368:323–342

Hamberg J, Björklund M, Nordgren B, Sahlstedt B 1993 Stretchability of the rectus femoris muscle: investigation of validity and intratester reliability of two methods including X-ray analysis of pelvic tilt. Archives of Physical Medicine and Rehabilitation 74 (3):263–270

Hanus SH, Homer TD, Harter DH 1977 Vertebral artery occlusion complicating yoga exercises. Archives of Neurology 34:574–575

Harms-Ringdahl K, Brodin H, Eklund L, Borg G 1983 Discomfort and pain from loaded passive joint structures. Scandinavian Journal of Rehabilitation Medicine: 205–211

Harris ML 1969 Flexibility. Physical Therapy 49:591–601

Harvey C, Benedetti L, Hosaka L, Valmassy RL 1983 The use of cold spray and its effect on muscle length. Journal of American Podiatry Association 73:629–632

Harvey LA, Crosbie J, Herbert RD 2002 Does regular stretch produce lasting increases in joint range of motion? A systematic review. Physiotherapy Research International 7:1–13

Harvey LA, McQuade L, Hawthorne S, Byak A 2003 Quantifying the magnitude of torque physiotherapists apply when stretching the hamstring muscles of people with a spinal cord injury. Archives of Physical Medicine and Rehabilitation 84:1072–1075

Harvey VP, Scott PP 1967 Reliability of a measure of forward flexibility and its relation to physical dimensions of college women. Research Quarterly 38:28–33

Haut TL, Haut RC 1997 The state of tissue hydration determines the strain-rate sensitive stiffness of human patellar tendon. Journal of Biomechanics 30:79–81

Hennessy L, Watson AWS 1993 Flexibility and posture assessment in relation to hamstring injury. British Journal of Sports Medicine 27:243–246

Henricson A, Fredriksson K, Persson I 1984 The effect of heat and stretching on the range of hip motion. Journal of Orthopedic Sports Physical Therapy 6:110–115

Herbert R, Gabriel M 2002 Effects of stretching before and after exercising on muscle soreness and risk of injury: systematic review. BMJ 325:468–472
Highet WB, Sanders FK 1943 The effects of stretching nerves after suture. British Journal of Surgery 30:355–371
Hilyer JC, Brown KC, Sirles AT, Peoples 1990 A flexibility intervention to reduce the incidence and severity of joint injuries among municipal firefighters. Journal of Occupational Medicine 32:631–637
Hoeger WWK, Hopkins DR 1992 A comparison of the sit and reach and the modified sit and reach in the measurement of flexibility in women. Research Quarterly Exercise and Sport 63:191–195
Hoen TI, Brackett CE 1970 Peripheral nerve lengthening. Exper J Neurosurg 13:43–62
Holly RG, Barnett CR, Ashmore CR, Taylor RG, Moli PA 1980 Stretch-induced growth in chicken wing muscles: a new model of stretch hypertrophy. American Journal of Physiology 238:C62–71
Horowits R 1992 Passive force generation and titin isoforms in mammalian skeletal muscle. Biophysical Journal 61:392–398
Horten MR 1987 Muscle elasticity and human performance. Med Sports Sci 25:1–18
Hsieh C-Y, Walker JM, Gillis K 1983 Straight-leg-raising test: comparison of three instruments. Physical Therapy 63:1429–1433
Hubbard RP, Soutas-Little RW 1984 Mechanical properties of human tendon and their age dependence. Journal of Biomechanical Engineering 106:144–150
Hubley CL, Kozey JW Stanish WD. The effects of static stretching exercises and stationary cycling on range of motion. Journal of Orthopaedic and Sports Physical Therapy 6:104–109
Hunter JP, Marshall RN 2002 Effects of power and flexibility training on vertical jump technique. Medicine and Science in Sports and Exercise 34:478–486
Hutton RS 1992 Neuromuscular basis of stretching exercises. In: Komi PV (ed) Strength and power in sport. Blackwell Scientific, Cambridge, 29–38
Huxley AF, Simmons RM 1973 Proposed mechanism of force generation in striated muscle. Nature 33:533–538
Häkkinen K, Komi PV 1985 Changes in electrical and mechanical behavior of leg extensor muscles during heavy resistance strength training. Scandinavian Journal of Sports Science 7:55–64
Iashvili AV 1983 Active and passive flexibility in athletes specializing in different sports. Soviet Sports Review 18:30–32
International Anatomical Nomenclature Committee 1983 Nomina anatomica, 5th edn. Williams & Wilkins, Philadelphia
Jackson AW, Baker AA 1986 The relationship of the sit and reach test to criterion measures of hamstring and back flexibility in young females. Research Quarterly Exercise Sport 57:183–186
Jacobs SJ, Berson BL1986 Injuries to runners: a study of entrants to a 10 000 meter race. American Journal of Sports Medicine 14:151–155
Jaeger B. Reeves JL 1986 Quantification of changes in myofascial trigger point sensitivity with the pressure algorneter following passive stretch. Pain 27:203–210
Jami 1992 Golgi tendon organs in mammalian skeletal muscle: Functional properties and central actions. Physiology Review 72:623–626
Jesse EF, Owen DS, Sagar KB 1980 The benign hypermobile joint syndrome. Arthritis and Rheumatology 23:1053–1056
Järvinen M 1976 Healing of a crush injury in rat striated muscle. With reference to treatment by early mobilization and immobilization. Thesis. University of Turku, Turku
Kabat H, McLeod M, Holt C 1959 The practical application of proprioceptive neuromuscular facilitation. Physiotherapy 45:87–92
Kamibayashi LK, Richmond FJR 1998 Morphometry of human neck muscles. Spine 23:1314–1323
Kapandji IA [illegible] The physiology of joints. Churchill Livingstone, Edinburgh
Kendall HO, Kendall FP 1948 Normal flexibility according to age groups. Journal of Bone and Joint Surgery 30A:690–694
Kerner JA, D' Kerner JA, D'Amico JC 1983 A statistical analysis of a group of runners. Journal of the American Podiatry Association 73:160–164
King JW 1992 Static progressive splints. Journal of Hand Therapy 5:36–37
Kirkebe A, Wisnes A 1982 Regional tissue fluid pressure in rat calf muscle during sustained contraction or stretch. Acta Physiologica Scandinavica 114:551–556
Knapik JJ, Jones BH, Baumau CL, Harrsi J 1992 Strength, flexibility, and athletic injuries. Sports Medicine 14:277–288
Knudson D, Bennett K, Corn R, Leick D, Smith C 2001 Acute effects of stretching are not evident in the kinematics of the vertical jump. Journal of Strength and Conditioning Research 15:98–101
Kokkonen J, Eldredge C, Nelson AG 1997 Chronic stretching improves specific sport skills. Medicine and Science in Sports and Exercise 29:S63
Komi PV 1992 Stretch-shortening cycle. In: Komi PV (ed) Strength and power in sport. Blackwell Science, London, 169–179
Koslow RE 1987 Bilateral flexibility in the upper and lower extremities as related to age and gender. Journal of Human Movement Studies 13:467–472
Kottke FI, Pauley DL, Ptak RA 1966 The rationale for prolonged stretching for correction of shortening of connective tissue. Archives of Physical Medicine and Rehabilitation 47:345–352
Krahenbuhl GS, Martin SL 1977 Adolescence body size and flexibility. Research Quarterly 48:797–799
Kubo K, Kanehisa H, Fukunaga T 2003 Gender differences in the viscoelastic properties of tendon structures. European Journal of Applied Physiology 88:520–526
Kudina L 1980 Reflex effects of muscle afferents on antagonists studies on single firing motor units in man. Electroencephalography and Clinical Neurophysiology 50:214–221
Kutsuna T, Watanabe H 1981 Contractures of the quadriceps and hamstring muscles in healthy male adults. Journal of the Japan Orthopaedic Association 55:237–242
Labeit S, Kolmerer B 1995 Titins: giant proteins in charge of muscle ultrastructure and elasticity. Science 270:293–296
Laubach LC, McConville JT 1966 Muscle strength, flexibility, and bone size of adult males. Research Quarterly 37:384–392
Laubach LL, McConville JT 1966 Relationship between flexibility, anthropometry, and the somatotype of college men. Research Quarterly 37:241–251
Leighton JR 1955 An instrument and technic for the measurement of range of joint motion. Archives of Physical Medicine and Rehabilitation 36:571–578
Leighton JR 1956 Flexibility characteristics of males ten to eighteen years of age. Arch Phys Mental Rehabil 37:494–499
Levarlet-Joye H 1979 Relaxation and motor capacity Journal of Sports Medicine 19:151–156
Levine MG, Kabat H, Knott M. Relaxation of spasticity by physiological techniques. Archives of Physical Medicine 35:214–223
Levine MG, Kabat H 1952 Cocontraction and reciprocal innervation in voluntary movement in man. Science 116:115–118
Lewit K, Simons D 1984 Myofascial pain: relief by post-isometric relaxation. Archives of Physical Medicine and Rehabilitation 65:452–456
Lieber RI 1991 Frog semitendinosis tendon load-strain and stress-strain properties during passive loading. American Journal of Physiology 261:C86–C92
Lieber RL, Woodbourn TM, Friden J 1991 Muscle damage induced by eccentric contractions of 25% strain. Journal of Applied Physiology 70:2498–2507
Lieber RR, Friden J 1993 Muscle damage is not a function of muscle force but active muscle strain. Journal of Applied Physiology 74:520–526
Liebesman JL, Cafarelli E 1994 Physiology of range of motion in human joints: a critical review. Crit Rev Physic Rehabil Med 6:131–160
Light KE, Nuzik S, Personius W 1984 Low-load prolonged stretch vs. high load brief stretch in treating knee contractures. Physical Therapy 64:330–333
Locke JC 1983 Stretching away from back pain. Occup Health Sci 52:8–13
Loebel WY 1972 The assessment of mobility in the metacarpophalangeal joints. Rheumatology and Physical Medicine 9:365–379
Logan GA, Egstrom GH 1961 Effects of slow and fast stretching on the sacro-femoral angle. Journal of the Association for Physical and Mental Rehabilitation 150:85–89
Lund JP, Donga R, Widmer CG, Stohler CS 1991 The pain adaptation model: a discussion of the relationship between chronic musculoskeletal pain and motor activity. Canadian Journal of Physiology and Pharmacology 69:683–694
Lundborg G, Rydevik B 1973 Effects of stretching the tibial nerve of the rabbit. Journal of Bone and Joint Surgery 55:390–401
Lundborg G 1993 Peripheral nerve injuries: pathophysiology and strategies for treatment. Journal of Hand Therapy 6:179–188
Lustig S, Ball T, Looney M 1992 A comparison of two proprioceptive neuromuscular facilitation techniques for improving range of motion and muscular strength. Isokinetics and Exercise Science 2:154–159
Maganaris CN, Paul JP 1999 In vivo human tondon mechanical properties. Journal of Physiology 521:307–313
Magnusson SP, Aagaard, P, Nielsson JJ 2000 Passive energy return after repeated stretches of the hamstring muscle-tendon unit. Medicine and Science in Sports and Exercise 32:1160–1164

Magnusson SP, Aagaard P, Simonsen EB, Bojsen-Møller F 1988 A biomechanical evaluation of cyclic and static stretch in human skeletal muscle. International Journal of Sports Medicine 19:310–316

Magnusson SP, Simonsen EB, Aagaard P, Kjaer M 1996 Biomechanical responses to repeated stretches in human hamstring muscle in vivo. American Journal of Sports Medicine 24:622–628

Magnusson SP, Simonsen EB, Aagaard P, Sorensen H, Kjaer M 1996. A mechanism for altered flexibility in human skeletal muscle. Journal of Physiology 497:291–298

Magnusson SP, Simonsen EB, Dyhre-Poulsen P, Aagaard P, Mohr T, Kjaer M 1996 Viscoelastic stress relaxation during static stretch in human skeletal muscle in the absence of EMG activity. Scandinavian Journal of Medicine and Science in Sports 6:323–328

Magnusson SP 1998 Passive properties of human skeletal muscle during stretch maneuvers. A review. Scandinavian Journal of Medicine and Science in Sports 8:65–77

Mair S, Seaber AV, Glisson RR, Garrett WE 1996 The role of fatigue in susceptibility to acute muscle strain injury. American Journal of Sports Medicine 24:137–142

Mallik AK, Ferrell WR, McDonald AG, Sturrock RD 1994 Impaired proprioceptive acuity at the proximal interphalangeal joint in patients with the hypermobility syndrome. British Journal of Rheumatology 33:631–637

Marcos PD 1979 Ipsilateral and contralateral effects of proprioceptive neuromuscular facilitation technique on hip motion and electromyographic activity. Physical Therapy 59:1366–1373

Marras WS, Wongsam PE 1986 Flexibility and velocity of the normal and impaired lumbar spine. Archives of Physical Medicine and Rehabilitation 67:213–217

Maruyama K 1986 Connectin, an elastic filamentous protein of striated muscle International Review of Cytology 1048–1115

Massey BA, Chaudet NL 1956 Effects of systematic, heavy resistance exercise on range of joint movement in young adults. Research Quarterly 27:41–51

Mathews DK, Shaw V, Bohnen M 1957 Hip flexibility of college women as related to body segments. Research Quarterly 28:352–356

Mathews DK, Shaw V, Woods JW 1959 Hip flexibility of elementary school boys as related to body segments. Research Quarterly 31:297–302

Mayerson NH, Milano RA 1984 Goniometric measurement reliability in physical medicine. Archives of Physical Medicine and Rehabilitation; 65:92–94

Mayhew TP, Norton BJ, Sahrmann SA 1983 Electromyographic study of the relationship between hamstring and abdominal muscles during unilateral straight leg raise. Physical Therapy 63:1769–1773

McAtee RE 1999 Facilitated stretching, 2nd edn. Human Kinetics, Champaign, IL

McCue BF 1963 Flexibility measurements of college women. Research Quarterly 24:316–324

McDonald CM 1998 Limb contractures in progressive neuromuscular disease and the role of stretching, orthotics, and surgery. Med Rehabil Clin North Am 9:187–211

McHugh MP, Kjaer M 1995 Viscoelastic response to repeated static stretching in the human hamstrings muscle. Scandinavian Journal of Medicine and Science in Sports 5:342–347

McHugh MP, Magnusson SP, Gleim GW, Nicholas JA 1992 Viscoelastic stress relaxation in human skeletal muscle. Medicine and Science in Sports and Exercise 24:1375–1382

McKenzie R 1981 Mechanical diagnosis and treatment of the lumbar spine. Spinal, New Zealand

McKenzie R 1983 Treat your own neck. Spinal, New Zealand

Mechelen W van, Mobil H, Kemper HCG, Voom WJ 1993 Prevention of running injuries by warm-up, cool-down, and stretching exercises. American Journal of Sports Medicine 21:711–719

Mellin G 1985 Physical therapy for chronic low back pain: correlations between spinal mobility and treatment outcome. Scandinavian Journal of Rehabilitation Medicine 17:163–166

Melzack R, Stillwell DM, Fox EJ 1977 Trigger points and acupuncture points for pain: correlations and implications. Pain 3:3–23

Merni P, Balboni M, Bargellini S, Menegatti G 1981 Differences in males and females in joint movement range during growth. Med Sport 15:168–175

Miglietta O 1973 Action of cold on spasticity. American Journal of Physical Medicine and Rehabilitation 52:198–205

Milne RA, Mierau R 1979 Hamstring distensibility in the general population: relationship to pelvic and low back stresses. Journal of Manipulative and Physiological Therapeutics 2:146–150

Milner-Brown HS, Stein RB, Lee RG 1975 Synchronization of human motor units: Possible roles of exercise and supraspinal reflexes. Electroencephalography and Clinical Neurophysiology 38:245–254

Minajeva A, Kulke M, Fernandez JM, Linke WA 2001 Unfolding of titin domains explains the viscoelastic behavior of skeletal myofibrils. Biophysical Journal 80:1442-1451

Mohan S, Radha E 1981 Age related changes in muscle connective tissue: acid mucopolysaccharides and structural glycoprotein. Experimental Gerontology 16:385–392

Moore MA, Kukulka CG 1991 Depression of Hoffmann reflexes following voluntary contraction and implications for PNF therapy. Physical Therapy 71:321–333

Moore MA 1979 An electromyographic investigation of muscle stretching techniques. Unpublished masters thesis, University of Washington, Seattle

Muir IW, Chesworth BM, Vandervoort AA 1999 Effect of a static calf-stretching exercise on the resistive torque during passive ankle dorsiflexion in healthy subjects. Journal of Orthopaedic and Sports Physical Therapy 29:106–115

Murphy DR 1991 A critical look at static stretching: Are we doing our patients harm? Chiropractic Sports Medicine 5:67–70

Murphy P 1986 Warming up before stretching advised. Physician and Sportsmedicine 14:45

Myklebust BM, Gottlieb GL, Agarwal GC 1986 Stretch reflexes of the normal human infant. Developmental Medicine and Child Neurology 28:440–449

Nagler W 1973 Mechanical obstruction of vertebral arteries during hyperextension of neck. British Journal of Sports Medicine 7:92–97

Noonan TJ, Best TM, Seaber AV, Garrett WE 1993 Thermal effects on skeletal muscle tensile behavior. American Journal of Sports Medicine 21:517–522

Nordschow M, Bierman W 1962 Influence of manual massage on muscle relaxation. Journal of the American Physical Therapy Association 42:653–657

Norkin CC, White DJ 1995 Measurement of joint motion. A guide to goniometry, 2nd edn. FA Davis, Philadelphia

Norton BJ, Sahrmann SA 1981 The effect of stretching procedures on EMG activity in the hamstring muscles. Physical Therapy 61:686–674

Ogata K, Naito M 1986 Blood flow of peripheral nerve effects of dissection, stretching and compression. Journal of Hand Surgery 11B:10–14

Osterning LR, Robertson RN, Troxel RK, Hansen P 1990 Differential responses to proprioceptive neuromuscular facilitation (PNF) stretch techniques. Medicine and Science in Sports and Exercise 22:106–111

Page SG, Huxley HE 1963 Filament lengths in striated muscle. Journal of Cell Biology 19:369–390

Petajan JH, Watts N 1962 Effects of cooling on the triceps surae reflex. American Journal of Physical Medicine Rehabilitation 41:240–251

Pollack GH 1990 Muscles and molecules: uncovering the principles of biological motion. Ebner, Seattle

Pousson M, Van Hoeck J 1990 Changes in elastic characteristics of human muscle induced by eccentric exercise. Journal of Biomechanics 21:343–348

Pratt M 1989 Strength, flexibility, and maturity in adolescent athletes. American Journal of Diseases of Children 143:560–563

Prentice WE, Kooima E 1986 The use of PNF techniques in rehabilitation of sport related injury. Athletic Training 21:26–31

Prentice WE 1982 An electromyographic analysis of the effectiveness of heat or cold and stretching for inducing relaxation in injured muscle. Journal of Orthopaedic and Sports Physical Therapy 3:133–140

Proske U, Morgan DL, Gregory JE 1993 Thixotropy in skeletal muscle and in muscle spindles: a review. Progress in Neurobiology 41:705–721

Provinciali L, Giattini A, Splendiani G, Logullo F 2000 Usefulness of hand rehabilitation after carpal tunnel surgery. Muscle Nerve 23, 211–216

Raab DM, Agre JC, Mcadam M, Smith EL 1988 Light resistance and stretching exercise in elderly women: effect upon flexibility. Archives of Physical Medicine and Rehabilitation 62:268–272

Radin EL 1989 Role of muscles in protecting athletes from injury. Acta Medica Scandinavica 711(Suppl) 143–147

Read M 1989 Over stretched. British Journal of Sports Medicine 23:257–258

Reimers J 1974 Contracture of the hamstrings in spastic cerebral palsy. Journal of Bone and Joint Surgery 56:102–109

Riddle DL, Rothstein JM, Lamb RL 1987 Goniometric reliability in a clinical setting: shoulder measurements. Physical Therapy 67:668–673

Roberts JM, Wilson K 1999 Effect of stretching duration on active and passive range of motion in the lower extremity. British Journal of Sports Medicine 33:259–263

Rodenburg JB, Steenbeek D, Schiereck P, Bar PR 1994 Warmup stretching and massage diminish harmful effects of eccentric exercise. International Journal of Sports Medicine 15:414–419

Rohen JW, Yokochi C, Lutjen-Drecoll E 2002 Anatomian värikuva-atlas. Medirehabook, Muurame

Rowe RWD 1981 Morphology of perimysial and endomysial connective tissue in skeletal muscle. Tissue Cell 13:681–690

Russell P, Weld A, Pearcy MJ, Hogg R, Unsworth A 1992 Variation in lumbar spine mobility measured over a 24-hour period. British Journal of Rheumatology 31:329–332

Sabbahi MA, Fox AM, Druffle C 1990 Do joint receptors modulate the motoneuron excitability. Electromyography and Clinical Neurophysiology l30:387–396

Sanjeevi R 1982 A viscoelastic model for the mechanical properties of biological materials. Journal of Biomechanics 15:107–109

Scott D, Bird HA, Wright V 1979 Joint laxity leading to osteoarthrosis. Rheumatology and Rehabilitation 18:167–169

Seabee AV, Garrett WE 1993 Thermal effects on skeletal muscle tensile behavior. American Journal of Sports Medicine 21:517–522

Segal RL, Wolf SL 1994 Operant conditions of spinal stretch reflexes in patients with spinal cord injuries. Experimental Neurology 130:202–213

Shellock FG, Prentice WE 1985 Warming-up and stretching for improved physical performance and prevention of sports-related injuries. Sports Medicine 2:267–278

Shephard RJ, Berridge M, Montelpare W 1990 On the generality of the 'sit and reach' test: an analysis of flexibility data for an aging population. Research Quarterly Exercise and Sport 61:326–330

Shirado O, Ito T, Kaneda K, Strax TE 1995 Flexion relaxation phenomenon in the back muscles. American Journal of Physical Medicine & Rehabilitation 74:139–144

Shorten MR 1987 Muscle elasticity and human performance. Med Sport Sci 25:1–18

Shrier I 1999 Stretching before exercise does not reduce the risk of local muscle injury: a critical review of the clinical and basic science literature. Clinical Journal of Sport Medicine 9:221–227

Shyne K, Richard H, Dominguez MD 1982 To stretch or not to stretch? Physician and Sportsmedicine 10:137–140

Sihvonen T, Partanen J, Hanninen O, Soimakallio S 1991 Electric behavior of low back muscles during lumbar pelvic rhythm in low back pain patients and healthy controls. Archives of Physical Medicine and Rehabilitation 72:1080–1087

Silman AJ, Haskard D, Day S 1986 Distribution of joint mobility in a normal population: results of the use of fixed torque measuring devices. Annals of The Rheumatic Diseases 1986; 45:27–30

Smith CA 1994 The warm-up procedure: to stretch or not to stretch. Journal of Orthopaedic and Sports Physical Therapy 19:12–17

Smith JL, Hutton RS, Eldred E 1974 Post contraction changes in sensitivity of muscle afferents to static and dynamic stretch. Brain Research 78:193–202

Solveborn SA 1997 Radial epicondyalgia ('tennis elbow'): treatment with stretching on forearm band. A prospective study with long-term follow-up including range of motion measurements. Scandinavian Journal of Medicine and Science in Sports 7:229–237

Stevens A, Stijns H, Roselle N, Stappaerts K, Michels A 1974 Slowly stretching the hamstrings and compliance. Electromyography and Clinical Neurophysiology 14:495–496

Stolov W, Weilepp TG, Riddell WM 1970 Passive length-tension relationship and hydroxyproline content of chronically denervated skeletal muscle. Archives of Physical Medicine and Rehabilitation 51:517–525

Stromberg DD, Wlederhielm C 1969 Viscoelastic description of a collagenous tissue in simple elongation. Journal of Applied Physiology 26:857–862

Summers TB, Hines HM 1951 Effects of immobilization in various positions upon the weight and strength of skeletal muscle. J Neurophys 245–251

Sunderland S, Bradley KC 1961 Stress-strain phenomena in human spinal nerve roots. Brain 84:102–119

Sutro CJ 1947 Hypermobility of bones due to 'overlengthened' capsular and ligamentous tissues. Surgery 21:67–76

Svantesson U, Ernstoff B, Bergh P, Grimby G 1991 Use of a Kin-Com dynamometer to study the stretch-shortening cycle during plantar flexion. European Journal of Applied Physiology 62:415–419

Tardieu C, Tabary JC, Tabary C, Tardieu G 1982 Adaptation of connective tissue length to immobilization in lengthened and shortened positions in cat soleus muscle. Journal of Physiology Paris 78:214–220

Taunton JE 1982 Pre-game warm-up and flexibility. New-Zealand Journal of Sports Medicine 10:14–18

Taylor DC, Brooks DE, Ryan JB 1997 Viscoelastic characteristics of muscle: passive stretching versus muscular contractions. Medicine and Science in Sports and Exercise 29:1619–1624

Thompson DB, Chapman AE 1988 The mechanical response of active human muscle during and after stretch. European Journal of Applied Physiology 57:691–697

Tomanek RJ, Lund DD 1974 Degeneration of different types of skeletal muscle fibres. II. Immobilization. Journal of Anatomy 118:531–541

Troup JDG, Hood C, Chapman AE 1968 Measurement of the sagittal mobility of the lumbar spine and hips. Annals of Physical Medicine 9:308–321

Urban LM 1981 The straight-leg-raising test: a review. Journal of Orthopaedic and Sports Physical Therapy 2:117–134

Vandervoort AA, Chesworth BM, Cunningham DA, Patterson DH 1992 Age and sex effects on mobility of the human ankle. Journal of Gerontology 47:M17–21

Viidik A, Danielson CC, Oxlund H 1982 On fundamental and phenomenological models, structure and mechanical properties of collagen, elastin and glycoasaminolycan complexes. Biorheology 19:437–451

Voss DE, Ionta MK, Myres BJ 1985 Proprioceptive neuromuscular facilitation. Harper and Row, Philadelphia

Vujnovich AL, Dawson NJ 1994 The effect of therapeutic muscle stretch on neural processing. Journal of Orthopaedic and Sports Physical Therapy 224:231–244

Wall EJ, Massie JB, Kwan MK, Rydevik BJ, Myers RR, Garfin SR 1992 Experimental stretch neuropathy: changes in nerve conduction under tension. Journal of Bone and Joint Surgery 7413:126–129

Walter J, Figoni SF, Andres FF, Brown E 1996 Training intensity and duration in flexibility. Clin Kines 50:40–45

Warren CG, Lehmann JF, Koblanski JN 1976 Heat and stretch procedures: an evaluation using rat tail tendon. Archives of Physical Medicine and Rehabilitation 57:122–127

Wear CR 1963 Relationship of flexibility measurements to length of body segments. Research Quarterly 34:234–238

Wilby J, Linge K, Reilly T, Troup JDG 1987 Spinal shrinkage in females: circadian variation and the effects of circuit weight-training. Ergon 30:47–54

Wiliams PE 1988 Effect of intermittent stretch on immobilized muscle. Annals of the Rheumatic Diseases 47:1014–1016

Williams PE, Catanese T, Lucey EG, Goldspink G 1988 The importance of stretch and contractile activity in the prevention of connective tissue accumulation in muscle. Journal of Anatomy 158:109–114

Williams PE, Goldspink G 1984 Connective tissue changes in immobilised muscle. Journal of Anatomy 138:342–350

Wilson GJ, Elliot BC, Wood BA 1992 Stretch shorten cycle performance enhancement through flexibility training. Medicine and Science in Sports and Exercise 24:116–123

Wilson GJ, Murphy AJ, Pryor JF 1994 Musculotendinous stiffness: its relationship to eccentric, isometric, and concentric performance. Journal of Applied Physiology 76:2714–2719

Wilson GJ, Wood GA, Elliot BC 1991 The relationship between stiffness of the musculature and static flexibility: an alternative explanation for the occurrence of muscular injury. International Journal of Sports Medicine 19:403–407

Wisnes A, Kirkebo A 1976 Regional distribution of blood flow in calf muscles of rat during passive stretch and sustained contraction. Acta Physiologica Scandinavica 96:256–266

Witvrouw E, Mahieu N, Danneels N, McNair P 2004 Stretching and injury prevention. An obscure relationship. Sports Medicine 34:443–449

Wolf SL, Segal RL 1990 Conditioning of the spinal stretch reflex: implication for rehabilitation. Physical Therapy 70:652–656

Wolpaw JR, Noonan PA, O'Keefe JA 1984 Adaptive plasticity and diurnal rhythm in the primate spinal stretch reflex are independent phenomenon. Brain Research 33:385–391

Wonell TW, Smith TL, Winegardner JW 1994 Effect of hamstring stretching on hamstring muscle performance. Journal of Orthopaedic and Sports Physical Therapy 20:154–159

Woo SL-Y, Matthews JV, Akeson WH 1975 Connective tissue response to immobility: correlative study of biomechanical and biochemical measurements of normal and immobilized rabbit knees. Arthritis and Rheumatism 257–264

Worrell TV, McCullough M, Pfeiffer A 1994 Effect of foot position on gastrocnemius/soleus stretching in subjects with normal flexibility. Journal of Orthopaedic and Sports Physical Therapy 19:352–356

Worrell TW, Perrin DH, Gansneder BM, Gieck JH 1991 Comparison of isokinetic strength and flexibility measures between hamstring injured and noninjured athletes. Journal of Orthopaedic and Sports Physical Therapy 13:118–125

Wortman M, Blanke D 1982 Flexibility training: ballistic, static or proprioceptive neuromuscular facilitation? Archives of Physical Medicine and Rehabilitation 63:261–263
Wyke B 1972 Articular neurology. Physiotherapy 58:94–99
Wyke B 1979 Neurology of the cervical spinal joints. Physiotherapy 65:72–76
Yamashita T, Ishii S, Oota I 1992 Effect of muscle stretching on the activity of neuromuscular transmission. Medicine and Science in Sports and Exercise 24:80–84
Ylinen J, Airaksinen O, Kolari P 1993 Digital tissue compliance meter. Acup Electr Ther Res 18:169–174
Zito M, Driver D, Parker C, Bohannon R 1997 Lasting effects of one bout of two 15-second passive stretches on ankle dorsiflexion range of motion. Journal of Orthopaedic and Sports Physical Therapy 26:214–221
Zuurbier CJ, Everard AJ, Wees P, Huijing PA 1994 Length-force characteristics of the aponeurosis in the passive and active muscle condition and in the isolated condition. Journal of Biomechanics 27:445–453
Öberg, B. Evaluation and improvement of strength in competitive athletes 1993 In: Harms-Ringdahl K(ed) Muscle strength. Churchill Livingstone, Edinburgh 167–185

INDEX

Notes: Page numbers in *italics* refer to figures, those in **bold** refer to boxes and tables

A

B

C

J

K

L

M

N

O

P

Q

R